Surgical Techniques for Cutaneous Scar Revision

BASIC AND CLINICAL DERMATOLOGY

1. Cutaneous Investigation in Health and Disease: Noninvasive Methods and Instrumentation, *edited by Jean-Luc Lévêque*
2. Irritant Contact Dermatitis, *edited by Edward M. Jackson and Ronald Goldner*
3. Fundamentals of Dermatology: A Study Guide, *Franklin S. Glickman and Alan R. Shalita*
4. Aging Skin: Properties and Functional Changes, *edited by Jean-Luc Lévêque and Pierre G. Agache*
5. Retinoids: Progress in Research and Clinical Applications, *edited by Maria A. Livrea and Lester Packer*
6. Clinical Photomedicine, *edited by Henry W. Lim and Nicholas A. Soter*
7. Cutaneous Antifungal Agents: Selected Compounds in Clinical Practice and Development, *edited by John W. Rippon and Robert A. Fromtling*
8. Oxidative Stress in Dermatology, *edited by Jürgen Fuchs and Lester Packer*
9. Connective Tissue Diseases of the Skin, *edited by Charles M. Lapière and Thomas Krieg*
10. Epidermal Growth Factors and Cytokines, *edited by Thomas A. Luger and Thomas Schwarz*
11. Skin Changes and Diseases in Pregnancy, *edited by Marwali Harahap and Robert C. Wallach*
12. Fungal Disease: Biology, Immunology, and Diagnosis, *edited by Paul H. Jacobs and Lexie Nall*
13. Immunomodulatory and Cytotoxic Agents in Dermatology, *edited by Charles J. McDonald*
14. Cutaneous Infection and Therapy, *edited by Raza Aly, Karl R. Beutner, and Howard I. Maibach*
15. Tissue Augmentation in Clinical Practice: Procedures and Techniques, *edited by Arnold William Klein*
16. Psoriasis: Third Edition, Revised and Expanded, *edited by Henry H. Roenigk, Jr., and Howard I. Maibach*
17. Surgical Techniques for Cutaneous Scar Revision, *edited by Marwali Harahap*

ADDITIONAL VOLUMES IN PREPARATION

Drug Therapy in Dermatology, *edited by Larry E. Millikan*

Cosmetic Surgery: An Interdisciplinary Approach, *edited by Rhoda S. Narins*

Surgical Techniques for Cutaneous Scar Revision

edited by

Marwali Harahap

University of North Sumatra Medical School
Medan, Indonesia

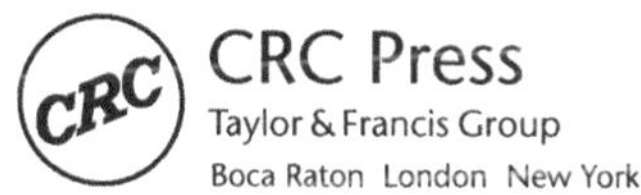

CRC Press is an imprint of the
Taylor & Francis Group, an **informa** business

CRC Press
Taylor & Francis Group
6000 Broken Sound Parkway NW, Suite 300
Boca Raton, FL 33487-2742

Visit the Taylor & Francis Web site at
http://www.taylorandfrancis.com

and the CRC Press Web site at
http://www.crcpress.com

Series Introduction

Since the initiation of this series there has been an increasingly large body of new information relating to the art and science of dermatology and fundamental cutaneous biology. Furthermore, this information is no longer of interest only to the small but growing specialty of dermatology. Scientists from a wide variety of disciplines have come to recognize both the importance of skin and fundamental biological processes and the broad implications of understanding the pathogenesis of skin disease. As a result there is now multidisciplinary and worldwide interest in the progress of dermatology.

With these factors in mind, we have continued to expand this series of books which is specifically oriented to dermatology. The series has been purposely broad in focus and has ranged from pure basic science to practical, applied clinical dermatology. Thus, while there is something for everyone, all editions in the series should ultimately prove to be valuable additions to the dermatologist's library. The latest addition to the series, edited by Marwali Harahap, is both timely and pertinent. Dr. Harahap has assembled an internationally renowned list of contributors who are well known authorities in the field of dermatologic surgery. We believe that this volume compliments earlier volumes in the series and trust that it will be of broad interest to physicians interested in the care of skin.

Alan R. Shalita
David A. Norris

Foreword

Why a book on scar revision? The importance of such a book cannot be understated. All physicians who perform skin surgery encounter patients who have scars that have been produced by trauma or surgery. Many of these patients are physically and/or psychologically deformed by the scars. They are anxious for treatment that will normalize them again. Consequently, it is important for physicians to study and perfect the time-tested techniques for scar revision. The ability of a cutaneous surgeon to camouflage and revise scars defines his/her ability as a surgeon. Fundamental skills in scar revision are essential for success in skin surgery. Without these skills, patients with scars will turn to other physicians and also attorneys for assistance.

There are many varieties of scars. The physician who is experienced in scar revision can analyze a scar and apply the appropriate techniques to modify it. The chapters in this book delineate the many modalities that are currently available.

Professor Marwali Harahap is an ideal person to edit a new book on surgical techniques for cutaneous scar revision. He is an international editor in dermatologic surgery with extensive experience. Well-known experts from the specialties of dermatology/dermatologic surgery, facial plastic surgery, plastic surgery, and radiation oncology are included in the list of contributors. Their combined expertise and creativity have resulted in a book that physicians from many specialties will read and reread.

Eckart Haneke, Ph.D., M.D.
Department of Dermatology,
Wuppertal Hospitals Ltd.;
Clinical Health Center,
University of Witten/Herdecke;
and Academy Teaching
Hospital of Heinrich,
Heine University of Dusseldorf,
Wupertal, Germany

Preface

The treatment of scars is one of the most important problems that confront dermatologists and other physicians. With increased demand for more specialized and comprehensive treatments, scar revision will clearly occupy a significant portion of a dermatologist's future practice.

Surgical Techniques for Cutaneous Scar Revision has an entirely practical purpose: to show how to avoid scars and, once they are there, how to repair or remove them.

The book is designed to provide the latest and most comprehensive information related to cutaneous scar revision, including some new and innovative methods and techniques. No previous or contemporary monograph on scar revision discusses the relatively recent treatments, such as laminar dermal reticulotomy, scalpel sculpting technique, subcutaneous incisionless technique, and laser treatment for scars.

The first part of the book presents fundamental principles. The opening chapter is an overview of the mechanisms of scar tissue formation, problems caused by an overgrowth of scar tissue, and complications presented by scars. Chapter 2 discusses the biomechanical properties of skin that have an important influence on surgical decision. They provide insight in planning elective incision, excision, or scar revision. Information on facial scarring is the subject of Chapter 3. Chapter 4 covers the cultural and psychological aspects of skin defects caused by scars. Chapter 5 discusses prevention and minimization of scars by proper management of the initial wound.

The subsequent 19 chapters present the clinical applications of scar revision, resurfacing, elevation, excision, irregularization, and other scar removal techniques. Operative techniques are well illustrated and explained in step-by-step detail, and complications and postoperative problems are discussed with recommendations for their avoidance. The contributors have included many drawings and photographs to illustrate their points.

This book is designed to be comprehensive in scope by providing much useful information for both the beginning dermatological surgeon and the more experienced practitioner. The contributors were carefully selected for their technical skill and their long experience. They are well known for their publications and contributions to the field.

Marwali Harahap

Contents

Other Techniques

Contributors

Abdel-Fattah M. A. Abdel-Fattah, M.D. Plastic Surgery Section and Burns Unit, Faculty of Medicine, University of Alexandria, Alexandria, Egypt

Tina S. Alster, M.D. Washington Institute of Dermatologic Laser Surgery and Georgetown University Medical Center, Washington, D.C.

Mitchell S. Anscher, M.D. Radiation Oncology Department, Duke University Medical Center, Durham, North Carolina

Steven Burres, M.D School of Medicine, University of California, Los Angeles, Los Angeles, California

Judith A. Carr, BSOT, OTR/L Westchester Burn Center, Westchester Medical Center, Valhalla, New York

Brian Cook, M.D. Department of Dermatology, Northwestern University School of Medicine, Chicago, Illinois

Terence M. Davidson, M.D., F.A.C.S. Division of Otolaryngology–Head and Neck Surgery, Department of Surgery, University of California, San Diego, and VA Health Care, San Diego, California

Michael H. Gold, M.D. Gold Skin Care Center, Nashville, Tennessee

Greg J. Goodman, M.B.B.S., F.A.C.D. Skin and Cancer Foundation of Victoria, Melbourne, Victoria, Australia

Edmond I. Griffin, M.D. Department of Dermatology, Dermatology Associates of Atlanta, P.C., Atlanta, Georgia

Eckart Haneke, Ph.D., M.D. Department of Dermatology, Wuppertal Hospitals Ltd.; Clinical Health Center, University of Witten/Herdecke; and Academic Teaching Hospital of Heinrich, Heine University of Dusseldorf, Wuppertal, Germany

Marwali Harahap, M.D. Department of Dermatology, University of North Sumatra Medical School, Medan, Indonesia

Giuseppe Hautmann, M.D. Department of Dermatology, University of Florence, Florence, Italy

Shinichi Hirabayashi, M.D. Department of Plastic Surgery, Teikyo University, Tokyo, Japan

David B. Hom, M.D., F.A.C.S. Division of Facial Plastic and Reconstructive Surgery, Department of Otolaryngology, University of Minnesota and Hennepin County Medical Center, Minneapolis, Minnesota

Drew M. Horlbeck, M.D. Division of Otolaryngology–Head and Neck Surgery, Department of Surgery, University of California, San Diego, and VA Health Care, San Diego, California

George J. Hruza, M.B.A., M.D. Departments of Medicine (Dermatology), Surgery, and Otolaryngology, Washington University, St. Louis, Missouri

Azim J. Khan, M.D., M.A.C.P. Department of Dermatology, Northwestern University School of Medicine, Chicago, Illinois

Maurice Morad Khosh, M.D. Department of Otolaryngology–Head and Neck Surgery, St. Luke's–Roosevelt Hospital Center, New York, New York

Wayne F. Larrabee, Jr., M.D. Department of Otolaryngology–Head and Neck Surgery, University of Washington, Seattle, Washington

L. Scott Levin, M.D., F.A.C.S. Plastic/Reconstructive/Maxillofacial and Oral Surgery Division, Duke University Medical Center, Durham, North Carolina

M. Reza Perkasa Marwali, M.D. Department of Internal Medicine, Wayne State University, Detroit, Michigan

Aaron J. Mayberry, M.D. Duke University Medical Center, Durham, North Carolina

Michel McDonald, M.D. Mohs Micrographic Surgery, Vanderbilt University Medical Center, Nashville, Tennessee

Larry E. Millikan, M.D. Department of Dermatology, Tulane University Medical Center, New Orleans, Louisiana

John C. Murray, M.D. Department of Medicine, Duke University Medical Center, Durham, North Carolina

Rick M. Odland, Ph.D., M.D. Department of Otolaryngology–Head and Neck Surgery, University of Minnesota and Hennepin County Medical Center, Minneapolis, Minnesota

Fumio Ohkubo, M.D., Ph.D. Department of Plastic and Reconstructive Surgery, Showa University School of Medicine, Tokyo, Japan

Takuya Onizuka, M.D., Ph.D. Showa University School of Medicine, Tokyo, Japan

David Scott Orentreich, M.D. Orentreich Medical Group, LLP, New York, New York

Norman Orentreich, M.D., F.A.C.P. Orentreich Medical Group, LLP, New York, New York

Constantin E. Orfanos, M.D. Department of Dermatology, University Medical Center Benjamin Franklin, The Free University of Berlin, Berlin, Germany

Howard A. Oriba, M.D. Departments of Dermatology and Pathology, University of Southern California School of Medicine, Los Angeles, California

Emiliano Panconesi, M.D. Department of Dermatology, University of Florence, Florence, Italy

Harold E. Pierce, M.D. Pierce Cosmetic Surgery Center, Philadelphia, Pennsylvania

Timothy J. Rosio, M.D., F.A.A.C.S. Cosmetic, Laser and Dermatologic Surgery Institute and Department of Dermatology, University of California Davis Medical Center, Sacramento, California

Hisakazu Seno, M.D. Department of Plastic Surgery, Juntendo University, Tokyo, Japan

Stephen N. Snow, M.D., MBA Department of Surgery, University of Wisconsin Hospital and Clinics, University of Wisconsin Medical School, Madison, Wisconsin

Thomas Stasko, M.D. Mohs Micrographic Surgery, Vanderbilt University Medical Center, Nashville, Tennessee

Akira Yanai, M.D. Department of Plastic Surgery, Juntendo University, Tokyo, Japan

Christos C. Zouboulis, M.D. Department of Dermatology, University Medical Center Benjamin Franklin, The Free University of Berlin, Berlin, Germany

Surgical Techniques for Cutaneous Scar Revision

1
Wound Healing and Scar Formation

Azim J. Khan and Brian Cook
Northwestern University School of Medicine
Chicago, Illinois

I. INTRODUCTION

Wound healing has been one of the most actively researched areas of medicine in the past several years. Availability of highly sophisticated molecular and cellular biology techniques has given us the opportunity to better understand the intricate and complex mechanisms involved in wound healing. In the lower forms of life, healing involves regeneration of the tissue that retains all the anatomical and physiological capabilities of the healthy uninjured organ. For example, amphibians heal extremity wounds by regeneration, a process whereby injured tissues are reconstituted entirely without scar formation (1). Instead of restoration of the native tissue to its preinjury state, wound healing in adult mammals result in a fibrotic scar. While the scar mends the injured tissue by putting a patch on the broken area, it does not completely restore all the anatomical and physiological capabilities lost during injury. Thus, the ideal repair for the injured tissue is the regeneration, not the scarring. Damaged organs such as the myocardium or liver can only restore their function to normal by regeneration. Scarring in these circumstances heals the tissue but does not bring the function back to normal. This is also true for cutaneous wounds. Ideal cutaneous wound repair should involve regeneration of the skin, bringing all the anatomical as well as physiological capabilities back to normal. Scarring can be prevented if we can make the cutaneous wounds heal by regeneration, but this never happens in adult mammals. The wound healing process is markedly different in a fetus as compared to its adult counterpart (2,3). Interestingly, mammals are capable of regenerative healing of cutaneous wounds without scarring in the first two trimesters of development (4–6), however, by the time of birth, cutaneous wound repair is accompanied by scar formation. The mechanisms involved in scarless, regenerative fetal wound healing are being studied extensively to help modulate the adult wound healing into a scarless and regenerative process (7).

Cutaneous wound healing can result either in a normal scar or an abnormal scar formation. Abnormal scarring leads to hypertrophic scar or keloid formation. Keloids are locally aggressive and, in contrast to the hypertrophic scars, they can invade the healthy tissue (8). Differences between keloids, hypertrophic scars, and normal scars include distinct scar appearance, histologic morphology, and cellular function in response to growth factors (9). This chapter is intended to share a small part of the vast information that has become available in recent years about the biological processes involved during the healing of the

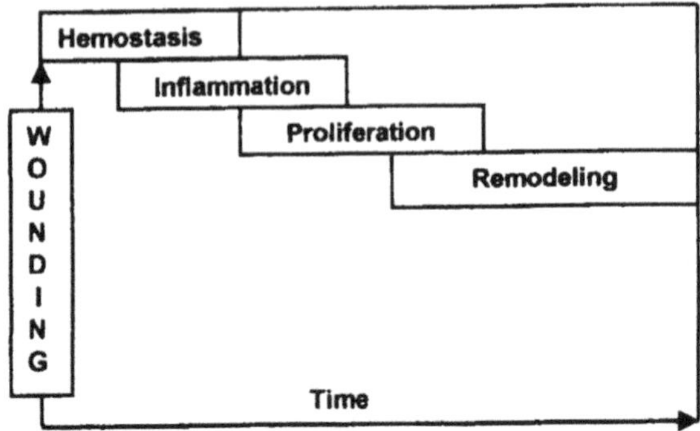

Figure 1 Four phases of wound healing. The distinction is conceptual for understanding purposes only. These phases overlap in time.

wound. It also describes some of the differences in adult and fetal wound healing that might be responsible for the scarless wound healing in fetal life.

Cutaneous wound healing involves dermal and epidermal repair. Both processes are concurrent, and the distinction is meant only to understand them more clearly. Epidermal wound healing is discussed mainly in the section on reepithelialization. Again, dermal wound healing has been temporally divided into different phases for the purpose of understanding (10,11). We can divide the wound healing process into hemostasis, inflammatory, granulation or proliferation, and tissue remodeling phases (Fig. 1). The distinction between these phases is only conceptual and they overlap in time.

II. COAGULATION OR HEMOSTASIS

Blood vessel damage by dermal injury causes the plasma and other blood elements to extravasate into the wounded area. The blood coagulation starts with clot formation through activation of intrinsic and extrinsic pathways. The outcome of both these pathways is the production of thrombin (12). Thrombin causes conversion of fibrinogen to fibrin, which serves the main purposes of coagulation and formation of a provisional extracellular matrix. Thrombin also activates platelets (13) in the blood vessel lumen. A thrombus is formed by the interaction of fibrin, von Willebrand factor, and platelets (14), and hemostasis is restored. The fibrin clot within the wound space, in conjunction with fibronectin, provides a provisional extracellular matrix for the migration of keratinocytes (15), fibroblasts (16), and monocytes (17) (Fig. 2). Termination of blood coagulation starts with the removal of clotting stimuli. Clot formation is restricted to the focus of injury by the production of prostacyclin (18), antithrombin III (19), protein C (20), and plasminogen activator (21).

A. Platelets

Platelets are the most important cells immediately after injury. The two major functions of platelets are achieving homeostasis by adhesion and aggregation in the blood clot and pro-

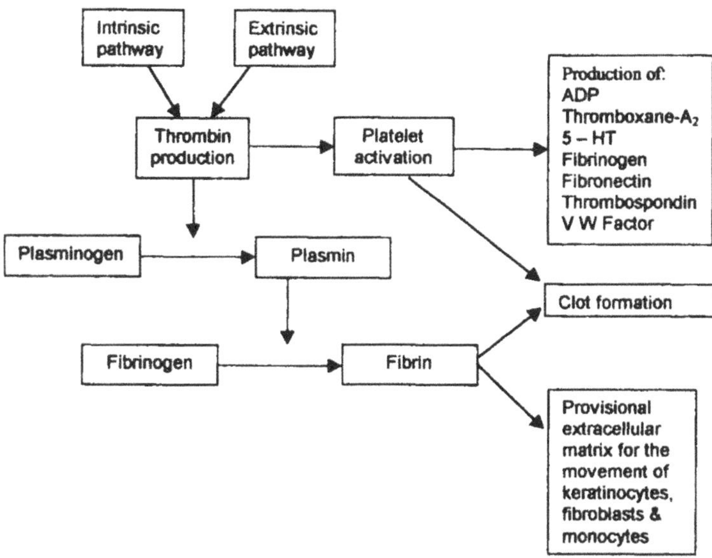

Figure 2 Hemostasis during wound healing. (5-HT, 5-Hydroxytryptophan; ADP, Adenosine diphosphate; VW factor, von Willebrand factor VIII).

ducing cell mediators. Platelets are activated at the wound site by locally generated thrombin and exposed fibrillar collagen (22). Activated platelets release adenosine diphosphate (ADP), thromboxane A_2, 5-hydroxytryptophan, fibrinogen, fibronectin, thrombospondin, and von Willebrand factor (factor VIII) (23) (Fig. 2). The adhesive proteins fibrinogen, fibronectin, and thrombospondin act as ligands for platelet aggregation (24), and von Willebrand factor mediates platelet adhesion to fibrillar collagens. Platelet surface receptor GPIIb/IIIa (integrin $\alpha IIb\beta_3$) is used to attach these adhesive proteins (25). Moreover, platelets release very important growth factors such as platelet-derived growth factor (PDGF) (26), transforming growth factors α (TGF-α) (27) and β (TGF-β) (28) and chemotactic factors for leukocytes (29).

III. INFLAMMATORY PHASE

Inflammation is an essential part of the healing process. It has been demonstrated that suppressing inflammation with steroids at the time of wounding inhibits healing (30,31). Neutrophils and monocytes play the major role in this phase (Fig. 3).

A. Neutrophils

Neutrophils are the first cells to arrive at the wound site, possibly because of their greater number in the blood as compared with monocytes. Many substances produced during the coagulation cascade act as chemoattractants for leukocytes. Some are general leukocyte chemoattractants, whereas others are specific chemoattractants for neutrophils or specific for monocytes. Fibrin degradation products, fibrinopeptides from fibrinogen cleavage by

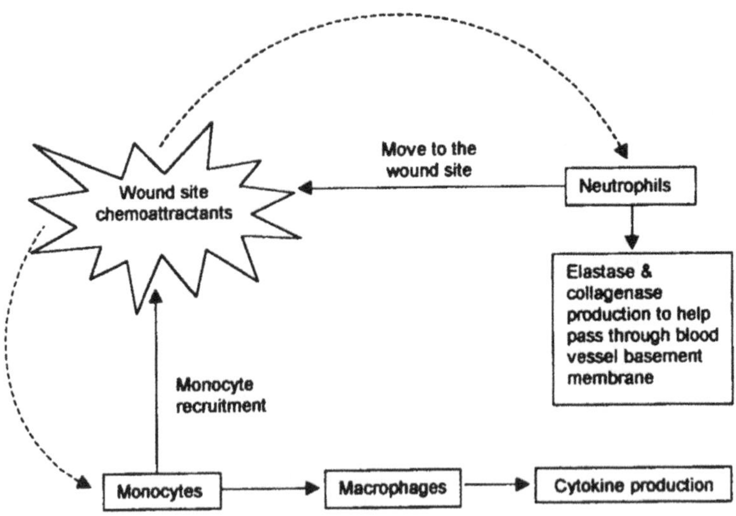

Figure 3 General leukocyte as well as cell specific chemotactic factors produced at the wound site are the main source of neutrophil and monocyte attraction to the wounded area. Monocytes, once activated, change their morphology to macrophages, which are the major source of cytokine production during wound healing.

thrombin, leukotriene B_4 released from neutrophils, some bacterial proteins, PDGF, and platelet factor 4 all act as general leukocyte chemoattractants. In addition to attracting the neutrophils, these chemotactic factors upregulate the expression of some receptors on the neutrophil surface that increase neutrophil adherence to the blood vessel endothelium (32). Elastase and collagenases are released by neutrophils in response to chemoattractant stimulation. These enzymes help neutrophils to pass through the basement membrane of blood vessels (33) (Fig. 3). Once at the wound site, neutrophils kill and phagocytose the contaminating bacteria and other debris. The neutrophil recruitment of the wound area stops within a few days, and the neutrophils that have done their part of the job in wound healing are entrapped in the eschar and sloughed off during the regeneration process or phagocytosed by macrophages (34). Prolonged stay of neutrophils in the wound in the case of continued infection may cause impaired wound healing.

B. Monocytes

Initially, monocytes invade the wounded area with neutrophils in response to general leukocyte chemoattractants (Fig. 3). Once in the tissue, they change their morphology to that of macrophages. Later, monocytes continue to invade the wound area in response to selective monocyte chemoattractants including collagen fragments (35), elastin (36), fibronectin (17), thrombin (37), and TGF-β (38). It has been demonstrated in animal studies that macrophage depletion can cause impaired wound healing (39). This is probably because of their extremely important role in synthesizing and secreting cytokines that are important for inducing cell migration and proliferation as well as matrix production. The cytokines produced by macrophages include PDGF, fibroblast growth factor (FGF), TGF-β, and TGF-α (40). The production and release of growth factors as well as some enzymes (41,42) required for debris and microorganism digestion is turned on when macrophages come in contact with extracellular matrix of the wound area.

C. Lymphocytes

Lymphocytes are not required for the initiation of wound healing, but an intact cellular immune response is essential for a normal outcome of the tissue repair (43). Injury produces generalized immunosuppression by affecting T-cell activity. Although the exact origin of post-traumatic immunosuppression is not exactly understood, stress hormones and immunosuppressive factors, such as inflammatory cytokines, prostglandin E-2 and nitric oxide, affect lymphocyte function adversely. Since decreased immunity increases host susceptibility to infection and sepsis, the healing process can be affected as a result of these factors.

IV. PROLIFERATIVE PHASE

The proliferative phase of wound healing can be divided into epidermal and dermal wound healing, for a better understanding. Both, epidermal and dermal repair proceed simultaneously. While keratinocytes are the major cells responsible for the epidermal repair (reepithelialization), dermal wound healing is a joint effort of fibroblasts, macrophages and endothelial cells Table 1 summarizes the major players and their roles during the proliferative phase of wound healing.

Table 1 Role of Different Cell Types[a]

Cell type	Function
Keratinocytes	Reepthelialization
	Cytokine production
	Protease release
	Provisional matrix & basement membrane formation
Fibroblasts	Growth factor production
	Granulation tissue formation
	Protease release
	Extracellular matrix production
	Extracellular matrix remodeling
	Tissue contraction
Macrophages	Phagocytosis of microorganisms & tissue debris
	Growth factor production
Endothelial Cells	Limit coagulation
	Clot lysis
	Growth factor production
	Angiogenesis

[a] Role of different cell types during proliferative phase of wound healing. Functions described are the major roles played by these cells. There are numerous other less significant functions of these cells at different stages of wound healing.

A. Reepithelialization

Coverage of the wound bed with keratinocytes is referred to as reepithelialization. Keratinocytes from surrounding epidermis and residual hair follicles in the wound area, begin to migrate laterally onto the fibrin and fibronectin clot of the wound bed within hours of wounding (44). The morphology of the migrating keratinocytes changes from that of their stationary counterparts, in that they flatten out, retract their hemidesmosomes from their plasma membrane, increase their number of gap junctions, express actin cables within cytoplasm, and project lamellipodia in the direction of migration (45). The induction signals for the migratory keratinocyte phenotype are not yet fully understood but different possibilities have been suggested. In the normal intact skin, keratinocytes rest on the lamina lucida, which is made mainly of laminin. As laminin has been shown to decrease the motility of keratinocytes in vitro (46), it is speculated that laminin may act as a "stop" signal for kertinocytes in the state of intact healthy skin. On the other hand, when wounding occurs, the lamina lucida and thus laminin are disrupted and keratinocytes come in contact with the basement membrane collagens (type IV and VII) or fibronectin. Type IV collagen and fibronectin have been demonstrated to increase keratinocyte motility in vitro (47). On the basis of these observations, it is thought that fibronectin and collagen may act as a signal for keratinocytes to migrate to a wound. Heparan sulfate proteoglycan, albumin, type V collagen, and type III collagen matrices do not stimulate keratinocyte migration to any significant extent (46). Type I native or denatured collagen, however, highly stimulates keratinocyte migration.

Cells interact with the extracellular matrix through specialized cell surface receptors called integrins. Integrins play a significant role not only in cell movement but also in modulating the cell behavior in response to different extracellular matrices. Keratinocytes move over the fibronectin matrix with the help of integrin receptor $\alpha_5\beta_1$ (48). Growth factors TGF-β and epidermal growth factor (EGF) have been shown to increase keratinocyte migration in vitro (49,50). Moreover, topical application of EGF has been demonstrated to promote cutaneous wound repair in human beings (51). Keratinocytes migrating over the nonviable dermal collagen produce collagenases that degrade type I and type IV collagens (52). This helps the movement of keratinocytes as they travel through the wound separating viable from nonviable tissue (15). One to 2 days after injury, keratinocytes at the wound margin begin to divide and contribute additional cells to the neoepithelium, covering the wound bed (48). Although the stimulus for the cells undergoing rapid proliferation is not known, several growth factors may be involved, including EGF and TGF-α.

As described earlier, basement membrane proteins, laminin, and type IV collagen are disrupted during injury. As the reepithelialization progresses, these proteins start to make basement membrane in an orderly fashion (15). Keratinocytes change to their stationary phenotype and attach to the newly formed basement membrane through hemidesmosomes.

B. Dermal Wound Healing

While the keratinocytes are busy with epidermal repair by the reepithelialization process, dermal repair proceeds with the help of macrophages, fibroblasts, and blood vessels as they migrate into the wound as a unit (53). These events will be described under Proliferative Phase. Proliferation of fibroblasts and endothelial cells is the hallmark of this phase. Granulation tissue formed in this phase of wound healing consists of newly formed blood vessels, macrophages, fibroblasts, and loose connective tissue. The newly formed capillaries give this tissue a granular appearance on gross examination, hence it is called granulation tissue.

1. *Neovascularization*

During the proliferation phase, macrophages, fibroblasts, and blood vessels forming endothelial cells are very much dependent on each other. Macrophages, as described earlier, are important for cytokine production, to stimulate fibrosis, and for new blood vessel formation (neovascularization). Fibroblasts are important for the production of extracellular matrix, and endothelial cells are important as they form new blood vessels to deliver oxygen and nutrients to keep these macrophages and fibroblasts alive.

New blood vessel formation or neovascularization is also called angiogenesis. On the second day after injury, the process starts with migration of the endothelial cells. The endothelial cells lining the blood vessels adjacent to the wound cavity migrate through the fragmented basement membranes and enter the perivascular space. By the second or third day, the endothelial cells in the parent vessel begin to proliferate to provide the large number of cells required for new blood vessel formation. The endothelial cells located at the capillary tip, however, do not divide (54). This finding suggests that the endothelial cell replication could be a secondary event to cell migration (54), as the soluble factors that stimulate angiogenesis in the wound environment are as yet unknown. Several factors, however, have been shown to have angiogenic activity, including acidic and basic fibroblast growth factors (aFGF and bFGF) (55), TGF-α, TGF-β (56), angiogenin, and TNF-α (57). Heparin, fibronectin, and platelet factors known to stimulate endothelial cell migration into the wound may also stimulate endothelial cell proliferation directly or indirectly (58–60). Recently, it has been shown that, in surgical wounds, an initial angiogenic stimulus is supplied by fibroblast growth factor-2 (FGF-2), followed by a subsequent and more prolonged angiogenic stimulus by vascular endothelial growth factor (VEGF).

2. *Fibroplasia*

Fibroplasia is the formation of a mixture of fibroblasts and extracellular matrix components made by fibroblasts. The most important cell for the production of dermal matrix is the fibroblast. During cutaneous wound repair, fibroblasts progress through four phenotypes: proliferating fibroblasts, migrating fibroblasts, fibroblasts that synthesize extracellular matrix, and myofibroblasts, which cause the wound to contract (62). Fibroblasts from the surrounding uninjured tissue proliferate for the first 3 days and then migrate into the wound site on day 4. PDGF and latent transforming growth factor-β (TGF-β) are produced by activated platelets and macrophages at the wound site. PDGF is the most potent mitogen in the serum for fibroblasts (26). It is presumed that PDGF produced by platelets during the early phase of wound healing induces the fibroblast proliferation around the wounded area. TGF-β released from platelets and macrophages can be the other major signal for fibroblast proliferation (63). Both PDGF and TGF-β have potent chemotactic activities for cultured fibroblasts in vitro (64,65) and probably the same holds true in vivo. Fibroblasts migrate by pulling themselves along the fibronectin, vitreonectin, and fibrin matrix with the help of integrin surface receptors.

Once the fibroblasts reach the wound space, they perform several functions. They change their morphology to that of the matrix-synthesizing fibroblasts with peculiar endoplasmic reticula, and start producing large quantities of collagen, proteoglycans, and elastin (66). Adult dermis mainly contains type I collagen, whereas type III collagen is a major component of fetal dermis. During wound healing, however, predominantly type III collagen is synthesized (67). It is maximally secreted between 5 and 7 days. TGF-β has been found to stimulate both type I and type III collagens in vitro and quite possibly also stimulates collagen synthesis in vivo (68). Enhanced expression of messenger RNA (mRNA) for TGF-β and type I, III, or VI collagen has been observed in tissues of patients with postburn hypertrophic scars (69).

Scar formation is a significant clicical problem, as it results in functional impairment and disfiguration. It has been known for some time that fetal wounds heal without scarring (70), and surgery on fetuses is now in limited use to repair defects with otherwise lethal outcomes (71). Collagen production by fibroblasts ceases when an abundance of collagen has been deposited in the wound (72). Hypertrophic scars, generally seen after delayed burn wound healing, are believed to be dermal pathology caused by an increased matrix production by dermal fibroblasts. Unhealed burn wounds lack an epidermis and some studies have shown the role of some soluble keratinocyte product on dermal fibroblast collagen synthesis, thus causing uncontrolled collagen production and hypertrophic scarring (73). The persistence of activated keratinocytes in hypertrophic scar epidermis causing abnormal epidermal-mesenchymal interactions has also been implicated as the cause of hypertrophic scar formation (74). Interferon-γ has also been shown to decrease collagen production by fibroblasts, in vitro as well as in vivo (75). In addition to collagen, the new connective tissue matrix contains glycosaminoglycans and proteoglycans (discussed later under Tissue Remodeling Phase). At this time, after laying down extracellular matrix, fibroblasts change their phenotype to that of myofibroblasts, which perform the important function of wound contraction (76).

3. *Wound Contraction*

During the second and third weeks of healing, fibroblasts begin to change their phenotype to that of myofibroblasts. This phenotype is characterized by actin-containing microfilaments along the plasma membrane and establishment of cell-to-cell and cell-to-matrix linkages (77). Myofibroblasts have electron microscopic characteristics of both smooth muscle cells and fibroblasts and are responsible for wound contraction. These fibroblasts attach to extracellular fibronectin and collagen matrix proteins through specialized integrin receptors and to each other through direct adhesion junctions (77). The collagen bundles produced during wound healing attach to the collagen bundles at the edge of the wound in an end-to-end manner and join each other through covalent links. Once these cell-matrix, matrix-matrix, and cell-to-cell firm attachments are in place, traction caused by myofibroblast contraction can be transmitted across the wound (78). Myofibroblasts within the wound align along the lines of contraction and differ from other cells that take part in wound healing, including leukocytes and endothelial cells, which do not exhibit such organized orientation (79). Now these myofibroblasts probably need some signal to start contraction. In in vitro studies, PDGF has been shown to stimulate fibroblasts to contract collagen matrices. The isoforms of PDGF produced by platelets (AB) and macrophages (BB) have been found to have this activity, (80) and it is speculated that macrophage-produced PDGF at the wound site starts the wound contraction about 1 week after injury. The myofibroblasts contract their pseudopodia, causing the wound to contract. Wound contraction depends on the depth of the wound. Superficial wounds contract little compared with deeper wounds. In full-thickness wounds, the contraction can cause up to a 40% decrease in the wound size (81) and plays an important role in wound healing.

V. TISSUE REMODELING PHASE

The third phase of wound repair is called the remodeling phase and involves extracellular matrix remodeling, cell maturation, and cell apoptosis (programmed cell death). As mentioned previously, like other phases of wound healing, this phase is only conceptual and the processes involved in this phase overlap those in the other phases of wound healing. The deposition of extracellular matrix materials and their subsequent change is a dynamic process that starts with the deposition of provisional matrix (15) (the name given to any extracellular matrix that is transiently present and has a provisional function) that transforms into a collagenous scar over a period of time. Figure 4 compares the composition of extracellular matrix at different stages of wound healing. The original blood clot, which contains fibrin, fibronectin, vitreonectin, von Willebrand factor, thrombospondin, and growth factors such as PDGF and TGF-β, serves as the first provisional matrix. This cell-derived provisional matrix gradually replaces this provisional matrix initially deposited by the plasma-derived constituents, as the cells migrate to the wound and start making extracellular matrix (77). For example, plasma fibronectin is first deposited in conjunction with fibrin, but after clot lysis, cellular fibronectin is deposited by a variety of wound cells (15,82). This fibronectin deposited mainly by fibroblasts serves as a second-order provisional matrix (77). In addition to its role in fibroblast, keratinocyte, and endothelial cell adhesion and movement (15,47,83,84) fibronectin serves as a template for collagen deposition (85) during later stages of wound healing.

The composition of the extracellular matrix changes as the wound heals. For the first 3 days the blood clot produced by plasma and platelets, containing fibrin, fibrinogen, vitreonectin, and thrombospondin, serves as a provisional matrix. From day 4 to day 6 (early granulation tissue), fibronectin, hyaluronic acid (HA), tenascin, and SPARC (secreted protein acidic and rich in cysteine) are the main components of the extracellular matrix (86).

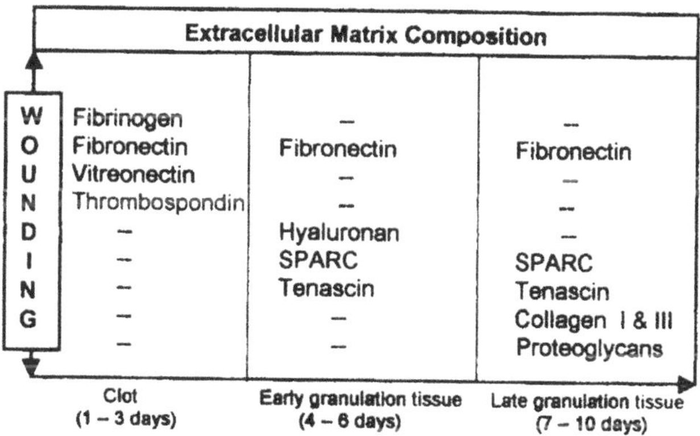

Figure 4 Comparison of extracellular matrix at different stages of wound healing. (—) denotes an absent or quantitatively insignificant component. (SPARC, secreted protein acidic and rich in cysteine).

Fibroblasts and macrophages are the source of their production. From day 7 to day 10, the late granulation tissue is deposited by fibroblasts and contains mainly collagen types I and III, fibronectin, proteoglycans, SPARC, and tenascin (86).

Another important and major component of early granulation tissue is hyaluronic acid. It is a gycosaminoglycan and is extremely hydrophilic. Because of this hydrophilic property, the expanded interstitial space at its deposition site might allow more cell recruitment and cell proliferation in these areas (87). With the passage of time, the HA content in extracellular matrix gradually falls from day 5 to day 10, whereas the proteoglycan level increases steadily during this time (88). In contrast to adult wound healing, the HA level does not fall during fetal wound healing, and this has been proposed to be one of the factors that may account for scarless repair of fetal wounds (89). Proteoglycans deposited by mature scar fibroblasts (90) in the late granulation tissue regulate collagen fibrillogenesis (91), modulate cell adhesion (92), possibly have some role in regulating cell proliferation, and may act as a reservoir for cytokines (10).

The deposition of granulation tissue matrix occurs in an ordered sequence of fibronectin followed by type III collagen and eventually type I collagen (93). As discussed before, type III collagen is the major type of collagen synthesized by wound fibroblasts (67). The dermis in the wound returns to the normal preinjury state containing type I collagen, over a long period of time. This task of converting a dermis containing predominantly type III collagen to one with a majority of type I collagen is accomplished through tightly controlled synthesis of new collagen with lysis of old collagen. Collagenolysis is performed by collagenases that are produced by wound granulocytes, macrophages, epidermal cells, and fibroblasts. Three major enzymes called metalloproteinases have the ability to degrade and digest collagens. Matrix metalloprotease 1 (MMP-1) or interstitial collagenase can cleave type I, II, III, XIII, and X collagens (94); MMP-2 or gelatinase can degrade denatured collagens of all types and native type V and XI collagens (95); and MMP-3 or stromelysin can degrade type III, IV, V, VII, and IX collagens as well as glycoproteins and proteoglycans (96). Their inhibitors, called tissue inhibitors of matrix metalloproteases (TIMP), control the activity of these MMPs. During the first 3 weeks after injury, the fibrillar collagen accumulates rapidly, followed by slower collagen deposition as well as collagen remodeling. In an attempt to return the tensile strength back toward normal, the scar tissue attains about 40% of its final strength in the first month and the strength continues to increase for as long as a year after injury (97) but never attains more than 80% of the preinjury strength (11).

REFERENCES

1. Brockes JP. Amphibian limb regeneration: rebuilding a complex structure. Science 1997; 276:81–87.
2. Burrington JD. Wound healing in the fetal lamb. J Pediatr Surg 1971; 6:523–528.
3. Rowlatt V. Intrauterine wound healing in a 20-week human fetus. Virchows Arch 1979; 381:353.
4. Longaker MT, Adzik NS. The biology of fetal wound repair: a review. Plast Reconstr Surg 1991; 87:788–798.
5. Lorenz HP, Longaker MT, Perkocha LA, Jennings RW, Harrison MR, Adzik NS. Scarless wound repair: a human fetal skin model. Development 1992; 114:253–259.
6. Martin P. Wound healing—aiming for perfect skin regeneration. Science 1997; 276:75–81.

7. Krummel T, Nelson J, Diegelmann R, et al. Fetal response to injury in the rabbit. J Pediatr Surg 1987; 22:601–664.
8. Saed GM, Ladin D, Olson J, Han X, Hou Z, Fivenson D. Analysis of p53 mutations in keloids using polymerase chain reaction-based single-strand conformational polymorphism and DNA sequencing. Arch Dermatol 1998; 134:963–967.
9. Tuan TL, Nichter LS. The molecular basis of keloid and hypertrophic scar formation. Mol Med Today 1998; 4(1):19–24.
10. Clark RAE. Biology of dermal wound repair. Dermatol Clin 1993; 11:647–660.
11. Kirsner RS, Eaglstein WH. The wound healing process. Dermatol Clin 1993; 11:629–640.
12. Werner R. Blood coagulation. In: Werner R, ed. Essentials in Modern Biochemistry. Boston: Jones & Bartlett, 1983:270–273.
13. Clark RAF. Cutaneous wound repair: molecular & cellular controls. Prog Dermatol 1988; 22:1–12.
14. Parker RI, Gralnick HR. Fibrin monomer induced binding of endogenous platelet von Willebrand factor to the glycocalcin portion of platelet glycoprotein IB. Blood 1987; 70:1589–1594.
15. Clark RAF, Lanigan JM, DellaPelle P, Manseau E, et al. Fibronectin and fibrin provide a provisional matrix for epidermal cell migration during wound re-epithelialization. J Invest Dermotol 1982; 70:264–269.
16. Grinnell F, Feld M, Minter D. Fibroblast adhesion to fibrinogen and fibrin substrate: requirement for cold-insoluble globulin (plasma fibronectin). Cell 1980; 19:517–525.
17. Clark RAF. Potential roles of fibronectin in cutaneous wound repair. Arch Dermatol 1988; 124:201–206.
18. Moncada S, Gryglewski R, Bunting S, Vane JR. An enzyme isolated from arteries transforms prostaglandin endoperoxides to an unstable substance that inhibits platelet aggregation. Nature 1976; 263:663–665.
19. Stern DM, Naworth PP, Marcum J, Handley D, Kisiel D, et al. Interaction of antithrombin III with bovine aortic segments. J Clin Invest 1985; 75:272–279.
20. Loedam JA, Meijers JCM, Sixma JJ, et al. Inactivation of human factor VIII by activated protein C: cofactor activity of protein S and protective effect of von Willebrand factor. J Clin Invest 1988; 82:1236–1243.
21. Loskutoff SE, Edgington TS. Synthesis of a fibrinolytic activator and inhibitor by endothelial cells. Proc Natl Acad Sci USA 1977; 74:3903–3907.
22. Santaro SA. Identification of a 160,000 dalton platelet membrane protein that mediates the initial divalent cation–dependent adhesion of platelets to collagen. Cell 1986; 46:913–920.
23. Plow EF, McEver RP, Coller BS, et al. Related binding mechanisms for fibrinogen, fibronectin, von Willebrand factor, and thrombospondin on thrombin stimulated human platelets. Blood 1985; 66:724–727.
24. Terkeltaub RA, Ginsberg MH. Platelets and response to injury. In: Clark RAF, Henson PM, eds. Molecular and Cellular Biology of Wound Repair. New York: Plenum, 1988:35–55.
25. Ginsberg MH, Du X, Plow EF. Inside-out integrin signaling. Curr Opin Cell Biol 1992; 4:766–771.
26. Ross RR, Rainer EW. Platelet-derived growth factor and cell proliferation. In: Sara VR et al. Growth Factors: From Genes to Clinical Application. New York: Raven, 1990:193–199.
27. Dernyk R. Transforming growth factor-α. Cell 1988; 54:593–595.
28. Sporn MB, Roberts AM. Transforming growth factor-β: recent progress and new challenges. J Cell Biol 1992; 119:1017–1021.
29. Weksler BB. Platelets. In: Gallin JI, Goldstein IM, R. Snyderman R, eds. Inflammation: Basic Principles and Clinical Correlates. New York: Raven, 1992:727–746.
30. Sanberg N. Time relationship between administration of cortisone and wound healing in rats. Acta Chir Scand 1964; 127:446.
31. Savlov ED, Dunply JE. The healing of disrupted and restructed wounds. Surgery 1954; 36:362.

32. Albelda SM, Buck CA. Integrins and other adhesion molecules. FASEB J 1990; 4:2868–2880.
33. Hibbs MS, Hasty KA, Seyer IM, et al. Biochemical and immunological characterization of the secreted forms of human neutrophil gelatinase. J Biol Chem 1985; 260:2493–2501.
34. Newman SL, Henson JE, Henson PM. Phagocytosis of senescent neutrophils by human monocyte derived macrophages and rabbit inflammatory macrophages. J Exp Med 1982; 156:430–442.
35. Postlethwaite AE, Kang AH. Collagen and collagen peptide–induced chemotaxis of human blood monocytes. J Exp Med 1976; 143:1299–1307.
36. Senior RM, Griffin GL, Mecham RP. Chemotactic activity of elastin-derived peptides. J Clin Invest 1980; 66:859–862.
37. Bar-Shavit R, Kahn A, Fenton JW, Wilner GD. Chemotactic response of monocytes to thrombin. J Cell Biol 1983; 96:282–285.
38. Wahl SM, Hunt DA, Wakefield LM, McCartney-Francis N, et al. Transforming growth factor type β induces monocyte chemotaxis and growth factor production. Proc Natl Acad Sci USA 1987; 84:5788–5792.
39. Leibovich SJ, Ross R. The role of macrophage in wound repair: a study with hydrocortisone and antimacrophage serum. Am J Pathol 1975; 78:71–100.
40. Falanga V, Zitelli JA, Eaglstein WH. Wound healing. J Am Acad Dermatol 1988; 19:559–563.
41. Werb Z, Gordon S. Elastase secretion by stimulated macrophages. J Exp Med 1975; 142:361–377.
42. Werb Z, Gordon S. Secretion of a specific collagenase by stimulated macrophages. J Exp Med 1975; 142:346–360.
43. Schaffer M, Barbul A. Lymphocyte function in wound healing and following injury. Brit J Surg 1998; 85(4):444–460.
44. Woodley DT, Chen JD, Kim JP, Sarret Y, et al. Re-epithelialization. Dermatol Clin 1993; 11:641–646.
45. Stenn KS, Depalma I. Re-epithelialization. In: Clark RAF, Hensen PM, eds. The Molecular and Cellular Biology of Wound Repair. New York: Plenum, 1988:3321–325.
46. Woodley DT, Bachmann PM, O'Keefe EJ. Laminin inhibits human keretinocytes migration. J Cell Physiol 1988; 136:140–146.
47. O'Keefe EJ, Payne RE, Russell N, et al. Spreading and enhanced motility of human keretinocytes on fibronectin. J Invest Dermatol 1985; 85:125–130.
48. Kim JP, Zhang K, Chen JD, et al. Mechanism of human keratinocyte migration on fibronectin: unique roles of RGD site and integrins. J Cell Physiol 1992; 151:443–450.
49. Sarret Y, Woodley DT, Grigsby K, et al. Human keratinocyte locomotion: the effect of selected cytokines. J Invest Dermatol 1992; 98:12–16.
50. Chen JD, Kim JP, Sarret Y, et al. Recombinant human epidermal growth factor (rEGF) promotes keratinocyte locomotion. J Invest Dermatol 1992; 98:614.
51. Brown GL, Nanney LB, Griffen J, et al. Enhancement of wound healing by topical treatment with epidermal growth factor. N Engl J Med 1989; 321:76–79.
52. Woodley DT, Kalebec T, Banes AJ, et al. Adult human keratinocytes migrating over non-viable dermal collagen produce collagenolytic enzymes that degrade type I and type IV collagen. J Invest Dermetol 1986; 86:418–423.
53. Hunt TK. Wound Healing and Wound Infection: Theory and Surgical Practice. Appleton-Century-Crofts, New York: 1980.
54. Folkman J: Angiogenesis: initiation and control. Ann N Y Acad Sci 1982; 401:212–217.
55. Folkman J, Klagsburn M. Angiogenic factors. Science 1987; 235:442–448.
56. Iruela-Arispe M, Sage H. Endothelial cells exhibiting angiogenesis in-vitro proliferate in response to TGF-β. J Cell Biochem 1993; 52:414–430.
57. Folkman J, Shing T. Angiogenesis. J Biol Chem 1992; 207:10931–10934.
58. Azizkhan RG, Azizkhan JC, Zetter BR, Folkman J. Mast cell heparin stimulates migration of capillary endothelial cells in-vitro. J Exp Med 1980; 152:931–944.

59. Raju KS, Allessandri G, Gullino PM. Characterization of a chemoattractant for endothelium induced by angiogenesis effectors. Cancer Res 1984; 44:1579–1584.
60. Weisman DM, Polverini PJ, Kamp DW, Leibovich SJ. Transforming growth factor beta (TGF-β) is chemotactic for human monocytes and induces their expression of angiogenic activity. Biochem Biophys Res Commun 1988; 157:793–800.
61. Nissen NN, Polverini PJ, Koch AE, Volin MV, Gamelli RL, Dipietro LA. Vascular endothelial growth factor mediates angiogenic activity during the proliferative phase of wound healing. Am J Path 1998; 152(6):1445–1452.
62. Clark RAF. Regulation of fibroplasia in cutaneous wound repair. Am J Med Sci 1993; 306:42–48.
63. Clark RAF, McCoy G, Folkvord JM. TGF-β stimulates extracellular matrix–dependent stratified growth of cultured human fibroblasts. Clin Res 1989; 37:229A.
64. Seppa HEJ, Grotendorst GR, Seppa SI, Schiffmann E, Martin GR. Platelet-derived growth factor is chemotactic for fibroblasts. J Cell Biol 1982; 92:584–588.
65. Postlethwaite AE, Keski-Oja J, Moses HL, Kang AH. Stimulation of the chemotactic migration of human fibroblasts by transforming growth factor-β. J Exp Med 1987; 165:251–256.
66. Woodley DT, O'Keefe EJ, Pruniers M. Cutaneous wound healing: a model for cell-matrix interactions. J Am Acad Dermatol 1985; 12:420–423.
67. Gabbiani G, Lelous M, Bailey AJ, et al. Collagen and myofibroblasts of granulation tissue: a chemical, ultrastructural and immunologic study. Virchows Arch Cell Pathol 1976; 21:133–145.
68. Varga J, Jimenez SA. Stimulation of normal human fibroblast collagen production and processing by transforming growth factor beta. Biochem Biophys Res Commun 1986; 138:974–980.
69. Ghahary A, Shen YJ, Scott PG, Gong Y, Tredget EE. Enhanced expression of mRNA for transforming growth factor-beta, type I and type III pro-collagen in human post-burn hypertrophic scar tissues. J Lab Clin Med 1993; 122:465–473.
70. Adzik NS, Lorenz HP. Cells, matrix, growth factor and the surgeon. The biology of scarless fetal wound repair. Ann Surg 1994; 220:10–18.
71. Adzik NS, Harrison MR. Fetal surgical therapy. Lancet 1994; 343:897–902.
72. Clark RAF, Nielsen LD, Welch MP, McPherson JM. Collagen matrices attenuate the collagen synthetic response of cultured fibroblasts to TGF-β. J Cell Sci 1995; 108:1251–1261.
73. Garner WL. Epidermal regulation of dermal fibroblast activity. Plast Reconstr Surg 1998; 102(1):135–139.
74. Machesney M, Tidman N, Waseem A, Kirby L, Leigh I. Activated keratinocytes in the epidermis of hypertrophic scars. Am J Path 1998; 152(5):1133–1141.
75. Granstein RD, Murphy GF, Margolis RJ, Byrne MH, Amento EP. Gamma interferon inhibits collagen synthesis in vivo in the mouse. J Clin Invest 1987; 79:1254–1258.
76. Majno G, Gabbiani G, Hirschel BJ, Ryan GB, Statkov PR. Contraction of granulation tissue in vitro: similarity to smooth muscle. Science 1971; 173:548–550.
77. Welch MP, Odland GF, Clark RAF. Temporal relationships of F-actin bundle formation, collagen and fibronectin matrix assembly, and fibronectin expression to wound contraction. J Cell Biol 1990; 110:133–145.
78. Singer II, Kawka DW, Kazazis DM, Clark RAF. In-vivo co-distribution of fibronectin and actin fibers in granulation tissue: immunofluorescence and electron microscope studies of the fibronexus at the myofibroblast surface. J Cell Biol 1984; 98:2091–2106.
79. Gabbiani G, Hirschell BJ, Ryan GB, et al. Granulation tissue as a contractile organ. J Exp Med 1972; 135:719–735.
80. Clark RAF, Folkvord JM, Hart CE, Murray MJ, McPherson JM. Platelet isoforms of platelet-derived growth factor stimulate fibroblast to contract collagen matrices. J Clin Invest 1989; 84:1036–1040.
81. Falanga V, Eaglstein WH. Wound healing: practical aspects. Prog Dermatol 1988; 22:1–10.

82. Brown LF, Lanir N, McDonagh J, Tognazzi K, Dvorak AM, et al. Fibroblast migration in fibrin gel matrices. Am J Pathol 1993; 142:273–283.
83. Grinnell F, Feld MK. Initial adhesion of human fibroblasts in serum-free medium: possible role of secreted fibronectin. Cell 1979; 17:117–129.
84. Clark RAF, Folkvord JM, Nielsen LD. Either exogenous or endogenous fibronectin can promote adherence of human endothelial cells. J Cell Sci 1986; 82:263–280.
85. McDonald JA, Kelley DG, Broekelmann TJ. Role of fibronectin in collagen deposition: Fab 1 antibodies to the gelatin-binding domain of fibronectin inhibit both fibronectin and collagen organization in fibroblast extracellular matrix. J Cell Biol 1982; 92:485–492.
86. Gailit J, Clark RAF. Wound repair in the context of extracellular matrix. Curr Opin Cell Biol 1994; 6:717–725.
87. Toole BP: Glycosaminoglycans in morphogenesis. In: Hay ED, ed. Cell Biology of Extracellular Matrix. New York: Plenum, 1981:259–294.
88. Bently JP. Rate of chondroitin sulphate formation in wound healing. Ann Surg 1967; 165:186–191.
89. Longaker MT, Chiu E, Adzik NS, Stern M, Harrison M, Stern R. Studies in fetal wound healing v. prolonged presence of hyaluronic acid in fetal wound fluid. Ann Surg 1991; 213:290–296.
90. Bronson RE, Argenta JG, Bertolami N. Interleukin-1 induced changes in extracellular gycosaminoglycans composition of cutaneous scar–derived fibroblasts in culture. Coll Relat Res 1988; 8:199–208.
91. Scott JE. Proteoglycan-fibrillar collagen interactions in tissues: dermatan sulphate proteoglycans as a tissue organizer. In: Scott JE, ed. Dermatan Sulphate Proteoglycans: Chemistry, Biology, Chemical Pathology. London: Portland, 1993:165–181.
92. Toole BP. Proteoglycans and hyaluronan in morphogenesis and differentiation. In: Hay ED, ed. Cell Biology of the Extracellular Matrix. New York: Plenum, 1991:305–341.
93. Kurkinen M, Baheri A, Roberts PJ, Stenman S. Sequential appearance of fibronectin and collagen in experimental granulation tissue. Lab Invest 1980; 43:47–51.
94. Grant GA, Eisen AZ, Marmer BL, Roswit WT, Goldberg GI. The activation of human skin fibroblast procollagenase. Sequence identification of the major conversion products. J Biol Chem 1987; 262:5886–5889.
95. Hibbs MS, Hoidal JR, Kang AH. Expression of a metalloproteinase that degrades native type V collagen and denatured collagens by cultured human alveolar macrophages. J Clin Invest 1987; 80:1644–1650.
96. Sans J, Quinones S, Otani Y, Nagase H, et al. The complete primary structure of human matrix-metalloproteinase III. Identity with stromelysin. J Biol Chem 1988; 263:6742–6745.
97. Levenson SM, Geever EG, Crowley LV, et al. The healing of rat skin wounds. Ann Surg 1965; 161:293–308.

2
Biomechanical Properties of Skin

Maurice Morad Khosh
St. Luke's–Roosevelt Hospital Center
New York, New York

Wayne F. Larrabee, Jr.
University of Washington
Seattle, Washington

I. INTRODUCTION

Successful treatment of wounds and favorable scar formation require an understanding of the biomechanical properties of skin. Such understanding will aid in the design and execution of skin closure methods. Surgeons have long been able to use experience and intuition in determining surgical technique for wound closure. Physical parameters that dictate scarring outcome and wound closure results are now better defined. Advances in experimental designs and measurement techniques have furthered our understanding of the biomechanical properties of skin. The complex composition of skin and the interaction of its components, however, still present a challenge in making in vivo measurements and applying mathematical approximations in predicting skin behavior.

II. STRUCTURAL BASIS OF SKIN BIOMECHANICS

Biomechanical properties of skin are most commonly attributed to the structural properties of the dermis. It has become evident however, that the epidermis, dermal-epidermal junction, and subcutaneous and deeper structures also contribute to skin biomechanical properties, albeit to lesser degrees.

Epidermis has a thickness of 0.07 to 1.4 mm and serves to protect the body surface against physical and ultraviolet injury, to provide a barrier to water and chemicals, and to resist microbial penetration. The presence of disulfide bonds within the keratin layer and the desmosomal attachments between the epithelial cells give the epidermis mechanical strength and relative water impermeability. Studies of the effects of water and emollients on skin indicate that epidermal hydration has a significant effect on maximum skin distention and accommodation to tension (1,2). Protective effects of melanin in maintaining skin extensibility and viscoelasticity have also been proposed (3).

Dermis is a connective tissue matrix that contributes the most to the biomechanics of skin. Dermal thickness varies from 1 to 3 mm. In terms of volume, dermis is composed of

27 to 39% collagen, 0.2 to 0.6% elastin, 0.03 to 0.35% glycosaminoglycans, and 60 to 72% water.

Collagen, the principal load-bearing component of the dermis, provides most of the mechanical strength of skin. Collagen molecules are produced by fibroblasts as three polypeptide chains that wrap around one another in a triple helix. In the extracellular space, collagen molecules are cross-linked with covalent bonds between lysine residues, thus forming fibrils. The fibrils are arranged in staggered fashion with one-fourth length overlap. Collagen fibers are woven in a multidirectional array and in the relaxed skin seem distributed in a seemingly haphazard way. The cross-linkage between collagen molecules has a significant effect on tissue strength. This cross-linkage is minimal at birth and increases with age (4). The ultimate tensile strength of skin is positively correlated with the mass average diameter of collagen fibrils (5). In general, skin subject to continual high-tension loads contains collagen fibrils of larger diameter than skin under low-tension loads (4,6).

Elastin is a fibrous protein that forms a meshlike network in dermis. Elastin fibers loop around collagen fibers and attach at multiple points along each bundle. Elastin is proposed to function as a type of energy storage device, bringing stretched collagen back to a relaxed position (7). It is thus postulated to have an effect on the directionality of skin tension, as in relaxed skin tension lines (8). Selective digestion methods have demonstrated in rats that the elastic fibers undergo a progressive distortion from a relatively straight meshwork to a tortuous and distorted arrangement as the animals age. This has been proposed as an explanation for the decreased tissue compliance seen with aging (9,10).

Glycosaminoglycans, principally dermatan sulfate, hyaluronic acid, and chondroitin sulfate, make up the ground substance and with water contribute to the viscoelastic nature of skin. Glycosaminoglycans are covalently linked to peptide chains that form high-molecular-weight complexes called proteoglycans. The viscous properties of connective tissue are strongly correlated with the type and the amount of glycosaminoglycans (11).

III. SKIN AS A VISCOELASTIC MATERIAL

The complex composition of skin imparts biomechanical properties that typify elastic properties of solids and the viscous properties of fluids. The elastic properties relate force to tissue movement in the steady state, without considering changes that may occur over time. Time-dependent changes that occur in skin are a result of fluid displacement and viscous properties of skin. Thus, biomechanical properties of skin are best explained in terms of viscoelasticity. In order to simplify the evaluation of cutaneous mechanical properties, scientists and engineers have attempted to analyze the elastic and viscous parameters of skin separately.

In an idealized simple elastic solid material, elongation along a given axis is proportional to the applied force. This relationship is known as Hooke's law: stress = strain × Young's modulus. Here, stress is force per unit area, strain is change in length as a ratio of initial length, and Young's modulus is a constant of elasticity. Hooke's law is most accurately applied to very small uniaxial deformations of materials with a linear stress-strain curve. For three-dimensional solids, multiple elastic coefficients are needed to describe material behavior along different axes. This relationship is greatly simplified when the material is isotropic, i.e., when elastic properties are the same in all three axes. An isotropic planar solid material requires only two coefficients of elasticity, Young's modulus and Poisson's ratio. Young's modulus is the slope of the stress-strain curve, and Poisson's ratio is the amount of contraction that occurs in one axis divided by the elongation in the other axis, perpendicular to the first axis.

In an ideal viscous fluid, applied stress causes a change in the fluid strain at a rate proportional to the viscosity. Mathematically, this is expressed in Newton's law: $\sigma = \eta(\delta\epsilon/\delta\tau)$, where σ is the stress, η the viscosity, $\delta\epsilon$ the change in strain, and $\delta\tau$ the change in time. This relation implies that applied stress is proportional to the rate of change of strain over time. In contrast, in elastic solids the relationship between stress and strain is unaffected by time. It should be evident that mathematical formulations as described here can function only as an approximation of the true properties of skin. Derived data, as a result, are only an approximation of true skin behavior. In order to approximate skin flap behavior better, experts have utilized finite-element analysis (12,13). Finite-element analysis permits modeling of complex structures by considering them as an aggregate of small elements. In this form of analysis, the skin surface is divided into a large number of small triangles and the mechanical behavior of each small segment is calculated separately. Mechanical properties of the skin surface are then approximated by solving a matrix that represents these triangles.

IV. BIOMECHANICAL PROPERTIES OF SKIN

In evaluating wound closure and scar revision, the biomechanical properties that are most pertinent are related to the directionality of resting skin tension, tensile and elastic properties, plasticity, and expandability of skin.

A. Directionality

Skin demonstrates an orientation preference, also known as anisotropy. This resting skin tension varies with the anatomic position, subcutaneous fat, and underlying joints and musculature. The German anatomist Langer (14) first described the lines of skin cleavage in cadaver skin. Langer used a round awl to make stab incisions in the skin of fresh cadavers. He noted that the round stab incisions resulted in linear clefts in the skin. The pattern that these skin clefts made became known as Langer's lines. The orientation of Langer's lines is frequently distinct from the skin creases in living subjects when the limbs are placed in

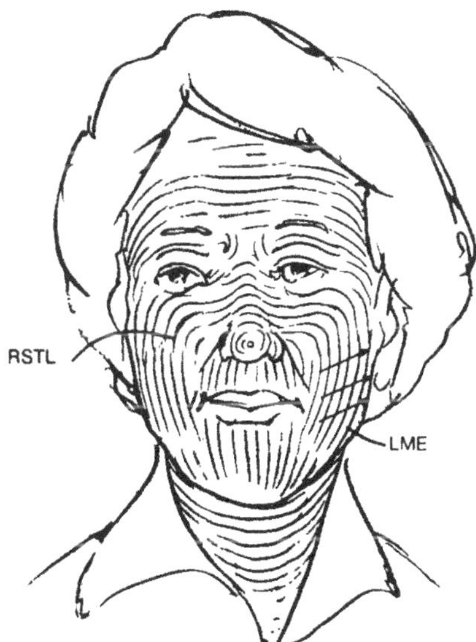

Figure 1 Relaxed skin tension lines (RSTLs) of the face. Lines of maximal extensibility (LMEs) are perpendicular to relaxed skin tension lines. (From Bailey BJ et al, eds. Head and Neck Surgery—Otolaryngology. Philadelphia: Lippincott, 1993:1917.)

a relaxed position. These creases are known as relaxed skin tension lines (RSTLs). RSTLs follow the longest and straightest furrows that form when skin is pinched (15) (Fig. 1). RSTLs are important to surgeons because they represent the desirable direction of skin incisions. Placing the long axis of a wound parallel to RSTLs will put the maximum closure tension along the lines of maximal extensibility (LMEs). The LMEs run perpendicular to the RSTLs and represent the direction of minimum tension in the wound (16).

Whether RSTLs and Langer's lines have a cellular anatomic basis or simply reflect the tension of underlying muscles, subcutaneous fat, and underlying joints remains a subject of controversy. Collagen and elastin fibers have been identified parallel to the RSTLs (8). The preferential orientation of these fibers in the direction of RSTLs suggests a possible causal relationship. It is not clear whether the collagen and elastin orientation is a primary event or is secondary to the forces of underlying structures. It seems reasonable to assume, however, that underlying muscles and joints exert the primary force that causes preferential alignment of collagen and elastin in skin.

B. Elasticity

A typical stress-strain curve for skin is shown in Fig. 2. The graph demonstrates the nonlinear nature of skin extensibility. The curve can be divided into three distinct regions: (I) an initial flat portion where elongation occurs without appreciable force, (II) an intermediate region of rapid transition, and (III) a terminal portion where little extension is possible despite a significant increase in applied force. Young's (elasticity) modulus can be calculated as the slope of this curve. The shape of the graph correlates with the clinical finding in wound closure that past a certain initial distance, wound edges cannot be reapproximated despite significant traction forces. This stress-strain relationship also points to the importance of wound closure design. It is evident that in wounds that are closed under moderate tension, small changes in strain have a large impact on skin tension and thereby on vascular perfusion of wound edges. It has shown that blood flow in a skin flap is inversely pro-

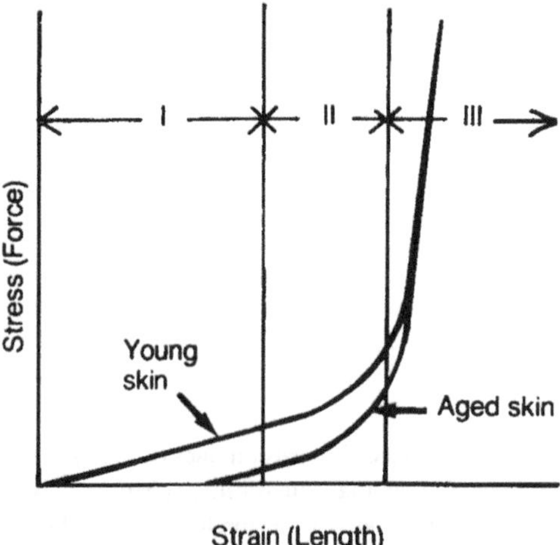

Figure 2 Stress-strain curve for skin divided into three separate regions. (From Larrabee WF. Immediate repair of facial defects. Dermatol Clin 1989; 7:662.)

portional to the tension placed across it (17). Tension-related decline in perfusion is not clinically significant in short flaps. In long cutaneous flaps, however, dimi-nished perfusion was crucial and resulted in flap necrosis (17).

Histologic evaluation of skin under tension reveals the microscopic corollary of the stress-strain curve. During the initial deformation, randomly arranged collagen and elastin fibers are stretched in the direction of force. Collagen fibers do not bear any burden until some of the fibers are completely straightened (18). As a result, there is little resistance to initial deformation and the stress-strain relationship is nearly linear. In the body, naturally occurring skin tensions due to joint movements correspond to this portion of the curve. As stress continues, additional collagen fibers are recruited into load bearing and resistance rises rapidly (region II of the stress-strain curve). At high stresses, nearly all collagen fibers are oriented in the direction of the force and fully extended (region III of the stress-strain curve). Skin nonextensibility past this level prevents further deformation and structural damage to the epidermis and dermal vascular structures (18).

Skin exhibits a rate-dependent resistance to applied force, which represents a viscous property of the skin. Breaking strain, therefore, is related to the rapidity of stress application. Breaking strain for rapidly stretched skin can be significantly lower than that for slowly stretched skin. Incremental increases in stress produce more consistent and reproducible results for the skin stress-strain curve. The tensile strength of human skin ranges between 5 and 30 N/mm^2 with a mean of about 28 N/mm^2 at age 8 and 17 N/mm^2 at age 95. The ultimate modulus of elasticity (determined from region III of the stress-strain curve) shows a moderate decline from a mean of 70 N/mm^2 at age 11 to 60 N/mm^2 at age 95. The ultimate skin strain before rupture varies from 35 to 115%. The mean value declines in linear fashion from 75% at birth to 60% at 90 years (19,20).

C. Shearing

Another factor that contributes to tension at wound edges is the resistance between the dermis and the underlying tissue (21). This shearing force varies according to the site of interest and age of the patient. Undermining reduces the shearing forces during wound closure by separating the subcutaneous attachments of the dermis. As undermining continues, the force required to advance a wound diminishes (21). However, the beneficial effects of undermining are not limitless. In fact, most of the benefit derived from wound closure occurs in the first 2 cm. In a study of undermining effects on wound closure tension, Larrabee and Sutton (22) showed that the most significant increase in elasticity occurred within the first 2 cm of undermining. There was a moderate increase in elasticity for the next 2 cm of undermining. Further undermining to 6 cm, however, occasionally resulted in a paradoxical increase in resistance (Fig. 3). The cause of this observation was not immediately apparent, but in light of these findings and the risk of adversely affecting vascularity of a flap, it can be concluded that excessive undermining may also be deleterious in wound closure.

D. Viscosity

Once the skin is stretched, it begins to modify its internal structure to minimize stress. Thus, the force necessary to maintain skin at a given length begins to decline; this is termed *stress relaxation*. Similarly, for a given amount of force, skin continues to stretch over time; this is referred to as *creep*. Stress relaxation and creep result from displacement of the interstitial fluid that exists in between collagen bundles. These viscous properties help explain an

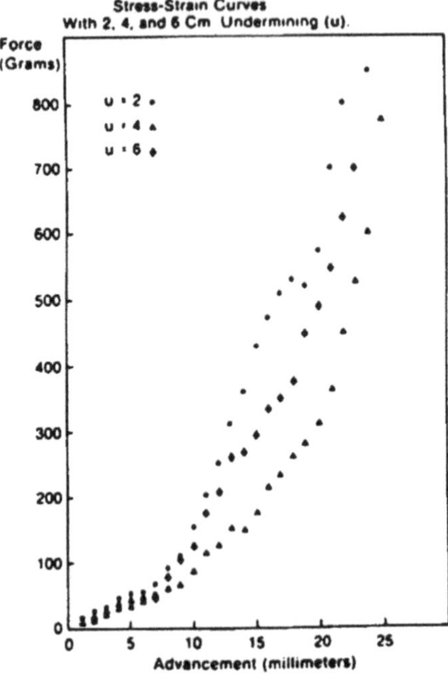

Figure 3 Stress-strain curves for pig skin advancement flaps after undermining 2, 4, and 6 cm. (From Ref. 22.)

apparent increase in the breaking strength of skin when it is stretched very slowly, as compared with rapid traction.

In a perfectly elastic tissue, the stress-strain curves for loading and unloading would coincide. In skin, however, the strain-stress curves for loading and unloading do not coincide. These divergent stress-strain curves are known as ***hysteresis loops*** (Fig. 4). In the hys-

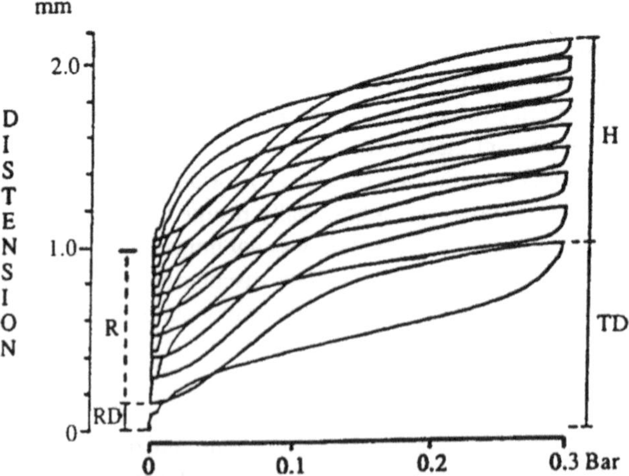

Figure 4 Hysteresis loops corresponding to skin deformation with repeated cycles of suction application to skin. H, hysteresis; TD, distensibility; R, elastic retraction; RD, resilient distensibility. (From Ref. 2.)

teresis loop, the area under the stress-strain curve represents the energy input into the system. The area between the two curves represents the energy loss, which is proportional to the viscosity of the system. Skin with large amounts of interstitial fluid, such as the skin of the young, shows a wide gap between the loading and unloading curves. The width of hysteresis loops becomes thinner as skin becomes less viscous. Skin viscosity closely correlates with the amount of glycosaminoglycans in the dermis. These substances contribute to the water-binding ability of the skin and the amount of interstitial fluid. In addition, it has been shown that epidermal hydration plays a role in viscous properties of skin. In experimental studies, skin plasticity increased with topical application of water and emollients to skin for short durations (1,2). In general, the viscosity of skin diminishes with age as the dermal and epidermal water content diminishes.

E. Skin Expansion

The viscoelastic properties of skin do not adequately explain the dramatic increases in skin surface area during skin expansion. Tissue expansion is the result of cellular proliferation and extracellular matrix production. The modern method of tissue expansion was popularized by Rodavan (23). Dermal thickness is decreased during the expansion period and for a variable time after expansion (Fig. 5). Collagen density, however, is not diminished during skin expansion (Fig. 6) (24). In physiologic tissue expansion, such as in obesity or pregnancy, dermal thickness and collagen content remain unaffected (25). Interestingly, epidermal thickness during skin expansion is preserved or increased. Tritiated thymadine labeling studies have shown an increase in keratinocyte proliferation that persists during the expansion period (26). This indicates a rapid proliferative potential in the epidermis as compared with a more gradual increase in dermal cellular proliferation and extracellular matrix production.

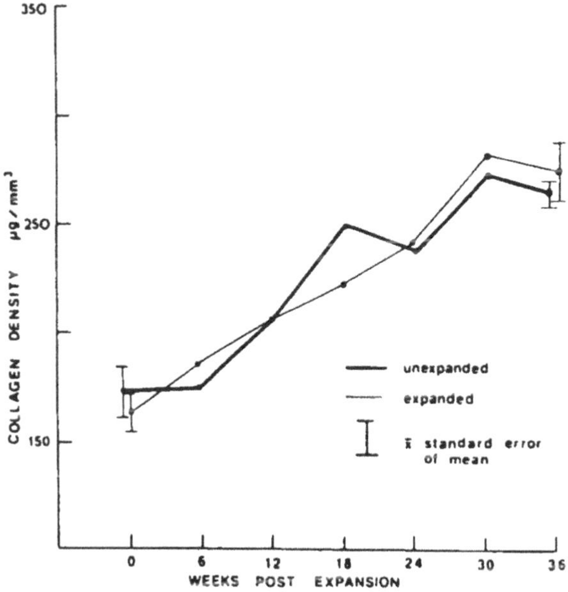

Figure 5 Dermal thickness following tissue expansion. (From Ref. 24.)

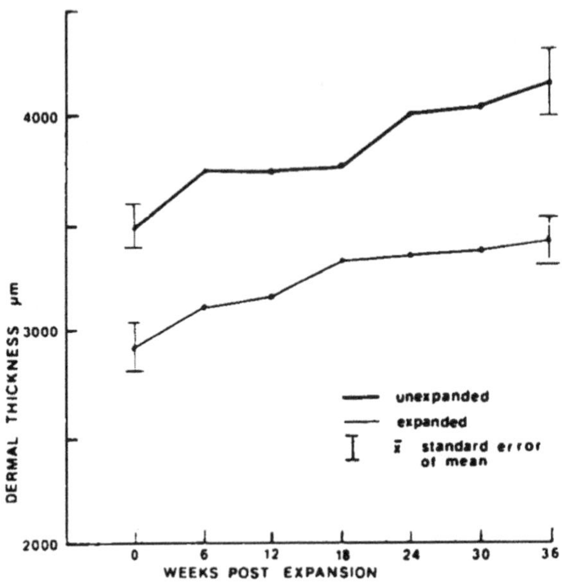

Figure 6 Collagen density of skin during tissue expansion. (From Ref. 24.)

Intraoperative skin expansion has been studied as a modality for increasing the amount of tissue available for wound closure. Studies of the effects of intraoperative tissue expansion indicate that it provides no added benefit compared with equivalent tissue undermining (27). This is intuitively logical, as no increase in dermal or epidermal proli-feration can be expected during acute tissue expansion.

V. CONCLUSION

The complex biomechanical properties of skin are related to the composition of the cutaneous tissue and its interaction with underlying fat, fascia, muscle, and skeleton. In order to achieve the best results in closing wounds or revising scars, the surgeon must have an understanding of these biomechanical properties. Directionality of skin tension and the corresponding RSTLs determine the direction of most favorable closure. Biomechanical skin properties offer a cellular and structural basis for the qualitative differences in skin according to site, age, and state of hydration. Appreciation of viscoelastic properties aids in designing skin flaps, minimizing ischemia at wound edges, and effectively reducing shearing forces in wound closure. Skin viscoelasticity and expandability together with scar maturation explain long-term results in wounds and flaps.

REFERENCES

1. Olsen LO, Jemec GBE. The influence of water, glycerine, paraffin oil and ethanol on skin mechanics. Acta Derm Venereol (Stockh) 1993; 73:404–406.

2. Jemec GBE, Jemec B, Jemec BIE, Serup J. The effect of superficial hydration on the mechanical properties of human skin in vivo: implications for plastic surgery. Plast Reconstr Surg 1990; 85:100–103.
3. Berardesca E, de Regal J, Leveque JL, Maibach HI. In vivo biophysical characterization of skin physiological differences in races. Dermatologica 1991; 182:89–93.
4. Parry DAD, Barnes GRG, Craig AS. A comparison of the size distribution of collagen fibrils in connective tissue as a function of age and a possible relation between fibril size distribution and mechanical properties. Proc R Soc Lond B Bio Sci 1978; 203:305–321.
5. Bailey AJ, Peach GRG, Fowler. In: Balazs EA, ed. The Chemistry and Molecular Biology of the Intercellular Matrix. Vol. 1. New York: Academic Press, 1970:385–404.
6. Craig AS, Eikenberry EF, Parry DAD. Ultrastructural organization of skin: classification on the basis of mechanical role. Connect Tiss Res 1987; 16:213–223.
7. Daly CH. The role of elastin in the mechanical behavior of human skin. Proceedings of the 8th International Conference on Med Bio Eng: 1969:18–27.
8. Pierard GE, Lapiere CM. Microanatomy of the dermis in relation to relaxed skin tension lines and Langer's lines. Am J Dermatopathol 1987; 9:219.
9. Imayama S, Braverman IB. A hypothetical explanation for the aging skin. Am J Pathol 1989; 134:1019–1025.
10. Daly CH, Odland GE. Age related change in the mechanical properties of the human skin. J Invest Dermatol 1979; 73:84–87.
11. Flint MH, Craig AS, Reilly HC, Gillard GC, Parry DAD. Collagen fibril diameter and glycosaminoglycan content of skin: indices of tissue maturity and function. Conn Tissue Res 1984; 13:69–81.
12. Larrabee WF, Sutton D. A finite element model of skin deformation (in three parts). Laryngoscope 1986; 96:399–417.
13. Pieper SD, Laub DR, Rosen JM. A finite element facial model for simulating plastic surgery. Plast Reconstr Surg 1995; 96:1100–1105.
14. Langer K. On the anatomy and physiology of the skin III (1862). Translated by Gibson T. Br J Plast Surg 1978; 31:185–199.
15. Borges AF. Relaxed skin tension lines. Dermatol Clin 1989; 7:169.
16. Borges AF. The rombic flap. Plast Reconstr Surg 1981; 67:458.
17. Larrabee WF, Holloway GA, Sutton D. Wound tension and blood flow in skin flaps. Ann Otol Rhinol Laryngol 1984; 93:112.
18. Daley CH, Odland GF. Age-related changes in the mechanical properties of human skin. J Invest Dermatol 1979; 73:84.
19. Vogel HG. Age dependence of mechanical and biochemical properties of human skin. Part I: Stress-strain experiments, skin thickness and biochemical analysis. Bioeng Skin 1987; 3:67–91.
20. Vogel HG. Age dependence of mechanical and biochemical properties of human skin. Part II: Hysteresis, relaxation, creep and repeated strain experiments. Bioeng Skin 1987; 3:141–176.
21. Cox KW, Larrabee WF. A study of skin flap advancement as a function of undermining. Arch Otolaryngol 1982; 108:112.
22. Larrabee WF, Sutton D. Variation of skin stress strain curves with undermining. Surg Forum 1981; 23:553.
23. Rodovan C. Breat reconstruction after mastectomy using the temporary expander. Plast Reconstr Surg 1982; 69:195.
24. Johnson PE, Kernahan DA, Bauer BS. Dermal and epidermal response to skin expansion in the pig. Plast Reconstr Surg 1988; 81:390.
25. Black MM, Bottoms E, Shuster S. Skin collagen and thickness in simple obesity. Br Med J 1971; 4:149.
26. Olenius M, Dalsgaard CJ, Wickman M. Mitotic activity in expanded human skin. Plast Reconstr Surg 1993; 91:213.
27. Mackay DR, Saggars GC, Kotwal N, et al. Stretching skin: undermining is more important than intraoperative expansion. Plast Reconstr Surg 1990; 86:722.

3
Prognosis for Facial Scarring

David B. Hom and Rick M. Odland
University of Minnesota and Hennepin County Medical Center
Minneapolis, Minnesota

The prognosis for facial scarring is dependent on how the wound has healed and the characteristics of the scar. This chapter describes the factors that increase the probability that a larger scar will result from a wound. Later in this chapter, wound characteristics that make a scar more visible are discussed.

Cutaneous wound healing consists of a highly coordinated cellular response following tissue injury. If healing is impaired, scarring frequently results. Thus, factors that contribute to poor healing often result in scarring.

A healed wound is the result of several major processes: hemostasis, inflammation, angiogenesis, epithelialization, and collagen production and remodeling. In open wounds, contraction also plays an important role. All of these components must occur in an orderly sequence for optimal wound healing to occur. When one or more of these processes are hindered, a nonhealing wound results that frequently gives more scarring. If any preceding healing step is impaired, all subsequent healing steps are affected. For example, derangement of inflammation alters angiogenesis and collagen formation, leading to more scarring. Factors that impair healing can be classified into intrinsic causes and extrinsic causes (Table 1).

I. INTRINSIC PATIENT FACTORS

A. Age

At various ages from the fetus to the adult, scar formation occurs differently. Compared with adult wounds, many fetal wounds heal without scarring. The fetal wound environment is different from the adult environment in that fetal wounds are contained in amniotic fluid rich in growth factors, fibronectin, and hyaluronic acid. A major difference between adult and fetal wound healing is the decreased acute inflammatory reaction seen in fetal wounds (1). Inflammation is important in reducing infection; however, if prolonged (>7 days) it increases the risk of scar formation (2). However, not all fetal wounds heal without scarring. Whether a fetal wound results in a scar depends on the organ type, severity of tissue injury, gestational age, and animal species. After a critical fetal age in utero, fetal wound healing becomes more similar to that of the adult with scar formation. Scarring does not occur in human fetal skin younger than 22 weeks old when it is transplanted to athymic mice (3).

Table 1 Factors That Impair Healing

Intrinsic factors	Extrinsic factors
Age	Malnutrition
Fetus	Protein-calorie
Child	Vitamins
Adult	Minerals
Immune status	Infection
Hypertrophic scarring and keloids	Insufficient oxygenation or perfusion
Psychophysiological stress	Hypoxemia
Stress	Hypoxia
Pain	Anemia
Noise	Hypovolemia
Hereditary healing diseases	Smoking
Ehlers-Danlos syndrome	Cancer
Epidermolysis bullosa	Radiation
Marfan's syndrome	Chemotherapy
Osteogenesis imperfecta	Medications
Werner's syndrome	Steroids
Disease states	Anticoagulants
Chronic pulmonary disease	Penicillamine
Chronic cardiac disease	Cyclosporine
Chronic liver disease (cirrhosis)	
Uremia	
Alcoholism	
Diabetes	
Peripheral vascular disease	

In children, wound contraction takes place more rapidly than in adults. As the body matures during adulthood, collagen density and fibroblasts decrease with elastin fiber fragmentation (4). In elderly individuals who do not have concurrent diseases, the rate of healing is slightly slower, with reepithelialization most effected (5,6). In addition, because the elderly often have associated chronic illnesses that can impair healing, older age is frequently considered a risk factor for additional scarring.

B. Immune Status

Immunosuppression is known to delay wound healing. This may be due to bacterial infections in immunosuppressed individuals or by the lack of specific cytokines necessary to complete healing. The inflammatory response plays an important role in preventing infections, and its derangement impacts wound healing and scar formation.

Acquired immunodeficiency syndrome (AIDS) delays wound healing, especially in advanced stages of the disease. In asymptomatic patients infected with human immunodeficiency virus (HIV), the risk of postoperative infections is probably no greater than that of the general population. However, as the disease progresses to AIDS and end-stage AIDS, a delay in wound healing becomes apparent. The average wound healing time in HIV-positive patients was 9 weeks, compared with 12 weeks in patients with advanced AIDS (7).

C. Hypertrophic Scars and Keloids

Hypertrophic scars and keloids are abnormal healing responses resulting in excessive collagen and glycoprotein deposition. Keloids grow beyond the boundaries of the original wound area and rarely involute. In contrast, hypertrophic scars do not extend beyond the limits of the original wound site. What determines whether a wound transforms into a keloid or hypertrophic scar remains undetermined.

Hypertrophic scars and keloids are present in all races. However, keloids have not been reported in albinos (8). Darker pigmented individuals appear to have a higher tendency for hypertrophic scars and keloids. Among the African-American population, keloids are found in 6–16% of individuals.

Body areas susceptible to keloid formation are the earlobes, mandibular angle, upper back, shoulders, upper arms, and anterior chest (9). When a wound is subjected to higher tension, keloid formation is more likely. Hormonal factors may also play a role in keloid formation in that keloids appear during puberty and frequently regress after menopause. Keloid fibroblasts have increased androgen binding compared with fibroblasts from normal tissue (10). Cutaneous disorders with an inflammatory or infectious component (cellulitis, pilonidal cysts, and foreign body reactions) have a greater risk for keloid formation.

During the early stages of wound repair, no histological distinction in a wound is present to determine whether it will become a keloid, hypertrophic scar, or normal scar. Each condition goes through a similar inflammatory stage followed by fibroplasia (11). However, by the third week, keloids begin to have more progressive and continuous fibroplasia than normal wounds. In new keloids, collagen synthesis is increased, with relatively more type III collagen than type I collagen (12). The collagen within keloids remains less mature than that in normal skin. The bulk of a keloid consists of excessive extracellular matrix (water and glycoproteins).

Transforming growth factor-β (TGF-β) appears to play an active role in keloid formation. Studies have shown that TGF-β1 induces keloid collagen growth. In addition, keloid tissue has enhanced messenger RNA (mRNA) expression of TGF-β1 (13).

D. Diabetes

Diabetes predisposes patients to poor healing through atherosclerosis, neuropathy, and an increased risk of infection. Uncontrolled diabetes results in wounds with slower collagen accumulation and weaker breaking strength (14,15). In addition, collagen synthesis and angiogenesis are decreased (16). Collagen impairment in wounds can be improved by controlling the hyperglycemia with insulin (17,18). Peripheral atherosclerosis, prevalent in diabetes, causes tissue hypoxia, which in itself impairs healing.

E. Stress

Healthy, well-nourished young patients who have been involved in multiple trauma frequently have delayed wound healing. One study showed that circulating B cells from trauma patients had diminished immunoglobulin synthesis and secretion. This phenomenon was thought to be a direct result of the trauma (19). Steroids are anti-inflammatory and are known to delay all aspects of wound healing. Endogenous steroids are released during periods of stress, and this may play a role in wound healing delay. Stress of any form, including from mental health, has been suggested to affect wound healing (20,21).

The stress-mediated mechanism that influences wound healing is believed to be directed through the immune system; however, decreased oxygen transport may also play a role (22).

F. Hereditary Healing Diseases

Several hereditary disorders directly affect wound healing. However, not all inherited syndromes with skin involvement cause delayed healing. Examples are cutis laxa and pseudoxanthoma elasticum, in which skin is excessively mobile but healing is usually normal.

Patients with Ehlers-Danlos syndrome are unable to form normal collagen or elastin. The skin is thin, lax, and friable with "onion skin" scars covered by thin, silvery, atrophic epithelium commonly found on the knees and shins. Ehlers-Danlos syndrome should be considered in young patients who have soft skin that tears easily with an associated history of hernias and a coagulopathy. Ten variants of the syndrome exist with different severities (23).

Epidermolysis bullosa is a disease in which a tissue adhesion defect in the epidermis, basement membrane, or dermis causes tissue separation and blistering upon minimal trauma. The different subtypes are determined by the different anatomical levels within the skin that are involved. Bart's syndrome is believed to be a subtype of dominantly inherited dystrophic epidermolysis bullosa. Abnormal cutaneous scarring is one manifestation of the syndrome (24).

In Marfan's syndrome there is an undefined defect in collagen cross-linking. It is associated with a tall physique, arachnodactyly, lax ligaments, scoliosis, pectus excavatum, myopia, and dissecting aneurysms. Another disease, osteogenesis imperfecta, is associated with a deficiency in collagen maturation. These patients present with blue sclerae, thin skin, easy bruising, hernias, and bone abnormalities.

In Werner's syndrome, progeria, and homocystinuria, an accelerated atherosclerosis interferes with healing and increases the risk for skin ulcers. Patients with homocystinuria have poor collagen cross-linking. Atrophia maculosa varioliformis cutis is a rare but intriguing disease in which scars appear spontaneously on normal facial skin (25).

G. Disease States

Many chronic diseases are characterized by impaired wound healing. This is often a direct biochemical effect of the disease state or may result from a depletion of metabolic reserves. Chronic pulmonary and cardiac diseases impair circulation and oxygenation. Uremia, jaundice, and alcoholism also impair wound healing. Acute critical illness related to major surgical procedures, shock, respiratory failure, and sepsis involve decreased oxygen transport and lower tissue oxygenation, which can affect wound healing (22). Distant malignancy can affect wound healing, presumably because of the catabolic state of malignancy (26).

II. EXTRINSIC PATIENT FACTORS

A. Malnutrition

Malnutrition is associated with impaired healing and increased likelihood of infection. Loss of more than 20% of body weight impairs the tensile strength of incisions (27–29). In most cases, wound healing delay results from protein-calorie depletion rather than lack of a single nutrient (27,28). Specifically, decreased protein intake results in decreased fibroblast proliferation, decreased proteoglycan and collagen synthesis, decreased angiogenesis, and derangement of collagen remodeling (29,30). If carbohydrate intake is insufficient, body protein catabolism begins. This is because the protein normally used for wound repair is diverted to provide glucose for the body.

Insufficient vitamin C results in higher collagen lysis relative to collagen formation. In addition, the hydroxylation of proline and lysine within the collagen molecule requires vitamin C, iron, oxygen, and α-ketoglutarate. Decreased levels of these substances result in impaired cross-linking, leading to decreased wound strength. Vitamin A deficiency results in inadequate inflammation; however, the pathophysiology of vitamin A deficiency remains unknown. Thiamine (vitamin B_1) deficiency leads to decreased collagen formation. Iron, zinc, copper, and manganese are required for normal collagen formation. Zinc is the best characterized mineral deficiency that impairs healing and can be reversed with supplementation (31). Insufficient zinc is seen in elderly individuals who have chronic metabolic stress and persistent diarrhea.

B. Infection

Infection is an important cause of delayed wound healing and subsequent scar formation. Skin injury disrupts the protective epithelial layer and provides an opportunity for bacterial penetration. The risk of bacterial infection increases from a higher bacterial load greater than 100,000 bacteria per gram of tissue (32,33). Contamination of a wound by saliva or stool increases the likelihood of infection. Faulty closure of the wound, which delays epithelialization, can also be a factor in wound infection. Retained foreign bodies, such as dirt or debris, increase the risks for infection. Penetrating wounds from human and animal bites also have a higher incidence of wound infection.

C. Insufficient Oxygen and Perfusion

Decreased tissue oxygenation (<20 mm Hg) results in decreased collagen synthesis and decreased collagen cross-linking. However, collagen lysis continues. Clinically, this can cause a wound to break down in a hypoxic environment (28). Low tissue oxygen levels also impair phagocytic activity, which increases the risk for infection. Hypoxia stimulates fibroblast proliferation and the release of angiogenic growth factors from macrophages. On the other hand, adequate oxygenation does not inhibit these events (34,35).

Impaired circulation frequently results from hypovolemia or hypothermia after surgery. Rehydrating and warming the patient improve oxygenation to wounds (36,37). In addition, impaired circulation may be due to cardiac disease, large or small vessel disease, or defects at the microcirculatory level. Pressure sores are also caused by impaired circulation to the tissues (38).

Hyperbaric oxygen can improve wound healing in hypoxic wounds. Hyperbaric oxygen increases tissue oxygenation by increasing oxygen transport through the blood plasma. Breathing 100% oxygen at 3 atm absolute pressure increases the oxygen-carrying capacity of blood by 5 vol %. In addition to transiently elevating tissue oxygen levels, hyperbaric oxygen increases angiogenesis in hypoxic tissues. This has been demonstrated in irradiated tissue (39).

D. Smoking

Smoking delays wound healing, as well as decreases skin flap survival. This effect is due to vasoconstriction and higher levels of carboxyhemoglobin, which limits the oxygen-carrying capacity of blood (40). Results of a study aimed at blocking the vasoconstrictive effect of nicotine have been promising (41).

E. Cancer

Whenever a persistent nonhealing skin wound is present, a cutaneous malignancy needs to be ruled out. Basal and squamous cell carcinomas can arise from chronic wounds. Scar carcinomas, which can occur 30 years later in a scar (Marjolin's ulcers), behave more aggressively than usual skin cancers (42).

F. Radiation

Radiation impairs healing by causing microvasculature obliteration, excessive fibrosis, and a disruption of cellular replication. Its long-term effects are due to its influence on blood vessels. Specifically, radiation causes narrowing of the lumen of arteries, arterioles and capillaries by endothelial swelling and vessel wall degeneration (43).

G. Chemotherapy

Chemotherapeutic agents delay healing by decreasing the number of precursor cells (i.e., megakaryocytes, monocytes) responsible for mediating the wound-healing response (i.e., platelets, macrophages). In experimental conditions, nitrogen mustard, cyclophosphamide, methotrexate, and doxorubicin are inhibitors of wound healing; however, their clinical effects on wound healing have not been fully elucidated. 5-Fluorouracil specifically decreases wound contracture, which may have future therapeutic benefit (44).

H. Medications

Medications can either promote or inhibit wound healing and scar formation. Steroids are well known to delay wound healing. Patients who take steroids over long periods commonly have thin, fragile skin and impaired healing (45,46). Cortisone has its maximal impact on incisional breaking strength when it is given 3 days before wounding and 2 days after wounding. Steroids affect most aspects of wound healing by decreasing wound incisional strength (45,47), inhibiting epithelialization (48), and impairing wound contraction (48,49). Steroids reduce DNA synthesis and cause morphologic changes in fibroblasts. Vitamin A can reverse the steroid effects on wound healing except for contraction impairment (48). Other medications that can inhibit wound healing include anticoagulants, aspirin, colchicine, penicillamine, cyclosporine, and phenylbutazone.

III. WOUND CHARACTERISTICS THAT CONTRIBUTE TO SCAR VISIBILITY

A. Orientation and Location

Scars are concealed maximally by adhering to techniques of tensionless wound closure, wound edge eversion, and having the wound lie within the relaxed skin tension line (RSTL) of the face or at the border of facial aesthetic units (Fig. 1).

The six major facial aesthetic units are the forehead, eye and eyebrow, nose, lips, chin, and cheek (Fig. 2). These aesthetic units can be divided into additional anatomical

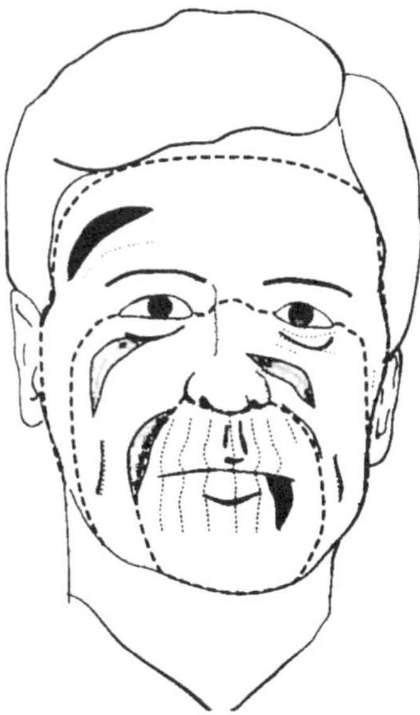

Figure 1 Relaxed skin tension lines on the face with optimal placement of fusiform excisions.

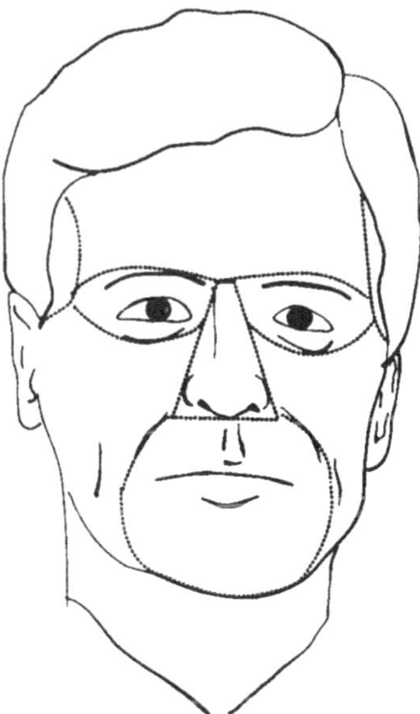

Figure 2 Boundaries of the facial aesthetic units (forehead, eye and eyebrow, nose, cheek, mouth, and chin).

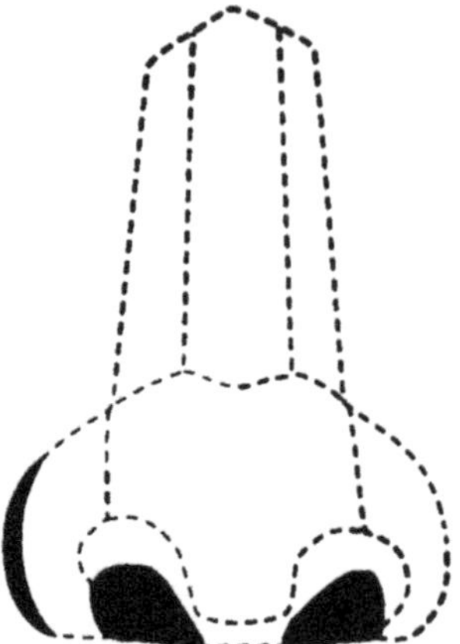

Figure 3 Aesthetic subunits of the nose (dorsum, sidewalls, nasal tip, nasal alae, soft tissue triangles, and columella).

subunit boundaries. Specifically, the nose can be divided into the dorsum, sidewalls, nasal tip, nasal alae, soft tissue triangles, and columella (Fig. 3) (50). These anatomical boundaries of the face represent areas in which scars lying on the borders appear less visible. This is because the facial aesthetic units and subunits are defined by light reflections and shadows.

With any wound, the extent of tissue loss in proximity to surrounding mobile facial structures (eyelids, nasal alae, nasal tip, auricle, vermilion, commissures, and philtrum) should be recognized. When closing the wound, one should avoid distortion of these neighboring structures, which can make the scar much more noticeable.

When a wound resulting from tissue loss cannot be adequately closed primarily without undue tension or vital structure deformity, planning for reconstruction is required. Reconstructive options include healing by secondary intention, local skin flaps, regional flaps, and skin grafts. For wound sites having the majority of a facial aesthetic unit missing, removal of the remaining aesthetic skin unit followed by local skin flaps or skin grafting can be considered. This technique can maintain uniformity of skin color and contour of the facial unit and make scars less visible by having them lie on the aesthetic unit boundaries. For defects encompassing more than one facial aesthetic unit, the units can be reconstructed independently of each other.

To determine the best method for reconstruction, the extent of the soft tissue defect must be clearly defined. The variables include the involved surface area, location, layers of tissue missing, and relationship to the facial units. Ideally, absent tissue should be repaired with tissue similar in color, texture, and thickness (Fig. 4). Missing supporting structures of bone and cartilage should be replaced, giving adequate support for natural contour.

IV. CHOICES FOR RECONSTRUCTION AND SCARRING POTENTIAL

A. Healing by Secondary Intention

The cosmetic appearance of a site healing by secondary intention depends on the facial area involved. Concave facial surface areas of the eye (medial canthus), nose (nasofacial crease

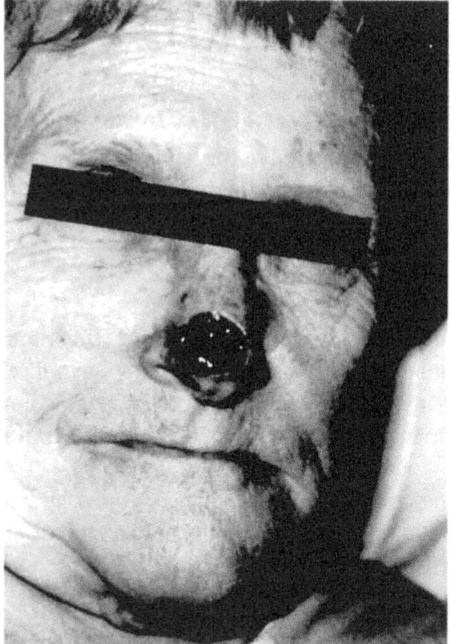

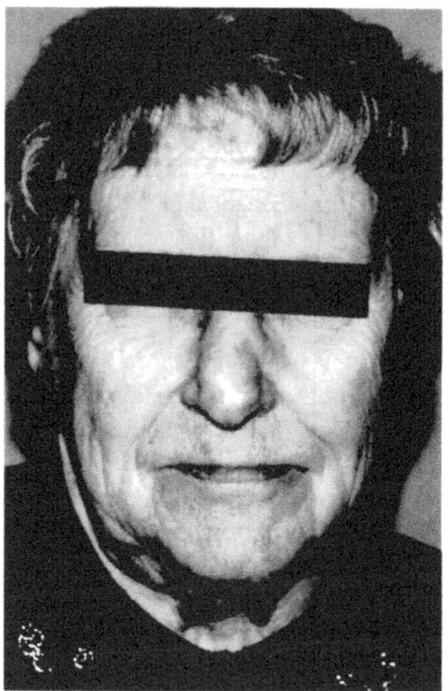

Figure 4 **(A)** A 78-year-old woman with a full-thickness nasal defect after basal cell carcinoma excision. **(B)** To maintain skin texture and color, an extended glabellar rotation flap was used. The photograph was taken 2 years after reconstruction.

and nasoalar grooves), ear, and temple heal very well by secondary intention. Healing by secondary intention is often used for small superficial wounds. The healing by secondary intention of convex surfaces on the cheek, lips, nose, chin, and helix frequently results in depressed or hypertrophic scars. Aesthetically, a reepithelialized scar healing by secondary intention appears more atrophic and hypopigmented and has more telangiectasia. Disadvantages of healing by secondary intention include a longer healing time and more contraction causing movement of surrounding structures. When multiple tissue layers and structural support are missing, secondary intention is not appropriate.

B. Skin Graft Repair

Skin grafts are often considered when local skin flaps cannot be used. Compared with skin flaps, skin grafts give a less optimal match of color and texture on the face.

Partial-thickness skin grafts (0.010 to 0.020 inch) can provide temporary coverage of soft tissue defects if adjacent soft tissue viability is uncertain or if a large amount of soft tissue coverage is required. However, they give a poor color and texture match with the surrounding skin, having a lighter, more atrophic, and glistening appearance. They also have less skin durability to infection and to future trauma with increased wound contracture.

Full-thickness skin grafts give a more acceptable facial color and texture match than split-thickness skin grafts if they are taken from the preauricular, postauricular, upper eyelid, or supraclavicular donor area.

C. Local Skin Flap Repair

For full-thickness defects of the face, skin flaps provide an excellent match of skin color and texture. When the flap incisions align along the aesthetic facial borders, subunit boundaries, and relaxed skin tension lines, optimal aesthetic results are obtained. Selecting the most appropriate skin flap is dependent on the size and location of the defect and the properties of the adjacent skin. If the defect is large, regional flap reconstruction or skin grafts may provide a more functional repair.

D. Wound Care

For wound cleaning, skin cleansers [hydrogen peroxide, povidone-iodine (Betadine), chlorhexidine gluconate (Hibiclens)] should not be routinely used in a wound to avoid cellular damage. Wound cleaning can be performed using normal saline or commercial wound cleansers. Moisture-retentive dressings or ointments should be maintained until reepithelialization of the wound is complete.

Local factors such as infection, hematoma, and seroma that impede wound healing increase the likelihood of scarring. Other factors that increase scarring potential include excessive pressure over the surgical site and increased wound tension. With careful preoperative planning and meticulous surgical technique, these risks can be minimized.

V. FUTURE RESEARCH

Scar-reducing therapy could improve function, mobility, and growth. In the future, it may be possible to reduce scarring by manipulating polypeptide growth factors within the wound.

One of the major growth factors studied in the scarring process has been transforming growth factor-β1 (TGF-β1). When TGF-β1 was administered intraperitoneally in the nude mouse model for 10 days, marked systemic fibrosis became evident (51). High levels of TGF-β have been found in human fibrotic diseases such as lung fibrosis, diabetic nephropathy, and glomerulonephritis (52–54).

For scar reduction, neutralization antibodies against TGF-β1, TGF-β2, and platelet-derived growth factor have given encouraging results (55–57). Wounds treated with neutralizing antibodies had a more organized dermal extracellular matrix. Injection of TGF-β1 neutralizing antibody into adult rat incisions resulted in reduced scarring and a decreased inflammatory response with less collagen, fibronectin, and blood vessels. The tensile strength of these treated wounds was similar to that of controls (55). Thus, scar formation may be related to active TGF-β1 levels at the wound site. Other studies in adult animal models have demonstrated that supplemental TGF-β3 or basic fibroblast growth factor can decrease scarring (56).

By modulating the inflammatory response, manipulating growth factor profiles, and modifying the extracellular matrix environment, progress in reducing scarring has been made. With further research, control of cutaneous scarring may be possible.

REFERENCES

1. Longaker M, Adzick N. The biology of fetal wound healing: a review. Plast Reconstr Surg 1991; 87:788–798.

2. Ferguson M, Whitby D, Shah M, Armstrong J, Siebert J, Longaker M. Scar formation: the spectral nature of fetal and adult wound repair. Plast Reconstr Surg 1995; 97:854–860.
3. Lorenz H, Longaker M, Perkocha L, Jennings R, Harrison M, Adzick N. Scarless wound repair: a human fetal skin model. Development 1992; 114:253–259.
4. Van de Kerkhof P, van Bergen B, Spruijt K, Kuiper J. Age-related changes in wound healing. Clin Exp Dermatol 1994; 19:369–374.
5. Holt D, Kirk S, Regan M, et al. Effect of age on wound healing in healthy human beings. Surgery 1992; 111:293–297.
6. Olerud J, Odland G, Burgess E, et al. A model for the study of wounds in normal and elderly adults and patients with peripheral vascular disease or diabetes mellitus. J Surg Res 1995; 59:349–360.
7. Luck J. Orthopedic surgery on the HIV-positive patient: complications and outcome. Instr Course Lect 1994; 43:543–549.
8. Omo-Dare P. Genetic studies on keloids. J Natl Med Assoc 1975; 76:428–432.
9. Ketchum D. Hypertrophic scars and keloids. Clin Plast Surg 1977; 4:301–310.
10. Ford L, King D, Lagasse L, et al. Increased binding in keloids: a preliminary communication. J Dermatol Surg Oncol 1983; 9:545–547.
11. Mancini R, Quaife J. Histogenesis of experimentally produced keloids. J Invest Dermatol 1962; 38:143–150.
12. DiCesare P, Chang D, Perelman N. Alteration of collagen composition and cross-linking in keloid tissue. Matrix 1990; 10:172.
13. Peltonen J, Hsiao L, Jaakkola S, et al. Activation of collagen gene expression in keloids: co-localization of type I and VI collagen and transforming growth factor beta-1 mRNA. J Invest Dermatol 1991; 97:240–248.
14. Goodson W, Hunt T. Studies of wound healing in experimental diabetes mellitus. J Surg Res 1977; 22:221–227.
15. Prakash A, Pandit P, Sharma L. Studies in wound healing in experimental diabetes. Int Surg 1974; 59:25–28.
16. Arquilla E, Weringer E, Nakajo M. Wound healing: a model for the study of diabetic microangiopathy. Diabetes 1976; 25(suppl):811–189.
17. Yue D, McLennan S, Marsh M. Effects of experimental diabetes, uremia, and malnutrition on wound healing. Diabetes 1987; 36:295–299.
18. Weringer E, Kelso J, Tamai I, et al. Effects of insulin on wound healing in diabetic mice. Acta Endocrinol 1982; 99:101–108.
19. Richter M, Jodouin C, Moher D, Barron P. Immunologic defects following trauma: a delay in immunoglobulin synthesis by cultured B cells following traumatic accidents but not elective surgery. J Trauma 1990; 30:590–596.
20. Selye H. Ischemic necrosis. Science 1967; 156:1262–1263.
21. Waldorf H, Fewkes J. Wound healing. Wound Healing Dermatol 1995; 10:77–96.
22. Dasta J, Brackett C. Defining and achieving optimum therapeutic goals in critically ill patients. Pharmacotherapy 1994; 14:678–688.
23. Uitto J, Murray L, Blumberg B, et al. Biochemistry of collagen diseases. Ann Intern Med 1986; 105:740–756.
24. Bart B, Gorlin R, Anderson V, Lynch F. Congenital localized absence of skin and associated abnormalities resembling epidermolysis bullosa: a new syndrome. Arch Dermatol 1966; 93:296–304.
25. Kolenik S, Perez M, Davidson D, Morganroth G, Kohn S, Bolognia J. Atrophia maculosa varioliformia cutis: report of two cases and review of the literature. J Am Acad Dermatol 1994; 30:837–840.
26. Holroyde C, Reichard G. General metabolic abnormalities in cancer patients: anorexia and cachexia. Surg Clin North Am 1986; 66:947–956.

27. Daly JM, Vars H, Dudrick S. Effects of protein depletion on strength of colonic anastomoses. Surg Gynecol Obstet 1972; 134:15–21.
28. Goodson W, Hunt T. Wound healing. In: Kinney J, Jeejeebhoy K, et al, eds. Nutrition and Metabolism in Patient Care. Philadelphia: Saunders, 1988, pp 635–642.
29. Irvin T. Effects of malnutrition on wound healing. Surg Gynecol Obstet 1978; 146:33–37.
30. Albina J. Nutrition in wound healing. JPEN 1994; 18:367–376.
31. Sandstead H, Henriksen L, Greger J, et al. Zinc nutriture in the elderly in relation to taste acuity, immune response, and wound healing. Am J Clin Nutr 1982; 36(suppl 5):1046–1059.
32. Kligman A. The bacteriology of normal skin. In: Wolcott B, Rund D, eds. Skin Bacteria and Their Role in Infection. New York: McGraw-Hill, 1965, pp 13–21.
33. Edlich R, Rodeheaver G, Morgan R, et al. Principles of emergency wound management. Ann Emerg Med 1988; 17:1284–1302.
34. Van FL, Hunt T. Oxygen and wound healing. Clin Plast Surg 1990; 17:463–472.
35. Falanga V, Grinnel F, Gilcrest B, et al. Experimental approaches to chronic wounds. Wound Rep Reg 1995; 3:132–140.
36. Radkin J, Hunt T. Local heat increases blood flow and oxygen tension in wounds. Arch Surg 1987; 122:221–225.
37. Jonsson K, Jensen J, Goodson III W, et al. Assessment of perfusion in postoperative patients using tissue oxygen measurements. Br J Surg 1987; 74:263–276.
38. Eaglstein W, Falanga V. Chronic wounds. Surg Clin North Am 1997; 77:689–700.
39. Marx R, Ehler W, Tayapongsak P, Pierce L. Relationship of oxygen dose to angiogenesis induction in irradiated tissue. Am J Surg 1990; 160:519–524.
40. Astrup P, Kjeldsen K. Carbon monoxide, smoking and atherosclerosis. Med Clin North Am 1973; 58:323–350.
41. Karlen R, Maisel R. Terazosin blockade of nicotine induced skin flap necrosis in the rat. Arch Otolaryngology 1997; 123:837–840.
42. Arons M, Lynch J, Jewis S, et al. Scar tissue carcinoma. I. A clinical study with special reference to burn scar carcinoma. Ann Surg 1966; 161:170–188.
43. Anderson W, Kissane J, eds. Pathology. Vol. 1. 7th ed. St Louis: Mosby, 1977.
44. Khan U, Occleston N, Khaw P, McGrouther D. Single exposure to 5-fluorouracil: a possible mode of targeted therapy to reduce contractile scarring in the injured tendon. Plast Reconstr Surg 1997; 99:465–471.
45. Howes E, Plotz C, Blunt J, et al. Retardation of wound healing by cortisone. Surgery 1950; 28:177–181.
46. Taubenhaus M, Ambromin G. The effects of the hypophysis, thyroid, sex steroids, and the adrenal cortex upon granulation tissue. J Lab Clin Med 1950; 36:7–18.
47. McNamara J, Lamborn P, Mills D. Effect of short term pharmacologic doses of adrenocortical therapy on wound healing. Ann Surg 1969; 170:199–202.
48. Hunt T, Chrlich H, Garcia J, et al. The effect of vitamin A on reversing the inhibitory effect of cortisone on the healing of open wounds in animals. Ann Surg 1969; 170:633–641.
49. Stephens F, Dunphy J, Hunt T. Effect of delayed administration of corticosteroids on wound contraction. Ann Surg 1971; 173:214–218.
50. Burget G, Menick F. The subunit principle in nasal reconstruction. Plast Reconstr Surg 1985; 76:239.
51. Zugmaier G, Paik S, Wilding G, et al. Transforming growth factor β-1 induces cachexia and systemic fibrosis without an anti-tumor effect in nude mice. Cancer Res 1991; 51:3590–3594.
52. Broeklmann T, Limper A, Colby T, McDonald J. Transforming growth factor β1 is present at sites of extracellular matrix gene expression in human pulmonary fibrosis. Proc Natl Acad Sci USA 1991; 88:6642–6646.
53. Yoshioka K, Takemura T, Murakami K, et al. Transforming growth factor β and mRNA in glomeruli in normal and diseased human kidneys. Lab Invest 1993; 68:154–163.

54. Yamamoto T, Nakamura T, Noble N, Ruoslahti E, Border W. Expression of transforming growth factor β is elevated in human and experimental diabetic nephropathy. Proc Natl Acad Sci USA 1993; 90:1814–1818.
55. Shah M, Foreman D, Ferguson MW. Control of scarring in adult wounds by neutralizing antibody to transforming growth factor β. Lancer 1992; 339:213–214.
56. Shah M, Foreman D, Ferguson MW. Netralization of TGFβ1 and TGFβ2 or exogenous addition of TGFβ3 to cutaneous rat wounds reduces scarring. J Cell Sci 1995; 108:985–1002.

4
Cultural and Psychological Aspects of Patients with Scars

Emiliano Panconesi and Giuseppe Hautmann
University of Florence
Florence, Italy

Perhaps no one more than the attentive dermatologist notices the enormous differences in how important esthetic (disesthetic, unesthetic) aspects are for different individuals. The value of esthetic factors and appearance in general must lie very deep in the individual ego. It seems to depend on that "esthetic ego," which we have often proposed as a not indifferent and very real part of living in the world. It comes into play with minimal but not negligible changes due to external influences. These include in particular cultural factors, such as the figurative arts, cinema, and television, and personal taste, which are all conditioned, even subliminally, by the pressures of advertising and publicity, especially in relation to the fashion and cosmetics industries. The latter, in particular, may produce undue pressures in favor of bad taste and poor esthetic judgment. We present examples from our everyday clinical experience as points for reflection.

- A 15-year-old girl had experienced about 6 months of acne, which was clinically cured but had left three tiny hole like scars (one of which was invisible without a magnifying lens). The girl obsessively insisted on undergoing treatment, finally done with a 70% glycolic acid peel, despite our disapproval. After only a few days she decided that the treatment was useless. All our attempts to convince her that the "scars" were practically nonexistent and certainly overvalued were in vain, and she could not be convinced to continue the glycolic acid treatment or, better, wait for a spontaneous improvement per *vis medicatrix naturae*. She insisted that she wanted to undergo plastic surgery or at the very least dermabrasion. We refused to assist in favoring either procedure and managed finally to schedule an interview in liaison consultation with a psychiatrist. The patient underwent short-term psychoanalytically oriented psychotherapy associated with a topical placebo. Her psychological situation improved noticeably; the three tiny scars remained, but they began to be tolerated and accepted and were finally forgotten. A year later they have practically disappeared and are not noticeable unless one looks for them.

- A young woman presented with a nodular melanocytic nevus–like lesion in the right nasal fold that was diagnosed as potentially malignant. The lesion was excised together with a margin of 1 cm of surrounding unlesioned skin. Histological examination confirmed a final diagnosis of junctional compound nevus. The excision left a raised scar that was still very noticeable 2 months afterward, and even the surgeon considered it "unesthetic" and proposed surgical correction. The patient, instead, declared that she was satisfied; she was extremely happy that the lesion was not a malignant melanoma and was satisfied with the consoling idea that with time the appearance of the scar might improve.

- A 60-year-old German man presented to the dermatologist with a raised, blackish-gray lesion about 1 cm in diameter and with a rough surface. It had first appeared about a year previously and had slowly increased in size. The diagnosis was simple seborrheic wart. The dermatologist reassured the man that the lesion was benign, reinforcing the fact by saying that the man could leave it be, as it was not particularly noticeable and therefore objectively did not constitute a problem, either healthwise or esthetic. The patient insisted that he wanted it removed because it was ugly. The dermatologist was somewhat surprised, because the man had on his other cheek a very evident dyschromic scar, about 1 cm wide and 5 cm long, that extended from the cheekbone down to the jawbone, which did not appear to bother him in any way. When asked what the scar was, the man replied, boldly and smiling, that it was nothing of importance, that it presented no problems. He said it was a mensur, that it had actually been done to order by a barber in Heidelberg. The word mensur (from the Latin *mensura*, meaning measure, in this case in reference to the distance between the two participants in a duel) in German signifies the wound, and thus the scar, produced in a duel, an old German ritual obligatory for admission to a student university corporation. The cheeks and forehead were the only parts of the face that remained free from the protection of a mask and were thus the areas struck during a duel with swords. The resultant scar was a sign of courage, from medieval times, but the practice has slowly been abandoned. Naturally, as with our patient, the duel came to be considered often too dangerous and the scar was procured by more sterile, safer methods.
- In many peoples (especially in Africa and in the past in Central America) hypertrophic scars (or keloids) are still provoked purposely to form sometimes elaborate geometric designs (see Fig. 1). These were often an indication that the person had reached sexual maturity or were inflicted in ceremonies of magic-religious exorcisms; they are still today, although somewhat less frequently, considered esthetically pleasing to the groups that practice this custom.

We have gone rapidly from practically invisible scars that provoke psychic suffering and feelings of inadequacy to very evident scars produced on purpose and worn with pride.

The skin is the envelope of the self, representing its maintenance and control. The residual evidence of interruption (imperfection) in the perfect continuum of the body surface (i.e., a scar) implies profound motives insofar as it is considered an important mark that alters the perfect homogeneity of the skin surface. It is a "historic" sign, a visible reminder of the past; it can incite fantasies of monstrosity and perfection through magical restoration, such as that which is achieved in psychoanalysis, where one tries to cancel (elaborate, work out) a bereavement, a memory, a "scar of the spirit." However, we all know that it is often impossible to cancel a fact or event completely, and one must learn to live with the memory and the mark(s) left by the event(s). Thus, such scars are experienced as ugly, signs of irregularity, ambiguity, imperfection, unworthiness, and even guilt. In

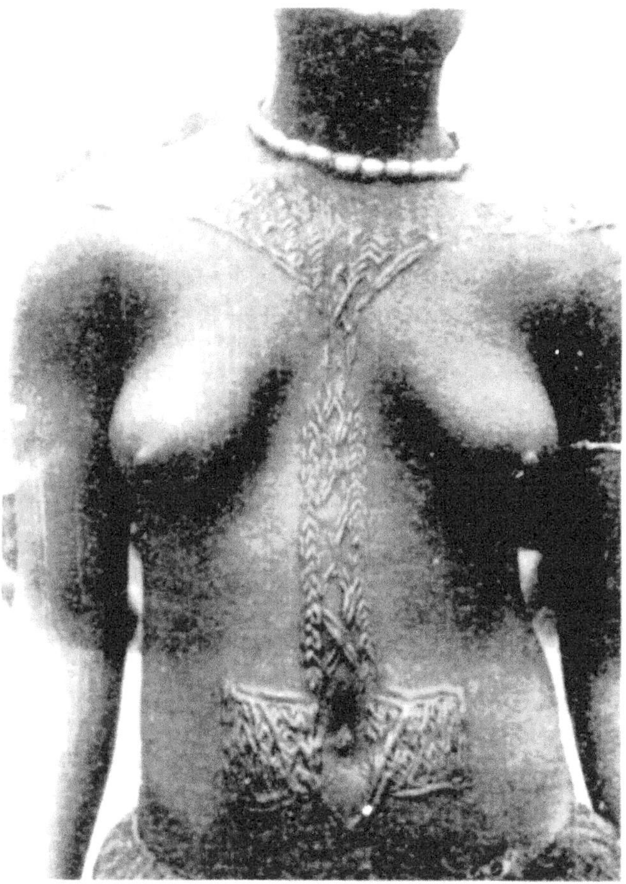

Figure 1 Bidiogo woman (Bijagos Island) with an elaborate, decorative scar produced purposely in a sexual rite. Note that the design follows the natural lines of the body: wide and necklace-like around the neckline, then narrow between the breasts and straight down to encircle the belly button, which is free of markings and remains set off as a central focal point in the overall design.

many modern cultures, especially in the Caucasian Occidental world, a scar is usually the source of negative perception of one's *body ego*. In Freudian terms this means the part of the ego that derives from the self's self-perception ("the ego is first and foremost a body ego, i.e. the ego is ultimately derived from bodily sensations, chiefly from those springing from the surface of the body," Freud, 1927). It belongs to individual *body image*, the psychological term that the dermatologist often uses to refer to self-conception of one's own body.

To our knowledge, the only case of positive value of a scar in our Western culture is related to the mensur (see case discussed earlier), as true or false testimony of courageous behavior in the old student tradition in Germany. This ritual of self-aggressive behavior, which dermatologists associate, for example, with excoriated acne and neurotic excoriations, may have some relationship with the Freudian superego, dependent also, according to Rycroft, on internalization of one's parents.

Even the mutilations and scars on a father's body can be experienced dramatically by relatives, in one known case by a daughter to the point that she presented in the same areas on her own body a cutaneous affection manifested by discolorations (an affection that some authors consider "psychosomatic"). In this regard we wish to recount the peculiar case reported by Roberto Bassi of a daughter who identified with her father through his scars. A 22-year-old woman, married and with a 2-year-old child, was in good health but requested hospitalization for relatively minor vitiligo because she was afraid the white areas would spread to her face. The lesions were limited to the fingers of her right hand and three spots on her trunk and abdomen. Clinical examination and psychological interview did not evidence any pathological findings of note, but a curious fact was brought out, which the patient had not been aware of previously. The spots of vitiligo corresponded exactly to the scars her father had from grenade wounds received in his fighting as a partisan during World War II (he had lost the same fingers as the ones on which she had vitiligo on her right hand and had scars on his trunk and abdomen in the same spots as her vitiligo). He was, in the young woman's own words, a fine, good father, a quiet man. The process of identification with her father, with the white areas of vitiligo on the same spots on her body as those marred by scars on his own, is noteworthy.

The theme of how a disfiguring scar can cause psychological problems and, thus, become the central point around which a narrative develops is clear in the novel *Schach von Wuthenow*, published in 1882 by the German writer Theodor Fontane (1816–1898).

> The protagonist is a well-known officer in the prestigious regiment "Gensdarmes" in Berlin in 1806, just before the battle of Jena that determined the fall of Prussia. Schach is a regular visitor to the drawing room of the beautiful widow Josephine von Carayon, with whom he is said to have an affair. Victoria, the widow's intelligent and sensitive daughter, has inherited her mother's beauty, marred by residual scarring from smallpox. In part influenced by the Prince of Prussia, Louis Ferdinand, who exalts the disquieting fascination which this young *beauté du diable* emanates, Schach seduces Victoria and begins an affair that leads to jokes and malicious comments in Berlin high society. Victoria becomes pregnant, but Schach seems reluctant to marry her, especially because he fears that he will cut a bad figure with a physically unattractive wife, notwithstanding her fine intellectual and spiritual qualities. Only when the king, Federick William III, requests personally that Schach marry Victoria to save the honor of the regiment, does he agree to do so. However, only a few hours after the wedding Schach commits suicide. As an aside, we note that with this novel Fontane denounces the false concept of honor that reigned in old Prussia before the defeat at Jena.

There is another example in the German language literature that indicates how scars may be related to sorcery, how they can be considered seductive and, as in Fontane's novel, even fatal signs of destiny. These aspects are evident and artistically presented in the short story "The Greek Dancer" (Die Grieschiche Tanzerin) by the famous Austrian writer Arthur Schnitzler, a Viennese physician and contemporary of Freud, who was an admirer of his work.

> A famous Viennese sculptor, adored by women, unscrupulous, and cynical, and his wife, who is very much in love with her husband and tries to overcome and hide her inevitable jealousy, are at the Moulin Rouge in Paris. During the evening a very pretty and apparently experienced young woman comes to their table and tells them the story of her adventurous life, including a suicide attempt. At this point in her story she bares her left breast, evidencing a small red scar, which she impudently asks the man to kiss. The man, who has not paid much attention to her until then, having preferred to talk with his

> friends at the table, consents and brushes his lips over the scar of this unknown young woman. The group of friends and the young woman continue their evening in various places until dawn, and when they break up the sculptor appears to be very much taken by the young woman with the scar and proposes that she model for him. They become lovers, and not long after the wife dies, officially of heart attack, but the narrator presumes suicide. The "Greek Dancer" of the title is the name of a statue for which the sculptor's young lover was the model.

The theme of sorcery can be connected to the medieval concept of witch's marks or devil marks, which were any anomalies or alterations of the skin. Extra nipples, warts, moles, tumors, protuberances (particularly those that secreted any liquid or blood), discolorations of the skin or mucosae, cavities, red spots, lumps, birthmarks (in Italian called *voglie*, meaning wants or desires in reference to the unsatisfied cravings of a pregnant woman; for example, a naevus flammeus is a *voglia di vino* = unsatisfied desire for wine), bumps under the tongue, and fleshy bumps and folds in the vagina were all seen as proof that the individual was a witch in witchcraft trials. However, because fear led some persons to excise such marks or lesions from the skin, even scars, often from wounds of other origin, became considered proof of witchcraft or possession by the devil. Another proof was numb insensitive areas or marks that did not bleed that the "prickers" tried to discover by pricking the skin of the subject with pins, needles, or bodkins; in fact, a scar that is pricked superficially often does not bleed. One famous pricker–witch hunter of the 17th century in Newscastle upon Tyne (England) earned from 20 shillings to 3 pounds for each witch captured who confessed, and before finally being hanged himself he confessed to having falsely accused 220 women of being witches.

The ritual scarification that leads to hypertrophic keloid-like, decorative, ornamental, mystical-religious scars that Dominique D. Verut (1973) presented in sculptures of the Mayan civilization (see Fig. 2) and similar ones still found in some contemporary African cultures has not penetrated Western culture, which has instead adopted, albeit in limited, often marginal groups, tattooing and piercing.

The example of the mensur as a socially accepted scar, to be exhibited with pride as an ostentatious sign of courage, has no equals in meaning, although it can be classified generically with the scars from war wounds, which veterans present unashamedly, especially in military and political circles. We note also that child psychologists have reported cases of children who, in the spirit of imitation and as signs of courage, show their scars caused by even minor injuries while playing or procured in sports events.

Only the navel scar (the umbilicus, belly button) is physiologically present from birth (the only *physiological* scar that man presents—like original sin, man's innate spiritual defect, or scar, according to Christian religions) (see Fig. 3). The symbolic importance of this particular scar is discussed later in this chapter. We all live with it, mostly without problems, until death, although there are cases in which an individual requests surgical correction of a navel that is particularly unsightly or thought to be so. All other scars are provoked by a traumatic or pathological process. Today, the majority of such events are treated pharmacologically and/or surgically.

Plastic surgery plays a major role in the correction of unesthetic or alteration of undesired physical appearance or manifestations, including the revision of scars. It is precisely in focusing attention on the psychological aspects of such cases that one realizes the importance that the individual may place on a scar, including residual or new, changed scars after surgical scar revision. In fact, surgeons in general, and plastic surgeons in particular, must be especially wary with subjects who request surgical scar revision.

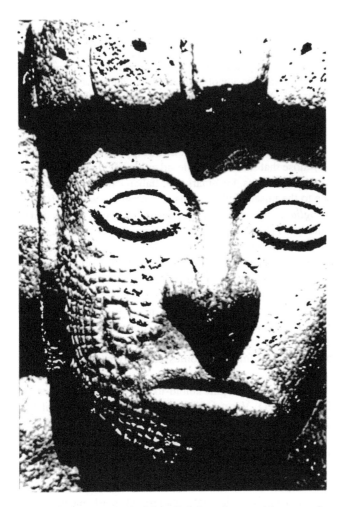

Figure 2 The head of a Maya-Toltek sculpture with geometric scars of unknown ritual significance.

One could say, paradoxically, that in all cases of request for surgery that involves correction of an esthetic problem, the surgeon should in turn request psychological-psychiatric examination of the patient before deciding whether to accept the task and should obtain the consent of the patient, preferably in writing and in the presence of witnesses. We make this forceful statement on the basis of personal conviction and supported by various reports and articles, including the article "Plastic Surgery: When the Patient Is Dissatisfied" by the well-known American plastic surgeon Robert M. Goldwyn. It has been estimated that only about 5% of subjects are dissatisfied with the results of plastic surgery and that teenagers (who in the majority of cases have insisted on nose reshaping against the wishes of their parents) are the most satisfied, perhaps partly because having won the fight to have the operation reinforces satisfaction with the results or because teenagers do not yet have a fully formed self-image. Dissatisfaction can arise irrespective of the actual results of the operation, whether they are objectively poor, excellent, or in some cases even better than expected or agreed upon beforehand. Neither the patient nor the surgeon consciously expects

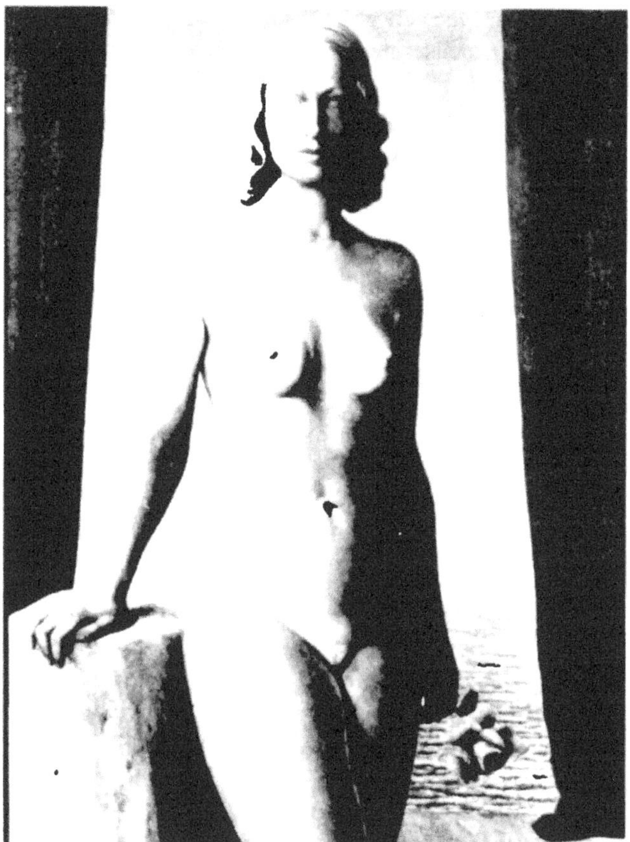

Figure 3 *Les Fleurs du Mal*, painting by René Magritte. Note at the very center of the painting, the very center of the lovely nude, the belly button, the human being's unique physiological scar; the umbilicus represents one of the most important symbolic points in the imagination worldwide.

something to go wrong, but Goldwyn suspects that "for the patient the fear (perhaps unconscious) of a bad result no doubt lingers." Any operation, especially cosmetic plastic surgery or other procedures to alter cosmetic appearance, can result in the patient's dissatisfaction: face-lift; nose reshaping; eyelid surgery; breast reduction, enlargement, or lifting; ear pinning; "tummy tuck"; liposuction; or collagen injection. The list is long and certainly should include surgical scar revision. We believe, however, that especially in the latter case there is much less probability of postsurgical dissatisfaction if the patient is adequately informed, with detailed, excellent information before the surgery. Goldwyn's acute observations include a list of the types of patients who are most unlikely to be dissatisfied and unhappy with the results of plastic surgery.

1. The perfectionist (and if the surgeon is also a perfectionist, together the two may creat inflated expectations).
2. The "patient with minimal deformity" (including, we add, above all those with minimal scars that they want to have corrected and that often can be classified with minor pictures of cutaneous dysmorphophobia).

3. The patient who "overshops" (i.e., who consults numerous surgeons and finally, usually, decides on the one who promises the best results, independent of comparative cost considerations).
4. The patient who wants cosmetic surgery to please someone else, usually the partner.
5. The "plastisurgiholic," who goes from one voluntary surgery to another (usually rich women with poor body image and self-esteem who see the surgeon or physician as an authoritarian father or mother figure who will solve their problems); these subjects often need psychiatric help, as does the next patient.
6. The depressed patient, who, independent of the cause of the original depression, may become more depressed after surgery that was foreseen as a miracle-making event, notwithstanding correct and normally adequate presurgical information and explanations by the surgeon.
7. The "pushy" patient, who is insistent and rude with secretaries and nurses and at first pleasant and courteous with the physician but then after surgery angry and complaining.
8. The older male patient who wants a new nose (and who is often dissatisfied with the results because what he really wants is youth and the sexual vigor of his youth).

Most cases of esthetic treatments, including surgical scar revision, in particular when the procedure is costly and the subject is no longer young, have a psychological undercurrent that the treatment is superfluous, vain, unnecessary (medically not necessary), frivolous, or even foolish or that it is against God's will or one's destiny, which should not be opposed. A bad esthetic result (or one considered so by the individual involved) may be experienced by a psychologically disturbed patient as a punishment. A hypertrophic scar or a keloid (which sometimes could have been foreseen) that replaces a previous flat, more acceptable scar is often experienced more or less consciously as a reminder or sign that one is guilty of vanity. The fact of having succombed to the false promises of media-promoted miracles increases the unhappiness of the dissatisfied individual, just like having followed the advice of an unqualified physician.

Dermatological surgeons must pay special attention to these considerations because they are in direct competition with the corporation of plastic surgeons. The patient can complain and accuse the surgeon of malpractice, saying that he should have been referred to a more specifically competent colleague for surgery.

The scars provoked by burns require special attention, perhaps more than the scars produced by any other specific cause. There are always specific circumstances related to the different pathological events that lead to a scar that requires revision, such as tuberculosis, leprosy, a tumor, all involving trauma with its own dynamics. In the case of burns, this is related above all to the scar as a reminder or sign of a precise event, e.g., fire, the flaming or burning hot liquid. In many cultures fire is a sign of purification and sublimation, but also related to fire produced by the friction of two bodies rubbing together sexuality and fertilization, as well as intellectual deviance, exalted imagination, subterranean cavities (the subconscious) and hell (fire in general). To be marked by fire may leave the individual bound in the scar with certain specific meanings. The accident of burning has been connected with "premorbid psychiatric disorders" and "alcohol-related problems" and can lead to residual anxiety (in about one third of cases), posttraumatic stress, significant intrusion symptoms, depression related to the visibility of the scar or visible disfigurement (especially on the face) with all the relative effects and influence on behavior, social integration, self-esteem, adaptation on returning to work, and emotional and sexual adjustments (Williams and Griffiths, 1991). This all indicates the need both before and after surgery (also in cases of scar revision) for practical advice, precise information, adequately prepared nursing staff, and psychological assistance on call. One extreme example of the severely scarred patient is proposed with artistic immediacy in the protagonist in the film *The English Patient*, which won many Oscars. This patient was not concerned about his terrible, disfiguring scars or with possible scar revision, because he was so overcome by physical suffering, memories, and the burden of living from one day to the next. He certainly benefited, however, from dedicated, tender care and the company of his most precious belonging, the book by Herodotus.

The scars left by a mastectomy are of special significance. The breast or breasts are laden with symbolism from ancient times. For the Jews, *bath* means young girl and is a measure for liquids and the word *amah* young girl and a measure of length. The breast in fact refers to "female principle," which is measure or limit (in contrast to "male principle," which is without limits). The right breast symbolizes the sun, the left breast the moon. The breasts also symbolize, obviously, maternity, nutriment, gifts, sweetness, security, intimacy, regeneration, and refuge (Abraham's breast—no matter whatever else is meant by this expression, according to Saint Augustine—is the resting place of the just, even after death, where there is neither pain, nor suffering, nor sighs). Breast or breasts signify fertility, fruitfulness, and milk and are even considered an overturned cup from which life gushes forth, as if from the heavens. It is easy to understand how important psychological rebound is after an operation that alters a woman's sexuality, her identity, and her body image, which regards both beauty and the integrity of the surface, all also modulated and conditioned by the customs and fashion of the time. The physician, the surgeon, the plastic surgeon, and later the dermatologist must pay close attention to these psychological implications, even before the operation, and must assist the patient with appropriate psychological or psychiatric liaison whenever necessary and support postmastectomy reconstructive surgery, including the application of skin expansion techniques and protheses to restore the integrity of the woman's skin surface and her body image.

We also wish to mention that in recent years surgeons in general have shown more attention to the esthetic aspects of the scars left by surgery. One of the first indications of such attention was the practice of doing abdominal incisions, especially in females, as low down in the abdominopelvic region as possible, so that the scars do not show when the subject is in a two-piece bathing suit, even a bikini. A young girl or woman who wants to lie in the sun or merely show off her body wants to present a perfect, unscarred body. The exception to this rule is the umbilicus.

"Eros is, of all the gods, the one most friendly to man because he is the one who brings succor and assistance when things go wrong, those wrongs that if they were corrected would give mankind the greatest happiness," said Aristophanes. Some of our readers will certainly have identified the magnificent philosophical work that contains this statement. It will be even more clear with the following concerning the "original nature of men": "the genders of man were three, and not two like now, that is male and female, but there was also a third gender, the androgen." The text continues with a description of the latter gender of human beings, round, ball-shaped figures with four hands, four legs, and two faces. "The male originated from the sun, the female from the earth, and the third sex, which shares the male and female natures, from the moon, which shares the natures of the sun and the earth." . . . "They were terrible in their strength and figure, 'the men', and had great pride, such that they tried to attack the gods." Now you have all recognized Plato's *Symposium* (which was held presumably around 400 B.C. in Athens, at the home of Agathon). Zeus cuts these beings in half, and while Apollo turns the face he "pulls the skin from all around to the part that is now called the belly/abdomen, and just as one does to close a bag, he ties it (the skin pulled together) in the middle of the belly, making a kind of mouth, which is now called *umbilicus*" (the italics are ours).*

The precise reason for mentioning this story here is that it deals with that primordial scar present on all humans, the *omphalos*. Apollo smoothed out the residual folds on the abdomen, leaving just a few around the center as "a reminder of the ancient punishment." Thus does Plato begin the series of symbolical meanings related to that unique physiological scar that is on all our bodies, the only one that man does not desire (cannot, out of respect for Apollo, to whom the omphalos of Delphi is dedicated) to cancel or change (requests for revision are almost always based on medical considerations).

Omphalos, umbilicus, or navel, commonly called belly button in English. It is a universal symbol for the center of the world, the umbilicus of incest in the Rig Veda; the lotus germinates in the umbilicus of Visnù; it is the *beith-el* erected by Jacob, the omphalos of the Holy Sepulcher; the Bod Ghaya tree under which Buddha finds illumination. The vedic altar is the *umbilicus of immortality*; for Yoga the umbilicus is the image of *return to the center*, and omphaloscopy is contemplation of the navel. In symbolic art a white egg-shaped stone standing upright represents the omphalos, which links mankind on earth, the subterraneous domain of the dead, and the divinity. Finally, for the Nordic peoples (Finns, Samoyedi, Estonians) the North Star is the umbilicus of the sky, and for the Scandinavians the umbilicus of the world (Chevalier and Gheerbraut).

Finally, in the reports of psychoanalysts the umbilicus represents (a) the idea, dream, and infantile fantasies of returning to one's most profound prenatal past by attempting to go through, beyond this insuperable scar-door, as well as (b) the fear, terror that it could open, allowing the unbearable emptying of the self.

The cinema, the most recent of the "arts" chronologically speaking, presents mostly facial scars in the stories narrated. There is often some psychological reference, with an anthropological-cultural meaning or symbolization. We will give a very brief comment on some of the most representative of these films.

There have been several versions of *The Phantom of the Opera* both in the cinema and on stage. In the first film production (R. Julian, 1925, USA) the protagonist has terrible scars on his face caused by acid. In *The Son of the Sheik* (G. Fitzmaurice, 1926, USA) (see Fig. 4) the famous actor Rudolph Valentino is the protagonist, who has scars on his chest, proof of his courage and value: the hypertrophic-keloid aspect of the scars is typical of that part of the body, the sternal region. We all remember the film *Scarface* (H. Hawks, 1932, USA and B. De Palma, 1983, USA). This is the story of Chicago gangs, and in the latter version Al Pacino is the protagonist, who has a noticeable scar on his face. In the original version of *The Man Who Knew Too Much* (A. Hitchcock, 1934, Great Britain) (see Fig. 5) involving a kidnapping, the chief of the ruthless group of spies is nicknamed for the scar on his face.

The Swedish film *En Kvinnas Ansikte* (G. Molander, 1938, Sweden) is about a gang of blackmailers headed by a woman with a badly scarred face. *A Woman's Face* (G. Cukor, 1941, USA) stars Joan Crawford, who was praised for having spent much of the time dur-

* Freely translated by the authors.

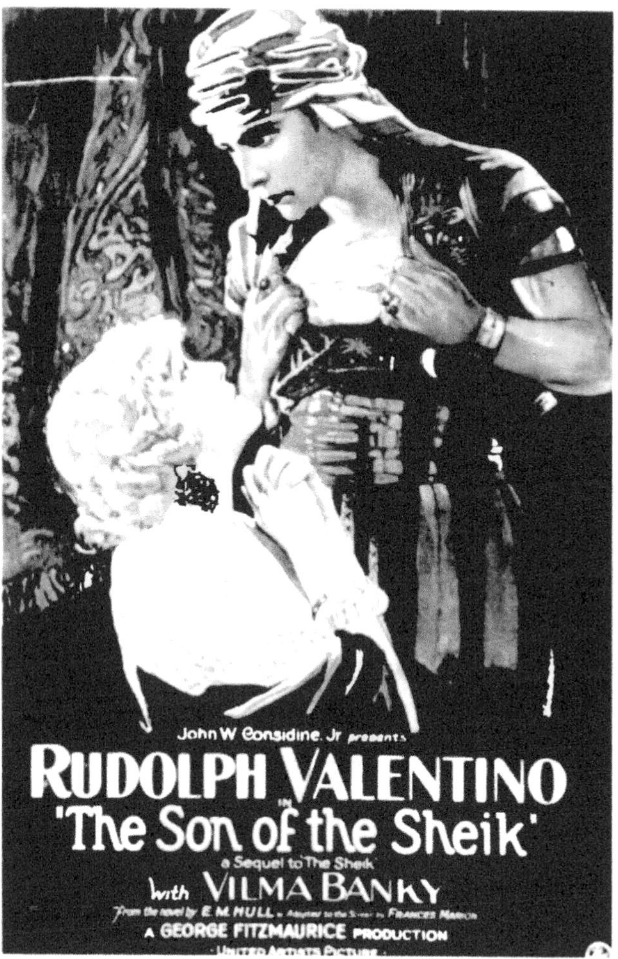

Figure 4 The poster of the film *The Son of the Sheik* (G. Fitzmaurice, 1926, USA) with a picture of the famous star Rudolph Valentino proudly showing the scars (hypertrophic, keloids?) on his chest, a sign of his difficult and courageous life.

ing the filming "disfigured," although she tried to avoid having pictures of herself like this distributed; the story is about a nanny with disfiguring scars on her face who leaves a terrible life of blackmail and murder for one of love and righteousness when she undergoes plastic surgery.

In *Hollow Triumph*, sometimes referred to as "The Scar" (S. Skely, 1948, USA), a confidence man in hiding kills a psychiatrist who looks like him and then assumes his identity; having studied some medicine, the crook even manages to reproduce a scar on his face to ensure his new identity, but working with a mirror he mistakenly scars the wrong cheek. The Apache chief in *The Searchers* (J. Ford, 1956, USA) is named Scar for a scar on his face. In the first production of *Witness for the Prosecution* (B. Wilder, 1957, USA), Marlene Dietrich appears as a perfidious woman, who presents a disfiguring scar on her face in one scene to save her husband from conviction in a murder trial.

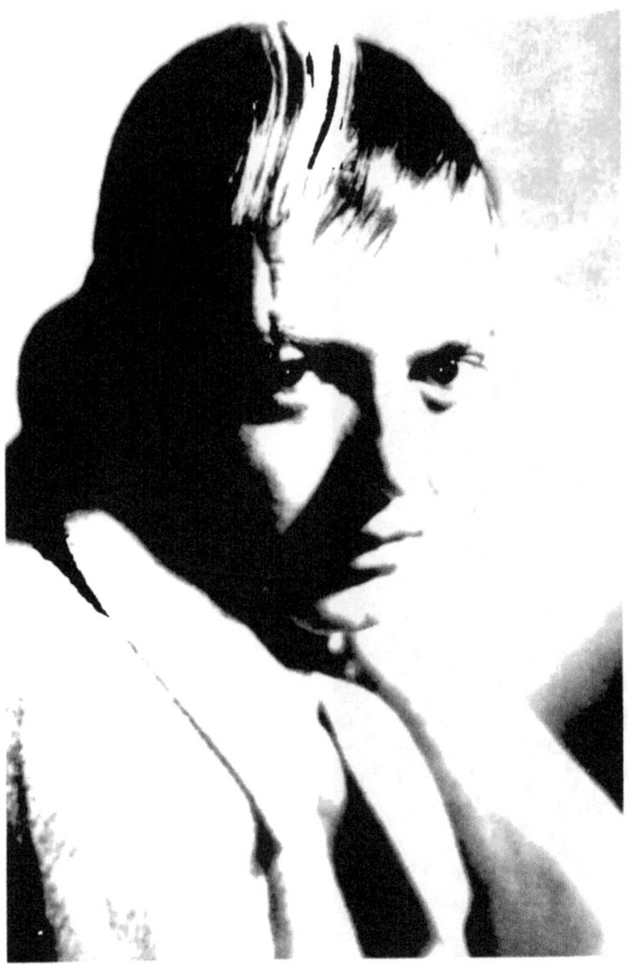

Figure 5 The actor Peter Lorre, the chief of a group of spies in the film *The Man Who Knew Too Much* (A. Hitchcock, 1934, Great Britain), with the ugly scar that singles him out from the others.

Tell Me That You Love Me, Junie Moon (O. Preminger, 1969, USA) is the touching story of three friends who are social outcasts because of their handicaps; one is a homosexual paraplegic, one an introverted epileptic, and one a girl with facial disfigurations. In *The Arp Statue* (A. Seckers, 1971, Great Britain), a model whose arm is eaten by a lion finds her life in crisis. *Johnny Got His Gun* (D. Trumbo, 1971, USA) is a not well known but very emotion-producing film about a World War I hero who was left deaf, dumb, and blind and without limbs and face; he lives a nonexistence in the back room of a hospital, where he learns to communicate by tapping Morse code with his head on his pillow, and his request that he be allowed to die if people cannot come to see him is refused. The horror film *The Abominable Dr. Phibes* (R. Fuest, 1971, Great Britain) involves a composer, disfigured by scars, who wants to avenge the death of his wife during surgery by murdering the doctors, In *Frances* (G. Cliffom, 1982, USA) J. Lang plays the part of a lovely, intelligent young actress whose career is destroyed, in part because of her uncompromising nature; the film ends with her mental destruction, due to a forced lobotomy, symbolized by a scar on her forehead. In *Edward Scissorhands* (T. Burton, 1990, USA) the protagonist provokes several self-inflicted scars on his own face. The *Man Without a Face* (M. Gibson, 1993, USA) is the story of the friendship between a disfigured, severely scarred outcast (nicknamed "Hamburger Head") and a 12-year-old boy who is not bothered by the man's physical appearance.

In most of these films, the presence of scars or other disfugurations is essential to the story or the character of the protagonist (see Fig. 6) and often heightens the emotional impact on the spectator, because we are all concerned about our appearance, especially in today's world of mass media and advertising with its emphasis on the canons of physical beauty promoted by the cosmetic and fashion industries.

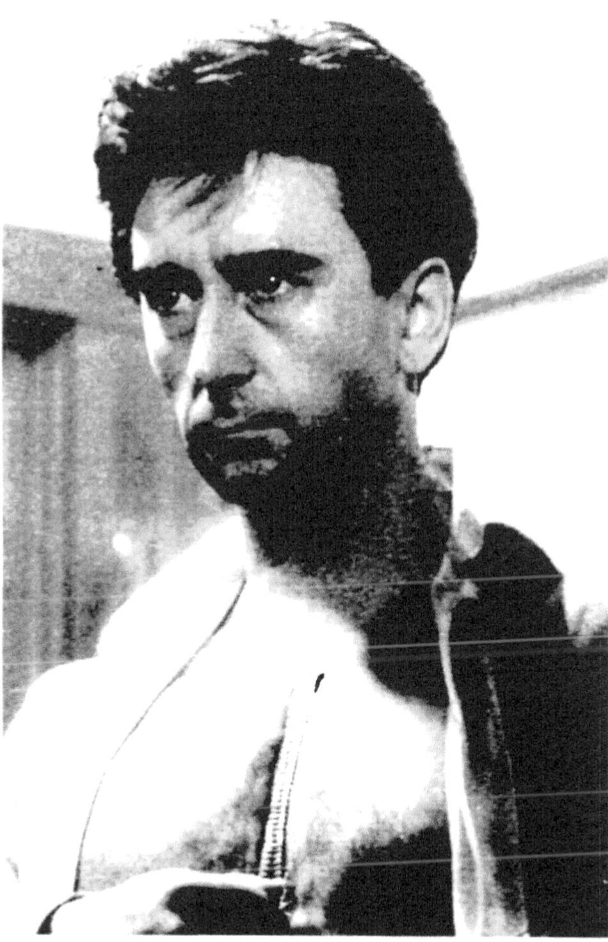

Figure 6 The protagonist of the film *The Zip* (J. Kaplan, 1987, Great Britain) closing the zipper on his chest that replaces a scar (maybe avoiding an ugly keloid, so common in scarring on the sternal region, perhaps to signify the possibility of easily entering and exiting the inside of the body).

In the Western tradition, the figurative arts, painting and sculpture, present few examples of scars with symbolic or anthropological-cultural significance. One important example, however, is the figure of Goliath in Caravaggio's painting *David with the Head of Goliath* (Galleria Borghese, Rome), in which Goliath is actually a self-portrait of the painter, who had a large scar on his forehead from a serious injury received in a brawl in Rome (during which he killed an opponent in a game of "pallacorda," which led to his fleeing from the city), one of the many unpleasant events in his very turbulent life.

An even more dramatic example is the paintings of Leonardo da Vinci, known to present hidden figures from the time of Freud's discovery, suggested by Pfister, of a vulture in the lap of the Virgin in the famous painting *The Virgin and Child and Saint Anne* (Louvre, Paris). Cesare Marchetti and Emiliano Panconesi have found myriads of tiny figures and often pathological alterations hidden in the persons represented in the splendid "Adoration of the Magi" by Leonardo (Uffizi Gallery, Florence). In fact, many of these secret lesions (hidden from the eye at one's first superficial view of the painting as a whole, with its appearance of peace and beauty) are in fact residual *scarring* from destructive pathological processes. This is what Leonardo had seen in the long hours spent in hospitals observing the patients and dissecting cadavers, and he painted it all, masked by the delicate theme and superficial beauty of the painting, with scars that signify historic body memory of the pain and suffering in human life.

REFERENCES

Bassi R. La ragazza che odiava gli specchi. Turin: Bollati Boringhieri, 1996.

Chevalier J, Gheerbrant A. Dictionaire des symboles. Paris: Laffont-Jupiter, 1969.

Cinotti M. Caravaggio: la vita e l'opera. Bergamo: Bolis, 1991.

Fontane T. Storia di un ufficiale prussiano. (Original title: Schach von Wuthernow.) Milan: Mondadori, 1981.

Goldwin RM. Plastic surgery: when the patient is dissatisfied. Med Health Annu Encyc Britt 1991; 403–407.

Guiley RE. The Encyclopedia of Witches and Witchcraft. New York: Facts on File, 1989.

Marchetti C, Panconesi E. Leonardo da Vinci: beauty or human suffering in the world. Notes on pathological cutaneous alterations in the "Adoration of the Magi." J Eur Acad Dermatol Venereal 1997; 8:101–111.

Panconesi E, ed. Stress and Skin Diseases: Psychosomatic Dermatology. Clinics in Dermatology. Philadelphia; Lippincott, 1984.

Plato. Platone: Tutti gli scritti. G. Reali, ed. Milan: Rusconi, 1991.

Pym J. Time Out Film Guide. London: Penguin, 1995.

Rycroft C. A Critical Dictionary of Psychoanalysis. Middlesex: Penguin, 1985.

Scarpa A. Etnomedicina. Milan: Lucisano, 1980.

Schnitzler A. Die Griechische Tanzerin. In: Die Brzahlenden Schriften. Vol. 2. Frankfurt Am Main: Fischer-Verlag, 1961.

Torczyner H. Magritte: The True Art of Painting. New York: Abrams, 1979.

Verut DD. Precolombian Dermatology and Cosmetology in Mexico. New York: Chanticleer, 1973.

Williams EE, Griffiths TA. Psychological consequences of burn injury. Burns 1991; 17:478–481.

5

Prevention of Unsatisfactory Scarring

Michel McDonald and Thomas Stasko
Mohs Micrographic Surgery, Vanderbilt University Medical Center
Nashville, Tennessee

The cutaneous surgeon must be aware that any procedure involving the skin has an inherent risk of scarring. With cutaneous surgery, unlike surgery on other organs, the scar is readily apparent to the patient.

The prevention of unsatisfactory scarring begins before the initial incision with planning of the orientation of the excision. Subsequently, certain surgical techniques performed intraoperatively can be beneficial in scar prevention. Good postoperative care is vital to ensure the best final result. Finally, complications may lead to an increased risk of scarring. This chapter is divided into four segments: planning the initial excision, surgical techniques, postoperative wound care, and the management of complications.

I. INFORMED CONSENT

A key part of the preoperative discussion is informed consent. Informed consent requires that the patient have adequate information to make a decision regarding a procedure. The indications for the procedure, followed by alternative treatment options, risks of the procedure, and potential adverse outcomes, need to be discussed with the patient. Possible adverse outcomes are especially important with elective procedures so that the patient may weigh the potential risks and benefits. Informed consent requires that the patient is competent. In cases in which the patient is not competent or is younger than 18, informed consent must be obtained from the patient's parent or legal guardian. With regard to scarring, the patient should be aware preoperatively of potential scarring that may occur.

II. PREOPERATIVE EVALUATION

The preoperative evaluation is an essential part of the entire operative procedure. This section focuses on preexisting conditions that can affect postoperative scarring. The acceptable postoperative risks often depend on whether the procedure is elective or medically necessary. For larger excisions, Mohs micrographic surgery, laser resurfacing, or trichloracetic acid peels, it is preferable to see the patient in consultation before scheduling the actual procedure. The initial evaluation begins with a thorough medical history.

A. Preoperative History Pertaining to Risk of Scar Formation

Factors that can have particular bearing on postoperative scarring include a previous history of hypertrophic scarring or keloid formation. Specific ethnic groups deserve special mention regarding possible adverse postoperative effects. African-American patients have a higher incidence of keloid formation. Being aware that a patient has a history of keloid formation can facilitate postoperative planning. If patients have such a history, it is helpful to discuss with them the possibility of similar problems with the current procedure in advance so that they may be prepared for such an eventuality. This will allow a discussion of possible postoperative intervention such as steroid injections. Other techniques, such as use of the pulsed dye laser, can also be used postoperatively (1).

It is important to consider preoperatively which areas of the body are more prone to scarring. Excisions on the upper chest, shoulders, and upper arms are much more likely to form hypertrophic scars or spreading scars. The patient needs to be fully aware of this. With regard to resurfacing procedures, the neck area most often should be avoided, as this area is more likely to scar. Areas with decreased numbers of adnexal structures such as the dorsal hand are also more likely to scar if treated with any procedure deeper than superficial resurfacing.

A factor that can have a particular impact on the healing of flaps and grafts is smoking. The quantity of cigarettes smoked may influence wound healing (2). Although it is best to convince patients to stop smoking, it is often difficult in practice to do so. If they will not quit, we suggest that they decrease consumption to less than a pack per day for 1 week preoperatively and 3 to 4 weeks postoperatively.

Another consideration with extensive facial resurfacing procedures such as chemical peels, dermabrasion, or laser resurfacing is a history of herpes simplex labialis. Patients with this history should be treated with oral antiviral agents beginning 2 to 5 days preoperatively and continuing 5 days postoperatively (3). Some sources recommend treating all patients prophylactically, even those without a prior history.

Understanding the principles of wound contraction is also important in relation to postoperative scarring and in choosing closures for certain locations. Wound contraction is mediated by myofibroblasts and begins approximately 7 days postoperatively in secondary intention wounds. The importance of respecting free margins will be discussed at length later, and it is important to remember that contraction of a scar in areas such as the nasal tip or vermilion border can result in an unacceptable scar.

B. Preoperative Medications That May Affect Scar Formation

A preoperative history must also include an inquiry about previous difficulties with bleeding and the use of medications that may increase the risk of bleeding. Such drugs include, but are not limited to, aspirin, dipyridamole, Coumadin, nonsteroidal anti-inflammatory drugs (NSAIDS), and alcohol (Table 1). The duration of discontinuation of these drugs varies with the agent. Elective use of aspirin should be discontinued 2 weeks before a planned procedure that might involve significant bleeding or bruising. Many patients now

Table 1 Medications That May Affect Scar Formation

Oral anticoagulants
Coumarin derivatives: dicoumarol, phenprocoumon, nicoumalone
Indanedione derivatives: diphenadione, phenindione, anisindione
Oral antiplatelet agents
Aspirin
Nonsteroidal antiinflammatory medications
Dipyridamole
Ticlopidine
Prostaglandins
Other oral agents with antiplatelet activity
Beta-blockers
Beta-lactam antibiotics
Calcium channel blockers
Nitrates
Serotonin antagonists
Vitamin E
Heparin
Fish oil

take aspirin under a physician's direction for its anticoagulant properties in the prophylaxis of myocardial infarction and stroke, and discontinuance should be under the guidance of that physician. Coumadin should be discontinued only in conjunction with the originally prescribing physician, as the risk of even short periods without anticoagulation in this group of patients can be significant. If it is possible to discontinue Coumadin, it should be stopped 48 to 72 hours before the procedure and the prothrombin time and bleeding time checked immediately before the procedure. If there is no problem with bleeding during or after the procedure, the medication can be restarted the evening or morning after the procedure. Alcohol should be discontinued for at least 24 hours prior to the procedure and 48 hours after the procedure. If the use of drugs that increase the risk of bleeding cannot be stopped before a procedure, consideration must be given to forgoing elective procedures. Necessary, limited procedures could be considered if a preoperative bleeding time is within normal parameters (4).

Certain medications, such as retinoids, may have a negative impact on the final scar. It is particularly important to ask about the history of retinoid use, as many patients with Accutane present for dermabrasion or laser resurfacing. Retinoids are known to inhibit collagenase, making patients more prone to develop keloids. Most sources recommend that a patient discontinue these medications for 1 year before dermabrasion (5). Although it has not yet been documented by studies, this standard would also apply to carbon dioxide laser resurfacing.

Other medications that may complicate wound healing include glucocorticoids, immunosuppressives, and penicillamine (Table 2). Although these medications delay healing rather than increase scar formation, the physician should be aware of all of the patients' preoperative medications. This awareness will aid in planning postoperative care.

The patient must also be questioned about possible allergic reactions to any topical antibiotics or dressing materials. Postoperative allergic contact dermatitis can adversely af-

Table 2 Important Medications That Affect Potential Scarring

Retinoids
Glucocorticoids
Immunosuppressives
Penicillamine

fect the final scar. The antibiotic that most commonly causes an allergic reaction is neomycin; therefore, the authors routinely recommend polymyxin-bacitracin (Polysporin) ointment instead of the ubiquitously available polymyxin-neomycin (Neosporin) ointment. If the patient has an allergy to Polysporin (or bacitracin), mupirocin (Bactroban) ointment may be substituted postoperatively. Evidence suggests that plain petrolatum may be used in place of antibiotic ointments without a significantly increased risk of infection (6).

When the preoperative evaluation or discussion is concluded, there are still considerations that need to be addressed at the beginning of the procedure to decrease the possibility of postoperative scarring. When dealing with an excision, one of these considerations is the orientation and placement of the excision.

III. ORIENTATION OF THE INCISION

A. Preferred Sites for Incision Placement

The placement of the final scar in an orifice or within a hair-bearing area can decrease the visibility of the postoperative scar (Table 3). In areas such as the temple, the possibility of orienting the scar within or at the hairline should be considered. Another preferred site for the final scar is at the junction of two cosmetic units. On the face, this may include the forehead, as this larger unit can be subdivided into forehead, temple, and glabellar regions. The orbital region extends from the eyebrow superiorly to the infraorbital crease inferiorly, laterally to the temples, and medially to the nasal root. The nose is considered to have the root, dorsal nose, lateral nasal sidewalls, nasal alae, soft triangle, tip, and columella. The melolabial fold separates the lip region from the remainder of the cheek. The lip unit can be subdivided into the philtrum, cutaneous upper lip, vermilion, cutaneous lower lip, and chin.

In the excision of skin tumors, camouflaging the scar as described is often not possible because the tumor "chooses" the site of the excision. If an orifice, hair-bearing area, or cosmetic unit junction is not available, the scar should be oriented parallel to the relaxed

Table 3 Preferred Sites for Incision Placement

Within an orifice
In a hair-bearing area
At the junction of two cosmetic units
Parallel to relaxed skin tension lines

skin tension lines. The resulting scar is therefore less noticeable, as it melds with the already present lines. In a younger patient, these lines may not be as obvious. Having the patient contract muscles allows more adequate visualization.

B. Relaxed Skin Tension Lines

The planning of the initial excision can often have a large impact on the final scar. The biomechanics of the skin have already been addressed in detail in Chap. 2. The cutaneous surgeon should be familiar with these principles, including the location of skin tension lines.

Skin tension lines are the result of repeated contraction of the underlying muscles. These muscles contract perpendicular to the orientation of the resulting lines. On the forehead, the lines are transverse because of the underlying frontails muscle. In the glabellar area, the lines are vertical because of the action of the underlying corrugator muscles (Fig. 1).

In the periocular region, these lines are often described as crow's feet; they emanate initially horizontally and then obliquely from the lateral canthus because of the action of the underlying orbicularis oculi muscles (Fig. 2). As one progresses onto the cheek, these lines are oblique. However, in the preauricular region they are vertical. In the perioral region, the lines are radial.

C. Free Margins

The principle of free margins needs to be taken into account when planning an excision or repair. Free margins of importance on the face are the eyelids, the nasal rim, the helix, and

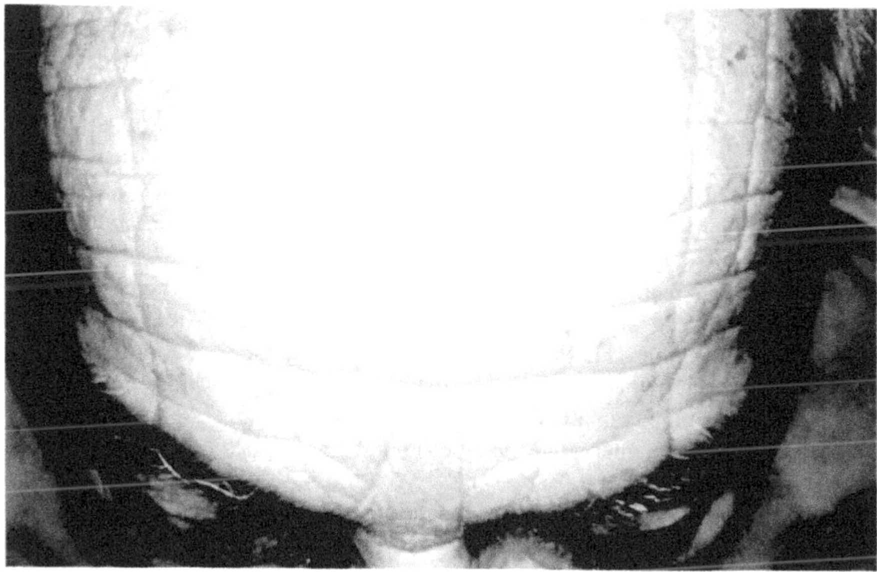

Figure 1 Transverse skin tension lines of the forehead and vertical skin tension lines of the glabella.

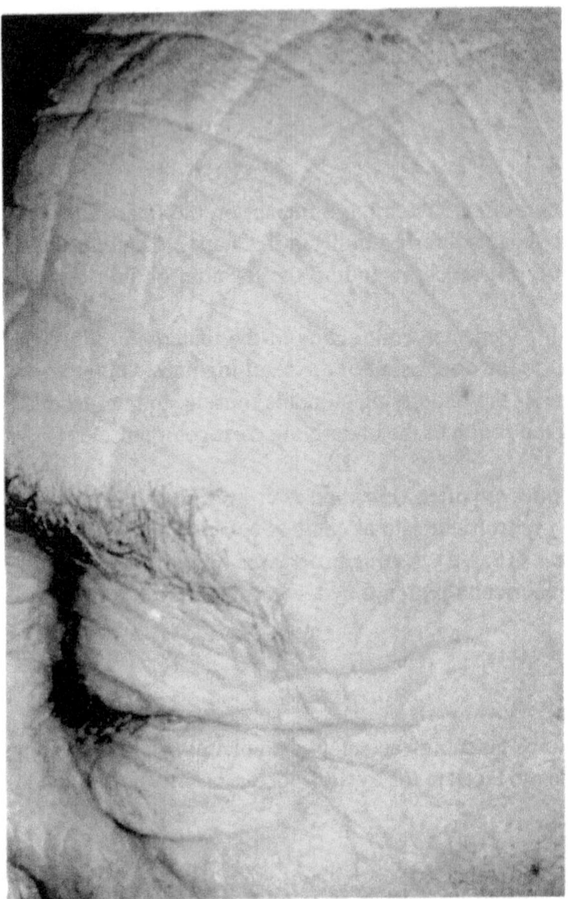

Figure 2 Horizontal skin tension lines radiating from the lateral canthus.

the lips. If these are distorted, the resulting scar will be much more noticeable. When planning a repair, these margins must be respected to prevent an unsatisfactory result (Fig. 3A and B).

When planning repairs in the eyelid region, especially for defects in close proximity to the lower eyelid, care needs to be taken to avoid ectropion. One should always test the closure before finishing. This can be done by utilizing skin hooks to bring the edges together and asking the patient to look as far upward as possible while opening the mouth. This test places the maximal pull on the lower eyelid. If this test causes dislocation of the lower eyelid, an alternative closure should be performed to avoid an unsatisfactory result.

As with the eyelid, the integrity of the nasal rim must be respected in order to avoid an unsatisfactory result. Lesions that are near the alar rim should be tested with skin hooks before closure. If primary closure would distort the rim or cause an upturn, a full-thickness skin graft or a flap taking advantage of loose skin from the glabellar or nasolabial regions is preferable.

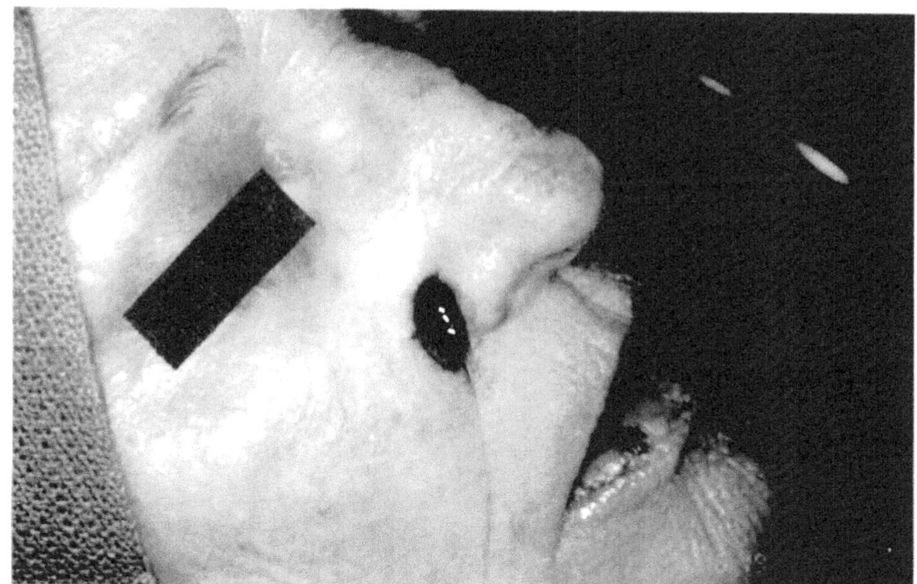

A

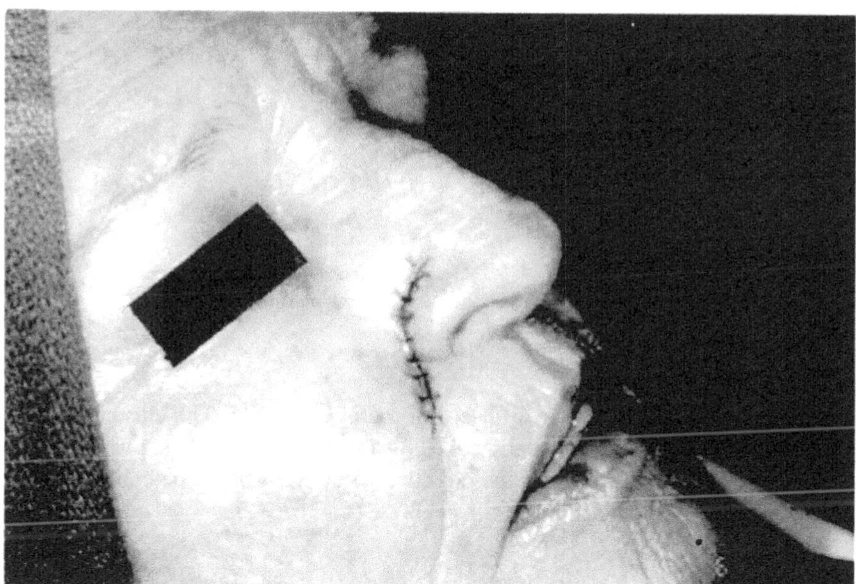

B

Figure 3 **(A)** Defect encompassing margin between the nasal rim and the cheek. **(B)** Perialar crescentic advancement flap preserving the free margin of the nasal rim.

The helix is another area where the contour needs to be respected. Although defects are often not as readily noticeable as with the eyelid or the nasal rim, malalignment should be avoided if possible (Fig. 4).

When repairing a defect of the lip, care should be taken to realign the edges of the vermilion border (Fig. 5A and B). If the defect does not involve the border but is in prox-

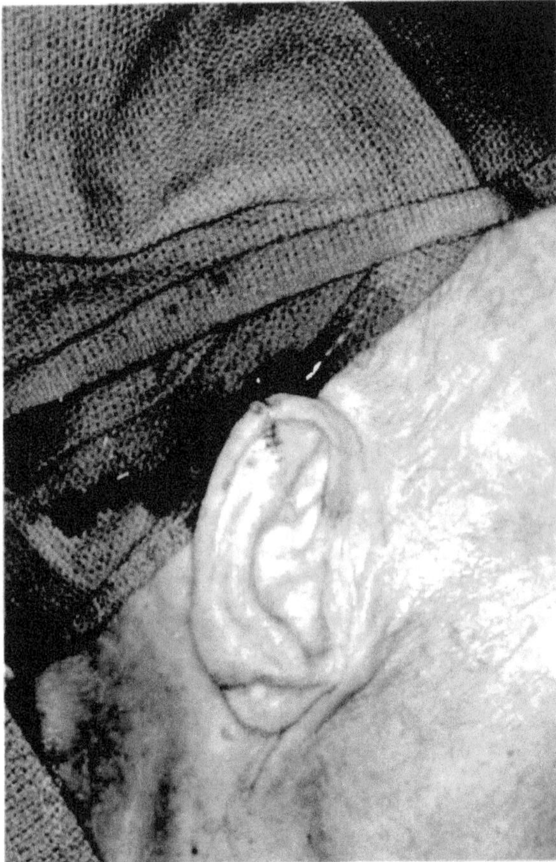

Figure 4 Ear wedge repair preserving the contour of the ear margin.

imity to the lower lip, rules similar to those for the eyelid apply. The closure should be tested to ensure that the lip is not malaligned. If distortion appears to be a possibility, then a flap such as an O to T that changes the direction of tension should be considered. This principle would also apply to defects of the eyebrow (Fig. 6A–C).

IV. INTRAOPERATIVE TECHNIQUE

A. Initial Preparation

Proper surgical technique is obviously essential in minimizing scarring. Preoperatively, the area should be cleaned with isopropyl alcohol or chlorhexidine. Care should be taken not to use chlorhexidine in the periocular region because of the risk of keratitis. Betadine may be used as a substitute in this area. The operative field should be delineated with sterile towels to create a sterile field.

Infiltration of anesthetic does not have a large impact on the final scar. However, edema may result from the anesthetic alone, especially in the periocular region. The patient needs to be made aware that this swelling will not be permanent.

B. Simple Excision Techniques to Minimize Scar Formation

When performing the excision, the blade should be angled perpendicular to the skin. If the edge is beveled inward, the deeper edges will be nearer each other than the superficial edges, causing a gap superficially unless the edges are pulled tightly. If the superficial epidermal

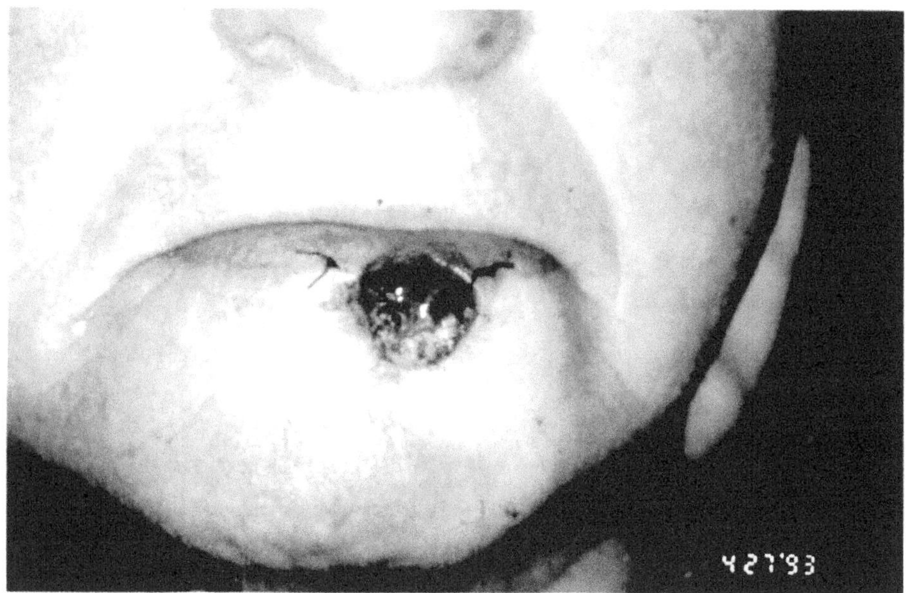

A

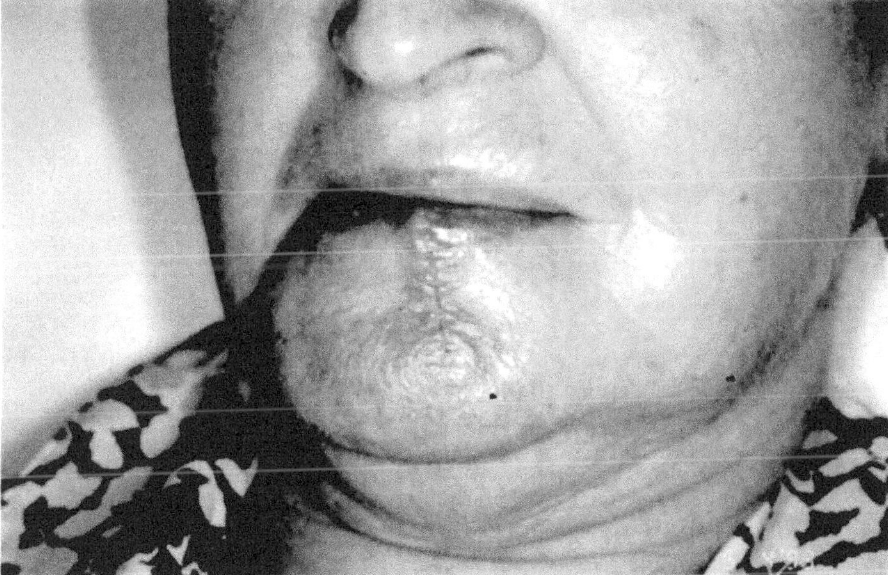

B

Figure 5 **(A)** Sutures placed to mark the border between the vermilion and the cutaneous lip. These help to align the vermilion when reconstructing the defect. **(B)** Postoperative picture of same patient demonstrating alignment of the vermilion after closure.

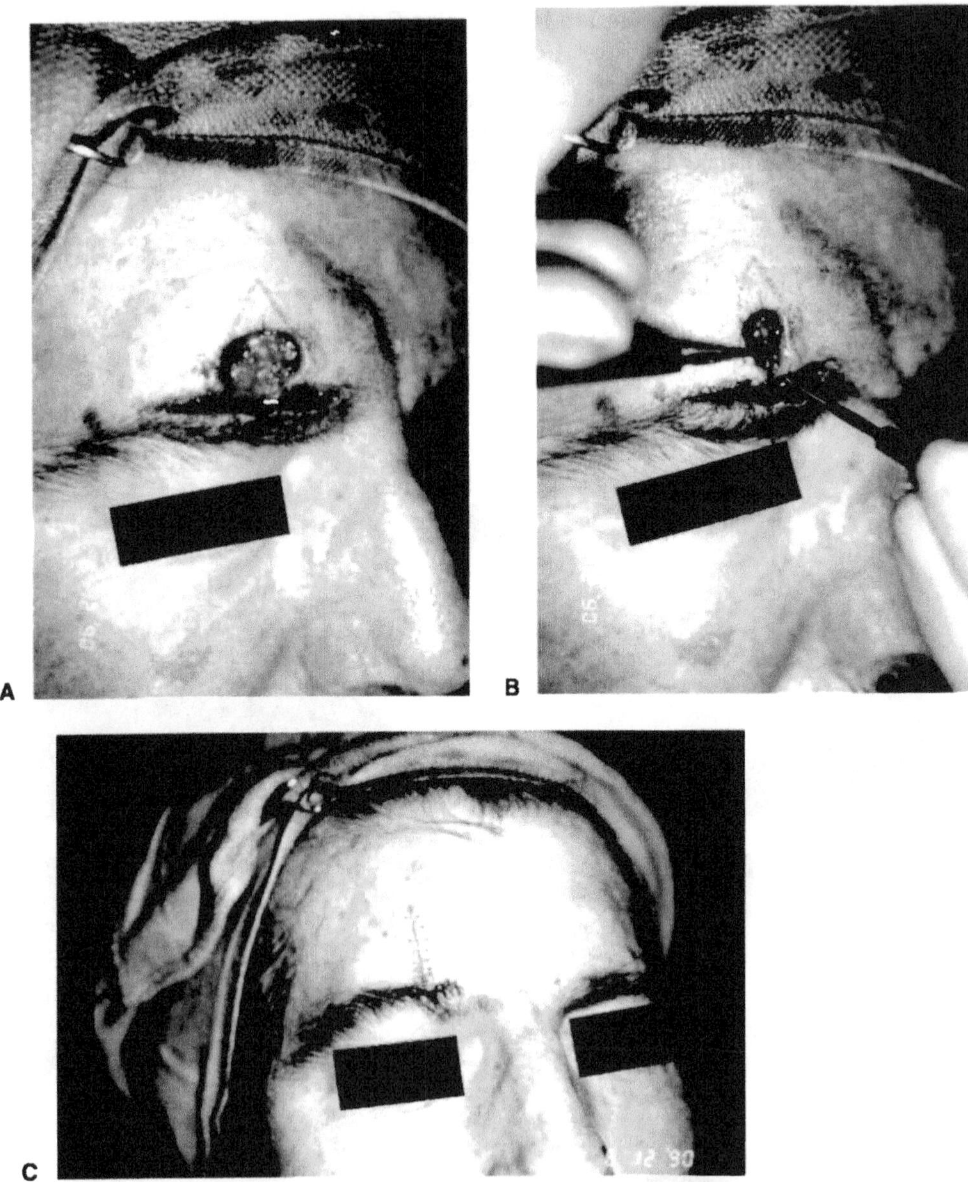

Figure 6 **(A)** Defect abutting up to the eyelid margin with planned O to T closure. **(B)** O to T closure above eyelid to preserve margin. **(C)** Postoperative picture demonstrating O to T closure.

edges are closed under too much tension, necrosis may occur; therefore, a straight edge is preferable to one that is beveled inward. The tissue is then removed with sharp scalpel or scissors dissection. This should be done at even plane throughout the specimen. If the edges are taken more superficially than the center, excess tissue at the edges will bunch.

After removal of the specimen, the edges must be undermined. The level of the undermining varies with anatomic location. On the face, undermining is usually performed in the superficial subcutaneous fat. On the scalp, it is preferable to undermine in the subgaleal plane. This is a relatively avascular plane, and it also avoids transection of the hair follicles. On the trunk or extremities, undermining is usually performed in the deep subcutaneous fat. We prefer to utilize skin hooks to grasp the tissue while undermining to minimize trauma to the skin edges (Fig. 7). If forceps are used, they should be used only to lift up tissue and not to grasp it (Fig. 8). Excess trauma to wound edges is more likely to result in necrosis.

Hemostasis is then achieved with electrocoagulation. Cauterizing only where necessary helps minimize tissue destruction and facilitates wound healing. The subcutaneous layer is reapproximated with absorbable suture to minimize tension of the epidermal edges. The cutaneous layer is then closed with nonabsorbable suture. The authors prefer Vicryl to close the subcutaneous tissue and Prolene for the cutaneous layer. Prolene is preferred as it facilitates suture removal. Table 4 shows nonabsorbable and absorbable sutures, with their duration, strength, and tissue reactivity.

The subcutaneous closure should reapproximate the edges, allowing the cutaneous sutures to be under minimal tension. Wound tension increases fibroblast activity, resulting in a more exuberant scar. Care should also be taken not to pull the cutaneous sutures too tightly to avoid necrosis. When placing the cutaneous sutures, the surgeon should also take into account that the tissue will swell postoperatively.

In certain areas of the body, wounds are inherently under tension and subject to increased activity postoperatively compared with other regions. These areas include the chest, shoulders, and back. The increased tension makes spreading of scars more likely. The patient should be aware that cutaneous surgery in these particular areas is more likely to result in a spread scar. Longer lasting subcutaneous sutures such as PDS help decrease

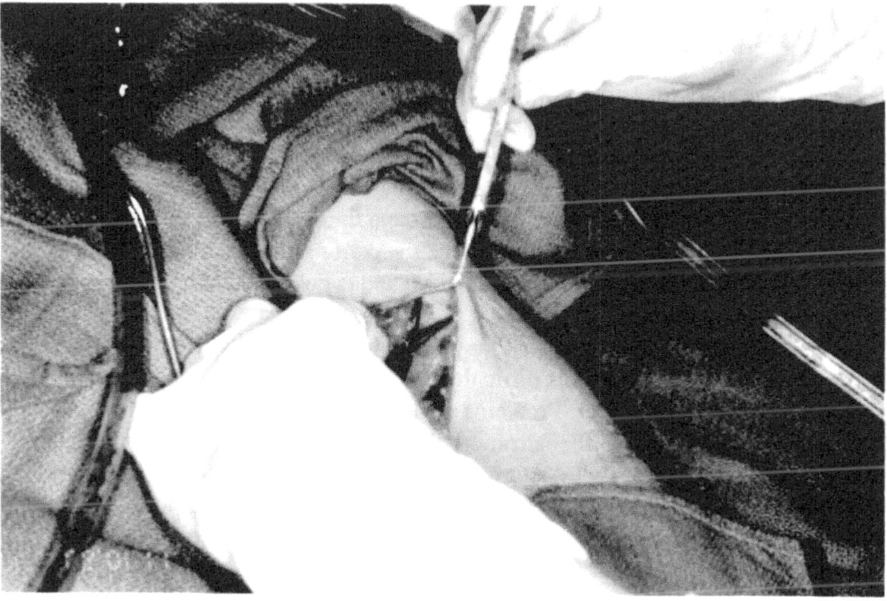

Figure 7 Use of skin hook to assist with visualization while undermining. Skin hooks minimize trauma to the skin edge.

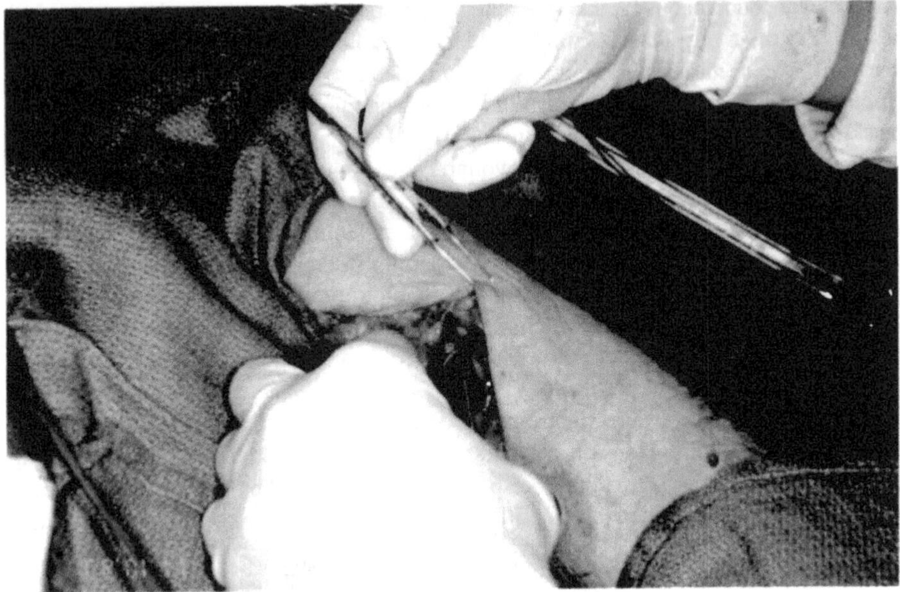

Figure 8 Use of forceps while undermining. Note the lifting rather than grabbing of the skin edge to minimize trauma to the tissue.

the probability of scar spread. A Z-plasty can also be used to revise a spread scar. Changing the direction of the tension may result in a more acceptable cosmetic result.

C. Suture Problems Related to Scar Formation

Sutures, while necessary for primary wound closure, can also be the cause of postoperative problems and scarring. Buried sutures are absorbable over a period of one to several months, as noted in Table 4. During this time, they are degraded by either proteolysis or hydrolysis. As this degradation occurs, a firm papule may be formed. If the suture is near the superficial aspect of this papule, it may project through the surface. It is thought that more superficially placed sutures or sutures tied on their superior rather than inferior aspect are more likely to "spit." If the suture can be visualized and is not adherent to the surrounding skin, it may be gently removed.

Another difficulty with sutures that may exacerbate scarring is due to the tract that they form within the epithelium. This difficulty arises with nonabsorbable sutures used to reapproximate the superficial layer. Problems are more likely to develop if sutures remain in place more than 8 days, as epithelialization of the suture tract is complete by this time (7). "Track marks" may occur with sutures left in beyond 8 days, especially if they are pulled too tightly. The potential for these marks increases with increasing suture duration; therefore, early suture removal is the most beneficial form of prevention. The use of absorbable buried sutures to reapproximate the wound and decrease the tension on the cutaneous sutures aids in early removal. In areas such an extremity or trunk where the sutures will stay in place for 2 weeks, a running subcuticular suture may be used instead to decrease the possibility of suture marks.

The epithelialization of the suture tract may also result in inflammation. This inflammation may lead to scarring around the suture tract, with the final result being pitted scars in these areas. Again, early suture removal lessens the chance of this occurring.

D. Techniques Regarding Flap or Graft Closure Related to Scar Formation

More extensive procedures such as those involving flaps have a unique problem in relation to scarring, which is the trap-door deformity. This deformity is described as having a pincushion appearance (Fig. 9). Although the etiology has not been completely elucidated, it is most likely due to contraction of the recipient wound below the flap combined with lymphatic obstruction and excess subcutaneous tissue. The cutaneous surgeon needs to be aware of several techniques for minimizing the trap-door effect. These include undermining the tissue surrounding the wound. Studies on guinea pigs demonstrated a trap-door effect only on wounds that were not undermined (8). A second technique is the use of straight lines and angles rather than circular lines. This is important for circular wounds such as those often created with Mohs surgery. If slightly more tissue can be removed from the defect to create a rhombic shape before the flap repair, the likelihood of trap-door deformity is minimized.

Understanding the principles of wound contraction is also important in relation to postoperative scarring and in choosing closures for certain locations. Wound contraction is particularly an issue with wounds that heal by second intention. Wound contraction is mediated by the myofibroblast, which is considered one of the most important cells in the wound-healing process. Contraction begins to occur at 7 days, but a noticeable decrease in wound size is not noted until 14 days. Choosing secondary intention healing for sites near a free margin may ultimately result in a poorer result because of contraction. Guiding sutures may aid in changing the direction of wound contraction. These sutures are useful near free margins. The direction perpendicular to the sutures has the least amount of contraction. For example, below the lower lip, horizontal sutures across a defect would minimize vertical tension and minimize pulling down of the lip margin.

Table 4 Absorbable and Nonabsorbable Sutures

Absorbable suture Name	Tensile strength	Reactivity
Catgut	60% lost at 1 week	Marked
Polyglycolic acid	45% lost at 2 weeks	Much less than catgut
Polyglycan 910	45% lost at 2 weeks	Same as polyglycolic
Polydioxanone	30% lost at 2 weeks	Minimal
Nonabsorbable suture Name	**Elasticity**	**Reactivity**
Silk	Minimal	Higher
Nylon	High	Less than silk
Polypropylene	Higher than nylon	Similar to nylon
Novafil	Highest	Minimal

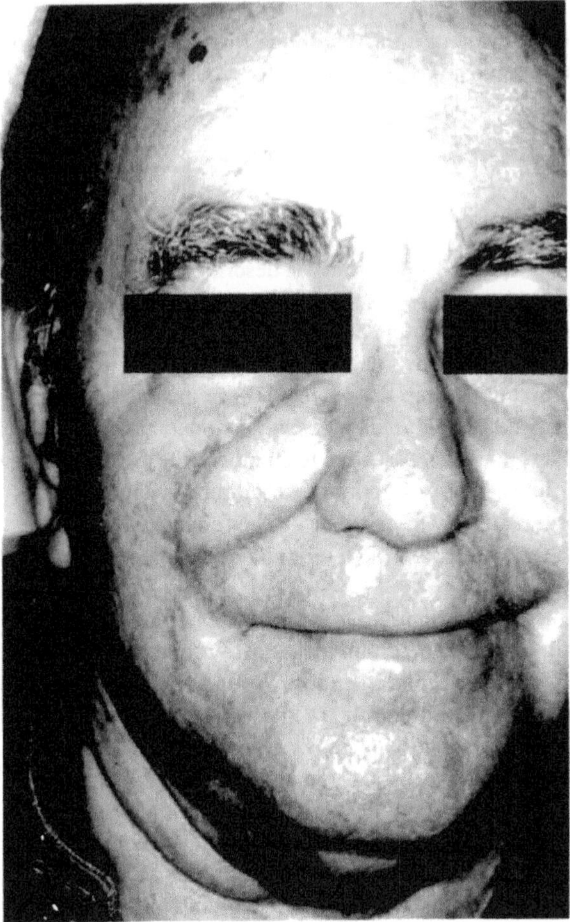

Figure 9 Example of trap-door deformity after flap repair.

When choosing to repair a defect with a skin graft, wound contraction also becomes a factor. The reticular dermis is a strong deterrent to wound contraction; therefore flaps and full-thickness skin grafts undergo minimal contraction. Split-thickness skin grafts undergo significant contraction. Again, areas near free margins or other sites where contraction adversely affects the final scar should not be repaired with split-thickness skin grafts.

V. COMPLICATIONS CAN LEAD TO SCARRING

When a procedure is beset by complications, the risk of less acceptable scar formation increases. The problems of bleeding, infection, necrosis, and dehiscence form an interrelated series of events that has been referred to as the "terrible tetrad" (9). These complications, by disrupting the normal sequence of wound healing, can lead to scars of less desirable size, texture, and color. Some complications are the direct result of a single event in a procedure. Most often, complications result from a series of small events that interrelate to produce the final outcome. Each event is enabled by a previous event and provides the proper conditions for the development of the next step in the sequence (Fig. 10).

Prevention is the best way to avoid this increased risk of scarring. Through strict adherence to thorough preoperative screening procedures, the use of sound and conservative surgical planning, paying detailed attention to intraoperative surgical techniques, and providing optimal postoperative care, the series of events that may ultimately lead to a poor outcome can often be interrupted. Unfortunately, the human response to injury and disease is not always predictable, and some complications occur regardless of all attempts to prevent them. In this circumstance, minimization of the adverse effects is the primary goal.

A. Bleeding

Intraoperative bleeding can range from rare catastrophic events (exsanguination) to nuisance bleeding. Even nuisance bleeding can obscure the surgical site and make adherence to optimal surgical technique difficult. In addition, although any bleeding requires control before wound closure, each use of cautery or ligatures runs the risk of providing a site for increased inflammation or a small nidus of devitalized tissue that might potentiate infection. Therefore, it is critical to attempt to minimize bleeding by controlling as many potentially adverse factors as possible preoperatively. The patient should be evaluated for possible drug usage, hereditary factors, and disease states that might contribute to increased bleeding. These factors should be recognized preoperatively and controlled if possible. The almost ubiquitous use of aspirin in today's population of patients cannot be overemphasized. All possible efforts should be made to discontinue aspirin usage at least 14 days before an elective procedure.

Bleeding that persists into the postoperative period or develops after closure of the wound can also lead to problems with wound healing. Bleeding may develop as the vasoconstrictive effect of epinephrine utilized in the anesthetic injection wanes. Excessive activity and movement of the patient may dislodge fragile clots. Elevations in the patient's blood pressure may also contribute to postoperative bleeding. Effective bandaging and postoperative care instructions can often minimize bleeding. A properly applied pressure dressing can control minor bleeding and wick away small amounts of blood (10). Bulky dressings or splints may be useful in limiting movement of the operative site and thereby limiting the possibility of additional bleeding. In addition, a dressing may provide protection against inadvertent external trauma. The patient should be given explicit instructions

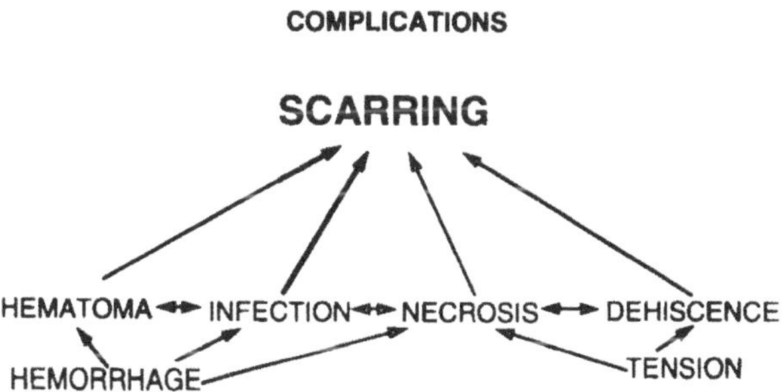

Figure 10 Complications may interrelate and lead to increased scarring.

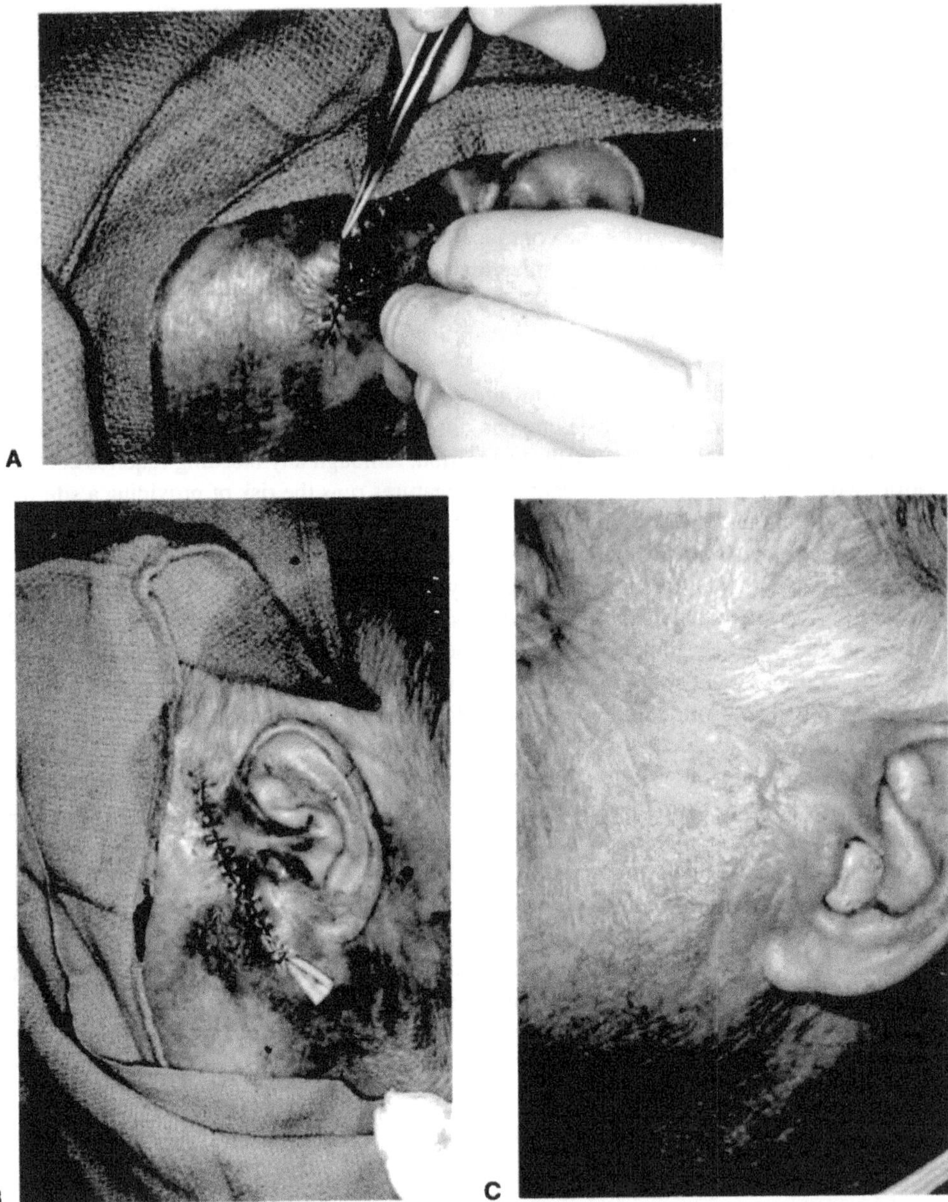

Figure 11 **(A)** Hematoma: a clot of gelatin-like material is removed from an acute hematoma. **(B)** A drain is placed at the inferior pole of the wound in the preauricular crease. **(C)** Approximately 1 month later with good healing and minimal increase in scarring.

for appropriately limiting activities in the postoperative period. Patients generally assume that they can engage in any activity that is not prohibited.

Minor bleeding onto the bandage can usually be controlled with direct pressure with few adverse consequences. However, persistent intraoperative or postoperative bleeding can require the placement of a drain to prevent hematoma formation. A simple drain may be fashioned from a sterilized rubber band or a fenestrated portion of Penrose tubing. More elaborate drains such a Jackson-Pratt device may also be utilized. Because the drain occupies subcutaneous space and prevents wound apposition at its exit site, the potential for increased scarring exists. The drain exit should be placed in the most inconspicuous portion of the wound possible. Such a site might be hidden by natural structures (such as the hairline) or might fall into natural skin folds such as the nasolabial fold or the preauricular crease (Fig. 11B). The drain should be removed as soon as its presence is no longer required. Immediate closure of the drain exit wound is not advisable, because in most circumstances there is continued slight drainage from the site. As a result, at least a small portion of the wound must heal by second intent. With good wound care, the site may heal well with a minimal increase in scarring (Fig. 11C).

A hematoma forms when postoperative blood collects in a wound. Bleeding through the wound may precede the development of a hematoma, and a small amount of bleeding may persist during its formation. The onset of hematoma formation is most often heralded by a deep pressure sensation or a new, throbbing pain. Examination of the wound usually reveals ecchymosis surrounding a firm yet fluctuant mass. Early or expanding hematomas should be evacuated to minimize potential adverse effects such as infection, dehiscence, or necrosis. Opening the wound by removing several or all sutures and exploring the dead space will yield gelatin-like clots of blood (Fig. 11A). Care should be taken to remove all of the clot fragments by carefully exploring the entire site. The wound should be irrigated and inspected for bleeding sites. Occasionally, a single bleeding vessel is located. Often, multiple bleeding points are located and require cauterization. The wound may be reclosed if good hemostasis can be obtained and there is no clinical evidence of infection. In most circumstances, placement of a drain is advisable and empirical use of antibiotics is justified. The procedure requires local anesthesia.

If left unattended over several days, a hematoma becomes organized. The clot develops a thick, fibrous texture and is difficult to remove from the surrounding wound (Fig. 12).

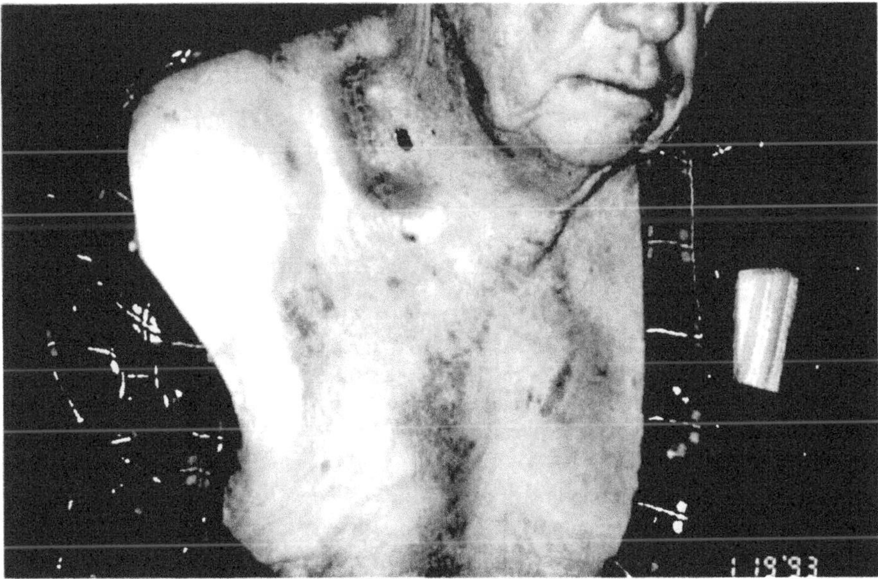

Figure 12 A well-organized hematoma in the supraclavicular area with extensive ecchymoses spreading to the upper abdomen.

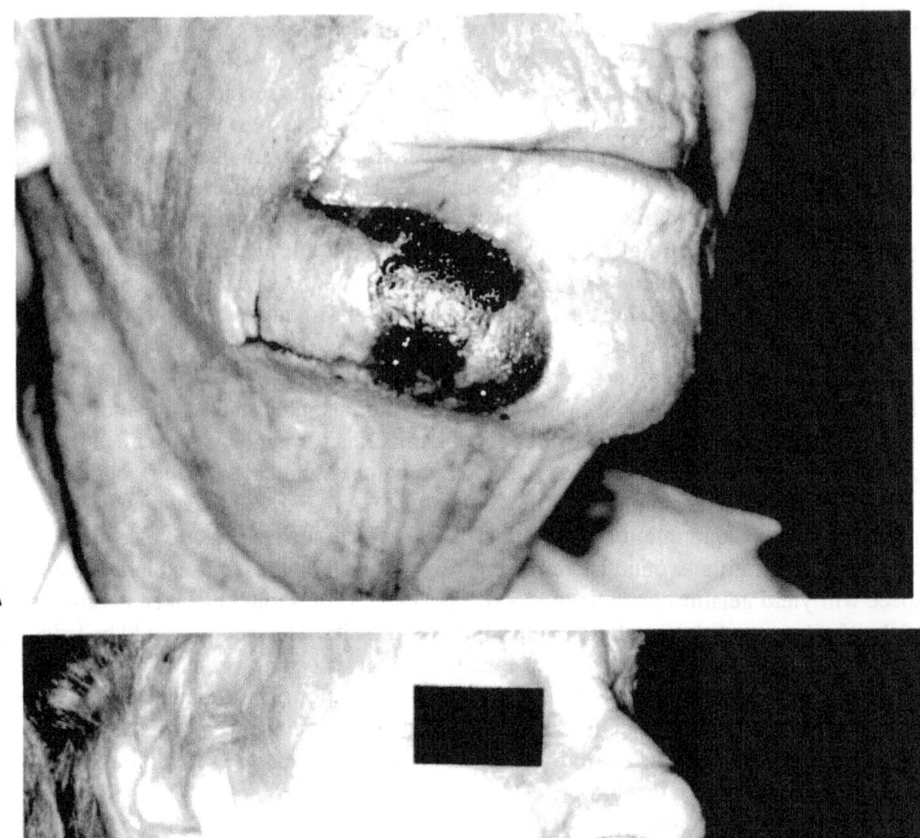

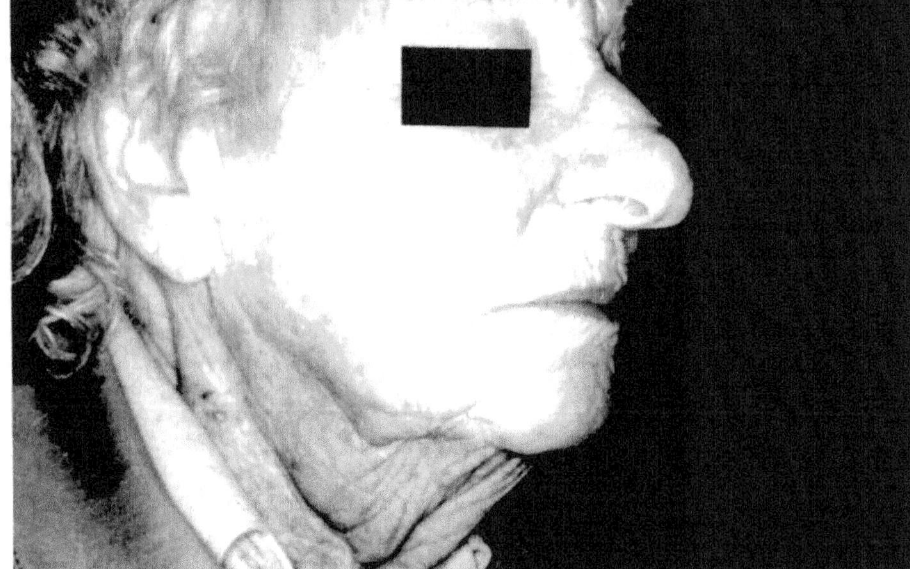

Figure 13 **(A)** An organized hematoma leading to necrosis. **(B)** The necrosis was allowed to self-demarcate and the area to heal by second intention.

At this stage, unless the hematoma is still expanding, it is best to allow natural resolution of the clot rather than attempt evacuation. The site is still at risk for infection, and the pressure of the hematoma may still lead to dehiscence or necrosis (Fig. 13A). Gentle heat may be applied to the wound several times a day to hasten liquefaction and reabsorption of the hematoma. With liquefaction, larger hematomas may develop into a fluctuant mass that requires aspiration. Without anesthesia, the serosanguineous fluid may be removed with a syringe and a 16- to 18-gauge needle. Such aspiration may have to be repeated several times.

Leaking of small amounts of blood into the interstitial space around the surgical site leads to ecchymosis. The development of ecchymoses after procedures, especially in areas of loose tissue, is common. Ecchymoses can spread quite widely around the surgical site or migrate away from the wound under the influence of gravity. Although the appearance of ecchymoses may be quite alarming, they usually resolve without sequelae (Fig. 12).

B. Infection

Although the risk of infection is low in most procedures, the development of a wound infection can increase the risk of poor healing and unacceptable scar formation. Again, prevention of wound infection beginning in the preoperative period is the best method of minimizing this risk. A number of factors may predispose a patient to the development of a wound infection (Table 5). A careful preoperative history may elucidate an increased risk of infection and provide the surgeon with the opportunity to alter the procedure or pre- and postoperative care in a manner that might minimize the risk. In elective procedures, the surgeon must consider the advisability of the procedure in the presence of increased risk of infection.

Table 5 Risk Factors for Infection

- Systemic
  - Immunosuppression
    - Acquired immunodeficiency syndrome (AIDS)
    - Leukemia, myeloma, lymphoma
    - Drugs
      - Corticosteroids
      - Immunosuppressants: cyclosporine, azathioprine, etc.
      - Cytotoxic agents
  - Diabetes
  - Liver failure
  - Renal failure
  - Malnutrition
- Local factors
  - Existing bacterial infection (28)
  - "Dirty" anatomic regions (groin, mouth, axilla) (11, 15, 29)
  - Impaired local defenses
    - Poor circulation
    - Previous therapeutic radiation
    - Surgical factors
      - Prolonged (>3 hours) surgical time [9]
      - Excessive wound cauterization
      - Traumatic tissue handling
      - Foreign bodies (including buried suture)
      - Excessive wound tension
    - Postsurgical factors
      - Hematoma
      - Necrosis+

Antibiotic prophylaxis is controversial because the true risk of infection is low [less than 5% (11) and perhaps as low as 1 to 2% (12)], and as a result few clear data are available to prove the efficacy of prophylaxis. If antibiotic prophylaxis is to be used because of increased risk factors, it is most effective if the agent is administered immediately before the beginning of the procedure (13,14). Parenteral antibiotics are now administered within 30 minutes of surgical wounding. Oral antibiotics should probably be administered about an hour before the procedure. The effectiveness of the prophylaxis may be reduced if the antibiotics are started several hours or days before the procedure. In prophylactic use, the duration of antibiotic administration can be brief. Administration beyond 24 hours is not supported by the current literature (15). Although not as effective as preoperative antibiotic prophylaxis, postoperative administration of antibiotics, which has been a common practice among cutaneous surgeons, may be able to reduce wound infections (11).

Once the decision to use antibiotic prophylaxis has been made, the choice of antibiotic should be based on the most likely causative organisms. Preoperative bacterial flora are not necessarily a good predicator of the organisms to be found in wound infections (16). Fortunately, the organisms encounter in typical wound infections are somewhat limited. A first-generation cephalosporin, such as cephalexin, has activity against the most common causative agents, *Staphylococcus aureus* and *Streptococcus viridans*, as well as activity against common gram-negative organisms including *Escherichia coli*, *Klebsiella*, and *Proteus mirabilis*. The usual dosage would be 1 g by month (PO) 1 hour prior to the procedure, with 500 mg 4 to 6 hours later. If the patient is sensitive to cephalosporins, macrolide antibiotics (erythromycin and newer agents), semisynthetic penicillins (oxacillin and the like), or amoxicillin–clavulanate potassium may be considered. If methicillin-resistant *S. aureus* is a concern, vancomycin may be the drug of choice. The usual dose is 500 mg intravenously (IV) 30 minutes before the procedure with 250 mg IV 6 hours later for prolonged procedures. *Pseudomonas aeruginosa* must be considered for prophylaxis against liquefying chondritis in external ear procedures. In that circumstance, the use of ciprofloxacin or a similar agent is necessary. The usual dosage is 1 g PO 1 hour before the procedure, followed by 500 mg in 12 hours. The use of antiviral prophylaxis for herpes simplex has already been addressed.

Prevention of infection is critical during preparation of the patient and the surgical procedure. Preparation should be appropriate to the procedure and rigorously applied according to protocol. Because of the great diversity in procedures, different preparations are required in different circumstances. In a similar manner, the degree of sterility maintained during a procedure depends on the procedure. Strict sterile technique should be adhered to during most incisional surgery, but destructive techniques without wound closure requires slightly less scrupulous aseptic technique.

Most wound infections begin during the operative session but become manifest 4 to 8 days after surgery (9). The first symptom is often increased wound pain. The wound may show increased erythema and edema (Fig. 14). The site may become warm. The redness and swelling may spread rapidly and regional lymphadenopathy may develop. The wound may become fluctuant and discharge purulent exudate. Wound infection may be accompanied by systemic symptoms such as fever, chills, and malaise.

Rapid treatment of a developing wound infection may reduce the associated potential for increased scarring. Treatment must be tailored to the site and type of infection. Infected incisional wounds should be treated according to the principles long established in general surgery-drainage, heat, elevation, and rest (17). If fluctuance and exudate are present, the wound should be opened and drained. Sutures, including subcutaneous sutures,

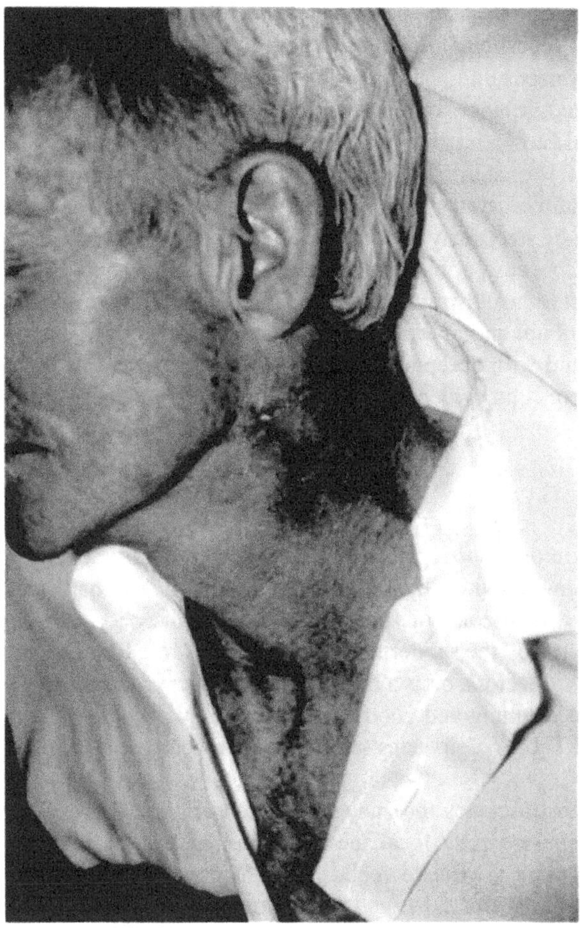

Figure 14 Wound erythema, induration, drainage, warmth, and tenderness present at suture removal are indicative of infection.

may have to be removed for the area of fluctuance to be drained. This procedure most often requires anesthesia. The wound should be left open, and packing with iodoform gauze may be needed to prevent self-sealing of deep cavities. The wound should be cleaned daily and the packing changed, if needed. If no fluctuance is present, it may not be necessary to open the wound. Gentle heat may provide comfort and hasten improvement of the infection by increasing local blood flow. The wound should be cultured, but antibiotic therapy should be instituted immediately based on the most probable organism. Gram stain may provide some guidance in selecting the initial antibiotic coverage. *S. aureus* is the most common causative organism. In most circumstances, a first-generation cephalosporin provides broad initial coverage. If another causative organism is suspected, therapy should be directed toward that organism. Changes in antibiotic therapy should be based on culture results and clinical response.

Extensive or rapidly progressing wound infection or infection with systemic symptoms may require hospitalization for aggressive wound care, parenteral antibiotics, and support of the patient. Patients with superficial infections of the skin may require different treatment. The area of infection may need additional cleansing to remove crust and exudate. If the area of involvement is limited, topical antibiotics such as mupirocin may be employed. In cases of excessive occlusion, with either ointments or dressings, infection with *Candida* must be considered. A KOH examination of scrapings from the area should be performed. If it is positive, the use of topical or systemic anti-*Candida* agents may be indicated. Drying the area and using acidic soaks may also be helpful in resolving the infection.

If the wound must be opened because of bacterial infection, it usually cannot be reclosed immediately and must be left to heal by second intent. This situation obviously has the potential for scarring in manners not anticipated before the procedure. With adequate wound care, most sites heal well and with acceptable scarring. Delayed closure of large wounds may be performed after there is no evidence of infection. Delayed scar revision is also an option.

C. Necrosis

If the blood supply to an area of skin or tissue is inadequate to support viability, necrosis results. The blood supply to the skin is provided by a subdermal arterial plexus that is derived from small segmental arteries. A horizontal dermal plexus with plexuses around hair follicles and eccrine glands is supplied by the subdermal arterial plexus (18). If this blood supply is lost because of disease, local factors, or as a by-product of surgery, necrosis may result. When possible, preoperative planning and good surgical technique should be employed to minimize such problems. Table 6 delineates some factors in necrosis and possible methods of prevention.

The earliest sign of vascular insufficiency that may lead to necrosis may be a pallor that persists after the effect of epinephrine in the local anesthetic has resolved. A cyanotic swelling of the wound or wound edge may indicate venous insufficiency. Early intervention may abort or limit the extent of the necrosis. Wound tension or tension on a flap pedicle may be relieved by judicious suture removal or replacement. Efforts to reduce edema, such as elevation, may improve venous return. Gentle heat may increase blood flow to the area. The use of hyperbaric oxygen may increase tissue survival (19).

Observation is often the most prudent course of action when necrosis is established. It is often impossible to predict the depth of the final necrosis. It may range from loss of only the epidermis, through full-thickness loss of the skin, to loss of skin and the underlying fat, fascia, and muscle. An eschar will form at the site of necrosis. As the ultimate extent of the tissue loss is difficult to predict, the area of necrosis should be allowed to demarcate with only minimal cleaning and débridement. Vigorous débridement may serve only to extend the area of necrosis. As the eschar separates from the wound, the site should be treated as any wound healing by second intent (9). Good wound care at this point may limit the extent of increased scarring (Fig. 13B).

D. Dehiscence

The wound edges may separate because of infection, necrosis, or hematoma. If there is excessive wound tension, the edges may also separate. Separation may be noted before suture removal but usually becomes more obvious after suture removal (Fig. 15). As the wound has only 3 to 5% of its original tensile strength at 2 weeks and is held together only by the

Table 6 Factors in Necrosis

Factors	Prevention
Systemic factors	
Arteriosclerotic vascular disease Systemic vasculitis Collagen vascular disease Diabetes	Good surgical planning to avoid undue stress on the vascular supply. Avoid elective procedures if the risk of necrosis is excessive. Optimal control of underlying disease process.
Smoking	Stop smoking or reduce smoking to less than one pack per day (26)
Local factors	
Location: lower extremities, acral Radiation dermatitis Lymphedema Stasis dermatitis	Modify procedures to provide optimal blood supply (i.e., avoid random flaps, split-thickness grafts instead of full-thickness grafts). Avoid elective procedures.
Wound factors	
Hematoma Infection Edema	Planning and prevention as discussed
Excessive wound tension Tight sutures	Allowance in closure for edema. Use of suture with some stretch (monofilament nylon or polypropylene) (9) Use of 1–2 mm loop stitch between first and second throws of the knot (27).
Excessive or superficial undermining	Good surgical technique
Inadequate blood supply to flap	Adequate pedicle width for random flaps (1:3, length:width). Delayed removal of dog ears created by flap rotation [24]. Use only arterial-based flaps in areas of marginal local perfusion. Handle pedicles with care to avoid excessive twisting.
Inadequate bed for graft	Avoid more than 1 cm^2 of bare cartilage or bone. Avoid sites previously exposed to therapeutic radiation. Assure no bleeding under the graft.

newly bridged epithelium, wound coagulum, and early neovascularization (9), dehiscence is a danger at the time of suture removal in most wounds. The practice of removing sutures in stages over a period of days may minimize the risk of dehiscence. The benefit of prolonged suture placement must always be weighed against the development of unsightly suture track marks. Many of the factors that lead to necrosis may also increase the risk of dehiscence. Cigarette smoking (20), advanced age of the patient, systemic infection, hypoproteinemia, uremia, hypertension, steroid usage, and pulmonary disease may all increase the risk of dehiscence (21). Rapid wound healing may also be inhibited by the presence of excessive char from anticoagulation (22) or the intraoperative use of the CO_2 laser (23). In addition, excessive postoperative activity or external trauma to the wound may cause dehiscence.

If the wound opens at suture removal as a result of excessive tension or before suture

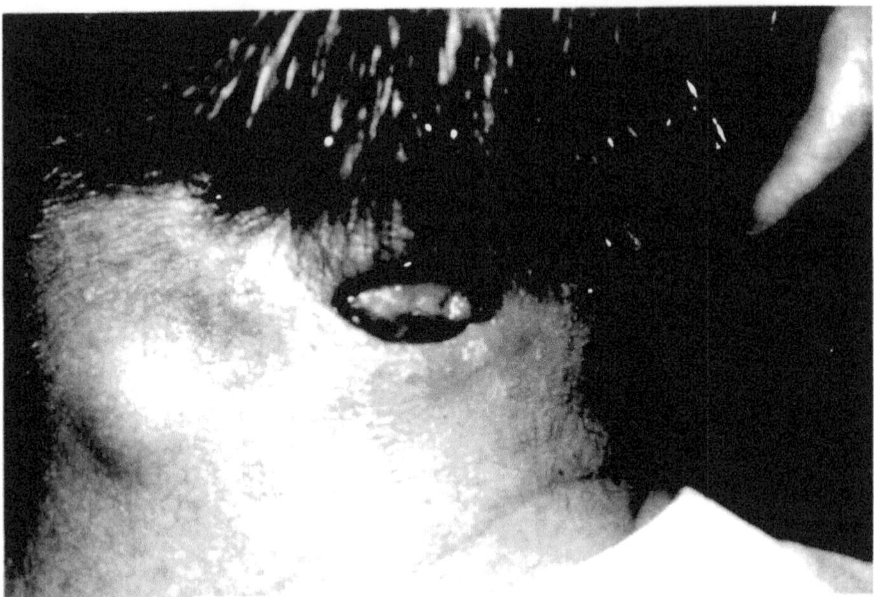

Figure 15 Dehiscence after suture removal. Enlarged lymph node suggests the additional complication of infection.

removal because of trauma or activity, immediate reapproximation of the wound edges can be considered if there is no evidence of infection, hematoma, or necrosis. Wound freshening should be kept to a minimum, as allowing the wound edges to remain as is may remove the lag period to fibroplasia and accelerate the development of wound strength (9). The wound should be reapproximated in a sterile fashion with nylon or Prolene (24). Such reclosure may greatly reduce the healing time (25) and provide an improved scar compared with allowing the site to heal by second intent.

If dehiscence is the result of hematoma, infection, or necrosis, the underlying cause must be treated and the wound left open to heal by second intent. Again, good wound care may limit the amount of additional scarring. After the underlying problem has resolved, a delayed closure can be considered.

Complications can certainly increase the risk of adverse scar formation. Early appropriate intervention can minimize the risk and most often lead to a favorable outcome (Fig. 16A–D).

VI. POSTOPERATIVE WOUND CARE

Prevention of postoperative scarring does not end with the conclusion of the procedure. Proper wound care postoperatively is essential. Key principles are keeping the wound moist, preventing secondary impetiginization, and protecting the sutures.

Multiple studies have shown that keeping a wound moist allows faster wound healing. This principle is most applicable to wounds that heal by second intention, as preventing eschar formation facilitates epidermal migration. Sutured wounds also benefit from occlusion. Postoperatively, a nonsensitizing antibiotic ointment should be placed. As

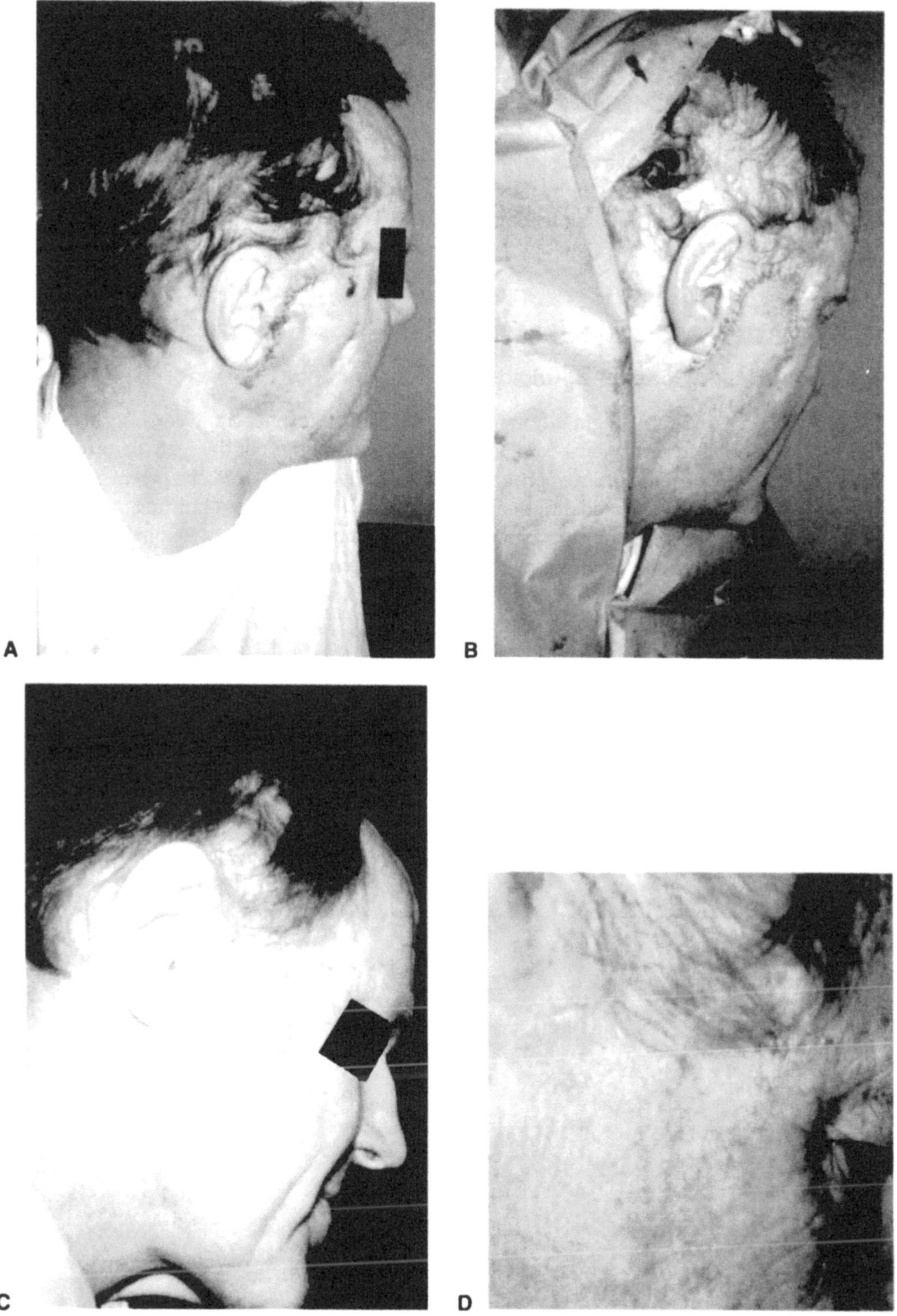

Figure 16 **(A)** Flap reconstruction on the cheek with hematoma formation on postoperative day 1. **(B)** After evacuation of the hematoma, strict control of bleeding and resuturing. **(C)** At the time of suture removal, 1 week after evacuation of the hematoma. **(D)** At 14 months after surgery with excellent overall appearance.

discussed earlier, Polysporin is preferable to Neosporin because of the high incidence of allergic contact dermatitis with neomycin. The wound is then covered by a nonadherent sterile dressing such as Telfa followed by gauze for extra protection and then tape.

The patient should be given detailed verbal and written wound care instructions. This step facilitates proper wound care by the patient as well as early intervention by the physician regarding postoperative complications. Frequent follow-up is also essential for the latter.

VII. POSTOPERATIVE PROBLEMS

A. Hypertrophic Scars and Keloids

Hypertrophic scars usually begin a few weeks after the sutures are removed (Fig. 17). In contrast to keloids, hypertrophic scars do not grow beyond the confines of the original wound. At the initial signs of a hypertrophic scar, intralesional steroids or potent topical steroids can be used. These modalities can also decrease the associated pruritus. As noted earlier, patients of specific ethnic backgrounds or with a family history of keloids are more prone to keloid formation. Keloids may require more extensive treatment including surgical therapy such as cryosurgery, laser surgery, or excision. Nonsurgical therapies include silicone gel, intralesional steroids, and pressure therapy.

B. Pigment Alterations

Pigmentary changes are largely a function of injury to the epidermis, because melanocytes reside in the epidermis. Procedures that result in epidermal damage that is then left to heal are most likely to lead to significant pigmentary changes postoperatively. These proce-

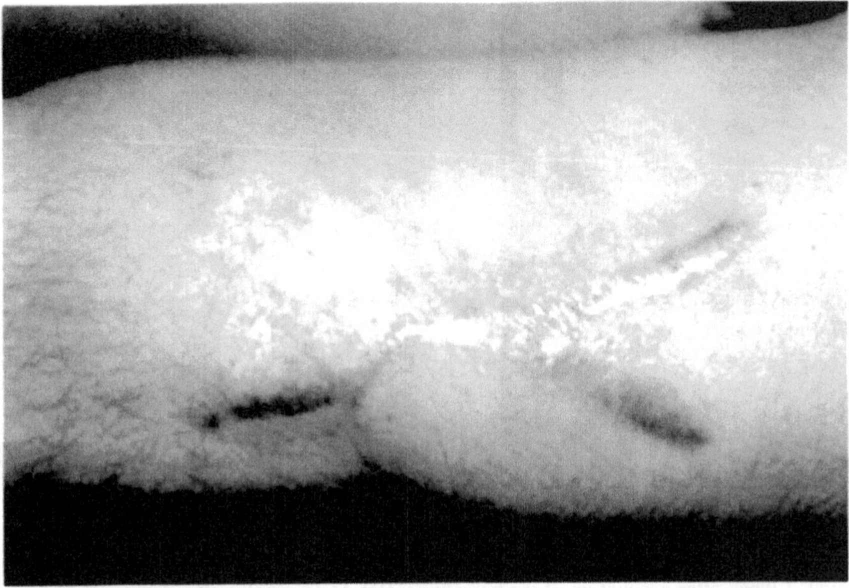

Figure 17 Hypertrophic scar.

dures include dermabrasion, cryosurgery, and chemical peels. The larger the area of the epidermis affected, the more likely pigmentary changes are to occur. Whether hyperpigmentation or hypopigmentation occurs is also a function of the depth of the epidermal damage. Deeper epidermal damage is more likely to result in hypopigmentation as a result of destruction of the majority of the melanocytes. More superficial epidermal damage is more likely to result in hyperpigmentation as the remaining melanocytes proliferate in the injured area.

REFERENCES

1. Dierckx C, Goldman MP, Fitzpatrick RE. Laser treatment of erythematous/hypertrophic and pigmented scars in 26 patients. Plast Reconstr Surg 1995; 95:84–90.
2. Smith JB, Fenske NA. Cutaneous manifestations and consequences of smoking. J Am Acad Dermatol 1996; 34:733–734.
3. Roenigk R. Chemical peel with trichloracetic acid. In: Roenigk and Roenigk, eds. Dermatologic Surgery Principles and Practice. New York: Marcel Dekker, 1996; 1121–1135.
4. Billingsley EM, Maloney ME. Intraoperative and postoperative bleeding problems in patients taking warfarin, aspirin, and nonsteroidal antiinflammatory agents. Dermatol Surg 1997; 23:381–383.
5. Rubenstein R, Roenigk HH, Stegman SJ, et al. Atypical keloids after dermabrasion of patients taking isotretinoin. J Am Acad Dermatol 1986; 15:280–285.
6. Smack DP, Harrington AC, Dunn C, et al. Infection and allergy incidence in ambulatory surgery patients using white petrolatum vs bacitracin ointment. JAMA 1996; 276:972–977.
7. Stasko T. Complications of cutaneous procedures. In: Roenigk and Roenigk, eds. Dermatologic Surgery Principles and Practice. New York Marcel Dekker, 1996; 149–175.
8. Kaufman AJ, Kiene KL, Moy RL, Role of tissue undermining in the trapdoor effect of transposition flaps. J Dermatol Surg Oncol 1993; 19:128–132.
9. Salasche SJ. Acute surgical complications: cause, prevention, and treatment. J Am Acad Dermatol 1986; 15:1163–1185.
10. Winton GB, Salasche SJ. Wound dressings for dermatologic surgery. J Am Acad Dermatol 1985; 13:1026–1044.
11. Bencini PL, Galimberti L, Signorini M, Crostic. Antibiotic prophylaxis of wound infections in skin surgery. Arch Dermatol 1991; 127:1357–1360.
12. Haas AF. Antibiotic prophylaxis. Semin Dermatol 1994; 13:27–34.
13. Classen DC, Evans RS, Pestotnik SL, Horn SD, Menlove RL, Burke JP. The timing of prophylactic administration of antibiotics and the risk of surgical wound infection. N Engl J Med 1992; 236:337–339.
14. Burke JF. The effective period of preventive antibiotic action in experimental incision and dermal lesions. Surgery 1961; 50:161–163.
15. Dellinger EP. Antibiotic prophylaxis of wound infections in skin surgery. Is 4 days too much? Arch Dermatol 1991; 127:1394–1395.
16. Becker G. Chemoprophylaxis for surgery of the head and neck. Ann Otol Rhinol Laryngol Suppl 1981; 90:8–12.
17. Burke JF. Infection. In: Hunt TK, Dunphy JE, eds. Fundamentals of Wound Management. New York: Appleton-Century-Crofts, 1979:170–240.
18. Wilkin JK. Diseases of the blood vessels: introduction. In: Demis DJ, ed. Clinical Dermatology. Philadelphia: Lippincott, 1993: Sec 7–0, p 1–8.
19. Pellitteri PK, Kennedy TL, Youn BA. The influence of intensive hyperbaric oxygen therapy on skin flap survival in a swine model. Arch Otolaryngol 1992; 118:1050–1054.
20. Jones JK, Triplett RG. The relationship of cigarette smoking to impaired intraoral wound heal-

ing: a review of evidence and implications for patient care. J Oral Maxillofac Surg 1992; 50:237–239.

21. Riou JP, Cohen JR, Johnson H. Factors influencing wound dehiscence. Am J Surg 1992; 163:324–330.
22. Rappaport WD, Hunter GC, Allen R, et al. Effect of electrocautery on wound healing in midline laparotomy incisions. Am J Surg 1990; 160:618–620.
23. Buell BR, Schuller DE. Comparison of tensile strength in CO_2 laser and scapel skin incisions. Arch Otolaryngol 1983; 109:465–487.
24. Maloney ME. Management of surgical complications and suboptimal results. In: Wheeland RG, Cutaneous Surgery. Philadelphia: Saunders, 1994:921–934.
25. Dodson MK, Magann EF, Meeks GR. A randomized comparison of secondary closure and secondary intention in patients with superficial wound dehiscence. Obstet Gynecol 1992; 80:321–324.
26. Goldminz D, Bennett RG. Cigarette smoking and flap and full-thickness graft necrosis. Arch Dermatol 1991; 127:1012–1015.
27. Bernstein G. The loop stitch. J Dermatol Surg Oncol 1984; 10:587.
28. Polk HC, Jr, Simpson CJ, Simmons BP, Alexander JW. Guidelines for prevention of surgical wound infection. Arch Surg 1983; 118:1213–1217.
29. Sebben JE. Prophylactic antibiotics in cutaneous surgery. J Dermatol Surg Oncol 1985; 11:901–906.

6

Scar Analysis and Treatment Selection: The "Geo-Topographic Approach"

Timothy J. Rosio
Cosmetic, Laser and Dermatologic Surgery Institute and University of California Davis Medical Center Sacramento, California

Marwali Harahap
University of North Sumatra Medical School Medan, Indonesia

The purpose of this chapter is to guide the reader through scar analysis and provide an overview of treatment selection. The goal is to show how to accomplish the greatest scar improvement through surgical techniques of scar revision or unsatisfactory scar prevention. We introduce the term "geo-topographic approach," coined by one of the authors (TR), as a conceptual tool for analyzing scars, their treatment, and prevention to achieve satisfying results. Thoroughly referenced sections on individual aspects of scars and revisionary techniques are included with the specific chapters in this book. Therefore, case examples from one author's (TR) practice will be used to demonstrate the geo-topographic approach. Diagrammatic medical illustrations of these cases may be found in prior publications (1). Progressive defects of various tissue strata will highlight procedure selection and implementation, as well as integration of the individual techniques, procedures, and methods presented in other chapters.

I. GENERAL APPROACH TO A SCAR AND PATIENT

A. Introduction

1. The "Geo-Topographic Approach"

The topographic approach to scars suggests that elevations, depressions, and texture changes are like hills and valleys in a contour map; these may be used qualitatively to focus on patients' dissatisfaction and to attempt reproducible descriptions and ratings (2, 3). This analysis alone is too superficial for planning adequate scar revision. The question remains of how much quantitative improvement can be achieved through various methods to ameliorate the defect. A geologic approach examines the characteristics of superficial and deep tissue strata in a scar, the tissues contiguous to them in adjacent anatomic units, and passive and dynamic stresses. Integrating the "geo" and the "topographic" into a "geo-topographic approach" helps maximally in analysis and planning (Fig. 1).

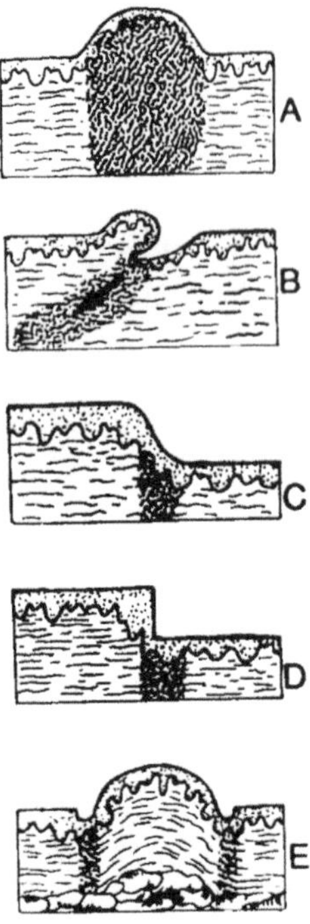

Figure 1 Elevated scars, geo-topographic perspective. **(A)** Hypertrophic scars or keloids have thinned epidermis and absence or paucity of adnexal elements. **(B)** Avulsion wound or oblique incision resulting in an inclined contraction scar. **(C)** Correctly apposed skin of different dermal thicknesses results in a sloping contour. **(D)** Inaccurately apposed wound margins result in a step-off deformity. **(E)** Trap-door or pincushion scars result from circumferential contraction along a semicircular incision line and may have a thickened fibrotic layer at the dermal subcutaneous junction. Narrow, peripheral, depressed scars simulate an ice-pick scar. (From Ref. 1.)

Scar revision decision making fits a neural net model with richly interconnecting parallel paths, rather than a linear branching algorithm. Therefore, this overview, within the space confines of the chapter, will emphasize a visual approach using case examples to illustrate procedural judgment. The reader is referred to other chapters in this book and previous publications (e.g., Ref. 1) for more extensive diagrams.

The general approach to analysis begins with some practical questions. How to define a scar will be followed by descriptive categories; these help in diagnosing the causative factors in scar formation and, therefore, their treatment and prevention. Scar revision objectives and regional and local factors that affect scar revision will be summarized. Keeping to a practical geo-topographic approach, scar revision techniques are broken into more invasive and minimally invasive groups and the affected strata. Eleven examples of patients, plus tables and figures, will be used to facilitate judgment in the selection and integration of scar revision techniques. Finally a few pearls and final conclusions will be provided.

B. Practical Questions

A significant question in scar analysis is "how old is the scar?" Scars are likely to mature over a period of 1 to 3 years. Many surgeons postpone treatment until a 6- to 12-month scar maturation period has passed. Earlier intervention may be indicated if the scar does not fall within relaxed skin tension lines. Because some scars are at their worst after 2 weeks and before 4 months, revision done within this period will result in improvement that is much greater and more obvious to the patient than that obtained by revising a mature scar (4).

The age of the patient is also a factor to be considered before attempting scar revision. In children and young adolescents, the scar maturation phase takes longer than in older individuals. The younger patient has greater overall skin tension with greater attendant risks of scar spreading and hypertrophy; therefore scars revised in older patients are almost always less noticeable than those in younger patients.

Some surgeons believe one should wait at least 6 months before revising a scar in children younger than 7 years. However, scar tissue may continue to improve through 12 months or more, so waiting until 6 to 12 months before attempting scar revision is justified. If there is functional deformity such as ectropion or difficulty in opening the mouth or in neck extension, early revision is definitely warranted (5).

Inquiring how the scar was caused may help in deciding the outcome of scar revision. An unsightly scar that results from a controlled surgical incision has a worse prognosis after scar revision than a raised, ragged scar caused by a dog bite that was not sutured. The former scar indicates the patient's poor reaction to surgical-type wounds, and the latter may be much improved by careful surgical revision.

The physician should also inquire about previous scar revision that was done without success. Approaching a keloid or hypertrophic scar using the same surgical technique as before without adjunctive treatment for wound healing risks producing a worse scar.

Analyze not only the scar but also the patient and yourself. Ask the patient what is most bothersome about the scar; is it the way it feels or looks, or does it interfere with normal function? Does it cause pain, or is it the elevation, depression, color, etc. that is most unsatisfactory? Does the scar interfere with the patient's work or social life? The surgeon and the patient should address the risk/benefit ratio for any contemplated scar revision procedure. The patient's expectations for the procedure as well as the results must be questioned thoroughly. Is the patient well prepared for a possible series of revisions, some of which may result in only limited improvement? Finally, physicians must examine their own personality and training to deal with uncertainty and assess their level of preparedness to perform other revisionary procedures if required for satisfactory surgical outcome.

C. Scar Definition

A scar is a previously injured area that has healed with fibrosis; it is distinct from the surrounding tissues in its contour, color, shape, length, width, direction, texture, or viscoelastic properties. Scar revision techniques are designed to prevent unsatisfactory scars before they form or to minimize or hide the features that make scars noticeable (Table 1).

D. Descriptive Categories of Scars

Descriptive characteristics that help categorize scars include contour, color, shape, length, width, direction (vis-à-vis relaxed skin tension lines), and consistency (texture, pliability, and viscoelasticity) (Table 2).

1. Contour

A scar may be elevated, flat, or depressed; if elevated, it is important to differentiate hypertrophy within the confines of the injury from keloidal growth past the noted areas of in-

Table 1 Scar Revision Objectives[a]

1. Hide scar
2. Improve scar direction
3. Redirect tension
4. Level contours
5. Narrow scar width
6. Shorten linear components
7. Camouflage scar

[a]These scar revision objectives aim to improve the contour, color, shape, length, width, direction, texture, or viscoelasticity of a scar.

jury. It is valuable to distinguish between scar depression due to a tissue deficiency and scar depression secondary to fibrotic retraction or lack of adequate wound support. The latter type of scar is referred to as an atrophic or a spread scar. "Atrophic" implies a relative loss of one or more of the tissue strata, e.g., because of involution or injury. A "spread scar" implies a separation of the original wound margins because of prolonged tension with inadequate support, often with rarefaction of strata resulting in depression but sometimes with a flat or elevated contour, atrophic or spread scars may show very subtle depression and may be more notable by pigmentary or textural changes.

Table 2 Descriptive Categories of Scars[a]

1. Contour
   a) Elevated
   b) Hypertrophic
   c) Keloid
   d) Depressed
   e) Atrophic or spread
2. Color
   a) Red-violaceous
   b) White
   c) Brown
3. Shape
   a) Linear or curved
   b) Trap-door semicircular
   c) Web or broken line
   d) Stellate or broken line
   e) Ice-pick or pitted
   f) Overhanging or avulsion
4. Length
5. Width
6. Direction (RSTLs)
7. Texture, consistency, extensibility

[a]This table summarizes morphological characteristics that are used to help categorize scars.
From Ref. 1.

Examination of elevated scar prototypes with a cross-sectional geologic view (Fig. 1) may be combined with clinical observations to obtain useful correlations. For example, in Fig. 1A, hypertrophic scars resulting from an unfavorable wound-healing milieu including high tension (or keloids secondary to genetic factors) have a thinned epidermis and absence or paucity of adnexal elements; conversely, an elevated scar with an otherwise normal-appearing surface texture may have primarily excess deep fibrotic or fatty tissue (central portion of profile in Fig. 1E). An "overhanging lip" profile (Fig. 1B) is frequently due to avulsion wounds or oblique incisions resulting in a diagonally contracting scar. Correctly apposed skin of different dermal thicknesses (Fig. 1C) results in a sloping contour, and inaccurately apposed wound margins (Fig. 1D) results in a step-off deformity. Trap-door or pincushion scars (Fig. 1E) result from circumferential contraction along a semicircular incision line and may have a thickened fibrotic layer at the dermal subcutaneous junction.

How can we proceed from the geologic perspective to therapeutic intervention? Before attempting to revise a scar, the criteria that render a scar ideal should be understood. Ideally, a scar should be (a) flat and level with no depressions; (b) a good match in color and texture with the surrounding skin; (c) narrow; (d) within or parallel to skin wrinkles, a contour junction, or a relaxed skin tension line (RSTL); and (e) without a bowstring or unbroken contracture line that catches the eye. Unfortunately, in scar revision practice, not all these criteria are always satisfied.

Myriad methods exist for scar treatment—so many, in fact, that it is challenging to recall and organize them. A schema that correlates degree of invasiveness, tissue strata, and type of procedure is offered (Table 3). A practical analysis of therapeutic approaches to scars drawing from this table follows.

Table 3 Scar Revision Techniques[a]

1. Invasive surgical methods
   a) Fusiform scar revision (FSR) and serial excision
   b) Broken line scar revision: Z-plasty, W-plasty, geometric broken line (GBL)
   c) Punch excision and elevation, subcision, laminar reticulotomy
   d) Skin grafting: punch excision and graft replacement, subepithelial flap (e.g., interleaving, advancement, plication)
   e) Excision and flap or graft coverage
   f) Dermabrasion, laserbrasion, scar and surround planing and injury
   g) Infrared laser (CO_2 or Nd:YAG) excision of keloids
   h) Subdermal augmentation fillers (autogenous, allogeneic synthetic)
      (1) Fat, dermal matrix, Gore-tex patches and tubes, silicone, $CaCO_3$ and other implants
2. Minimally invasive methods
   a) Vascular and pigment laser photothermolysis
   b) Dermal augmentation fillers (autogenous, allogeneic, synthetic)
      (1) Collagen, fibrel, hyaluronan
      (2) Gore-tex threads
   c) Silicone gel
   d) Physical modalities: compression, X-radiation, cryoinjury, laser injury, sclerotherapy, tissue injury
   e) Pharmaceutical medications: steroids, fibroblast and collagen synthesis or cross-linking inhibitors, low-energy photons, cell or tissue level processes catalyzed or inhibited, possibly cell receptor mediated

[a]A schema that organizes and correlates degree of invasiveness, tissue strata, and type of procedure is offered.
From Rosio TJ. Cosmetic Surgery and Scar Revision Workshops & Seminars, with permission.

Scars that are elevated because of excess deep fibrotic or fatty tissue may be debulked from beneath. One may reenter through the previous incision line or, if preferable, elect an incision along an adjacent cosmetic unit junction or RSTL.

Hypertrophic scars are likely to reform after scar revision attempts unless something can be done to alleviate the increased tension that predisposes to their formation (6–8). Attempts to resurface hypertrophic scars may provoke even thicker hypertrophic scars or leave a more irregular surface. Broken-line closures may result in a hypertrophic zigzag scar if high tension and inadequate wound support dominate; steroid injection may be elected in these instances and when the patient or surgeon decides against further surgical alternatives.

Simple fusiform scar revision (FSR) is often sufficient for small avulsion or overhanging lip scars and step-off scars. Superficial strata techniques such as resurfacing and blade planing may be sufficient for minor elevations. However, more prominent elevated scars are likely to worsen with resurfacing techniques alone; e.g., overhanging scars will leave a deep depression and step-off scars may result in a widened hypertrophic scar with undesirable texture and color.

Bigger step-off scars resulting from dermal or subcutaneous fat discrepancies may be treated with combinations of resurfacing of the bulkier side, broken line scar revision, and dermal fat or other filling substances to augment the thinner side (1, 9–11).

Trap-door scars are best treated with a running Z-plasty; in some cases, excision of the contracted scar line, wide undermining, and resuturing may be successful in the presence of substantially diminished wound tension since the original closure.

Keloid scars are discussed more thoroughly in a separate chapter. The prognosis for keloids varies tremendously depending on their location as well as the patient's genetic predisposition. Earlobe keloids often respond well to CO_2 laser excision, from the posterior aspect of the lobule, if possible. A course of intralesional incision line corticosteroids at increasing intervals is frequently necessary. Close follow-up for a minimum of 12 months is indicated.

Depressed scars can be analyzed by a simplified strategy proposed by one of the authors (TR) in which the scars are separated using a four-category grid (Table 4); the criteria are the presence or absence of superficial texture changes and, second, whether the depression is shallow versus moderate to severe.

Normal superficial texture and mild depression argue for techniques such as dermal fillers, subcision, laminar reticulotomy, or punch incision and elevation methods. If the superficial texture is abnormal and the depression is mild, any of the resurfacing methods may be used.

Table 4 Depressed Scar Decision Grid[a]

Degree of depression	Texture normal	Texture abnormal
Mild	Dermal filler, resurfacing Punch elevation	Subcision, resurfacing Punch transplantation
Moderate to severe	Deep filler or subepithelial flap	Excise and close; ± broken line

[a]A simplified strategy for selecting depressed scar treatment approaches uses presence or absence of superficial texture changes and degree of depression.

From Rosio TJ. Cosmetic Surgery and Scar Revision Workshops & Seminars, with permission.

If superficial texture is normal and the depression is quite deep, subdermal augmentation via fillers, subepithelial flaps, and implants (autogenous, allogeneic, or synthetic) may be indicated.

If the superficial texture is abnormal and the defect is deep, excision and closure are favored, possibly with a broken-line technique.

It is valuable to consider a wide variety of tissue augmentation and support strategies for the treatment of significantly depressed scars. These include the less commonly encountered subcutaneous transposition, interleaving, split-thickness advancement, tubing, trifolding, plication, and offset layered closing flaps (1, 12, 13).

Scars may also be atrophic or spread. Atrophic skin that is lax, whether it is due to a resolved hemangioma, inflammatory changes, or another disorder, may be excised and closed by the simplest method. There has been some mild improvement in treatment of atrophic scars and striae (14).

Lesional skin or existing scars that have a much greater risk for hypertrophic scar formation when excised include hypertrophic scars, spread scars, and tissues over a convexity or subject to high static or dynamic tension (e.g., over the sternum, shoulder, mandible, or neck). Prolonged tissue support and other measures can offset the higher risk of renewed hypertrophic scar formation (15).

2. *Color*

Distinguishing colors of scars are red to violaceous, white, and brown. Erythema does not always suggest an immature, hypertrophic, or keloidal scar. Mature scars may have simple surface telangiectasia or an arteriovenous malformation. Superficial laser photothermolysis is frequently effective for treating redness in immature scars and sometimes achieves slight flattening, especially if the scar is immature, erythematous, and on the face (16, 17). It is also effective for mature scar telangiectasia. Vascular laser pulse drilling is a valuable technique for superficial to mid-dermal small arteriovenous malformations (AVMs). Substantially elevated scars obviously need some other modality to improve them; if resurfacing is chosen, this would supersede primary use of superficial vascular lasers.

White is the color of a mature scar. Its other characteristics determine treatment selection.

Brown hyperpigmented scars may be due to either hypermelanosis or hemosiderin deposition. Nonsurgical treatment of postinflammatory hyperpigmentation is preferable, allowing gradual resolution with time or melanin formation inhibitors. Lack of improvement over time argues for a trial of pigment lasers such as Q-switched ruby, alexandrite, or yttrium aluminum garnet (YAG); although darkening can occur in pigment skin types III and above, it is usually temporary. One of the authors (TR) has successfully lightened some mature burn scars by 50% or more using a Q-Switched ruby laser. Hemosiderin deposits may gradually improve with time, but the poor absorption efficiency of currently available laser wavelengths hinders efficacy.

A Wood's lamp examination may be useful in determining whether the pigment has a superficial component. Late-occurring pigmentation warrants consideration of Addison's disease or other unusual systemic causes and pigments that are beyond the scope of this chapter.

3. *Shape*

"Shape" is a complex descriptor comprising contour, size, length, width, and pattern. Setting aside contour (discussed earlier), revision of a linear or curved scar is influenced more strongly by the direction of the scar with respect to the RSTLs (discussed later).

Trap-door semicircular scars produced by circumferential wound contraction are usually best approached with serial Z-plasties that have a leveling and lengthening effect on the contracted incision line.

If FSR within the RSTLs would sacrifice too much normal tissue or otherwise disturb function or aesthetics, then broken-line scar revision, grafting, or flaps are considered.

Web scars frequently occur across a concavity, and stellate scars may be due to either an irregular pattern of injury or centripetal wound contraction. A first choice for small web and stellate scars would be FSR when feasible. Alternatively, for large web or stellate scars or locations not conducive to FSR in RSTLs, broken-line closures with an outward local flap are considered. For smaller scars, a satisfactory result may be obtained with intralesional steroid injection and massage.

Ice-pick, broad pox, and pitted scars are generally treated according to the depressed-scar decision grid (Table 4). Simple resurfacing for shallow lesions, punch replacement or elevation or FSR for deeper lesions, and dermal and subcutaneous fillers for broad scars with softer edges are used (18).

4. Length and Width

Short narrow scars are less noticeable than long, wide ones. It is not necessarily intuitive, but an overall longer but discontinuous or broken line is less noticeable than an uninterrupted length. Broken-line scar revision techniques vary in their comparative features of lengthening, tissue sparing, cosmesis, and distortion (Table 5). The overall goal is to bring most of the incision line components as close to the RSTLs as possible. Greater incision line lengthening is the strength of Z-plasty; it is also subject to greater distortion. The reverse is true for W-plasty. Greater lengthening and leveling affects are ordinarily achieved with longer incision lines of the individual components of the broken-line closure; however, smaller components lead to better cosmesis and less local tissue distortion.

5. Texture and Consistency

The higher density, altered structure of collagen fibers, and lower water content of scars result in decreased pliability, extensibility, and altered texture. Rapid biochemical and structural changes, along with lengthening and reduced skin tension, have been documented to occur after broken-line closures, especially Z-plasty.

Table 5 Broken-Line Scar Revision Techniques[a]

Technique	Lengthening	Tissue sparing	Cosmesis	Distortion
Z-plasty	3+	3+	1+	3+
Planimetric Z-plasty	3+	1+	1+	1+
W-plasty	1+	1+	2+	1+
Geometric Broken Line (GBL) closure	1+	1+	3+	1+

[a]A personal comparative analysis rating features of common broken-line scar revision techniques.
From Ref. 1.

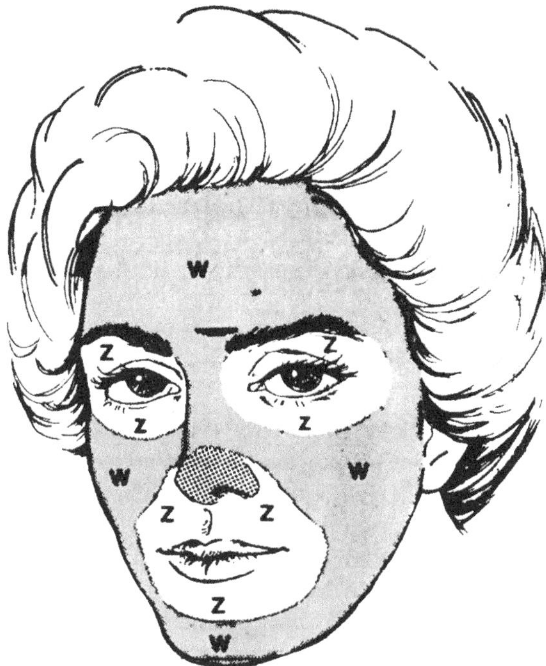

Figure 2 Preferred sites for W- or Z-plasty. Scars over relatively fixed broad or convex expanses such as forehead, chin, and cheek benefit from W-plasty; the normal landmarks around the nose, eyelids, and lips are easily distorted by scars and Z-plasties are the treatment of choice. (From Ref. 1.)

E. Scar Location, Systemic and Local Factors Affecting Scar Revision

Anatomic location, local skin tension, previous treatments or injuries, medications, nutrition, and general health affect the selection of a scar revision technique. Scar location is an important factor. Certain areas of the body are especially prone to scar thickening and widening after revision. Both shoulders, the sternum, and large breasts often react to scar revision with widened hypertrophic and keloidal scars (19). Scars tend to widen much more in nonfacial than in facial regions. Many descriptions of scar revision are most applicable to the face, and revisions on the trunk or extremities may heal with more noticeable scars. This is because, as a rule, the trunk and extremities have a higher degree of skin tension.

Altered vascularity resulting from prior surgery, radiation, diabetes, atherosclerosis, vascular stasis and edema, smoking, and other factors raise the risk/benefit ratio for more involved surgical revision procedures.

The interplay of anatomic structures, cosmetic units, and local skin tension is reflected in RSTLs, areas of laxity, and preferred locations for W- and Z-plasties (Fig. 2).

II. CASE EXAMPLES: SCAR REVISION TECHNIQUE SELECTION

A. Overview of Scar Revision Mechanisms

Most scar revision procedures may be grouped into three procedural categories: full-thickness tissue rearrangement with or without excision (e.g., FSR or broken-line closures); partial-thickness resurfacing and recontouring by ablation, abrasion, or superficial planing; and elevation of depressions with biologic or artificial substances.

B. Scar Revision Techniques

The wide array of scar revision modalities and techniques may be confusing. We have organized the procedures as "invasive" and "minimally invasive" methods and then grouped them according to the type of procedure and strata affected (Table 4).

Eleven cases will be used to illustrate scar and lesional analysis for either scar revision or prevention of unsatisfactory scar formation. These cases begin with a diagnosis, followed by a geo-topographic analysis of the problem and the surgical solution used.

Case 1: Nine-year-old girl with a mature hemangioma scar on the left cheek (Case 1A).

Analysis: Superficial atrophy and a full-thickness fibro-fatty scar characterize the medial cheek lesion. Debulking this scar alone and resuturing the atrophic surface, even if trimmed, would leave an unacceptable texture change. FSR is the best approach, with moderate cheek undermining and orientation of the incision line parallel to the RSTLs and meilonasal junction. Care should be taken not to skeletonize the incisional margins of all fat; rather, pronounced eversion is accomplished with a deep suture. Long-lasting support is desirable, and a slowly absorbable suture or permanently buried nonabsorbable suture may be considered here. Pronounced eversion prevents the mature scar from exhibiting a

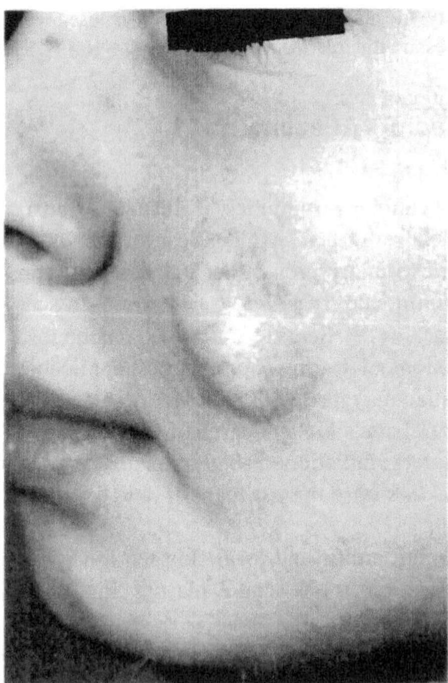

Case 1A Nine-year-old female with a fibro-fatty hemangioma scar of the left cheek. (From Rosio TJ. Cosmetic Surgery and Scar Revision Workshops & Seminars, with permission.)

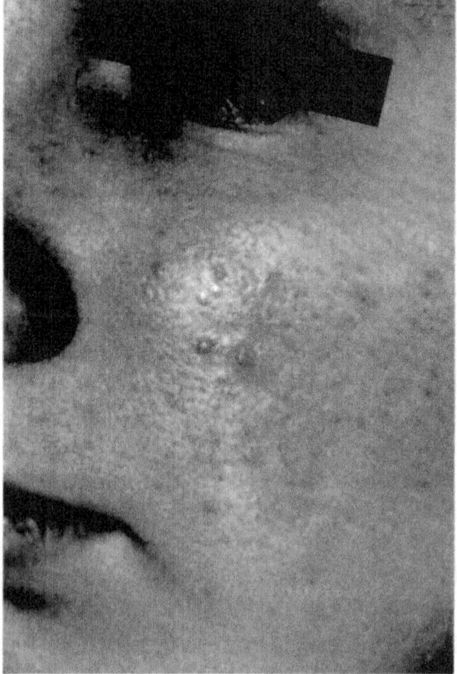

Case 1B Postoperative FSR followed by resurfacing. (From Rosio TJ. Cosmetic Surgery and Scar Revision Workshops & Seminars, with permission.)

linear depression. Early postoperative resurfacing at 4 to 8 weeks was performed in order to improve cosmesis. The result shown is approximately 12 weeks after FSR and 8 weeks after resurfacing (Case 1B).

Case 2: Ten-year-old girl with congenital hairy nevus of the temple (Case 2A).

Analysis: The large diameter of this lesion virtually fills the lower temple, extending from the brow into the hair-bearing scalp. An FSR in the RSTLs is not feasible because of tight skin in this region; furthermore, pulling the hair-bearing scalp inferiorly or elevating the brow is unacceptable.

Solution: First, an M-plasty removed the bulk of the lesion. Anterior incision lines approach the brow perpendicularly with branches running toward the lateral canthus and paralleling the brow at its junction with the forehead skin. The entire right forehead and upper lateral cheek were undermined to allow closure. The main body of the incision ran in an unfavorable antitension line (ATL) perpendicular to the RSTLs. Therefore, a running W-plasty was elected for the final revision step, placing incision lines more parallel to RSTLs (Case 2B). Even immediate postoperative pictures show only minor tissue distortion along the incision line and no abnormalities of the brow or hairline position. Resurfacing, e.g., with a CO_2 laser, reduces any residual scar irregularity once postoperative edema and flap settling has occurred (Case 2C and D).

Case 3: A 65-year-old man with a skin cancer defect (3A) closed with a cheek-neck rotation advancement flap.

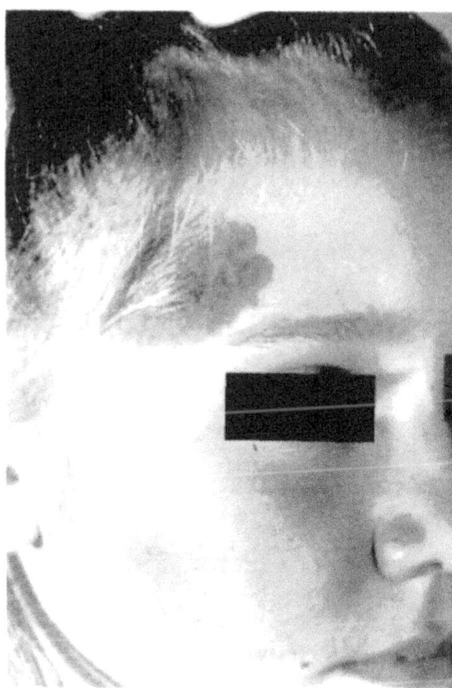

Case 2A Ten-year-old female with congenital hairy nevus filling the area between the lateral temple hairline and upper lateral canthus. (From Rosio TJ. Cosmetic Surgery and Scar Revision Workshops & Seminars, with permission.)

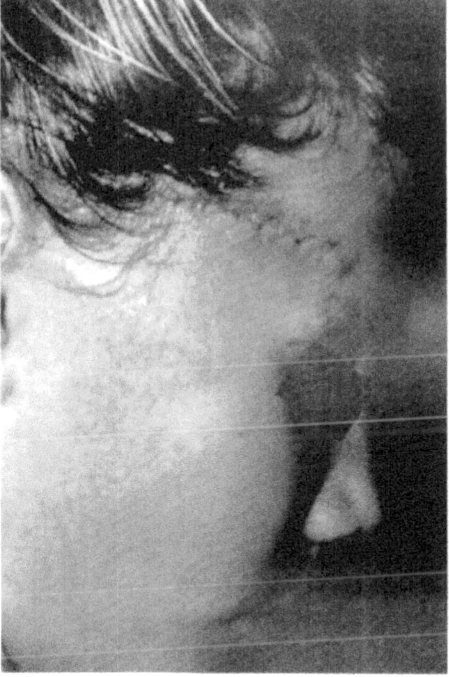

Case 2B Prior M-plasty followed by running W-plasty with forehead and upper lateral cheek mobilization was successful in lesion removal with prevention of an unsatisfactory scar. (From Rosio TJ. Cosmetic Surgery and Scar Revision Workshops & Seminars, with permission.)

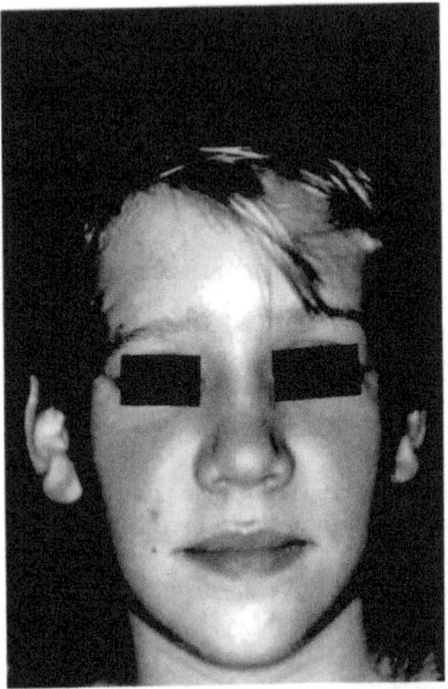

Case 2C Frontal view at 1 week demonstrates normal brow and scalp hair position. Early postoperative edema and slight tissue distortion from extreme tissue tension support measures are common. (From Rosio TJ. Cosmetic Surgery and Scar Revision Workshops & Seminars, with permission.)

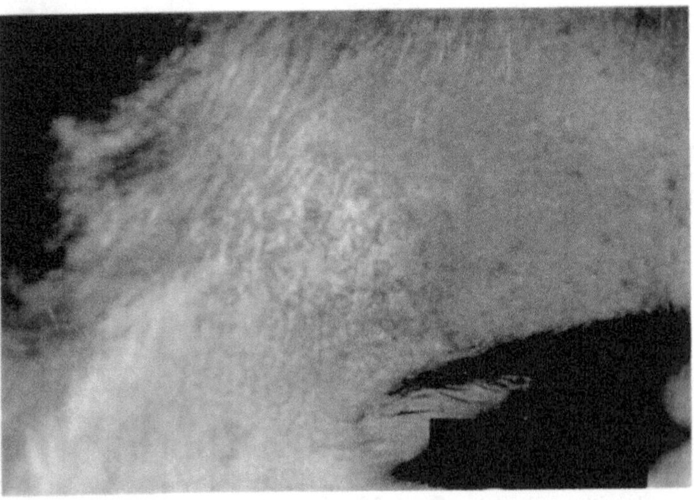

Case 2D Eight weeks after laser resurfacing, showing smooth texture and no perceptible scar line. (From Rosio TJ. Cosmetic Surgery and Scar Revision Workshops & Seminars, with permission.)

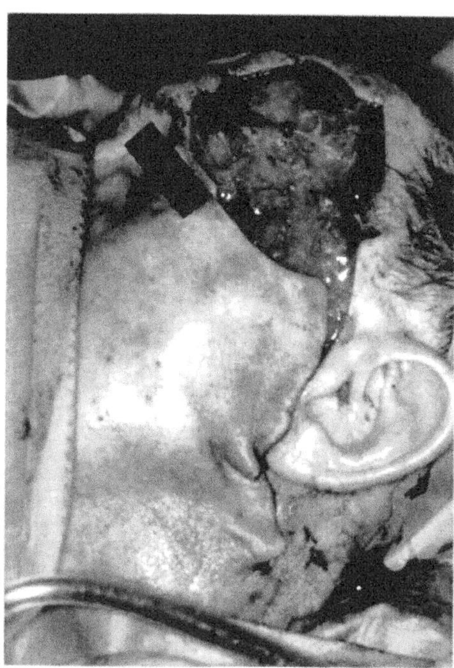

Case 3A Preoperative temple and lateral canthal defect. (From Rosio TJ. Cosmetic Surgery and Scar Revision Workshops & Seminars, with permission.)

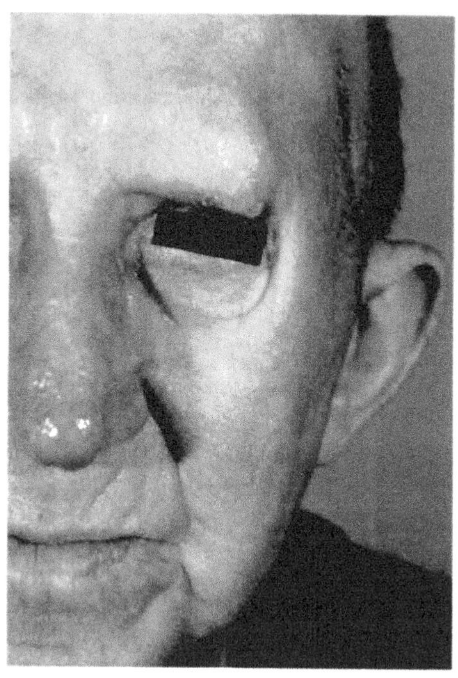

Case 3B Closure with cheek-neck rotation advancement flap. (From Rosio TJ. Cosmetic Surgery and Scar Revision Workshops & Seminars, with permission.)

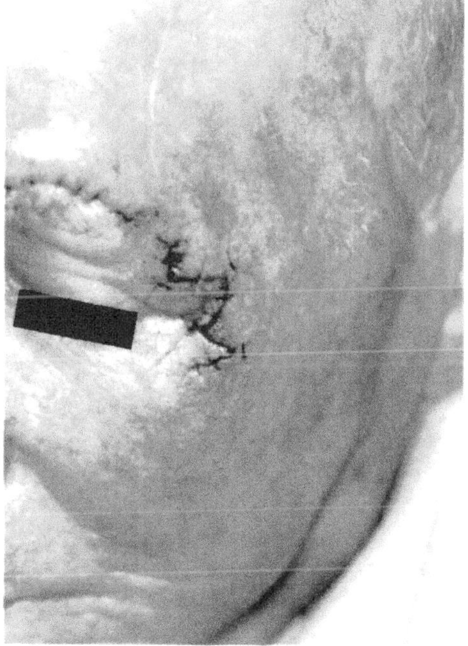

Case 3C Bridge scar over lateral orbital rim concavity with serial Z-plasty outlined. (From Rosio TJ. Cosmetic Surgery and Scar Revision Workshops & Seminars, with permission.)

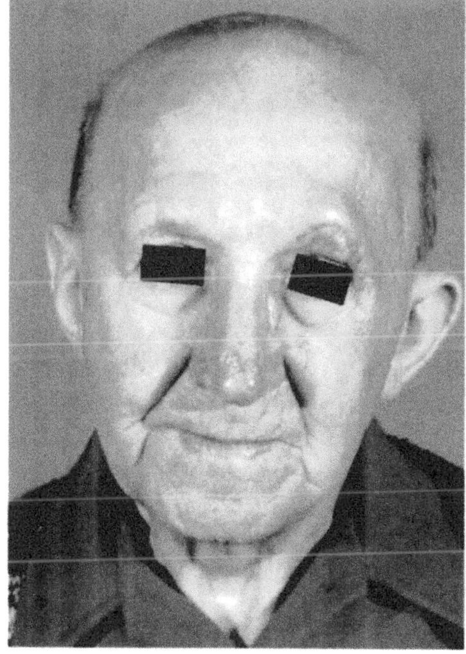

Case 3D Postoperative result (with suspension brow plasty due to prior nerve VII loss). (From Rosio TJ. Cosmetic Surgery and Scar Revision Workshops & Seminars, with permission.)

Analysis: A band scar resulting from linear scar contraction has bridged the lateral orbital rim concavity (Case 3B). A direct brow suspension was required in this patient because of sacrifice of the superior facial nerve branches at the original cancer surgery. The problem is how to lengthen such a scar, given its position immediately adjacent to the lateral canthus; furthermore, the potential donor skin is taut laterally because of the high tension in the prior reconstruction.

Solution: Scar lengthening is required. Serial Z-plasties allow smaller increments of donor skin to be taken from a more widely distributed area, which reduces closing tension (Case 3B and C). Small serial Z's also provide less distortion and better cosmesis. Short limb incision lines were an essential part of making Z-plasty possible here, because of proximity to the eye.

Case 4: A 70-year-old female with a large bilobe flap reconstruction of a lateral nasal defect (Case 4A).

Analysis: The curved incision line of this semicircular flap has undergone shortening and centripetal contraction, resulting in a classic trap-door or pincushion effect (Case 4B).

Solution: A semicircular oriented serial Z-plasty is performed to lengthen the contracted incision line and to redirect vectors centrifugally (Case 4C). Small amounts of redundant tissue may be removed from the flap with trimming. Flap components as small as

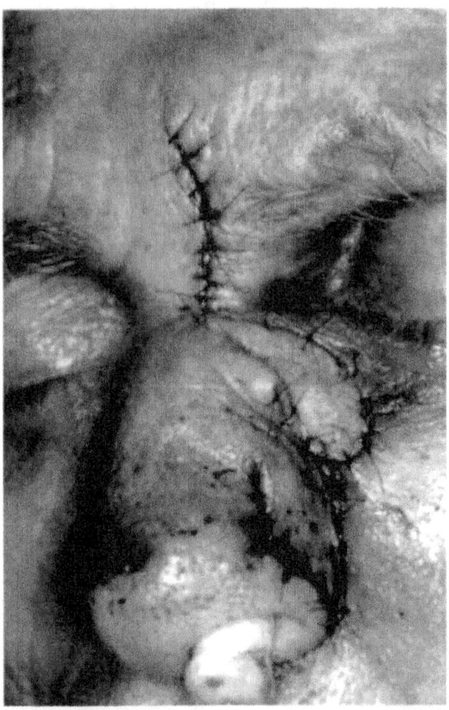

Case 4A Flap reconstruction. (From Rosio TJ. Cosmetic Surgery and Scar Revision Workshops & Seminars, with permission.)

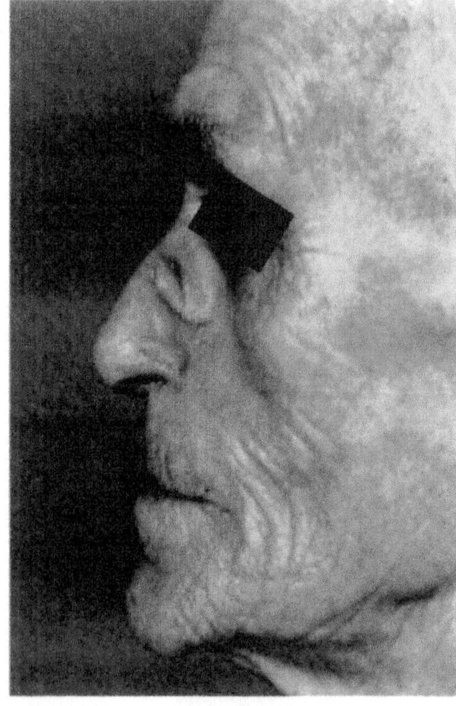

Case 4B Trap-door scar from semicircular incision line contraction. (From Rosio TJ. Cosmetic Surgery and Scar Revision Workshops & Seminars, with permission.)

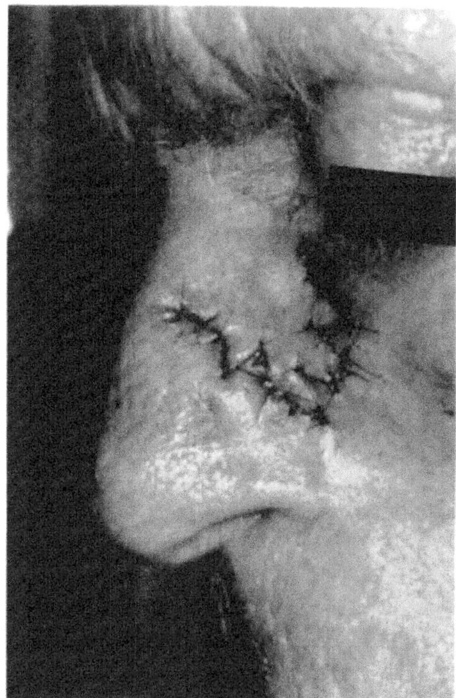

Case 4C Semicircular serial Z-plasty, immediate postoperative result. (From Rosio TJ. Cosmetic Surgery and Scar Revision Workshops & Seminars, with permission.)

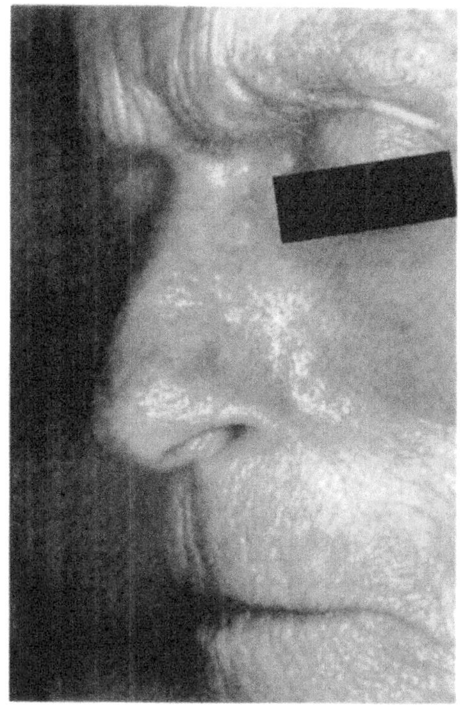

Case 4D Nine months postoperative result after semicircular serial Z-plasty. (From Rosio TJ. Cosmetic Surgery and Scar Revision Workshops & Seminars, with permission.)

4 to 5 mm may be used along with generous undermining to improve cosmesis. Force vectors now flatten the flap and produce a leveling effect. The semicircular Z's blended with a CO_2 laser result in an inconspicuous scar.

Case 5: A 68-year-old woman with a split-thickness skin graft (STSG) reconstruction of the forehead.

Analysis: Frontal and lateral views (Case 5A and C) show a prominent graft and scar with evident contour and texture differences. The notable thickness differential, the incurving of the normal junctional skin, and the graft's other disparities result in a disagreeable cyclopean appearance. Steroid injection into-marginal scars of the normal skin and graft would probably reduce deformity, but there would still be an abrupt color, texture, and tissue height difference.

Solution: CO_2 laser resurfacing was applied with a single pass to the split-thickness graft approximately 8 weeks after operation. The peripheral skin was selectively recontoured with many more passes. Results several months later demonstrate a more homogeneous appearance throughout the cosmetic unit and gradual transitions to adjacent units (Case 5B and D). The lateral temple skin required the fewest passes; the glabellar and suprabrow areas, being thickest, required greater recontouring.

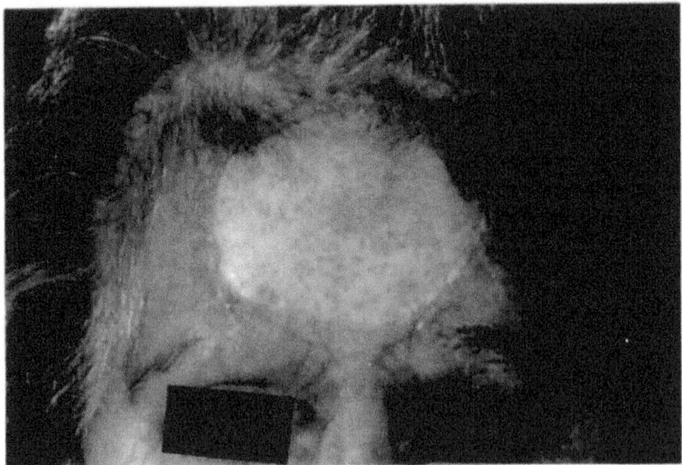

Case 5A Extensive forehead defect repaired with split-thickness skin graft (STSG). (From Rosio TJ. Cosmetic Surgery and Scar Revision Workshops & Seminars, with permission.)

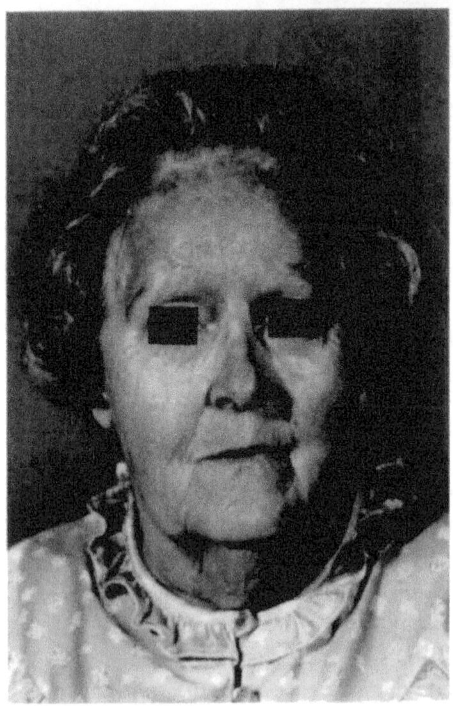

Case 5B Profile and frontal views show undesirable "cyclopean" cosmetic result. (From Rosio TJ. Cosmetic Surgery and Scar Revision Workshops & Seminars, with permission.)

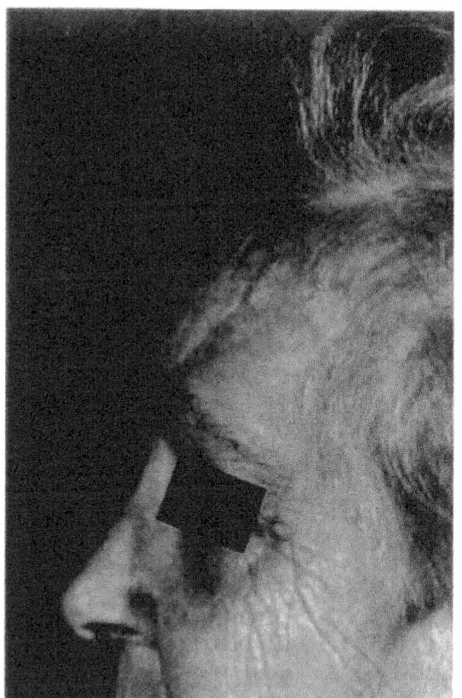
C

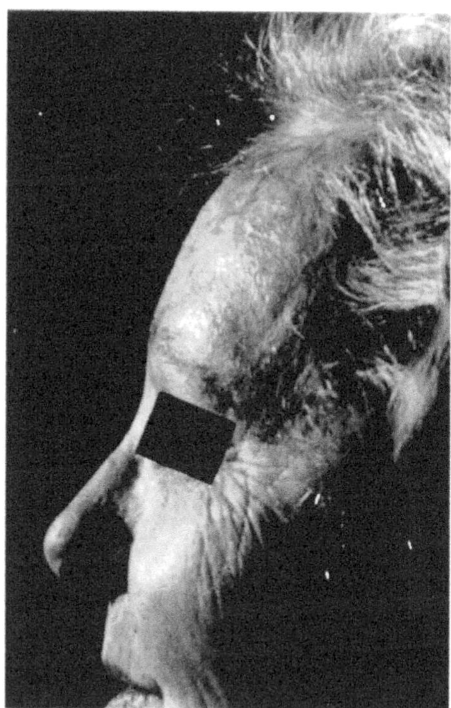
D

Case 5C and D Resurfacing with emphasis on nongraft skin results in greater homogeneity of color, texture, and graft versus adjacent skin in the cosmetic unit. Note gradual transition to adjacent cosmetic unit. (From Rosio TJ. Cosmetic Surgery and Scar Revision Workshops & Seminars, with permission.)

Case 6: Woman with a nasal tip graft.

Analysis: Elevation of a particularly full-thickness nasal tip graft is fairly common (Case 6A). The trap-door or pincushion phenomenon is implicated. A full complement of adnexal structures is present in full-thickness postauricular donor tissue. Nasal tip skin here is thin in this woman, and the difference in tissue thickness is relatively mild.

Solution: Resurface with emphasis on the graft while feathering to the surrounding tissue. In contrast to the previous forehead STSG case, the elevated graft will hold up well with multiple sculpting passes to obtain a more uniform contour (Case 6B). A small array of laser pulses or a small scan size of 3–5 mm is best suited to sculpting objects of this size.

Case 7: Mohs defect of skin and muscle down to (but not through) mucosa (Case 7A).

Analysis: Grafted defects of this nature and flap reconstructions routinely need scar revision. Revision is easier when the primary repair is done with a flap and prevents structural contraction, which is more severe with split-thickness than full-thickness skin grafts (STSG versus FTSG). A midline forehead flap replaces thickness from lost tissue in this case. Debulking the deep aspect of the flap, before or at the time of pedicle division, followed by resurfacing homogenizes height, texture, and color and minimizes incisional scars. A nearly imperceptible reconstruction results (Case 7B and C).

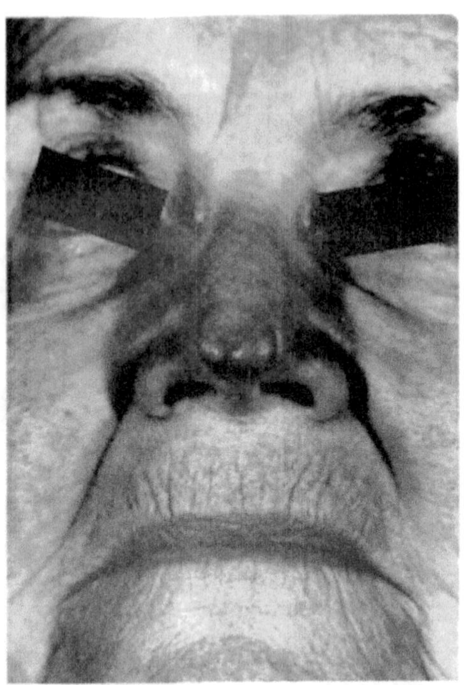

Case 6A Elevated full-thickness nasal tip graft. (From Rosio TJ. Cosmetic Surgery and Scar Revision Workshops & Seminars, with permission.)

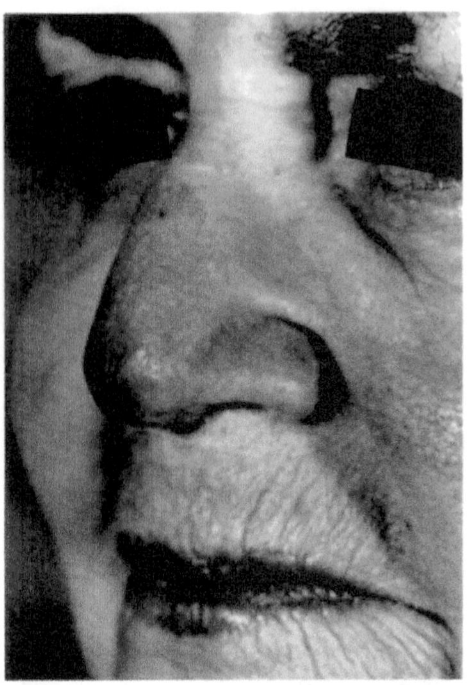

Case 6B Full-thickness nasal tip graft, postoperative CO^2 laser resurfacing. (From Rosio TJ. Cosmetic Surgery and Scar Revision Workshops & Seminars, with permission.)

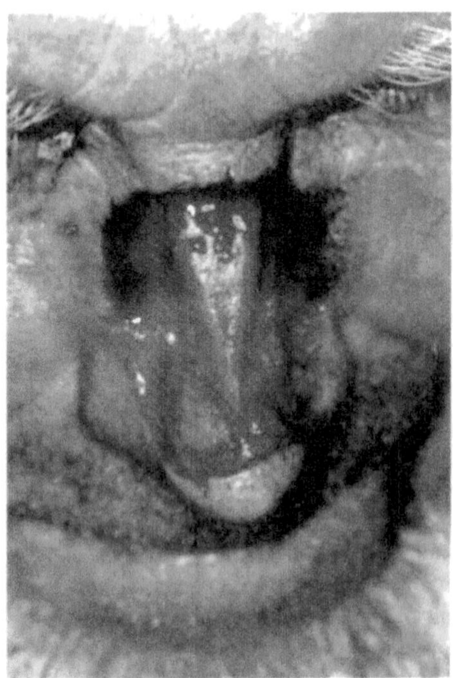

Case 7A Male with medial cheeks and complete dorsal nasal defect. (From Rosio TJ. Cosmetic Surgery and Scar Revision Workshops & Seminars, with permission.)

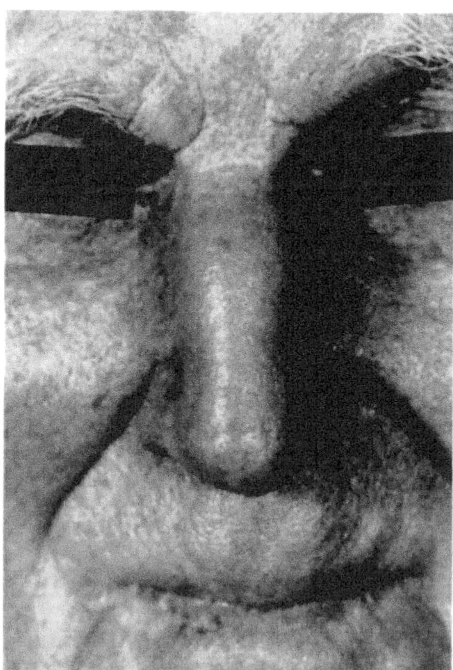

Case 7B Repaired with bilateral cheek advancement and paramedian forehead flaps. Frontal view result after forehead flap pedicle division, reinset, and postoperative CO_2 laser resurfacing of nasal and forehead cosmetic units. (From Rosio TJ. Cosmetic Surgery and Scar Revision Workshops & Seminars, with permission.)

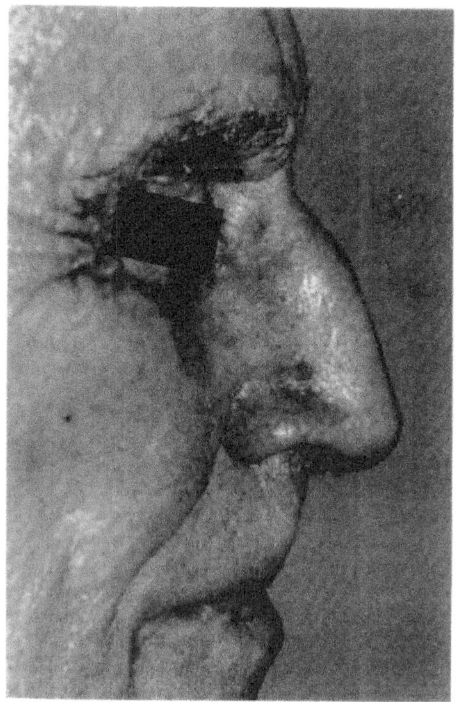

Case 7C Lateral view result after forehead flap pedicle division, re-inset and postoperative CO_2 laser resurfacing of nasal and forehead cosmetic units. (From Rosio TJ. Cosmetic Surgery and Scar Revision Workshops & Seminars, with permission.)

Case 8: Transnasal (skin through mucosa) defect (Case 8A).

Analysis: Obtaining a satisfactory scar may require deep and superficial layered flaps to reestablish the mucosal lining and adequate tissue bulk and circulation to optimize primary or revised scars. After a hinge flap for mucosal lining and bulk, a midline forehead flap was used to reconstruct the defect. At the time of pedicle division, undermining and debulking of the flap and adjacent tissues are performed before resuturing (Case 8B). Subsequently, minor differences in tissue thickness and texture may be approached with resurfacing methods. Here, CO_2 laser resurfacing of the adequately prepared tissue transformed a good result to an excellent one (Case 8C).

Case 9: Nasal tip loss with absence of composite tissue layers.

Analysis: Because of loss of mucosa, cartilage, fat, muscle, and cutaneous tissues, a satisfactory scar cannot be obtained without a composite tissue layer approach. Severe scarring and contraction prevention requires careful reconstitution of anatomic layers with thorough tissue support. Split turn-down flaps are prepared to replace mucosal linings in the right and left nostrils (Case 9A). Cartilage strut and shield grafts (Case 9B, C, and D) provide tissue support, shaping, and projection, followed by a midline forehead flap (Case 9D). Debulking of incision margin scar tissue followed by resurfacing refines contours and

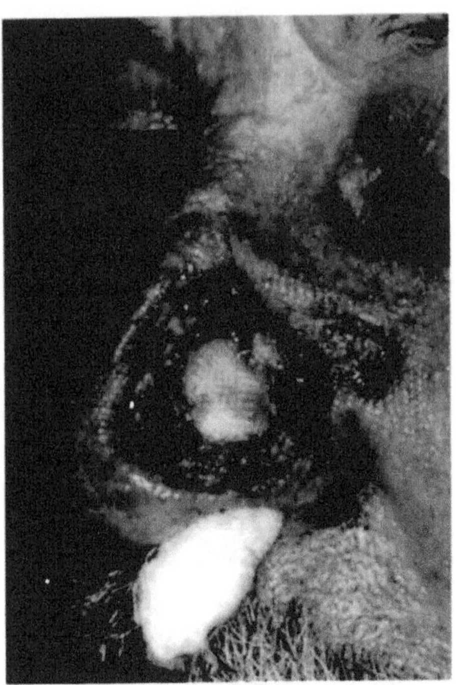

Case 8A Transnasal defect, from skin through mucosa, revealing intranasal gauze. (From Rosio TJ. Cosmetic Surgery and Scar Revision Workshops & Seminars, with permission.)

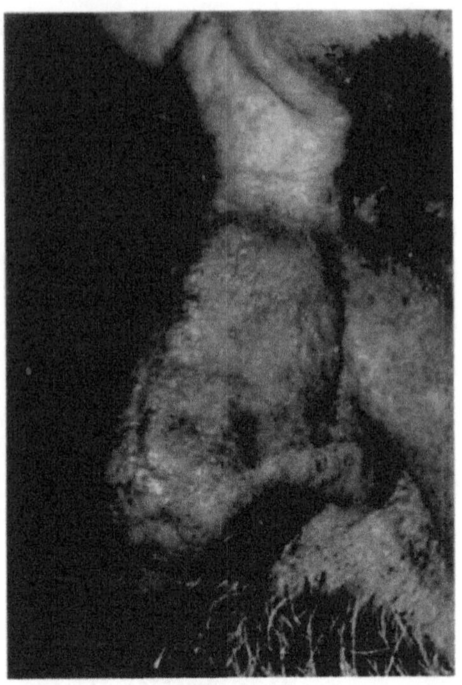

Case 8B After hinge flap and forehead flap debulking a division of pedicle. (From Rosio TJ. Cosmetic Surgery and Scar Revision Workshops & Seminars, with permission.)

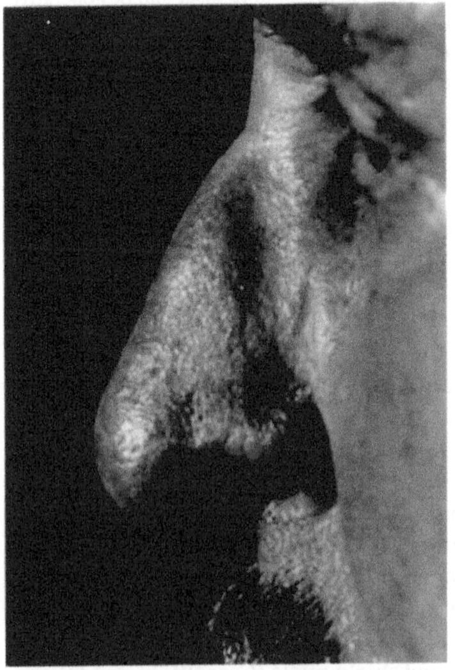

Case 8C After CO_2 laser resurfacing. (From Rosio TJ. Cosmetic Surgery and Scar Revision Workshops & Seminars, with permission.)

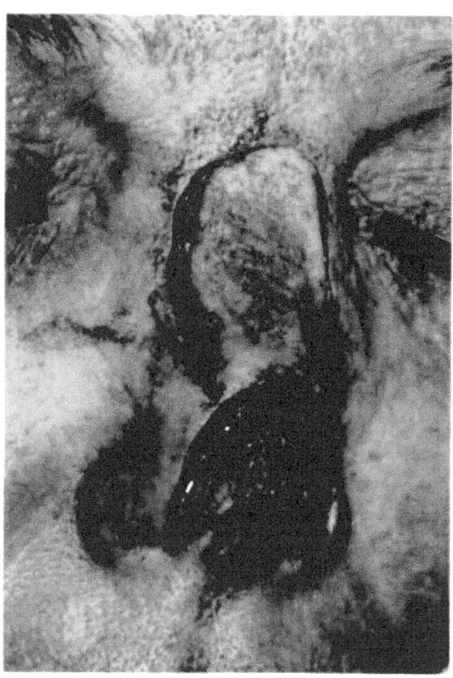

Case 9A Composite tissue loss of nasal tip. (From Rosio TJ. Cosmetic Surgery and Scar Revision Workshops & Seminars, with permission.)

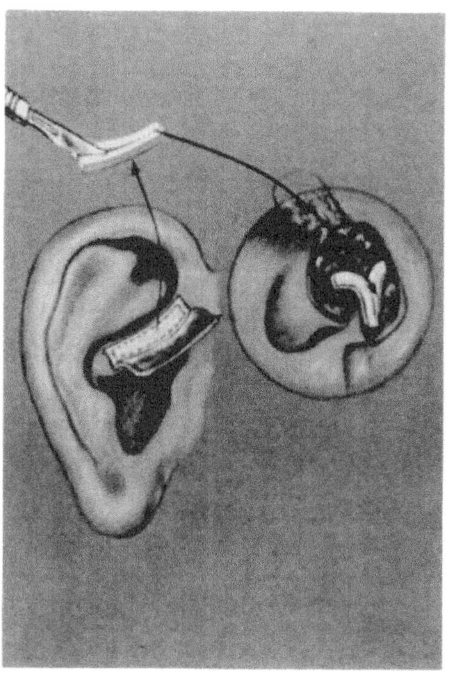

Case 9B Auricular cartilage strut graft. (From Rosio TJ. Cosmetic Surgery and Scar Revision Workshops & Seminars, with permission.)

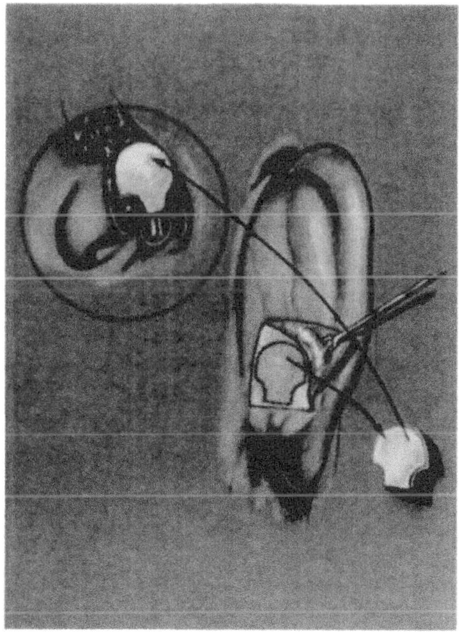

Case 9C Auricular cartilage shield graft. (From Rosio TJ. Cosmetic Surgery and Scar Revision Workshops & Seminars, with permission.)

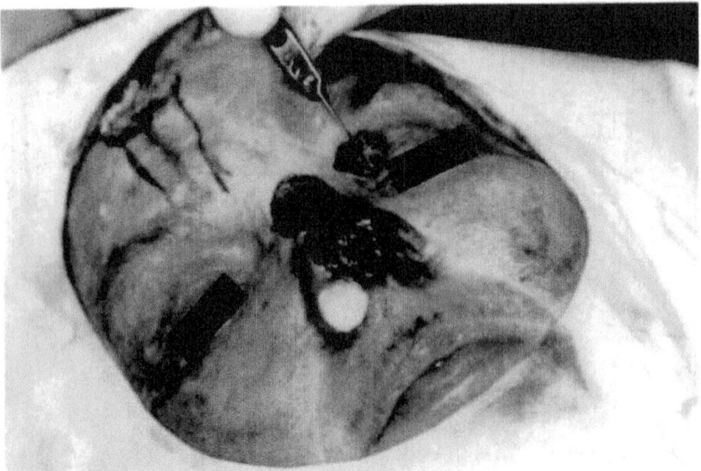

Case 9D Shield and strut graft placement after split hinge flaps reconstituted right and left nasal mucosal linings. (From Rosio TJ. Cosmetic Surgery and Scar Revision Workshops & Seminars, with permission.)

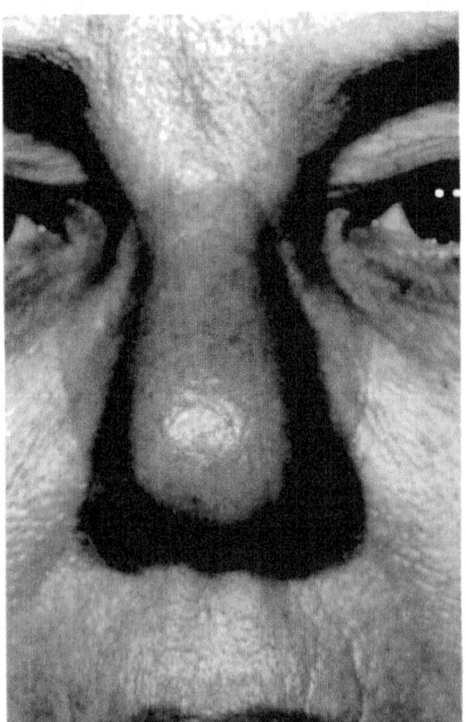

Case 9E Frontal result after forehead flap division and debulking followed by resurfacing. (From Rosio TJ. Cosmetic Surgery and Scar Revision Workshops & Seminars, with permission.)

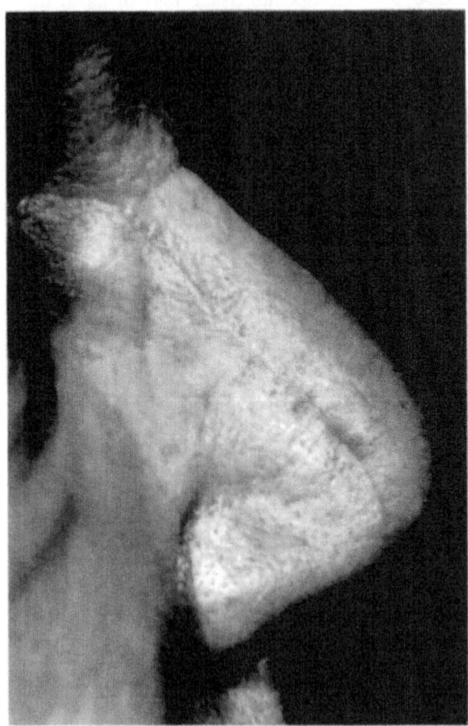

Case 9F Lateral view result after midline forehead flap division, debulking, and postoperative resurfacing. (From Rosio TJ. Cosmetic Surgery and Scar Revision Workshops & Seminars, with permission.)

blends textures (Case 9E and F). A repeated incision line revision with slight deep debulking and resurfacing would further improve the visible incision lines. This patient, however, found the result very satisfactory and declined further revision.

Case 10: Depressed scar of the left hemi-chin.

Analysis: A blunt traumatic injury 10 years before had resulted in subcutaneous muscular, dermal, and fat atrophy, perhaps accompanied by bone mass reduction. The resultant volume loss and wrinkling are evident in the preoperative photographs (Case 10A). Although resurfacing alone would improve the surface wrinkling, it would do nothing for the loss of soft tissue projection and normal cosmetic unit contours.

Solution: Layered injection lipotransplantation in a single session, followed by CO_2 laser resurfacing, resulted in the improvement seen in the 2 ½ month postoperative photographs (Case 10). Natural softness and very long correction are anticipated [Asaadi, 1993 #20; DeVore, 1994 #3]. Other deep augmentation material approaches include a silicone chin implant divided in half and contoured where needed. An expanded e-polytetrafluoroethylene (PFTE) implant has benefits comparable to those of silicone and the ease of subcutaneous pocket placement rather than a subperiosteal location. The e-PFTE undergoes some tissue integration and, therefore, even without wrapping around the chin, would probably hold its location.

Case 11: Extensive scalp, forehead, right nasal sidewall, alar, and intranasal linear verrucous epidermal nevus in a 13-year-old girl. Imagine facing the start of your teenage years known as "the girl with a black river running down her face."

A
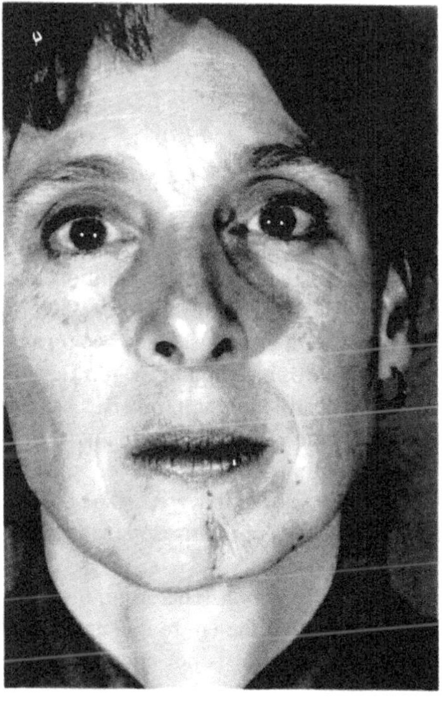

B
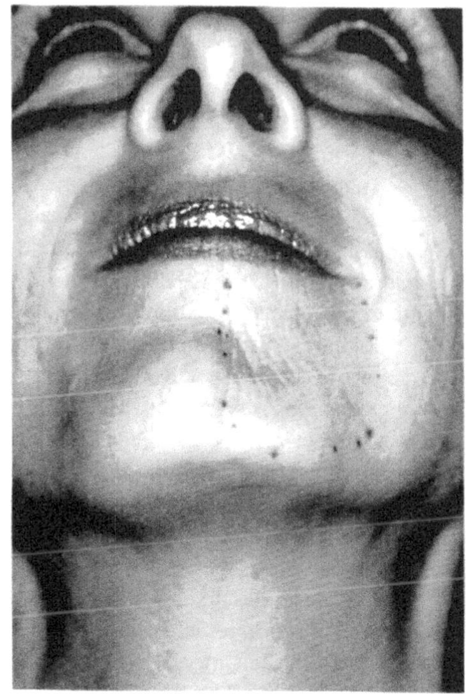

Case 10A–B Depressed scar with subcutaneous muscular and dermal atrophy with superficial wrinkling of left hemichin. (From Rosio TJ. Cosmetic Surgery and Scar Revision Workshops & Seminars, with permission.)

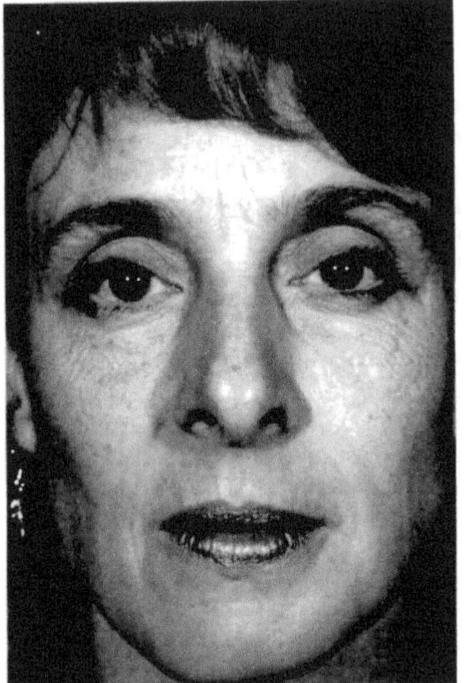
C

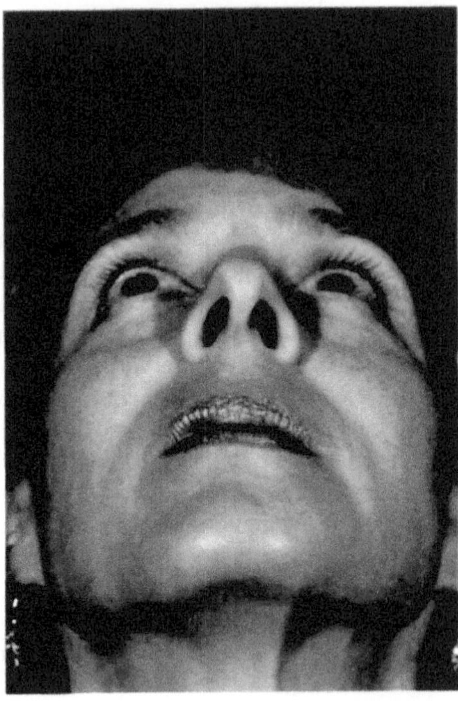
D

Case 10C–D After layered injection lipotransplantation and CO^2 laser resurfacing. The result integrates a high-percentage volume and texture correction. (From Rosio TJ. Cosmetic Surgery and Scar Revision Workshops & Seminars, with permission.)

Analysis: This case combines many principles and pitfalls of scar revision. First, the dramatic lesion beginning up in the scalp runs for the most part in the ATLs (Case 11A). Second, its verrucous surface and depth in a darkly pigmented patient preclude resurfacing measures alone (Case 11B). Third, it traverses multiple cosmetic units. In addition, the width of the lesion in the tight forehead skin of a young girl is a significant factor.

Solution: The lesion traverses the upper three fourths of the forehead between 60 and 90 degrees to the forehead RSTLs. Therefore, in the upper portion, a running W-plasty with 60-degree angles is selected (Case 11C). In the lower forehead, the lesion traverses briefly at an angle between 60 degrees and 30 degrees to the forehead RSTLs; in this portion a stair-step plasty is used with 90-degree angles. The preceding are all connected with an FSR of the medial suprabrow portion that traverses at 30 degrees to 0 degrees. The majority of the forehead and the temple is widely undermined to allow approximation in the high-tension area.

The lateral nasal sidewall lies close to the meilonasal junction. Therefore, the FSR technique is used here, undermining the right medial cheek and the entire dorsum of the nose over to the left medial cheek, to mobilize adequate tissue. It is not enough just to "close" the incision. Doing so increases the risk of dehiscence, a hypertrophic scar, and a hypopigmented spread scar.

The right alar lesion and the intranasal portion were resurfaced with a CO_2 laser (Case 11D). The deeper follicular structures of the nose were judged more likely to achieve repig-

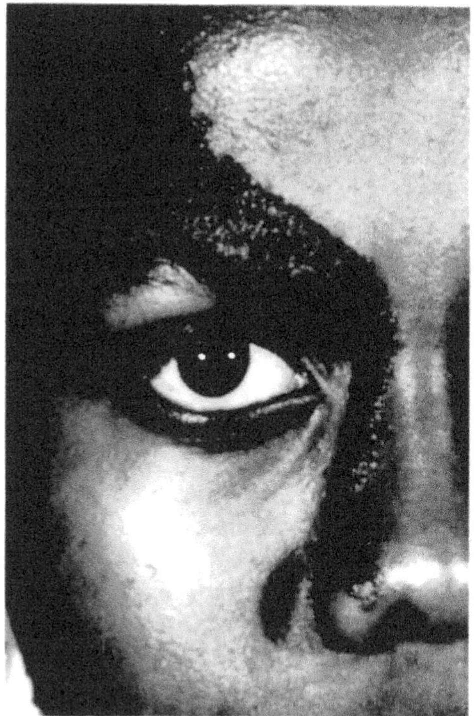

Case 11A Hyperpigmented linear verrucous epidermal nevus (LVEN) in a darkly colored child. (From Rosio TJ. Cosmetic Surgery and Scar Revision Workshops & Seminars, with permission.)

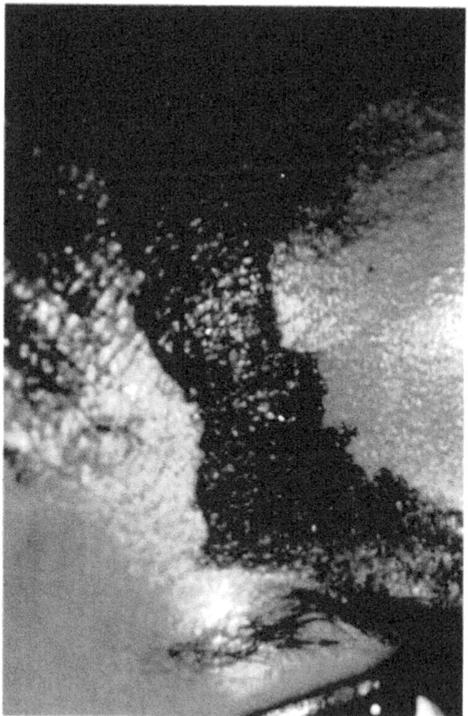

Case 11B LVEN close-up, three-fourths view. (From Rosio TJ. Cosmetic Surgery and Scar Revision Workshops & Seminars, with permission.)

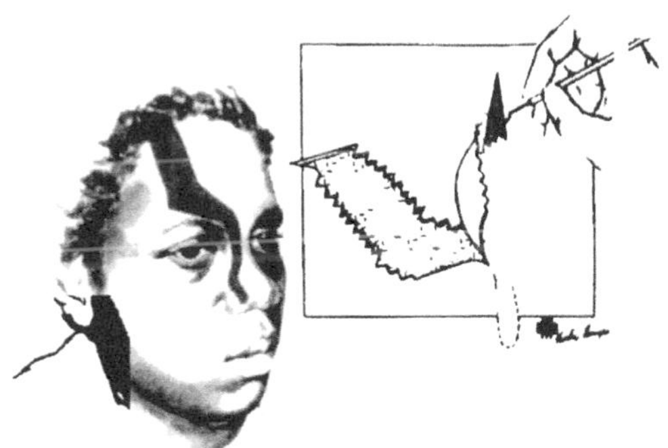

Case 11C Illustration of combined incisional techniques including running W-plasty, serial step-plasty, FSR, and focal laser resurfacing. (From Rosio TJ. Cosmetic Surgery and Scar Revision Workshops & Seminars, with permission.)

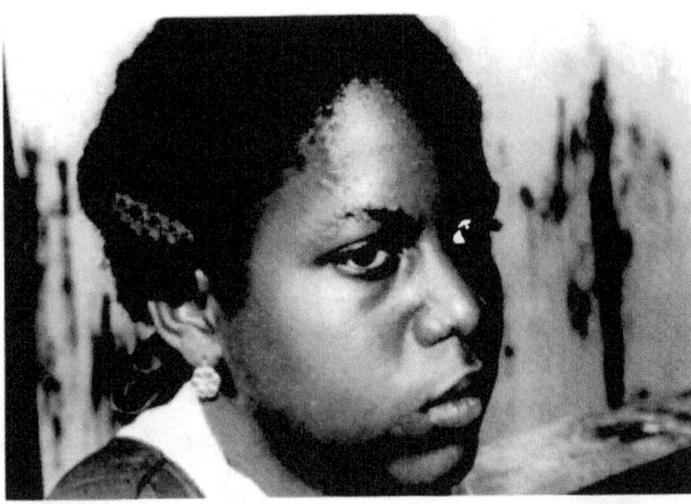

Case 11D Seven days postoperatively, demonstrating suture line and still reepithelializing ala. (From Rosio TJ. Cosmetic Surgery and Scar Revision Workshops & Seminars, with permission.)

mentation than the forehead after more than a superficial resurfacing. The risk/benefit ratio favored this approach over excision and grafting. According to the girl's priest and mother, her personality was transformed by the revision procedures.

C. Final Pearls

There are several reasons why unsatisfactory scars are not revised: "At times unsatisfactory scars are not revised because the surgeon may be ignorant of new scar revision modalities, there may be doubt as to the anticipated scar outcome, or it may be hoped that the patient will learn to accept the deformity, that gradual improvement will occur spontaneously as the scar matures or that the patient will seek treatment elsewhere, since his or her expectations are greater than what the surgeon can expect to achieve" (4).

In conclusion, to aid the reader in scar analysis and treatment selection, a geo-topographic approach to preventing and treating unsatisfactory scars has been presented. The analysis has included practical questions. Scar definitions and descriptive categories led to a review of scar revision objectives as well as regional and local factors affecting scar revision. A personal organization of scar revision techniques and procedures was provided that divides items into "invasive" and "minimally invasive" categories and assigns further groupings by the strata affected.

Eleven cases have been used to demonstrate scar prevention and revision analysis, with procedure selection discussed along with the solutions.

A few nontechnical practice pearls gleaned from the experience of working with scar revision patients are worth consideration. First, help the patient come to understand that we do not "remove" scars. Rather, we attempt to modify, adjust, reposition, improve, or minimize the scar that inevitably forms, in order to make it imperceptible or less obvious. Inform the patient that there is variability in the final outcome, but this is not as discouraging as unpredictability. Share the decision with the patient, always offering your willingness to support the patient's choice of simpler alternatives such as micropigmentation or makeup and clothing coverage (23, 24). Anticipate the challenging cases and have a backup plan. Network with specialty and interspecialty colleagues familiar with these techniques. After studying the techniques and alternatives thoroughly, you will be prepared to judge whether a case is challenging but within your purview or whether assistance is required.

Some day, progress in molecular biology, genetic engineering, and new drugs may solve or prevent many of the difficult scar problems we face (20–22). Until then, the authors sincerely believe that those interested in scar revision will find the geo-topographic approach helpful in preventing unsatisfactory scars, analyzing scars, and selecting methods most likely to yield superior results.

REFERENCES

1. Rosio T. Revision of acne, traumatic, and surgical scars. In: Cutaneous Surgery. Philadelphia: Saunders, 1992: 426–445.
2. Baryza MJ, Baryza GA. The Vancouver Scar Scale: An administration tool and its interrater reliability. J Burn Care Rehabil 1995; 16:535–538.
3. Siana JE, Rex S, Gottrup F. Comparison of self reported and observed length, width, and colour of scar tissue. Scand J Plast Reconstr Surg Hand Surg 1992; 26:229–231.
4. Borges AF. Timing of scar revision techniques. Clin Plast Surg 1990; 17:71–76.
5. Cook T. Use of local skin flaps for scar camouflage. Facial Plast Surg 1984; 1:226–239.
6. Asaadi M, Haramis HT. Successful autologous fat injection at 5-year follow-up (Letter). Plast Reconstr Surg 1993; 91:755–756.
7. Cacou C, Anderson JM, Muir IF. Measurements of closing force of surgical wounds and relation to the appearance of resultant scars. Med Biol Eng Comput 1994; 32:638–642.
8. Cacou C, Muir IF. Effects of plane mechanical forces in wound healing in humans. J R Coll Surg Edinb 1995; 40(1):38–41.
9. DeVore DP, Hughes E, Scott JB. Effectiveness of injectable filler materials for smoothing wrinkle lines and depressed scars. Med Prog Technol 1994; 20:243–250.
10. Orentreich DS, Orentreich N. Subcutaneous incisionless (subcision) surgery for the correction of depressed scars and wrinkles. Dermatol Surg 1995; 21:543–549.
11. Verardi G. Fat graft for the prevention of scar formation after laminectomy (macroscopic and microscopic findings in a case report). Chir Organi Mov 1990; 75(2):147–151.
12. Harahap M. Revision of a depressed scar. J Dermatol Surg Oncol 1984; 10:206–209.
13. Thomas JR, Ehlert TK. Scar revision and camouflage. Otolaryngol Clin North Am 1990; 23:963–973.
14. McDaniel DH, Ash K, Zukowski M. Treatment of stretch marks with the 585-nm flashlamp-pumped pulsed dye laser. Dermatol Surg 1996; 22:332–337.
15. Nordstrom R. Absorbable versus nonabsorbable sutures to prevent postoperative stretching of wound area. Plast Reconstr Surg 1986; 78:186–190.
16. Dierickx C, Goldman MP, Fitzpatrick RE. Laser treatment of erythematous/hypertrophic and pigmented scars in 26 patients. Plast Reconstr Surg 1995; 95:84–90.
17. Gaston P, Humzah MD, Quaba AA. The pulsed tuneable dye laser as an aid in the management of postburn scarring. Burns 1996; 22:203–205.
18. Johnson W. Treatment of pitted scars: punch transplant technique. J Dermatol Surg Oncol 1986; 12:260–265.

19. Musgrave R. The pitfall of surgical excision of vaccination scars in the deltoid area. Plast Reconstr Surg 1973; 51:198–199.
20. Adzick NS, Longaker MT. Scarless fetal healing. Therapeutic implications. Ann Surg 1992; 215:3–7.
21. Chang J, et al. Scarless wound healing: implications for the aesthetic surgeon. Aesthetic Plast Surg 1995; 19(3):237–241.
22. Khaw PT. Antiproliferative agents and the prevention of scarring after surgery: friend or foe? Br J Ophthalmol 1995; 79:627.
23. Guyuron B, Vaughan C. Medical-grade tattooing to camouflage depigmented scars. Plast Reconstr Surg 1995; 95(3):575–579.
24. Draelos ZD. Camouflaging techniques and dermatologic surgery. Dermatol Surg 1996; 22(12):1023–1027.

7
Dermabrasion

George J. Hruza
Washington University
St. Louis, Missouri

I. HISTORY

Kronmayer (1) reported on the use of rotating burrs and rasps under carbon dioxide snow and ether spray cryosthesia for the "scarless" removal of various skin lesions in 1905. Iverson successfully removed traumatic tattoos with sandpaper in 1947. This technique was complicated by the development of silica granuloma in some patients. Dermabrasion was reintroduced in 1953 by Kurtin (2), who used a wire brush with cryosthesia to improve acne scars and other superficial skin lesions. Orentreich, working with Kurtin, developed and refined much of the dermabrasion equipment in use today.

Dermabrasion's popularity has been on a roller-coaster ride during the past 45 years. Dermabrasion became widely used in the 1950s, but because of concerns about its safety and efficacy its popularity waned in the 1960s and early 1970s. Interest grew anew with increased demand of patients for cosmetic improvement in the late 1970s. The concern about transmission of human immunodeficiency virus (HIV) to health care workers dampened interest in performing dermabrasion in the late 1980s and resulted in the reintroduction of less bloody dermabrasion techniques such as manual dermasanding (3,4). Finally, in the 1990s, the development of laser skin resurfacing can be expected to reduce the popularity of dermabrasion even further (5,6). Notwithstanding these concerns, dermabrasion remains, in skilled hands, an effective time-tested technique for the improvement of scars and wrinkles and removal of superficial skin lesions.

II. SELECTION OF PATIENTS

The primary indication for dermabrasion is for the improvement of facial scars caused by acne, varicella, trauma, or surgery. Acne scars are the most common indication for full-face dermabrasion. Careful selection of patients is imperative to keep both patient and physician happy. Dermabrasion can improve scars, but they cannot be completely eliminated. During the initial consultation, the patient should be told that although the scars should improve, they will still be visible. Showing before-and-after photographs of excellent as well as only fair results can be helpful. The patient should be prepared for the 1- to 2-week healing period with swelling, bruising, drainage, and discomfort to be followed by a variable period of erythema.

All realistically possible complications, including scarring, hypopigmentation, hyperpigmentation, milia formation, acne exacerbation, and infection, have to be discussed at length with the patient (7). The patient must understand that white scars will remain white and dermabrasion will not improve enlarged pores. In fact, it can further enlarge them if it is carried out to a depth below the hair follicle infundibulum (8).

Ice-pick and deep bound-down scars have to be removed surgically with punch excision, punch elevation, or punch grafting 6 to 8 weeks before dermabrasion (9–11). Hypertrophic scars do not improve with dermabrasion and may, in fact, get worse. Acne scars off the face, especially on the neck, should not be treated with dermabrasion because of the very high risk of depigmentation and hypertrophic scarring.

Patients who have undergone previous skin resurfacing procedures including dermabrasion, deep chemical peel, or laser resurfacing should be warned that additional resurfacing procedures, while helpful, generally do not achieve the same degree of improvement as the initial resurfacing procedure and may have a somewhat increased risk of complications, as some dermal fibrosis is already present. The patient's skin should be carefully examined and any evidence of hypopigmentation, textural alteration, scarring, or lines of demarcation should be noted in the chart and pointed out to the patient.

Patients with acne scars often have active acne. Whenever possible, dermabrasion should be deferred until the acne is no longer active so that the patient does not develop new acne scars from continuing acne activity that may require future resurfacing procedures. If the acne activity is mild, it should be controlled with conventional acne treatments before dermabrasion. However, we prefer to avoid minocycline in the predermabrasion period because of the risk of dermal minocycline hyperpigmentation in areas of trauma and inflammation.

Dermabrasion is contraindicated in patients with deficient healing ability, such as patients with Ehlers-Danlos syndrome and patients who form keloids. Patients with scleroderma, ectodermal dysplasia, or x-ray–irradiated skin have reduced adnexal structures that make healing more difficult and result in increased risk of scarring from dermabrasion. Dermabrasion should not be performed on patients who are immunosuppressed, as the risks of infection, delayed healing, and scarring are significantly increased. Patients with vitiligo should not be dermabraded, as they may develop koebnerization of their vitiligo in the dermabraded skin.

As dermabrasion creates innumerable bleeding spots, patients with a bleeding diathesis such as hemophiliacs and thrombocytopenic patients are poor candidates; the bleeding will be difficult to stop and may require clotting factor or platelet transfusions.

Isotretinoin reduces sebaceous gland size and activity while the patient is taking it. Even though sebum production returns to normal after completion of isotretinoin treatment, there have been reports of atypical scarring in patients who have undergone dermabrasion before, during, and after taking isotretinoin (12–15). It is not clear when the skin has returned to normal after a course of isotretinoin. We prefer to wait at least 1 year after completion of isotretinoin treatment before proceeding with dermabrasion.

HIV poses a significant problem for personnel performing dermabrasion. Wentzell et al. (4) demonstrated that dermabrasion generates microdroplets of blood that stay suspended in the atmosphere for several hours after dermabrasion and are of a size that can settle on mucosal surfaces and be easily aspirated into lung alveoli. In addition, standard universal precautions including masks and eye protection are ineffective protection. Therefore, the surgeon, support staff, other patients, and even people passing by in the hall-

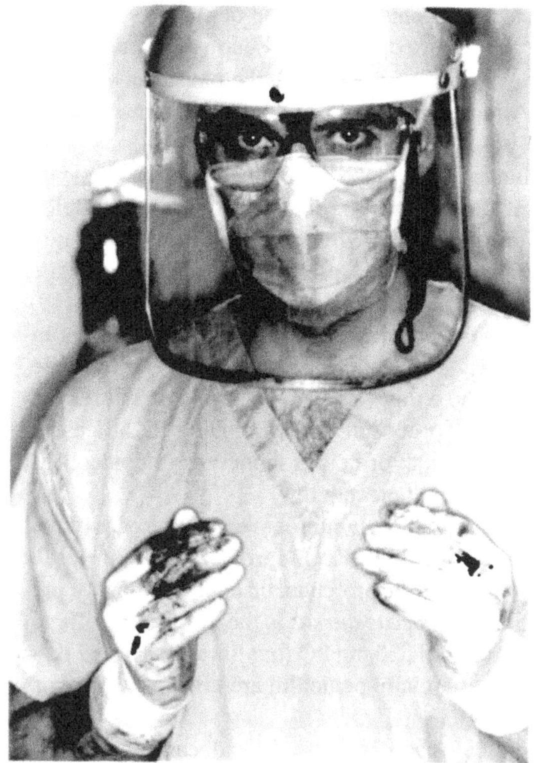

Figure 1 Universal precautions. The dermabrasion surgeon is wearing safety glasses, 0.1-μm particle filtration mask, cap, face shield, and gloves. Note blood on gloves and face shield (gown has been removed.).

way are potentially at risk. Fortunately, there have been no reports of HIV transmission to health care workers by dermabrasion.

HIV may not be detectable in the blood for a number of months after infection, so every patient has to be considered to be potentially HIV infected. In addition, testing of patients for HIV is not an option, as denial of the procedure based on a patient's HIV status is prohibited by federal statute. If the patient has acquired immunodeficiency syndrome (AIDS) or evidence of immunosuppression, then dermabrasion is contraindicated because of the increased risk of complications. Universal precautions including 0.1-μm filtration masks, goggles, face shields, gloves, and waterproof gowns should be worn by all personnel in the procedure room for all dermabrasion cases (Fig. 1). In regions of high HIV prevalence, a contained breathing apparatus to isolate the surgeon and assistants from the patient's tissue and body fluids may be advisable (16). Alternatively, sandpaper dermabrasion may be used, as no significant aerosol is produced (3,17,18). All personnel should have up-to-date hepatitis B vaccination.

III. PREOPERATIVE CONSIDERATIONS

Oral anticoagulants such as warfarin (Coumadin) should be stopped whenever possible for 3 days before dermabrasion and resumed 1 day after dermabrasion. Taking into account the

10-day half-life of platelets, aspirin with its irreversible inactivation of platelets should be stopped for 2 weeks before dermabrasion and restarted 2 days after dermabrasion. Any interruption of Coumadin or aspirin therapy should be cleared with the physician who prescribed it. Nonsteroidal anti-inflammatory drugs cause only reversible platelet inactivation. Therefore, they need to be stopped for only 2–3 days before dermabrasion.

Dermabrasion can trigger herpes labialis in patients carrying the virus. The patient's history is often not a reliable indicator if the patient is infected with herpes simplex. Dermabraded skin is also susceptible to primary herpes virus infection during the initial healing phase (6). If herpes simplex infection develops, it spreads rapidly from the trigger point to involve the entire dermabraded area, akin to Kaposi's varicelliform eruption (19).

Therefore, any time a large facial areas is to be dermabraded, even if it does not include the trigger zone, patients are given prophylactic antiherpes medication (20). We prescribe either acyclovir 400 mg by mouth (PO) three times a day or valacyclovir Valtrex 500 mg PO twice a day starting 0–2 days before the procedure and continuing for at least 10 days after dermabrasion. Patients are at greatest risk of herpes labialis development just when the skin is reepithelializing 7–10 days after the procedure.

Unlike skin treated with CO_2 laser resurfacing, which leaves behind significant necrotic tissue that serves as an ideal culture medium (21), dermabraded skin rarely becomes infected. However, we give all of our patients prophylactic antibiotics as we prefer to minimize any risk of infection. As *Staphylococcus aureus* is the most likely offending skin pathogen, we give our patients dicloxacillin 250 mg PO four times a day for 7 days starting on the day of the procedure. Patients allergic to penicillin are given azithromycin (Zithromax Z-pack).

Using prophylactic antibiotics also protects patients at risk for endocarditis or device infection because of valvular abnormalities or prosthetic devices, respectively. Patients who need prophylactic antibiotics are given 1 g of dicloxacillin as an initial dose, followed by 500 mg as a second dose. The rest of the antibiotic course is unchanged.

Tretinoin cream seems to "prime" the skin for faster healing after resurfacing. The use of 0.05% tretinoin cream for 2 weeks before dermabrasion has been found to speed reepithelialization from a maximum of 11 days down to only 7 days (22). We prescribe 0.02–0.05% tretinoin cream once a day for 4–6 weeks before dermabrasion in all patients who can tolerate the drying and skin irritation. Careful instruction about the proper use of tretinoin is important. The skin should be dry for at least 20 minutes before application, and a small, pea-sized amount is enough for the entire face.

Patients with Fitzpatrick skin type III or greater are at increased risk for postinflammatory hyperpigmentation after dermabrasion. To reduce this risk, we prescribe a bleaching cream such as Solaquin Forte for 4–6 weeks before the procedure. In addition, sun avoidance and the use of sun screens for several weeks before dermabrasion are advisable.

The use of oral corticosteroids after head and neck cosmetic surgery is controversial. Some studies have shown reduced postoperative edema, whereas others have shown no benefit of corticosteroids (23,24). No controlled studies of dermabrasion and corticosteroids have been reported. Anecdotally, a reduction in postoperative edema and discomfort has been reported by our patients. Therefore, we give a 4-day tapering course of prednisone starting, on the day of the procedure, with 60 mg for patients who have no contraindications for taking corticosteroids.

IV. ANESTHESIA

General anesthesia or even intravenous sedation is rarely needed but should be offered to especially anxious patients. In our office, the great majority of patients are given sublingual triazolam (Halcion, 0.25–0.5 mg) and meperidine hydrochloride 50 mg with prochlorperazine (Compazine, 10 mg intramuscularly) before anesthetizing the face. These medications relax the patient and reduce discomfort. Halcion often induces some degree of amnesia for the procedure. A pulse oximeter is helpful for monitoring the patient.

When dermabrasion is performed with a cryogen spray, local anesthesia may not be necessary. The spray freezes the skin, briefly anesthetizing it, so that the actual dermabrasion is not felt by the patient (25). We have found that the multiple freezing and thawing cycles when treating an entire face are distinctly uncomfortable for the patient. Therefore, at the very least, we anesthetize the central face with supraorbital, supratrochlear, infraorbital, infratrochlear, and mental nerve blocks (26). Some patients require additional local anesthetic infiltration into the lateral cheeks. The nerve blocks are achieved with 1% lidocaine with 1:100,000 epinephrine neutralized with sodium bicarbonate. The lateral cheek injections are done with 0.5% lidocaine with 1:400,000 epinephrine and bicarbonate neutralization. This reduces the amount of epinephrine injected. Large doses of epinephrine can lead to uncomfortable sinus tachycardia and palpitations.

An alternative to traditional anesthesia is the use of tumescent anesthesia. The dilute local anesthetic solution, 0.1% lidocaine with 1:1,000,000 epinephrine neutralized with sodium bicarbonate, is injected subcutaneously into the entire face with long spinal needles or anesthetic infiltration cannulas until tense tumescence has been achieved. Potential benefits include reduced bleeding because of epinephrine-induced vasoconstriction and a stiff surface that may be dermabraded without the use of a cryogen (27,28). Potential disadvantages include increased edema from the injected fluid, need for additional equipment, lengthening of the procedure, and distortion or obscuring of the target scars, which may make it difficult to achieve predictable results (29,30).

V. EQUIPMENT

A. Dermabrader

The choice of dermabrasion machine is a function of surgical technique and personal preference of the surgeon. The older dermabrasion machines consisted of electrical motor–driven cables that were able to generate rotational speeds up to 12,000 rpm. The machine and cable assembly was bulky and the large handpiece was somewhat awkward to use. The cable assembly was subject to breakage. Modern electrical dermabrasion machines, called hand engines, generate speeds up to 33,000 rpm with the speed controlled with a foot pedal. The hand engine consists of a base and a pen-shaped handpiece connected to the base with a coiled cord. The handpiece functions as a fast drill into which the various dermabrasion tips are placed. As with an electrical drill, the direction of rotation is reversible, making it easy to approach the face from different sides. Also, the left-handed surgeon is not at a disadvantage. Two popular hand engine brands are the Bell Hand Engine and the Osada models.

In order to achieve higher speeds, nitrogen-driven machines have to be used. The Stryker unit delivers 50,000 rpm or more. Such high speeds make dermabrasion without freezing the skin practical. However, at such high speeds one has to be cognizant of the significant heat that can be generated at the skin surface, which could cause a friction burn. The handpiece should not be allowed to dwell too long in one place. The nitrogen-driven Schreuss Derma III dermabrasion machine can achieve rotational speeds up to 60,000 rpm and newer machines can reach up to 85,000 rpm (31).

B. Diamond Fraise

The dermabrasion is performed by diamond fraises, wire brushes, or serrated wheels placed in the dermabrader handpiece tip. The diamond fraise consists of a wheel studded with industrial diamond chips of various degrees of coarseness ranging from fine and medium to coarse and extra coarse. The great majority of cases require coarse or extra coarse wheels in order to achieve sufficient speed as well as depth of tissue removal. We have found the coarse diamond fraise wheel to be the most versatile. The extra coarse wheels, because of the large number of diamond chips, are often somewhat unbalanced, resulting in a noisy hand engine with an unacceptable level of vibration. The finer textured wheels may be useful for the novice surgeon to get used to the feeling and handling of the equipment. The wheels come in various widths from 1 to 10 mm. Unlike the wire brush, the diamond fraise comes in various shapes, including bullet, pear, cylinder, and dome shaped. The special shapes are very useful for dermabrasion of curved areas such as the nose.

The diamond fraise is considered the easiest dermabrasion tool to use. It is the easiest to control, but also the slowest. It generally takes more passes with a diamond fraise than a wire brush to achieve equivalent depth of tissue removal. It is very difficult to create an undesirable gouge and relatively difficult to tear a free edge such as a lip or an eyelid accidentally with the diamond fraise. The skin does not have to be frozen as solidly when using a diamond fraise.

C. Wire Brush

The wire brush is the favorite dermabrasion tool of the most experienced dermabrasion surgeons. It gets to the desired depth very quickly, and some feel that the microlacerations created with the wire brush improve the final result of the procedure. The wire brush consists of a wheel with stiff stainless steel wires protruding around its circumference. The wires can be sticking straight out from the center or be slightly angled. If the wires are angled, the wheel can be rotated in only one direction. The wheels come in various widths. When using the wire brush, the skin surface has to be frozen solid in order to achieve efficient abrasion and to reduce the risk of gouging the skin.

The wire brush requires more practice and experience than the diamond fraise. The margin of safety is much less. It is relatively easy to gouge the skin or tear chunks of skin away, at times all the way into fat. The skin must be kept very taut and frozen hard to minimize these potential problems. Free margins have to be approached very gingerly, as there is a significant risk of a free edge such as the eyelid being caught up in the rotating wire brush.

D. Serrated Wheel

The serrated wheel was one of the earliest dermabrasion instruments. It consists of a wheel with serrations of varying degrees of coarseness. It is the least popular dermabrasion tool. It achieves tissue removal at a similar rate to a diamond fraise, but the increased spacing between the "teeth" on the wheel compared with a diamond fraise increases the risk of gouging and tearing of the skin. Therefore, only a select group of experienced surgeons still use it.

E. Sandpaper

With the spread of HIV infection, interest in manual dermabrasion using various kinds of abrasive paper has been rekindled (3,17,32). The most commonly used paper is one of several grades of sterilized silicone carbide sandpaper. In order to achieve abrasion into the dermis, relatively coarse grades of sandpaper have to be used. As the procedure is relatively slow, it is mostly reserved for spot dermabrasion of individual lesions or small cosmetic units. Alternatively, it has been used for full-face dermabrasion combined with mild trichloroacetic acid (TCA) chemical peels (33,34). The epidermis is abraded away with sandpaper and the acid is applied to the denuded surface, achieving greater depth of penetration than when it is placed on intact skin.

No cryogen is used with sandpaper, as the procedure is too slow and the skin thaws out before the abrasion has been completed in the frozen area. We have not found it useful for the treatment of acne scars. However, it has been quite helpful for improvement of post-surgical scars when the traditional dermabrasion equipment was unavailable. The sandpaper has to be wrapped around a finger, hard block, or tube, such as a 3- or 10-mL syringe, for stability, and the surface is abraded with a rapid back-and-forth sanding motion.

F. Cryogen Spray

For dermabrasion into the mid-dermis, a cryogen spray is usually necessary. Currently, the choice of spray is limited to Floro-Ethyl (Freon 114 ethyl chloride) and Frigiderm (Freon 114). These sprays can achieve a maximum of −40°C. A spray at this temperature, when applied to skin at body temperature, is unlikely to cool the skin much below freezing. Brief periods of freezing the skin with these sprays does not seem to cause irreversible tissue injury (35,36). However, caution should be exercised if multiple freeze-thaw cycles are performed on a given area (37). Cryogens that achieve colder temperatures such as Cryosthesia −30°C and Cryosthesia −60°C have been withdrawn from the market, because excessive cold injury with hypopigmentation and scarring has been reported (38,39).

Floro-Ethyl and Frigiderm both contain chlorofluorocarbons that have been shown to be damaging to the ultraviolet light–protective ozone layer. So far, no safe alternatives have been introduced, and the production of all chlorofluorocarbon sprays, including those used in medicine, is being phased out.

G. Instrument Care

Diamond fraises, serrated wheels, and wire brushes have to be carefully cleaned after use. Special wire brushes are available to clean debris from wire brush bristles. The various wheels can be steam autoclaved, and before each use they should be carefully inspected, looking for wear. For wire brushes, the bristles should be examined for alignment, proper direction, and presence of all wires.

The hand engine handpiece becomes contaminated with the patient's blood and has to be cleaned and sterilized as well (40). The handpiece contains a motor that can only be gas sterilized. Periodic lubrication of moving parts according to the manufacturer's instructions may be necessary. A spare hand engine and abrasion wheels should be available.

VI. TECHNIQUE

After the skin has been anesthetized and prepared with an antiseptic solution, a drape is wrapped around the patient's hair to keep it away from the rotating dermabrasion wheel lest it be caught up in it. Gauze is kept away from the field, as it can also be caught up in the spinning wheel.

Except for single isolated scars, dermabrasion of an entire cosmetic unit is done in order to avoid visible lines of demarcation. For most patients with acne scars, the entire face excluding the eyelids should be dermabraded. Patients with limited scarring can have the lower face including the cheeks and perioral region dermabraded without noticeable lines of demarcation. The dermabrasion is carried out into the hairline, to the orbital rim, and just below the mandible. So that any lines of demarcation will not be visible, the inferior extent of the dermabrasion is outlined with gentian violet just below the jawline with the patient sitting straight up and before any anesthetic has been infiltrated. When the patient lies down, the jawline skin will shift away from its natural position. Dermabrasion of the neck should not be undertaken, as scarring and hypopigmentation are likely outcomes.

Some surgeons paint the skin with gentian violet to help in determining the areas that have been dermabraded (Fig. 2). By painting the depths of the various acne scars, gentian violet can help to determine whether the depth of dermabrasion has been sufficient to get to the base of a given scar. As long as the violet color is visible, the base of the scar has not been abraded.

All personnel in the room wear gowns, masks, latex gloves, eyeglasses, and eye shields (Fig. 1). In addition, the operator and assistant can wear cotton gloves to make it easier to hold instruments and to stretch the patient's skin. The room is kept as cool as possible to make it easier to freeze the skin, and the patient is kept comfortable with warm blankets. The skin to be abraded can be prechilled with ice packs to enhance the efficiency of the cryogen spray.

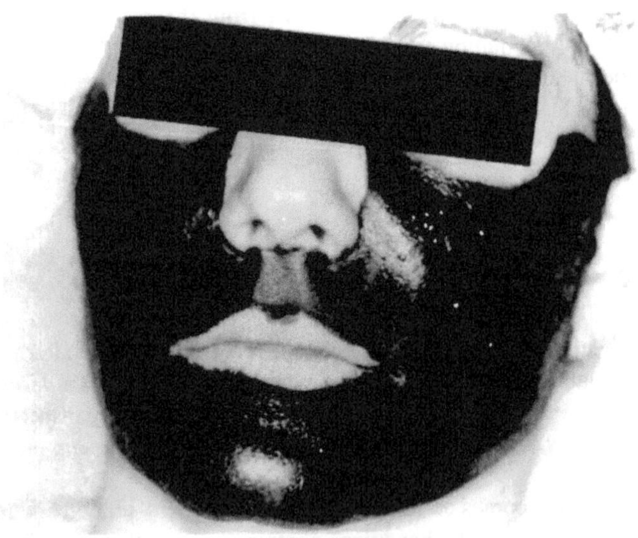

Figure 2 Proposed area of dermabrasion marked with gentian violet to orbital rim, hairline, ear, and below the jawline.

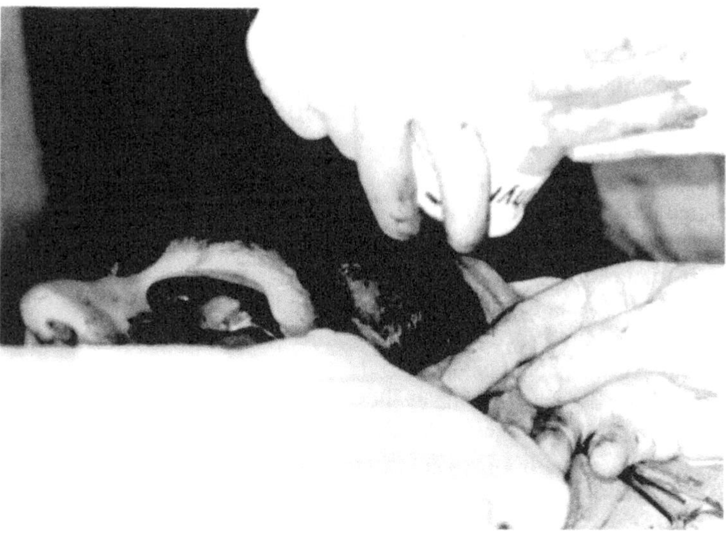

Figure 3 A 1–2-inch-square segment of skin being frozen with Floro-Ethyl cryogen spray while an assistant is protecting the eye with a teaspoon.

Dermabrasion is carried out in 1- to 2-inch-square segments. The skin of a segment is frozen solid with the cryogen spray (Fig. 3). The freezing takes approximately 10 seconds. The assistant usually does the spraying and then keeps the skin taut. Then the frozen area is dermabraded by rapidly moving the handpiece parallel to the skin surface and parallel to the long axis of the handpiece (Fig. 4). The wheel should press against the skin only

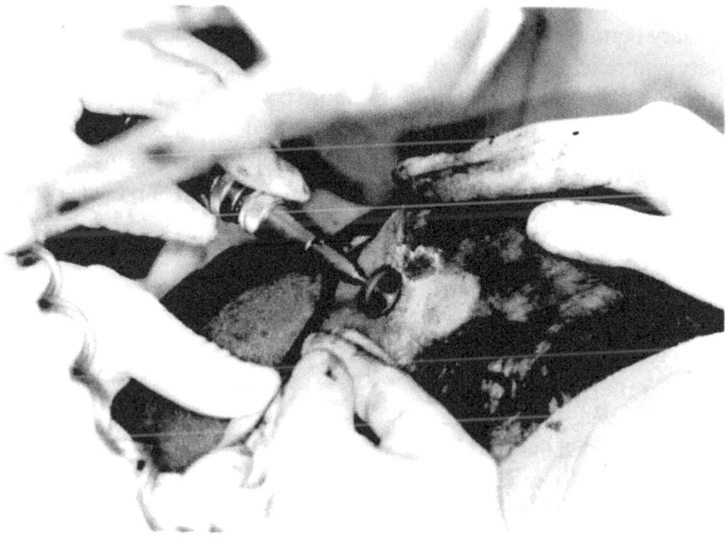

Figure 4 Frozen skin being abraded with a diamond fraise wheel while an assistant is protecting the eye with a teaspoon and providing traction.

while being pulled proximally along the direction of the handle of the handpiece. Circular or lateral motions should be avoided, as they increase the risk of catching skin and causing undesirable gouging or grooving of the skin as well as uneven results. This is especially true with the wire brush. When the site has thawed out, in about 10 seconds, an adjacent, overlapping segment is frozen and the process is repeated.

The number of freeze-thaw cycles for a given segment should be limited, as multiple freeze-thaw cycles increase the extent of cryoinjury and the risk of hypopigmentation and scarring. This is especially likely to happen in areas overlying bone, such as the mandible, malar cheek, and lateral forehead. The skin in these areas freezes very quickly as the skin is rather thin, and the dermabrasion proceeds deeply as the underlying bone stabilizes the skin, making it much easier to abrade deeply into the dermis. Therefore, a single freeze-thaw cycle and very light pressure should be used.

Dermabrasion near free edges such as the eyelids, lips, nasal alae, and earlobes has to be done cautiously. The free edge is approached with the long axis of the handpiece exactly perpendicular to the free edge. In this way, the free edge cannot be caught by the rapidly rotating wheel. Also, the free edge should be stabilized by the assistant. The vermilion border is approached with the dermabrader but should not be crossed, as the vermilion border is an area at high risk of scarring. When working in the periorbital area, the eyes can be covered with small tanning bed goggles or a metal teaspoon can be held over the eyelids by an assistant to protect the eyelids against inadvertent laceration with the dermabrader (Figs. 3 and 4) (41). When working in the perinasal area, the patient should be instructed to take a deep breath and hold it during the cryogen spraying in order to avoid inhaling the cryogen.

The pressure on the skin varies depending on the extent of the scars. In the periphery, the dermabrasion wheel barely touches the skin; in areas of deep and hard scars, the pressure is increased proportionately. When using the diamond fraise, the pressure required is significantly greater than with the wire brush.

When using the diamond fraise, the depth of dermabrasion can be gauged by carefully observing the skin surface. Stripping off the epidermis shows a slightly gray papillary dermis. In the midpapillary dermis, multiple small bleeding points become evident. At the junction of the papillary and reticular dermis, slightly yellowish sebaceous gland lobules become apparent. In the reticular dermis, the surface becomes coarser, and in the midreticular dermis larger, but fewer, bleeding points appear. Limiting the dermabrasion to the papillary dermis minimizes the risk of scarring and hypopigmentation but may be insufficient for improving deeper acne scars. Therefore, we keep the dermabrasion relatively superficial in the papillary dermis except in areas of significant scarring, where we may dermabrade into the upper reticular dermis.

With the wire brush, identifying the depth of dermabrasion is a little more subtle. The wire brush creates microlacerations of the surface. The lacerations appear very fine and uniform when the papillary dermis is being abraded. In the reticular dermis, the lacerations are somewhat coarser and less even.

The dermabrasion is carried out in a systematic fashion, starting with dependent areas to minimize the amount of blood that gets in the way of abrading each new section. Our sequence starts with the left lateral cheek, followed by left medial cheek, chin, lower lip, right medial cheek, right lateral cheek, upper lip, forehead, and finally nose.

After the entire treatment area has been dermabraded, the face is carefully examined for visible residual scars, and these are touched up further (Fig. 5). Special attention should

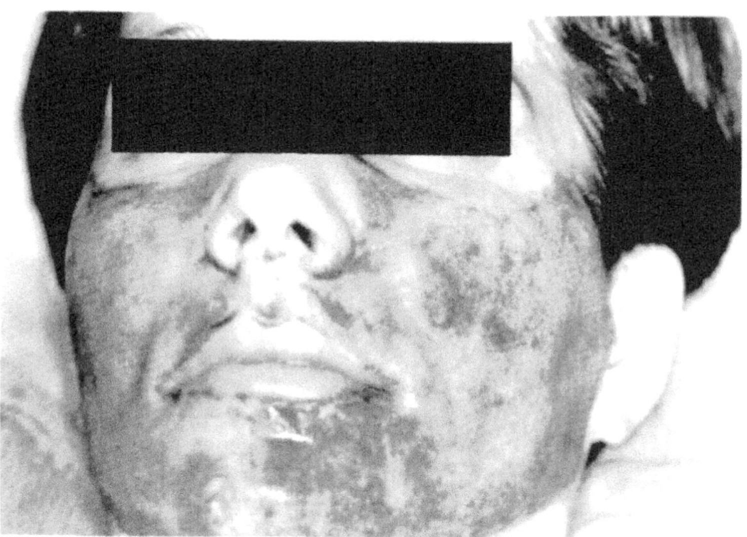

Figure 5 Skin at the conclusion of dermabrasion after removal of all visible scars.

be paid to the hard edges of scars. These should be sculpted away with the dermabrader. It may be helpful to switch from the wheel to a coarse pear-shaped diamond fraise for fine sculpting of scars and to abrade around the nasal alae.

Manual dermabrasion with sandpaper is carried out without a cryogen spray. The skin is held taut with one hand and the sandpaper, attached to a hard object such as a syringe, is moved rapidly across the skin surface. In general, this achieves abrasion only into the papillary dermis, as bleeding wets the sandpaper and skin surface, making deeper abrasion impossible. Because of this limitation, manual dermabrasion is often followed by application of 25% TCA to the dermabraded surface (34). The absence of the epidermis greatly enhances the effect of the TCA.

At the conclusion of dermabrasion, there is significant capillary bleeding, which is effectively stopped by applying 1% lidocaine with a 1:100,000 epinephrine-soaked gauze to the denuded surface (Fig. 6). The bleeding usually stops within 5 to 10 minutes and the skin surface becomes anesthetized (42).

VII. POSTOPERATIVE CONSIDERATIONS

Appropriate wound care after dermabrasion is often as important as the procedure itself in achieving good results. Moist wound healing is universally acknowledged to be far preferable to dry wound healing. After dermabrasion, one of the many bio-occlusive dressings available, in our case Vigilon (43), is applied to all dermabraded areas (Fig. 7). A great deal of gauze is placed around the periphery of the dressing, concentrating most of the gauze at dependent areas around the jaw. This allows the gauze to capture the copious drainage from the wound during the first few days. The dressing is held in place with tape or a cotton mask or surgical netting (Fig. 8).

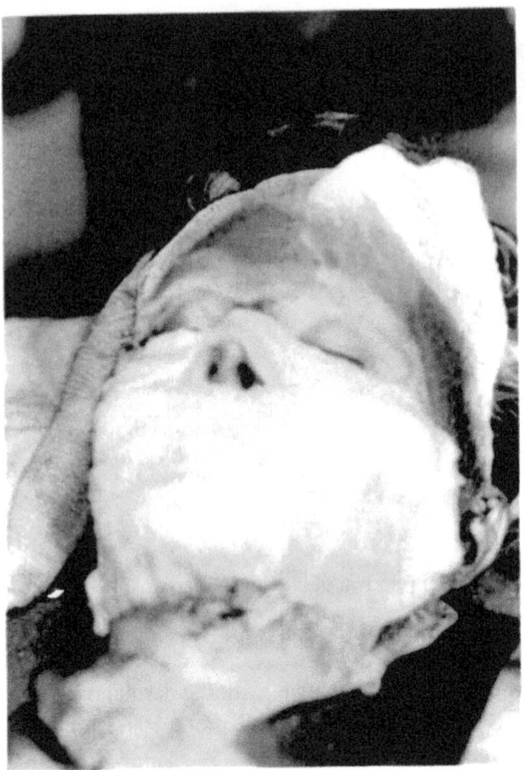

Figure 6 Patient's face is covered with 1% lidocaine with a 1:100,000 epinephrine-soaked gauze for hemostasis after the conclusion of dermabrasion.

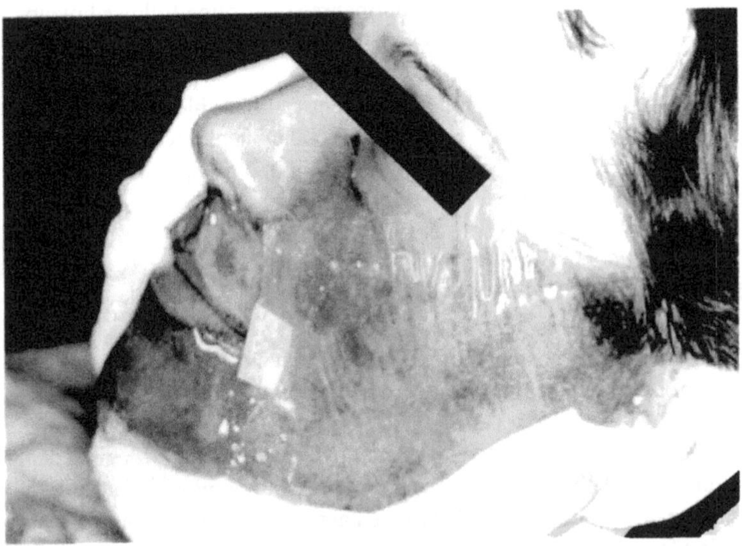

Figure 7 Vigilon bio-occlusive dressing in place. Absorbent gauze is being placed along the lower cheeks and neck in order to absorb the expected copious drainage.

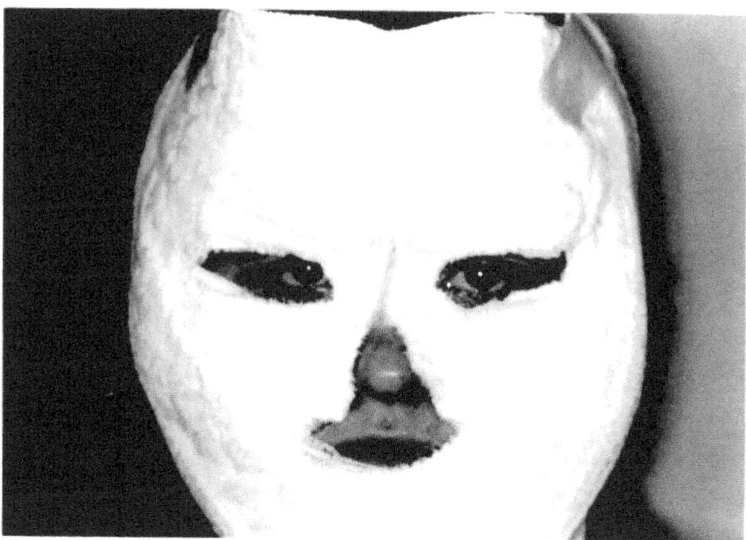

Figure 8 Cotton face mask to keep dressing in place.

The patient's companion is given careful wound care instructions and a prescription for pain medication such as acetaminophen with codeine (Tylenol No. 3). We have found that very few patients who have been given prednisone find a need to take the pain medication. A well-applied bio-occlusive dressing is also important in reducing postdermabrasion discomfort.

The patient returns to the office in 24 hours for cleansing of the wound with 0.25% acetic acid and reapplication of the bio-occlusive dressing. The patient removes the dressing 24 hours later at home and starts to cleanse the skin with multiple 0.25% acetic acid soaks per day followed by liberal use of Aquaphor Healing Ointment. We have found bacitracin, Polysporin, Neosporin, mupirocin (Bactroban), vitamin E (18), and aloe vera (18) to be associated with irritant and allergic contact dermatitis in recently resurfaced skin. Petrolatum seems to increase the frequency of folliculitis at the time of reepithelialization.

Bio-occlusive dressings have been found to speed wound reepithelialization significantly when used during the first 24 to 48 hours after injury. Some surgeons prefer to continue the use of dressings until the skin has healed over. If dressings are continued until reepithelialization, the dressings should be changed daily and the skin cleansed, as prolonged occlusion can lead to increased risk of infection. As the patients are already taking antibiotics, candidal infection is more likely to develop, causing delayed reepithelialization (44).

The skin should be reepithelialized within 7 to 10 days. The patient returns to the office 1 week after the procedure. All occlusive ointments should be stopped as soon as the skin has reepithelialized, as ointments on intact skin tend to promote the development of folliculitis. Shaving can be resumed when the skin surface is intact. Female patients are given instructions in how to cover the erythema, which may last from several weeks to several months. The key is to use green foundation to neutralize the redness. High-SPF sunscreens and sun avoidance during the period of erythema are recommended to reduce the risk of postinflammatory hyperpigmentation. Dermabrasion is best done in the fall and winter to help in reducing ultraviolet light exposure after the procedure.

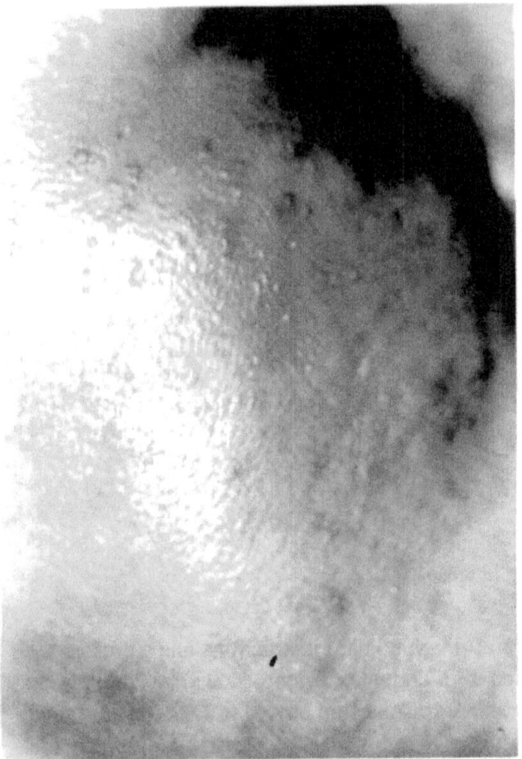

Figure 9 Milia formation and acne exacerbation 2 months after dermabrasion.

After dermabrasion, some patients develop acne exacerbation that may last for a number of weeks but responds to standard acne treatments (Fig. 9). Milia often develop 3 to 6 weeks after dermabrasion (Fig. 9). They are thought to be caused by implantation of epidermal fragments that continue to keratinize under the reepithelialized skin surface (45). The incidence of milia formation has been greatly reduced by the preoperative and postoperative use of tretinoin cream (22). If milia do form, they are usually self-limited and resolve spontaneously. Tretinoin can speed their resolution, and persistent and large milia can be incised and gently extracted with comedo extractors.

VIII. RESULTS

The improvement in scars after dermabrasion occurs in two phases. Initially, during the first few weeks, edema, erythema, and a very smooth and fresh skin surface make it seem that the scars have been almost completely eliminated. Once the edema has subsided, the scars reappear and the patient may become disappointed. However, collagen remodeling continues for 12 to 18 months, and it is during this time that gradual improvement in the scars becomes apparent (Figs. 10 and 11). Touch-up procedures may be needed for patients with moderate to severe scars but should be deferred for at least 12 or preferably 18 months to allow maximal improvement to become apparent.

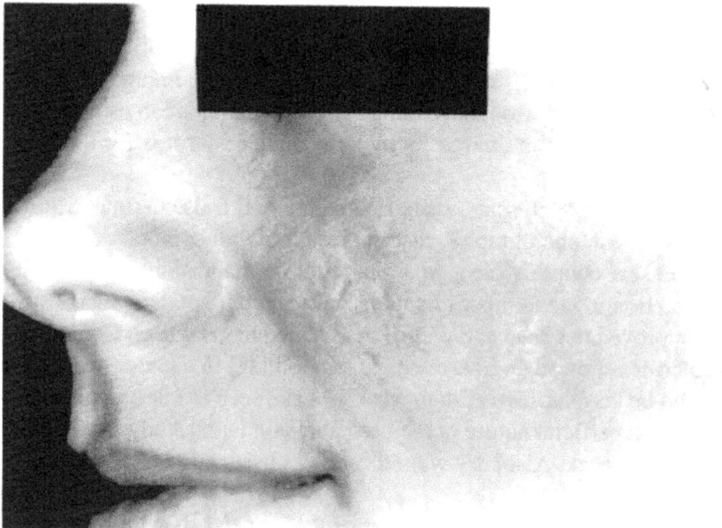

Figure 10 Cheek acne scars before punch grafts and dermabrasion.

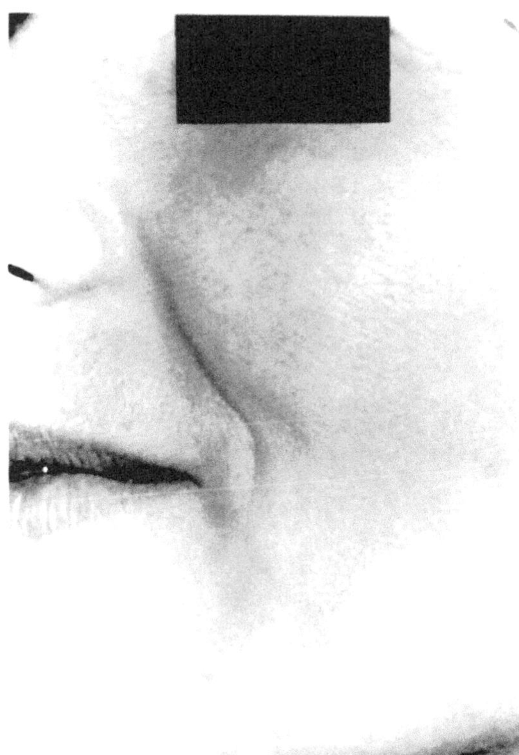

Figure 11 Cheek acne scars 18 months after punch grafts and dermabrasion.

The degree of improvement of acne scars after dermabrasion is difficult to measure. Most studies rely on before-and-after flash photographs, which are notoriously unreliable for assessing three-dimensional structures such as scars. In general, a 50% improvement in acne scars after one dermabrasion is a reasonable estimate. Female patients can usually tell how much improvement they achieved in their scars by how much easier it is for them to apply makeup to their skin.

In a study of 25 patients with acne scars treated with diamond fraise dermabrasion, the lesions were evaluated by flash photography, cast impressions with computer analysis of surface irregularities, and scar counting (46). At 1 year after dermabrasion, there was a statistically significant reduction in the number of superficial scars but not deep scars. Superficial and small scars improved but deep and wide scars seemed to get worse. Computer analysis of surface irregularities showed an improvement (smoothing) in about 50% of patients. These results seem to be less impressive than what we have seen in our practice and could be due to the relatively superficial nature of the dermabrasion in the study, as the patients were reepithelialized in 1 week. Also, dry wound care was used, allowing eschars to form.

Laser resurfacing has been introduced for the treatment of acne scars with results of up to 100% improvement reported (47). In our practice, we have found the degree of improvement after CO_2 laser resurfacing to be very similar to that achieved by dermabrasion and nowhere near 100%. The degree of improvement is probably related to the depth of tissue removal or destruction irrespective of the treatment modality employed.

IX. OTHER INDICATIONS

Other facial scars including traumatic, surgical (48), smallpox-induced (49,50), and varicella-induced scars are amenable to dermabrasion (Figs. 12–16) (51). If the scars are old, results similar to those for acne scars can be expected. If the scars are dermabraded ap-

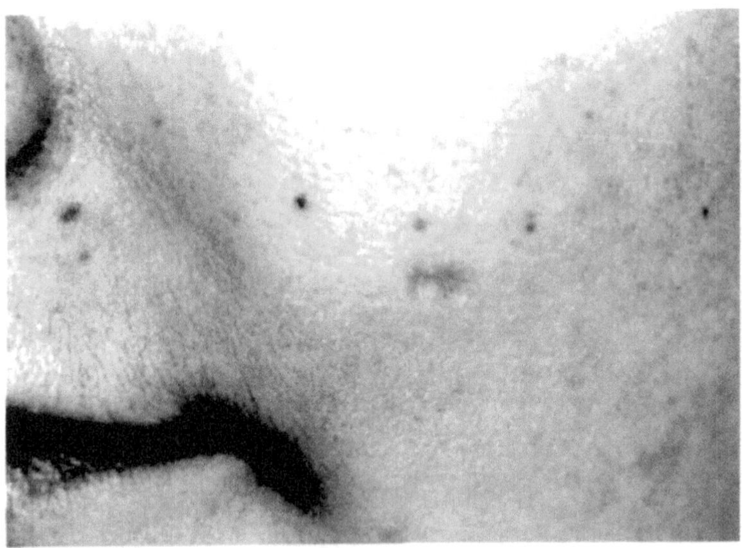

Figure 12 Varicella scar that is 2 months old before spot dermabrasion.

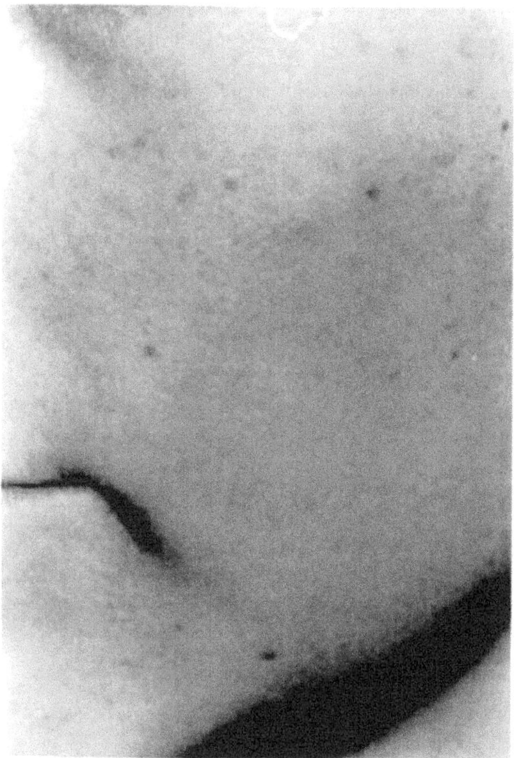

Figure 13 Varicella scar 6 months after spot dermabrasion.

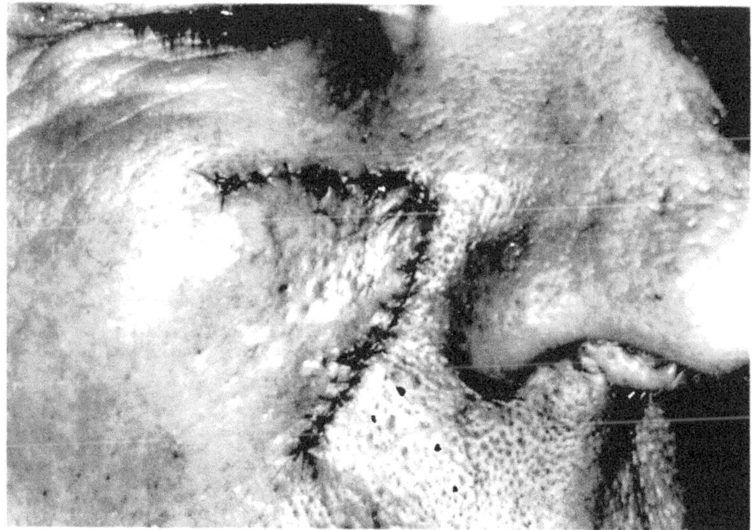

Figure 14 Cheek defect immediately after rotation flap repair.

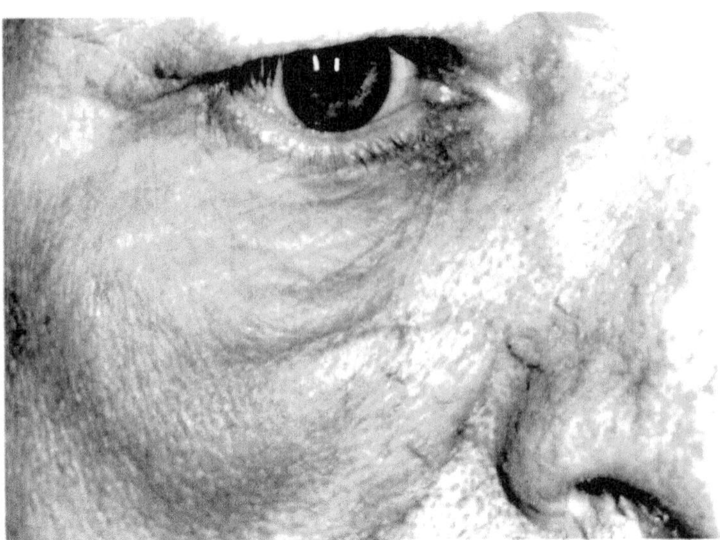

Figure 15 Cheek defect 6 weeks after rotation flap repair with moderate irregularity of suture line and trap-door deformity as well as mild lymphedema.

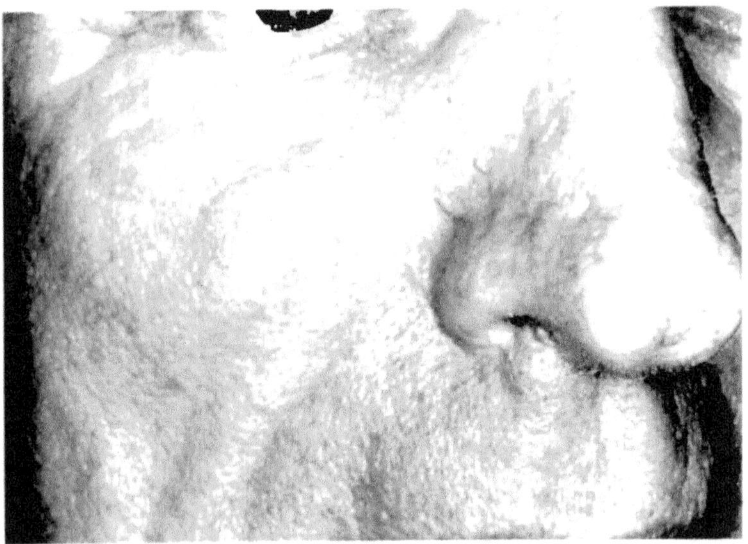

Figure 16 Cheek rotation flap 3 months after spot dermabrasion.

proximately 6 to 8 weeks after injury, the scars can often be almost completely effaced (52–55). If a scar is isolated, spot dermabrasion of the scar and the immediately surrounding area can be performed. Spot dermabrasion does not require any intralesional anesthesia as the cryogen spray provides sufficient anesthesia to the area (42).

Photodamage including actinic keratoses and rhytides can be effectively improved with dermabrasion (33,34,56,57), even though chemical peels and laser resurfacing are more popular. Dermabrasion has been used with the most success to improve perioral rhytides, but some residual hypopigmentation has been reported in two thirds of patients (58). When photodamaged skin is to be dermabraded, the entire face has to be treated in order to minimize color mismatch. Often perioral dermabrasion is combined with a medium-depth chemical peel to the rest of the face with satisfactory skin color blending.

Dermabrasion is often used to deepithelialize vitiliginous or piebald skin recipient sites for epidermal sheet grafts, cultured keratinocyte grafts, or melanocyte grafts as part of repigmentation procedures (59–62).

Before the advent of Q-switched lasers for the relatively scarless removal of tattoos (63), dermabrasion was used (64). However, removing tattoos with dermabrasion leaves the patient with, at best, a depigmented scar and, at worst, a hypertrophic or keloidal scar. Rhinophyma can be planed with dermabrasion (65), but the technique is extremely bloody and quite time consuming. We have found a CO_2 laser to be more effective and almost bloodless (66). Many other cutaneous lesions have been treated with dermabrasion with varying degrees of success, including epidermal nevi, adenoma sebaceum (67,68), lichen and nodular amyloidosis (69,70), granuloma faciale (71), congenital nevi (72), Hailey-Hailey disease (73), and psoriasis (74,75). All of these lesions have in common elevation above the skin surface.

X. COMPLICATIONS

A. Hyperpigmentation

Patients with Fitzpatrick skin type III–VI are at a significant risk of developing postinflammatory hyperpigmentation. Pretreatment with tretinoin and hydroquinones and sun avoidance may reduce the rate of hyperpigmentation but do not completely eliminate it. Postdermabrasion sun exposure during the period of erythema dramatically increases the rate of hyperpigmentation.

Hyperpigmentation usually develops 4 to 8 weeks after dermabrasion. At the first sign of hyperpigmentation, treatment with bleaching creams including hydroquinones (8), Kojic acid, or azelaic acid combined with tretinoin should be started and continued until all traces of hyperpigmentation have resolved. Resolution of hyperpigmentation may take 1 to 6 months. The sooner bleaching cream treatment and strict sun avoidance are instituted, the sooner the hyperpigmentation will fade. Skin types V and VI take the longest to fade.

B. Hypopigmentation

Permanent hypopigmentation of varying degree is a frequent sequela of dermabrasion (58). Noticeable hypopigmentation and even depigmentation are relatively infrequent. Hypopigmentation is related to the depth of tissue removal into the reticular dermis (8) and the extent of cryogen use. Melanocytes are especially sensitive to cold injury. Multiple freeze-thaw cycles and prolonged freezing increase the risk of hypopigmentation. Dermabrasion off the face invariably results in hypopigmentation or depigmentation. Delayed wound healing of any cause, including infection, poor wound care, or inadequate preoperative skin preparation with tretinoin, may increase the risk of hypopigmentation. Patients with history of vitiligo are at increased risk of developing depigmentation of the dermabraded areas. Patients with darker skin types do not develop hypopigmentation more often than those with lighter skin types, but the hypopigmentation is far more noticeable (76).

Subtle hypopigmentation is more evident if only a portion of a cosmetic unit is treated, as a line of demarcation may become noticeable. Patients with significant photodamage often develop lines of demarcation, as the dermabraded skin has the much lighter appearance of younger skin without photodamage compared with the variable hyperpigmentation of sun-damaged skin. Treating the entire face into the hairline and below the jawline eliminates visible lines of demarcation on the face but may, at times, make the skin of the photodamaged neck appear mismatched with the younger-looking facial skin.

Hypopigmentation may not develop until 12 months after dermabrasion and, once it has developed, the hypopigmentation is usually permanent (8). If only a limited facial area was dermabraded, the hypopigmentation can be made less noticeable by dermabrading the rest of the face or performing a medium-depth chemical peel with Jessner's solution and 35% TCA. Women can cover any noticeable hypopigmentation with makeup.

C. Scarring

Textural changes and scarring are related to the depth of dermabrasion, excessive freezing of the skin, and delayed wound healing. Careful selection of patients, conservative technique, especially in women with thin skin, preoperative skin preparation, and meticulous postoperative wound care should make scarring a very rare complication. Postoperative infections can lead to scarring. This is especially true in cases of herpes simplex reactivation. All patients should take prophylactic antiherpetic medication and continue taking it until the skin has completely reepithelialized, as herpes virus reactivation is most likely to lead to clinical lesions in epidermal cells. Any suspected herpes reactivation has to be treated aggressively.

Areas where bones are relatively superficial, especially the mandible, are at increased risk for scarring (Fig. 17). The bone support makes it easy to dermabrade too deeply, and the skin overlying bone also freezes very easily as the cold is removed more slowly than elsewhere by thermal conduction. Patients who have taken isotretinoin in the past are at increased risk of atypical scarring (13,15). The upper lip is another area at increased risk of scarring after dermabrasion. Dermabrasion off the face, because of the reduced number of adnexal structures and reduced superficial blood supply, invariably results in textural alteration, hypopigmentation, and often frank scarring.

If a developing scar is noted early and treated aggressively, the scar can often be almost completely eliminated. Early signs of possible scar development include areas of erythema that are darker and/or shinier than the surrounding dermabraded skin. At this point, treatment with high-potency topical corticosteroids, possibly combined with pulsed dye laser photocoagulation, can abort additional scar formation, and the site may heal uneventfully. The critical time is during the first 2 months after dermabrasion. If the area of erythema starts to develop any hint of hardening, intralesional corticosteroids, pulsed dye laser treatment, and silicone gel sheeting dressing (77) should be started and continued until the

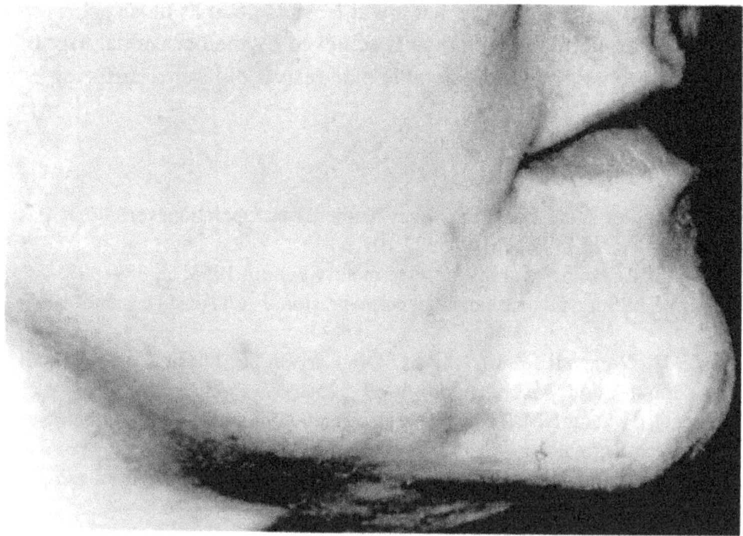

Figure 17 Jawline hypertrophic scar 6 months after dermabrasion.

skin has returned to normal. Pulsed dye laser treatments can be repeated every 4 to 6 weeks. The Silastic gel sheeting should be kept on the scar continuously or for at least 12 hours per day. Any residual scars tend to improve with time over the first 2 years after dermabrasion.

D. Test Spots

Performing a small dermabrasion spot test before dermabrading the entire face may be helpful in patients who are at high risk for complications or anxious about possible complications and efficacy (78). The test spot should be placed in an inconspicuous portion of the proposed dermabrasion area, such as the temple. Full-face dermabrasion should then be deferred for at least 6 months until final healing of the test spot is complete and efficacy and complications, if any, have had a chance to develop. However, a test spot can never be completely predictive of the outcome of full-face dermabrasion, as different areas of the face heal differently depending on the skin thickness and density of adnexal structures. Test spots off the face, such as on the postauricular scalp, are even less predictive.

XI. CONCLUSION

Dermabrasion is a time-tested, cost-effective resurfacing technique with a proven track record of moderate efficacy for facial scar improvement and a well-known side effect profile. The risk of bloodborne pathogen exposure to the surgeon and assistants is far greater with dermabrasion than other resurfacing techniques. The technique is very operator dependent, and expertise and reproductibility are achieved only with extensive experience. The learning curve is significantly longer than with laser resurfacing or chemical peels. In expert hands, dermabrasion can achieve results that are at least as good as those achieved with laser resurfacing. However, dermabrasion results achieved by the occasional user of the technique can be expected to be far less predictable than results of laser resurfacing.

REFERENCES

1. Kronmayer E. Die Heilung der Akne Durch in Neves Norbenlases Operationsverfahren: Das Stanzen. Illustr Monatsschr Aerztl Polytech 1905; 27:101.
2. Kurtin A. Corrective surgical planing of skin. Arch Dermatol Syphilol 1953; 68:389–397.
3. Zisser M, Kaplan B, Moy RL. Surgical pearl: manual dermabrasion. J Am Acad Dermatol 1995; 33:105–106.
4. Wentzell JM, Robinson JK, Wentzell JM Jr, Schwartz DE, Carlson SE. Physical properties of aerosols produced by dermabrasion. Arch Dermatol 1989; 125:1637–1643.
5. Fitzpatrick RE, Goldman MP, Satur NM, Tope WD. Pulsed carbon dioxide laser resurfacing of photo-aged facial skin. Arch Dermatol 1996; 132:395–402.
6. Waldorf HA, Kauvar AN, Geronemus RG. Skin resurfacing of fine to deep rhytides using a char-free carbon dioxide laser in 47 patients. Dermatol Surg 1995; 21:940–946.
7. Duffy DM. Informed consent for chemical peels and dermabrasion. Dermatol Clin 1989; 7:183–185.
8. Fulton JE Jr. The prevention and management of postdermabrasion complications. J Dermatol Surg Oncol 1991; 17:431–437.
9. Arouete J. Correction of depressed scars on the face by a method of elevation. J Dermatol Surg 1976; 2:337–339.
10. Johnson WC. Treatment of pitted scars: punch transplant technique. J Dermatol Surg Oncol 1986; 12:260–265.
11. Solotoff SA. Treatment for pitted acne scarring—postauricular punch grafts followed by dermabrasion. J Dermatol Surg Oncol 1986; 12:1079–1084.
12. Katz BE, MacFarlane DF. Atypical facial scarring after isotretinoin therapy in a patient with previous dermabrasion. J Am Acad Dermatol 1994; 30:852–853.
13. Rubenstein R, Roenigk HH Jr, Stegman SJ, Hanke CW. Atypical keloids after dermabrasion of patients taking isotretinoin. J Am Acad Dermatol 1986; 15:280–285.
14. Roenigk HH Jr, Pinski JB, Robinson JK, Hanke CW. Acne, retinoids, and dermabrasion. J Dermatol Surg Oncol 1985; 11:396–398.
15. Zachariae H. Delayed wound healing and keloid formation following argon laser treatment or dermabrasion during isotretinoin treatment. Br J Dermatol 1988; 118:703–706.
16. Weber PJ, Wulc AE. The use of a contained breathing apparatus to isolate the operator and assistant for aerosolizing procedures including dermabrasion and laser surgery. Ann Plast Surg 1992; 29:182–184.
17. Mokal NJ, Patel J, Thatte RL. Sandpaper mounted on a safety razor: a simple device for dermabrasion. Br J Plast Surg 1990; 43:502.
18. Hunter D, Frumkin A. Adverse reactions to vitamin E and aloe vera preparations after dermabrasion and chemical peel. Cutis 1991; 47:193–196.
19. Silverman AK, Laing KF, Swanson NA, Schaberg DR. Activation of herpes simplex following dermabrasion. Report of a patient successfully treated with intravenous acyclovir and brief review of the literature. J Am Acad Dermatol 1985; 13:103–108.
20. Perkins SW, Sklarew EC. Prevention of facial herpetic infections after chemical peel and dermabrasion: new treatment strategies in the prophylaxis of patients undergoing procedures of the perioral area. Plast Reconstr Surg 1996; 98:427–433.
21. Sriprachya-Anunt S, Fitzpatrick RE, Goldman MP, Smith SR. Infections complicating pulsed carbon dioxide laser resurfacing for photoaged facial skin. Dermatol Surg 1997; 23:527–535; discussion 535–526.

22. Mandy SH. Tretinoin in the preoperative and postoperative management of dermabrasion. J Am Acad Dermatol 1986; 15:878–879, 888–879.
23. Nordstrom REA, Nordstrom RM. The effect of corticosteroids on postoperative edema. Plast Reconstr Surg 1987; 80:85.
24. Echavez MI, Mangat DS. Effects of steroids on mood, edema, and ecchymosis in facial plastic surgery. Arch Otolaryngol Head Neck Surg 1994; 120:1137–1141.
25. Yarborough JM Jr. Dermabrasive surgery. State of the art. Clin Dermatol 1987; 5:75–80.
26. Abadir DM, Abadir AR. Dermabrasion under regional anesthesia without refrigeration of the skin. J Dermatol Surg Oncol 1980; 6:119–121.
27. Goodman G. Dermabrasion using tumescent anesthesia. J Dermatol Surg Oncol 1994; 20:802–807.
28. Coleman WP 3rd, Klein JA. Use of the tumescent technique for scalp surgery, dermabrasion, and soft tissue reconstruction. J Dermatol Surg Oncol 1992; 18:130–135.
29. Field LM. Problems of tumescent anesthesia for dermabrasion. Dermatol Surg 1997; 23:497–499.
30. Field LM. Problems of tumescent anesthesia for dermabrasion. Dermatol Surg 1996; 22:734–735.
31. Fulton JE. Dermabrasion by diamond fraises revolving at 85,000 revolutions per minute. J Dermatol Surg Oncol 1978; 4:777–779.
32. Lusthaus S, Benmeir P, Neuman A, Weinberg A, Wexler MR. The use of sandpaper in chemical peeling combined with dermabrasion of the face. Ann Plast Surg 1993; 31:281–282.
33. Cooley JE, Casey DL, Kauffman CL. Manual resurfacing and trichloroacetic acid for the treatment of patients with widespread actinic damage. Clinical and histologic observations. Dermatol Surg 1997; 23:373–379.
34. Harris DR, Noodleman FR. Combining manual dermasanding with low strength trichloroacetic acid to improve actinically injured skin. J Dermatol Surg Oncol 1994; 20:436–442.
35. Hanke CW, O'Brian JJ, Solow EB. Laboratory evaluation of skin refrigerants used in dermabrasion. J Dermatol Surg Oncol 1985; 11:45–49.
36. Hanke CW, O'Brian JJ. A histologic evaluation of the effects of skin refrigerants in an animal model. J Dermatol Surg Oncol 1987; 13:664–669.
37. Dzubow LM. Histologic and temperature alterations induced by skin refrigerants. J Am Acad Dermatol 1985; 12:796–810.
38. Strick RA, Moy RL. Low skin temperatures produced by new skin refrigerants. J Dermatol Surg Oncol 1985; 11:1196–1198.
39. Hanke CW, Roenigk HH Jr, Pinksi JB. Complications of dermabrasion resulting from excessively cold skin refrigeration. J Dermatol Surg Oncol 1985; 11:896–900.
40. Shelton RM, Grekin RC. Sterilization of the handengine. Is it a necessity? J Dermatol Surg Oncol 1994; 20:385–392.
41. Navarro-Gasparetto C, Jackson IT, de la Puente G. The spoon as a surgical instrument. Plast Reconstr Surg 1979; 63:853–854.
42. Hruza GJ. Spot dermabrasion for scar revision. Fitzpatrick's J Clin Dermatol 1995; 3(2):34–39.
43. Mandy SH. A new primary wound dressing made of polyethylene oxide gel. J Dermatol Surg Oncol 1983; 9:153–155.
44. Giandoni MB, Grabski WJ. Cutaneous candidiasis as a cause of delayed surgical wound healing. J Am Acad Dermatol 1994; 30:981–984.
45. Cohen BH. Prevention of postdermabrasion milia. J Dermatol Surg Oncol 1988; 14:1301.
46. Aronsson A, Ericksson T, Jacobsson S, Salemark L. Effects of dermabrasion on acne scarring. A review and a study of 25 cases. Acta Derm Venereol 1997; 77:39–42.
47. Alster TS, West TB. Resurfacing of atrophic facial acne scars with a high-energy, pulsed carbon dioxide laser. Dermatol Surg 1996; 22:151–154; discussion 154–155.
48. Robinson JK. Improvement of the appearance of full-thickness skin grafts with dermabrasion. Arch Dermatol 1987; 123:1340–1345.

49. Manchanda RL, Singh R, Keswani RK, Kaur G, Soni SK. Dermabrasion in small-pox scars of the face. Br J Plast Surg 1967; 20:436–440.
50. Vukas A. Smallpox-induced scars: treatment by dermabrasion. Dermatologica 1974; 148:175–178.
51. Roenigk HH Jr. Dermabrasion for miscellaneous cutaneous lesions (exclusive of scarring from acne). J Dermatol Surg Oncol 1977; 3:322–328.
52. Katz BE, Oca AG. A controlled study of the effectiveness of spot dermabrasion ('scarabrasion') on the appearance of surgical scars. J Am Acad Dermatol 1991; 24:462–466.
53. Harmon CB, Zelickson BD, Roenigk RK, et al. Dermabrasive scar revision. Immunohistochemical and ultrastructural evaluation. Dermatol Surg 1995; 21:503–508.
54. Yarborough JM Jr. Ablation of facial scars by programmed dermabrasion. J Dermatol Surg Oncol 1988; 14:292–294.
55. Wee SS, Hruza GJ, Mustoe TA. Refinements of nasalis myocutaneous flap. Ann Plast Surg 1990; 25:271–278.
56. Benedetto AV, Griffin TD, Benedetto EA, Humeniuk HM. Dermabrasion: therapy and prophylaxis of the photoaged face. J Am Acad Dermatol 1992; 27:439–447.
57. Nelson BR, Metz RD, Majmudar G, et al. A comparison of wire brush and diamond fraise superficial dermabrasion for photoaged skin. A clinical, immunohistologic, and biochemical study. J Am Acad Dermatol 1996; 34:235–243.
58. Niechajev I, Ljungqvist A. Perioral dermabrasion: clinical and experimental studies. Aesthetic Plast Surg 1992; 16:11–20.
59. Agrawal K, Agrawal A. Vitiligo: repigmentation with dermabrasion and thin split-thickness skin graft. Dermatol Surg 1995; 21:295–300.
60. Kahn AM, Cohen MJ. Vitiligo: treatment by dermabrasion and epithelial sheet grafting. J Am Acad Dermatol 1995; 33:646–648.
61. Olsson MJ, Juhlin L. Transplantation of melanocytes in vitiligo. Br J Dermatol 1995; 132:587–591.
62. Zachariae H. Autotransplantation in vitiligo: treatment with epithelial sheet grafting or cultured melanocytes (Letter; comment). J Am Acad Dermatol 1994; 30:1044.
63. Ashinoff R, Geronemus RG. Rapid response of traumatic and medical tattoos to treatment with the Q-switched ruby laser. Plast Reconstr Surg 1993; 91:841–845.
64. Clabaugh W. Removal of tattoos by superficial dermabrasion. Arch Dermatol 1968; 98:515–521.
65. Linehan JW, Goode RL, Fajardo LF. Surgery vs electrosurgery for rhinophyma. Arch Otolaryngol 1970; 91:444–448.
66. Simo R, Sharma VL. Treatment of rhinophyma with carbon dioxide laser. J Laryngol Otol 1996; 110:841–846.
67. Eichmann F, Blank A. Dermabrasion of lesions of adenoma sebaceum. J Dermatol Surg Oncol 1981; 7:884–887.
68. Earhart RN, Nuss DD, Martin RJ, Imber R, Aeling JL. Dermabrasion for adenoma sebaceum. J Dermatol Surg 1976; 2:412–414.
69. Lien MH, Railan D, Nelson BR. The efficacy of dermabrasion in the treatment of nodular amyloidosis. J Am Acad Dermatol 1997; 36:315–316.
70. Wong CK, Li WM. Dermabrasion for lichen amyloidosus. Report of a long-term study. Arch Dermatol 1982; 118:302–304.
71. Bergfeld WF, Scholes HT, Roenigk HH Jr. Granuloma faciale—treatment by dermabrasion. Report of a case. Cleve Clin Q 1970; 37:215–218.
72. Rompel R, Moser M, Petres J. Dermabrasion of congenital nevocellular nevi: experience in 215 patients. Dermatology 1997; 194:261–267.
73. Hamm H, Metze D, Brocker EB. Hailey-Hailey disease. Eradication by dermabrasion. Arch Dermatol 1994; 130:1143–1149.
74. Gold MH, Roenigk HH Jr. Surgical treatment of psoriasis: a review including a case report of dermabrasion of hypertrophic psoriatic plaques. J Dermatol Surg Oncol 1987; 13:1326–1331.

75. Olson ES. Abrasive treatment of psoriasis. Arch Dermatol 1972; 105:292–293.
76. Ship AG, Weiss PR. Pigmentation after dermabrasion: an avoidable complication. Plast Reconstr Surg 1985; 75:528–532.
77. Katz BE. Silicone gel sheeting in scar therapy. Cutis 1995; 56:65–67.
78. Swinehart JM. Test spots in dermabrasion and chemical peeling. J Dermatol Surg Oncol 1990; 16:557–563.

8
Laminar Dermal Reticulotomy

Harold E. Pierce
Pierce Cosmetic Surgery Center
Philadelphia, Pennsylvania

The need for revision of facial scars, whether such scars are preceded by disease or trauma or are acquired or self-inflicted, has posed aesthetic problems for years. Patients exhibiting facial scars seek surgical solutions to this problem from dermatologists and cosmetic plastic surgeons. Interestingly, no matter what the origin of the scars may be, patients are of the opinion that plastic or cosmetic surgery can remove these scars without leaving a trace.

The physicians evaluating these patients must be honest and forthright in explaining the mechanism to be utilized in an attempt to solve these problems and be most careful to assure the prospective patient that in many cases it may be possible to hide a surgical scar in a crease, a fold, or even a wrinkle and that some repairs lead to better aesthetic results than others. It must be clearly understood that any procedure that invades the integument covering the body will create a scar.

Many techniques have been devised to attempt to hide surgical scars, but the fact remains that one improves inappropriate, unattractive scars by using techniques that are designed to minimize the appearance of the resulting scar in terms of skin texture, color, and tissue remodeling. The experienced cosmetic surgeon assesses the scar characteristics presented to determine, first of all, whether the scar can be repaired. Prospective patients are made fully aware of the complications and risks associated with the surgical procedure. There is no better evidence than that seen after repairs of third-degree burns of the integument, which often require débridement and split- or full-thickness grafting procedures. Secondary procedures often require months or years of protracted scar revision techniques in an attempt to restore a normal aesthetic appearance. The procedure called escharotomy involves a surgical débridement technique. Burn surgeons perform this technique every day in an effort to restore function and a degree of normalcy with regard to the appearance of the patients (1).

Patients with severe postacne facial scarring are ideal candidates for the dermabrasion technique, an innovative dermatologic surgical procedure developed by Kurtin (2) in 1953. This original wire brush surgical technique was shortly followed by the use of a serrated steel cutting wheel intended for deeper scarring and a diamond abrasive wheel for less severe postacne scarring. At about the same time, there was interest in dermabrasion for tattoo removal. Sandpaper abrasion was in use, but at that early time the problem of silica granulomas became evident, and the technique was abandoned until much later when high-quality silicon carbide, better bonded to its cloth or paper backing, was developed. This was

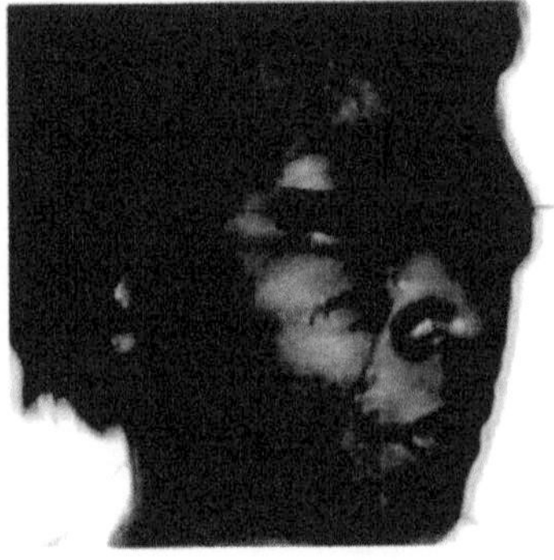

Figure 1 A black, 38-year-old female with facial discoid lupus scarring.

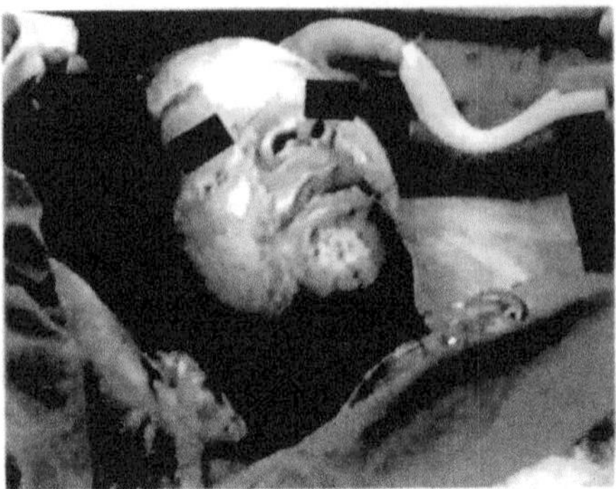

Figure 2 Intraoperative view—laminar dermal reticulotomy (LDR) for scarring from discoid lupus erythematosus (DLE).

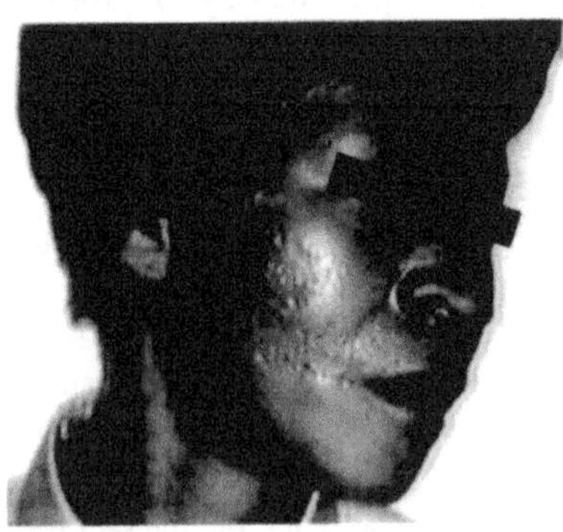

Figure 3 Six weeks after LDR.

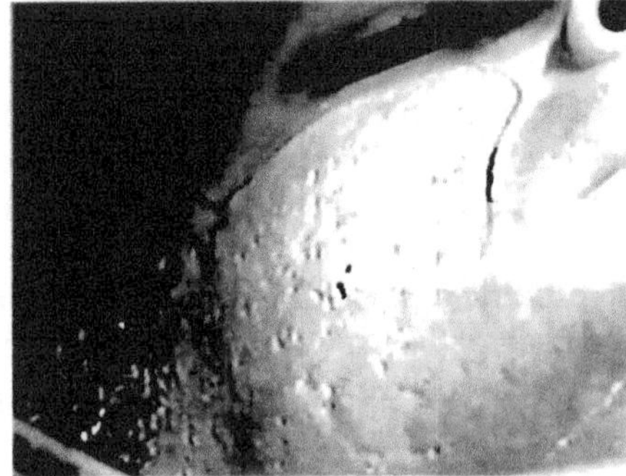

Figure 4 Postacne scarring prior to the LDR procedure in a 35-year-old black male.

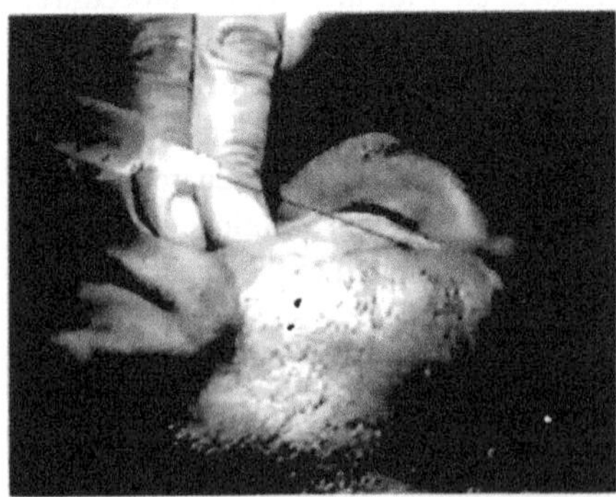

Figure 5 Infiltration xylocaine field block for LDR.

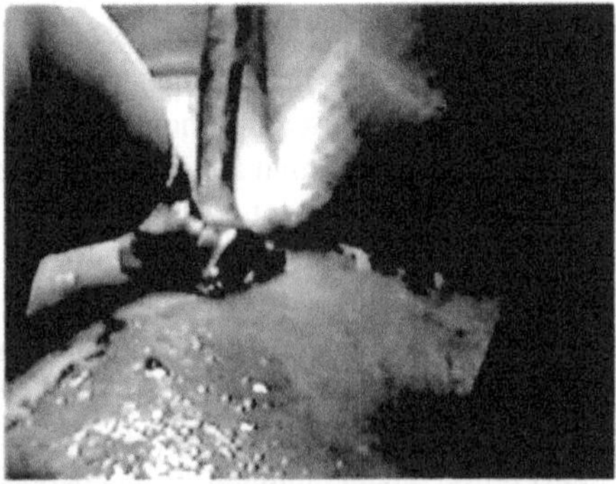

Figure 6 Dermaplaning with dermatome with the laminar dermal reticulotomy technique.

shortly followed by attempts to use sodium chloride (table salt) to accomplish the abrasion technique.

One cannot overlook the fact that dermabrasion, an imperfect surgical technique attempting to deal with an imperfect skin surface, left much to be desired in terms of the end cosmetic result. Estimates of improvement in most patients vary from as little as 10–15% to as much as 75–80%. Seven- to 14-day morbidities accompanied this procedure. Preplanning photographs often did not show significant improvement in the appearance of the dermabraded face. Discoloration in pigmented skins presented aesthetic problems for weeks to months after the procedure. Patients were reluctant to undergo a second or third procedure during a suitable follow-up time frame, either because of financial hardship or because they did not feel that the end justified the means.

During the 1980s, physicians were generally reluctant to perform dermabrasion and use of the technique, for the most part, decreased. For patients with severe acne, a revolution in antibiotics did much to reduce the severity of the condition, resulting in less severe postacne scarring. This really got a boost with the increased interest in isotretinoin introduced early enough in the management of recalcitrant facial acne, as well as the acne conglobata of the chest, shoulders, and back. Many patients had full recovery with a diminished tendency for the development of severe postacne scarring. Also during the 1980s, in addition to the need for better management of postacne and traumatic facial scarring, there was increased interest in the problems associated with dermatoheliosis and whether these problems were associated with the development of maturing skin in older patients. The "baby boomers" were arriving and with them the need to feel eternally young. More evidence was accumulated concerning skin cancer and associated actinic skin changes. The age of facial chemical peeling had arrived, utilizing the fruit acids trichloroacetic acid (TCA) and Baker's formula (3). The question arose of which modality was best designed for which condition.

The argon laser preceded the development of numerous CO_2 lasers, including the Ultra Plus, Silky Touch, neodymium yttrium aluminum garnet (YAG), and others claiming specific targets on a skin surface to be exact. There seemed to be a different laser for each skin problem. In reality, this meant that physicians performing laser surgery had to have available more than one laser, and a CO_2 laser might cost between \$50,000 and \$125,000. The question arose, "Will patients be able to pay for this?" Understandably, health maintenance and managed care organizations denied payment for what they considered cosmetic procedures.

Laser surgery became the most advanced cosmetic dermatologic technique of the 1990s, and eager manufacturers of this instrumentation sought a market share. In addition, a marketing blitz involving television, print, and Internet subjected the American public to much information that in many cases proved to be promotional publicity championing the outstanding achievements of this new technique. Certainly, although many good results were being obtained, there was a clinical downside that was downplayed by the purveyors of laser therapy. Meanwhile, a little-known German instrument manufacturer developed the infrared coagulator (4), which, in contrast to the laser, was reasonable in cost, and it seemed that this instrument or a modification of it might serve a useful purpose in resurfacing procedures. Known as the poor man's laser, this instrument may be an addition to our armamentarium worthy of further study.

In contemplating the possibility of cosmetic scar revision one must be aware of the patient's question, "What will the scar look like?" This may seem inconsequential in light of the medical necessity of a lifesaving procedure. However, once successful surgery is

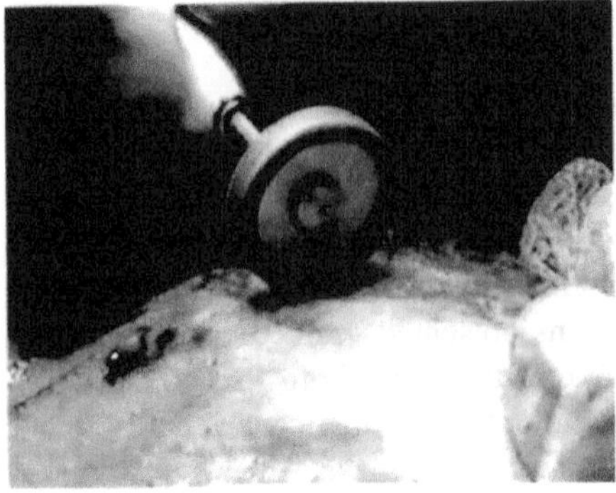

Figure 7 Fine-tuning the LDR procedure with speed dermabrasion.

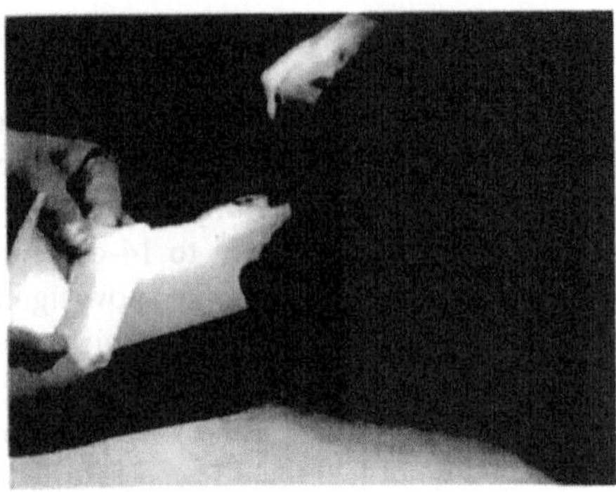

Figure 8 Application of opsite dressing.

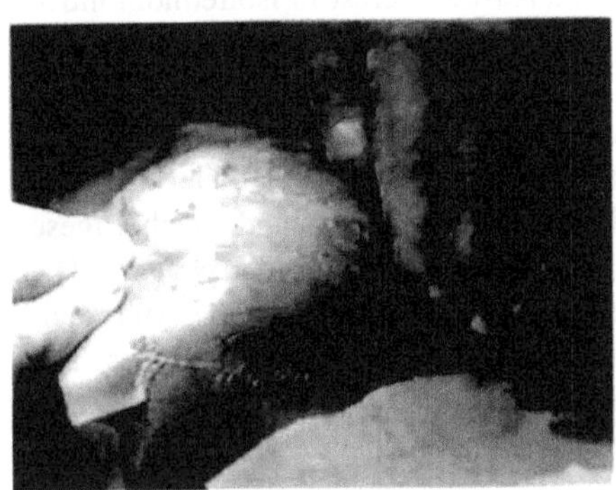

Figure 9 Application of dressing.

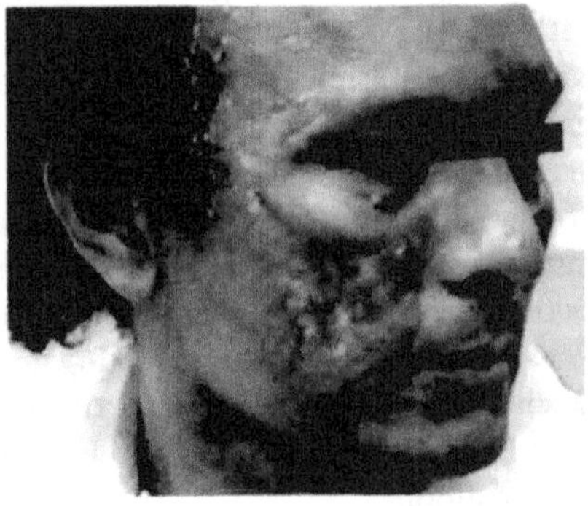

Figure 10 LDR scar revision at 2 weeks after operation.

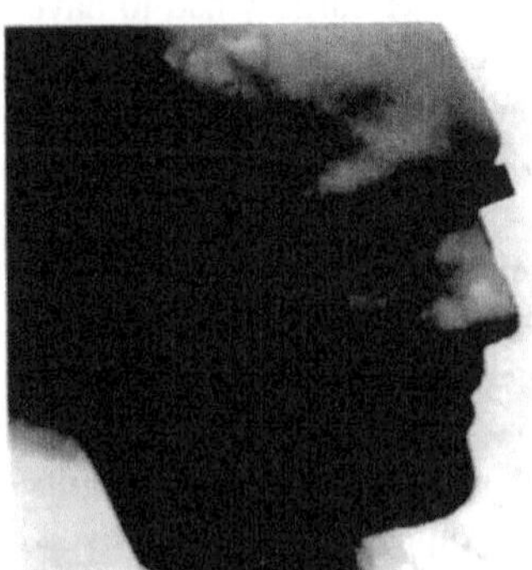

Figure 11 LDR scar revision at 6 weeks after operation.

over, aesthetic consequences become increasingly important to the patient. It is better to provide the patient with accurate expectations about surgery than to have to supply reasons for an unexpected unsatisfactory outcome. Depending on the nature of the original scar, it is now possible to select a procedure that will result in a scar with an improved appearance. The Z-plasty, M-plasty, W-plasty, and running W-plasty have their place for specific types of scars, but we are concerned primarily with improvement of the kinds of surgical scar defects that are particularly noted in postacne scarring. They are generally characterized by surface irregularities with typical hills and valleys suggesting the weather-beaten skin of a sailor or rancher.

DaSilva (5) was probably the first surgeon to perform dermal planing using the dermatome to smooth acne-scarred skin on the face. A special feature of the dermatome he used was a suction device connected to a vacuum pump that served to make the surface of the skin more uniform, particularly over the irregular contours of the face. Malherbe (6) used the dermatome successfully to treat cystic acne, which is generally conceded to be exceedingly difficult to treat with wire brushes. It became apparent that dermabrasion was not the final answer to postacne scar revision. There was a need for ancillary procedures to fine-tune the anticipated results of this cosmetic surgical procedure. It occurred to me that dermal planing was a good modality and that the work of Lloyd and Hight (7) on laminar escharotomy prior to skin grafting in burn cases might be applicable in the dermal planing procedure. These investigators performed their operations on patients under general anesthesia, and perhaps that is why their work did not attract dermatologic surgeons, who generally perform their surgical procedures on scars of the face using local anesthesia and topical refrigerants in office surgical suites.

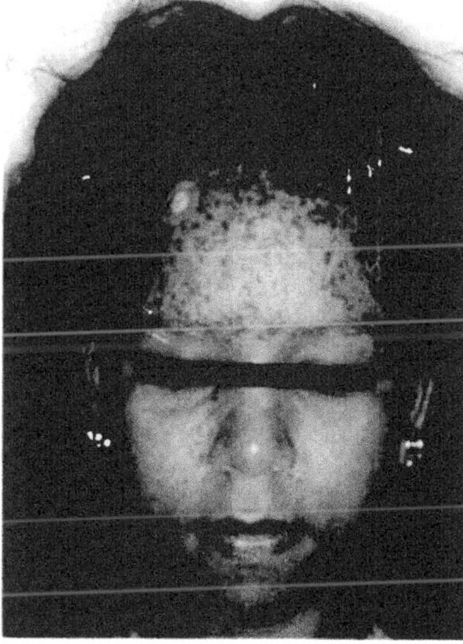

Figure 12 Black female with nevus of Ota with biopsy site on forehead.

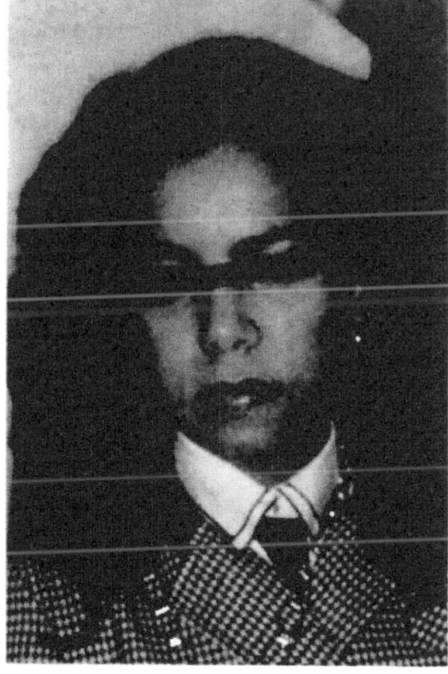

Figure 13 Three years after LDR of forehead and 35% TCA peel of face done concurrently.

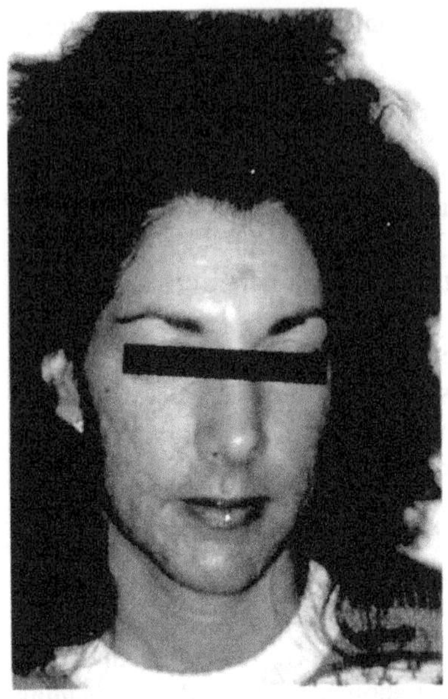

Figure 14 White female with postacne facial scarring.

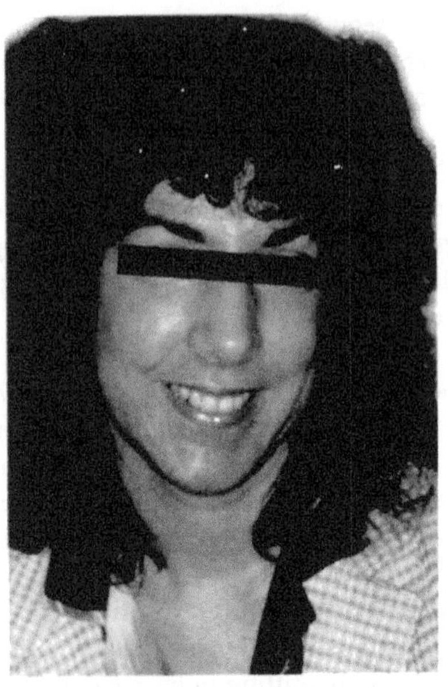

Figure 15 Six months after LDR of cheeks and chin and dermabrasion of forehead with persistent erythema.

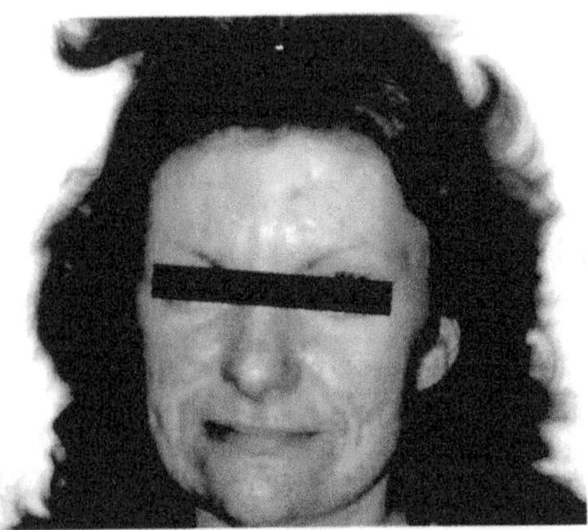

Figure 16 White female with postacne scarring.

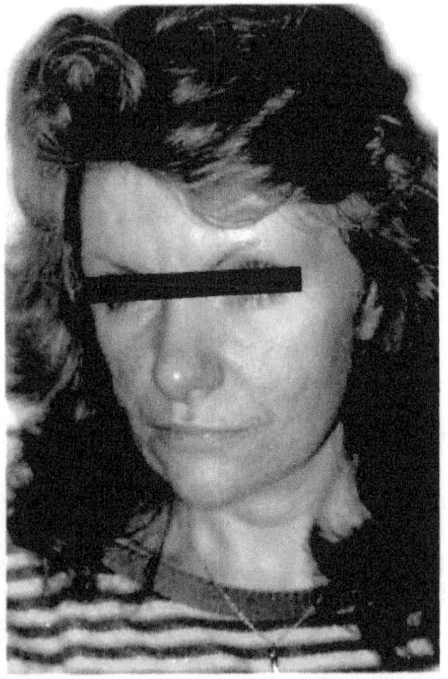

Figure 17 Nine months after LDR of face, forehead, and chin—feathering of cosmetic units with dermabrasion.

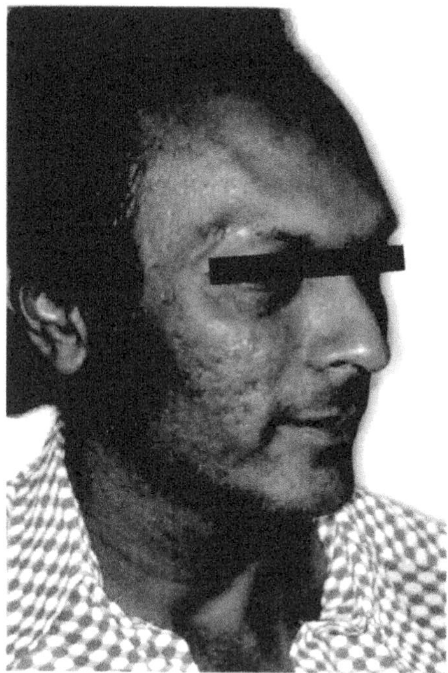

Figure 18 Black male with postacne scarring.

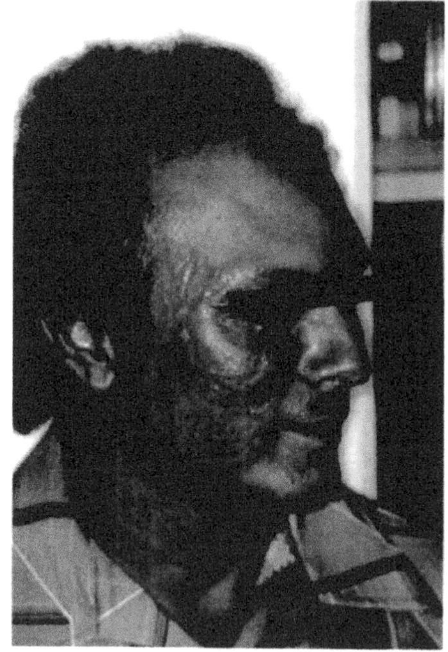

Figure 19 Four months after LDR and feathering of units with dermabrasion with benefit of cosmetic camouflage.

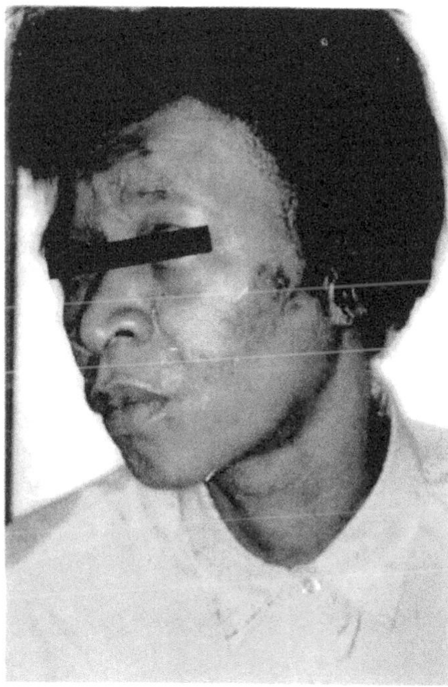

Figure 20 Black female with DLE scarring.

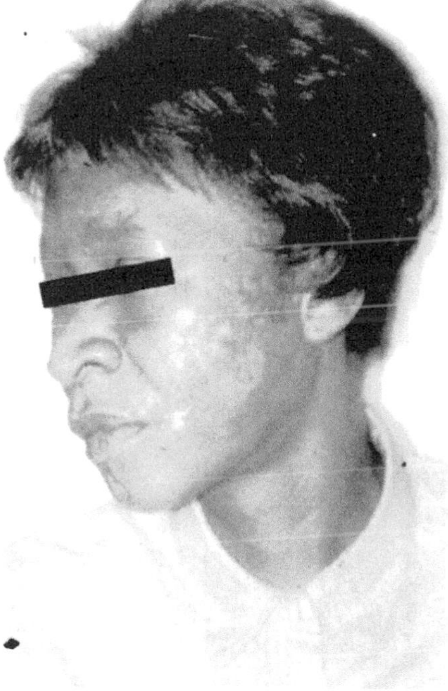

Figure 21 Six months after LDR and dermabrasion feathering.

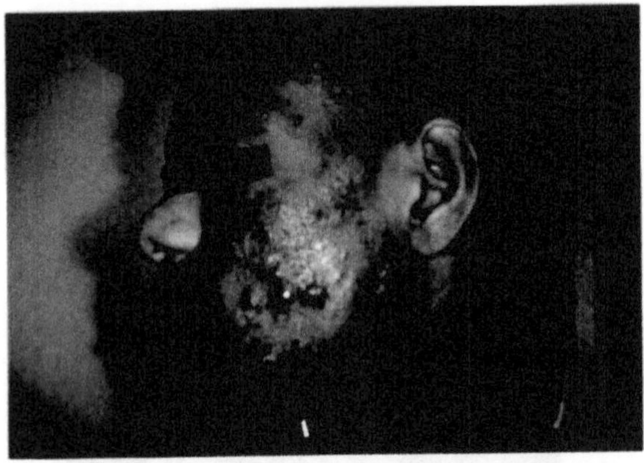

Figure 22 Black male with postacne scarring.

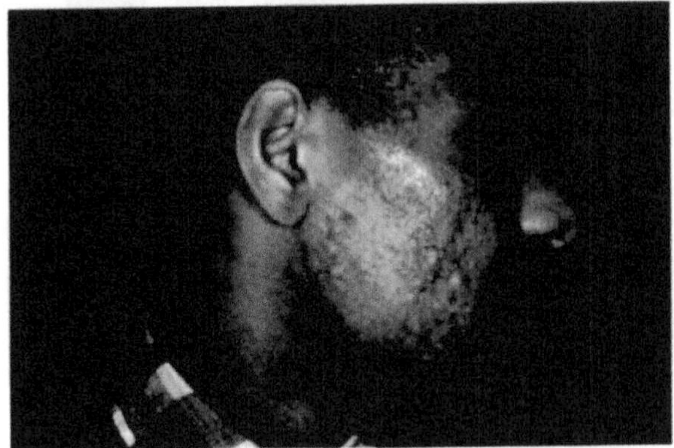

Figure 23 Six months after dermabrasion and marsupialization of cysts.

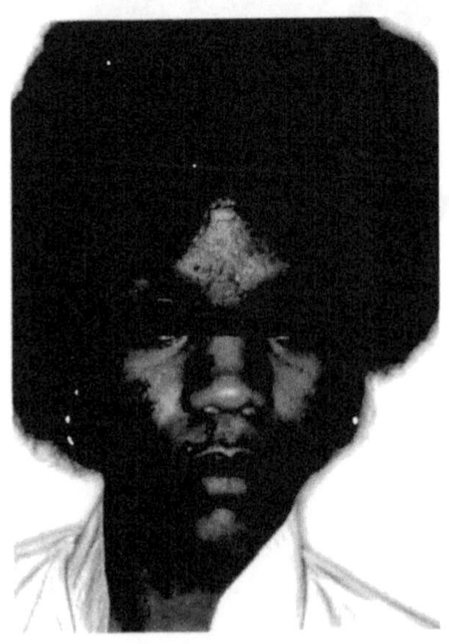

Figure 24 Black female with DLE scarring.

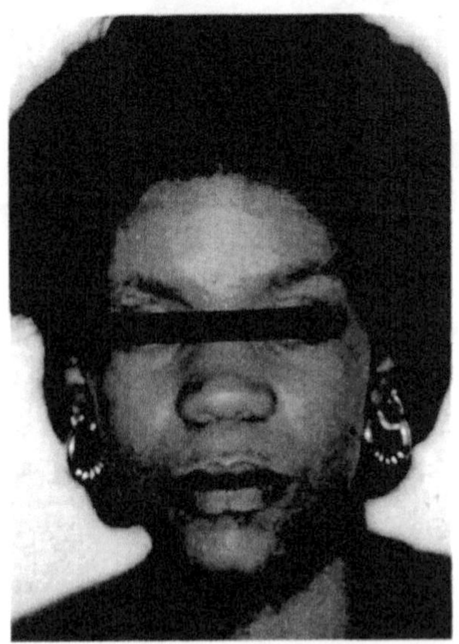

Figure 25 One year after LDR.

An early preoperative method for assessing the degree or depth of scarring of the face utilized a phototopographic technique involving a rubber roller impregnated with india ink. It was found helpful to place moistened 4 × 4 gauze pads in the mouth between the cheeks and teeth to bring out the surface that was to undergo laminar dermal reticulotomy. Observations in bold relief conveyed a sense of the improvement that was possible after the laminar dermal reticulotomy procedure and were compared with the postsurgical phototopographs (8). A technological improvement in this method of assessment today would involve computer imaging.

Laminar dermal reticulotomy, simply stated, is a technique involving precisely cut horizontal slabs of skin that encompass the ridges of the acne-scarred and traumatically scarred skin. It may be done before the dermabrasion procedure or after it for further improvement or, in some cases, used as the sole modality to improve the scarred skin. The patient is prepared for surgery appropriately sedated with hydroxyzine HCl (Vistaril, 25 mg) by mouth and diphenhydramine HCl (Benadryl, 25 mg) intramuscularly 20 minutes later. Meperidine (Demerol) may be given by mouth in a dose of 25–50 mg and an intravenous line established, and finally diazepam (Valium, 5–10 mg) is given intravenously. This is followed by a facial block, as described by Abadir, consisting of a regional block at the foramina at the exit of the supratrochlear, supraorbital, infraorbital, and mental nerves supplemented by radial injections of the area innervated by the auriculotemporal nerve from the point directly in front of the tragus of each ear. My preference is to use a 1% solution of lidocaine with 1:100,000 epinephrine to provide a facial field block and to use a spinal needle and 0.25% solution of lidocaine with 1:400,000 epinephrine to produce a profound anesthesia of these superficial tissues. It is wise to monitor the patient's vital signs while this is being performed. The tissue is hydrotomized further with infiltration of saline and 1:400,000 epinephrine to facilitate hemostasis. One then places saline-moistened gauze pads in the buccal space in a further effort to provide a dermal platform that is firm but not as rigid as that obtained with freezing.

I have generally used either the Davol-Simon Dermatome, which is preset to cut at 0.015 inch, or the Castroviejo Oculotome. Three or four passes of the instrument parallel to the relaxed skin tension lines are made carefully and palpably monitored each time with mineral-oiled gloved fingers to detect elevations that require more passes. In treating a complete face, generally the forehead is done first, followed by the temple and finally the cheeks. One works from the preauricular creases laterally to the nasolabial folds medially in the lower part of the infraorbital ridge superiorly and the skin overlying the mandible and the chin inferiorly. Feathering of the skin at the periphery of these areas around the nose, chin, and upper lips is best done with the course diamond fraise. No attempt is made to operate on the skin of the neck.

It should be noted that with a nonwhite patient the first step is to inform the patient that temporary dyschromic changes will result from such a technique, just as with dermabrasion. The typical sequence is one of hypopigmentation within 7–10 days during the early healing phase, followed by hyperpigmentation in the subsequent 2–4 months. The hypopigmentation cannot be avoided because of the mechanical removal of keratinocytes and melanocytes at the dermal-epidermal junctures. The hyperpigmentation, which is more of a postinflammatory phenomenon, can be modified with appropriate, timely dermatologic measures. To this end, epidermal regeneration can be facilitated by use of semiocclusive nonadherent dressings, and sunscreen with an SPF factor of 15 or more is recommended. In addition, bleaching agents such as hydroquinone or azaleic acid or kojic acid may be used for areas of patchy hyperpigmentation.

As with laser and other resurfacing procedures, a period of marked erythema may be managed with a low-potency topical corticosteroid, vitamin K, and vitamin C. The perioperative use of valacyclovir (Valtrex) is recommended for patients with a history of facial herpes simplex infections and for management of the periphery of treated areas requiring special attention. Here a feathering effect at the periphery of the aesthetic unit is created with either a chemical peel with 25% TCA or use of the diamond fraise.

In the completion of the laminar dermal reticulotomy procedure, the patient, upon recovery from anesthesia, has the face dressed with nonadherent dressing such as Opsite after the area has been cleansed with copious amounts of normal saline. The anticipated postoperative discomfort appears to subside rapidly, because the nerve endings are protected from the air and serous exudate quickly begins to bathe the traumatized surgical surface. The patient is permitted to shower and wash the hair the next morning and continue to do so at will for the next 6–8 days, during which time a concerted effort is made to prevent the formation of crusting. A smoother textured epidermis is evident. Frequent washing of the denuded face utilizing a lipophilic nonirritating facial cleanser followed by an aquaphor healing ointment serves to maintain the anticipated condition of the healing tissues.

In conclusion, dermabrasion, chemical face peel, and laminar dermal reticulotomy are cosmetic surgical procedures that, for the most part, because of lack of understanding on the part of the surgeon, have been regularly withheld in the management of acne scarring, rhytides, and posttraumatic scars in nonwhite patients with the admonishment that keloids or permanent pigmentary sequelae will result. Thirty years of experience has not proved this to be credible. Just as with white patients, selection of patients is of importance, taking into account history of scars and keloids, duration of previous dyschromia, and adequate motivation of the patient.

For discussion, one must consider the indications for a surgical plan that includes dermabrasion or laminar dermal reticulotomy (i.e., acne scars, active acne, Fox-Fordyce disease, senile rhytids, discoid lupus erythematosus traumatic scar, tattoos, dermatitis, papillaris capillitii, senile seborrheic keratoses, and adenoma sebaceum). Contraindications would include congenital ectodermal defects, radiodermatitis, keloids, burns, pyodermas, neurotic excoriations, and removal of identifying marks such as fingerprints. Complications of surgical planing techniques to be considered include hypertrophic scars, hyperpigmentation, hypopigmentation, autoeczematization, erythema, infection, and purpuric lesions.

It is noted that surgical planing is a viable therapeutic modality in the treatment of certain dermatologic conditions in nonwhite skin. Skin color in itself is not a contraindication to the use of this procedure. Indications, contraindications, and complications of surgical skin planing in dark-skinned patients are similar to those in white patients. Hypertrophic scarring and keloid formation are not complications to be feared with surgical planing of nonwhite skin, provided that on adequate history and examination have preceded the decision to perform these procedures. Patients may have keloids on one part of their body and have a successful surgical planing technique used on their face. Some dermatologists have a tendency to check a patient with keloids and hypertrophic scar formation by using a carbon dioxide applicator or planing an area the size of a dime or quarter on the abdomen or buttocks. This test may produce a hypertrophic scar because of the lack of dermal appendages in these areas. As one intends to utilize this technique as a preplaning procedure, it is reasonable that the pilot areas should be in the facial area, which is richly endowed with rapidly regenerative dermal appendanges. Furthermore, it is my opinion that if little or nothing is to be gained by surgical planing of a keloid or hypertrophic scar in ei-

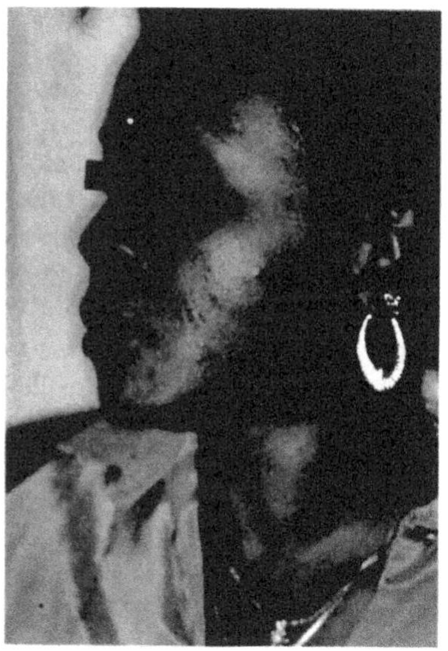

Figure 26 Black female with postacne scarring.

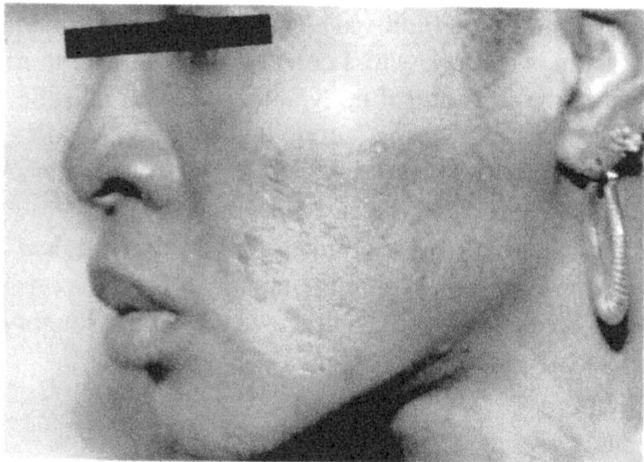

Figure 27 Six months after LDR and dermabrasion feathering of face.

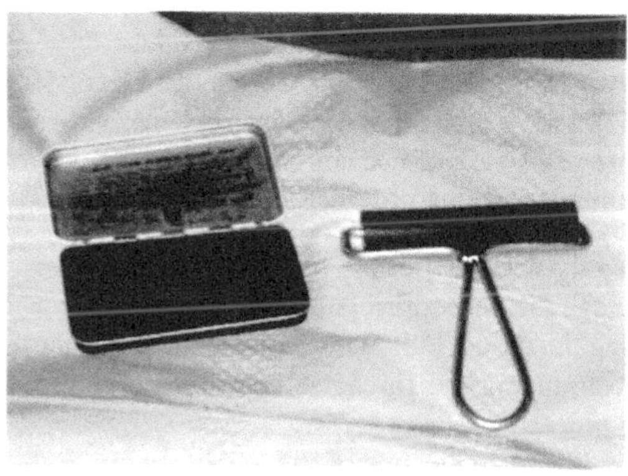

Figure 28 Rubber roller and ink pad used to scribe scar elevations before the LDR procedure.

ther white or nonwhite skin, dissuade the patient from pursuing this course. Pathologic studies of this tissue usually reveal a marked absence of these necessary regenerative dermal appendages. Healing of the skin following dermabrasion is accomplished by the proliferation of many adnexal epithelial cells derived from ectodermal buds, which are the remnants of dermal appendages. These spread out and coalesce, preserving their own anonymity as hair follicles and sweat and sebaceous apparatus in addition to the restoration of the normal protected epidermis.

Great care must be exercised in planing areas over bone prominences. Gouging must be avoided to preserve the integrity of the underlying dermal appendage so necessary to the healing process and prevention of scar formation. One must not attempt to plane the depth of ice-pick scars such as occur in some late acne scarring. It is advisable to resect and repair such scars before anticipated planing to obviate the necessity for planing too deeply. This procedure can reduce a four-stage operation to a one- or two-stage operation. Hyperpigmentation in light-skinned nonwhite patients, just as in white patients, is much more troublesome postoperatively than the depigmentation occurring in darker skinned patients. Judicious use of bleaching agents and avoidance of direct sunlight are helpful in achieving the desired cosmetic results.

Planing of facial lesions is a major surgical procedure. Due consideration must be given to the patient left with a completely denuded face. This area represents 5% of the total body surface. Although to date studies to determine fluid and electrolyte loss associated with this operation are lacking, the physician is dealing with a condition comparable to a severe second- or third-degree burn without the presence of nonviable tissue that must be phagocytized by the tissue and serum macrophages. It is my feeling that attention to postoperative management determines the degree of discomfort as well as the rate of recovery from the lymphedema and inflammation characteristic of the early healing phase.

My experience indicates that laminar dermal reticulotomy is a valuable surgical modality in the management of selected facial scarring of certain traumatic or postacne origin. It may be utilized as a primary or adjunctive procedure to maximize the benefit sought in remedying disagreeable scarring defects.

SUMMARY

The decision to use laminar dermal reticulotomy (LDR) for the cosmetic improvement of postacne or other suitable facial scars is preceded by a detailed physician-patient assessment of the risks, possible complications, and goals anticipated with the procedure.

LDR can be performed with a choice of instruments (i.e., the Coriotome, Davol Simon Dermatome, or Castroviejo Oculotome). I have used all of these instruments, and my choice is the Castroviejo instrument because of its ease of use and the ability to vary the thickness of the tissue removed by adjusting the shims provided with the instrument. Choice of tissue thickness may be limited by the depth of the midreticular skin layer.

Scribing of the skin includes outlining the scarred areas to be dermaplaned. Generally, the LDR procedure is designed to manage the deeper, irregular scars, and dermabrasion is suitable for fine tuning and feathering the tissue. Following suitable local anesthesia utilizing facial nerve blocks and hydrotomizing the forehead, cheeks, and chin to facilitate epidermal elevation, one can then proceed.

LDR is more easily accomplished after liberal application of sterile mineral oil. With moderate pressure on the skin, the instrument is observed to glide easily over the skin and a ribbon of skin emerges above the instrument. The assistant steadily grasps the tissue with Adson forceps. The surgeon may discontinue the cut by simply raising the cutting head. Hemostasis is controlled by increased pressure. Fine-tuning of the skin surface may be achieved with the dermabrader.

The patient's facial wounds are carefully irrigated with normal saline, and remaining debris is removed by manual damp gauze wiping. At this point, Opsite or Interface is applied to the raw surface and a Kling fluff dressing is applied for 24 hours.

Postoperative discomfort is remarkably minimal, probably because of the occlusive nature of the dressing. The dressing is removed, and postoperative care consists of frequent cleansing of the wound with warm water and soapless cleansers, such as Cetaphil or Aquanil, which suffices during recovery.

REFERENCES

1. Lloyd JR, Height DW. Early laminar excision: improved control of burn wound sepsis by partial dermatome debridement. J Pediatr Surg 1978; 13:698–706.
2. Kurtin A. Corrective surgical planing of the skin: new technique for treatment of acne scars and other skin defects. Arch Dermatol Syphilol 1953; 68:389–397.
3. Baker TJ, Gordon HL. The ablation of rhytids by chemical means, preliminary report. J Fla Med Assoc 1961; 48:451.
4. Colver GB. The infrared coagulator in dermatology. Dermatol Clin 1989; 7(1):155–167.
5. DaSilva G. Dermabrasion with the miniature electric suction dermatome. Plast Reconstr Surg 1962; 30:690–691.
6. Malherbe WDF. Dermatome dermaplaning and sycosis nuchae excision. Clin Plast Surg 1977; 4:289–296.
7. Lloyd JR, Hight DW. Early laminar excision: improved control of burn wound sepsis by partial dermatome debridement. J Pediatr Surg 1978; 13:698–706.
8. Pierce HE. Laminar dermal reticulotomy. J Dermatol Surg Oncol 1981; 7:43–49.

9
Scalpel Sculpting

Stephen N. Snow
University of Wisconsin Hospital and Clinics, University of Wisconsin Medical School
Madison, Wisconsin

Howard A. Oriba
University of Southern California School of Medicine
Los Angeles, California

I. INTRODUCTION

Scalpel sculpting refers to a variety of surgical techniques used to smooth the skin surface so that it blends seamlessly into the surrounding skin contours, using only the basic scalpel as the surgeon's tool. These sculpting techniques range from epidermal scraping of the skin surface to feather surface blemishes to intradermal planning of uneven postoperative scars of flaps and grafts. The following illustrations demonstrate the advantages of scalpel sculpting based on (a) the clinical assessment of the lesion itself; (b) low overall financial cost to the patient; (c) simplicity of instrumentality, time management, and execution; and (d) the likelihood of results that exceed the expectations of the patient.

Regardless of the scalpel technique, all wounds heal by second intention principally by reepithelialization over the exposed dermis. Knowledge of open-wound management is essential to optimize benefits from skin sculpting (see Chap. 1). Natural wound healing is especially suited for facial surgery, because the concentration of adnexal structures and underlying circulatory network are so extensive that wounds heal quickly with few complications. Second intention wound healing will be reviewed as it pertains to the clinical healing of superficial epidermal and dermal wounds with special emphasis on reducing the chances of dyschromasia and hypertrophic scars.

II. TECHNIQUES

Today, most dermatologic surgeons are trained in the traditional perpendicular incisions for standard side-to-side closures (Fig. 1). However, peeling away fine horizontal layers of skin is an art that requires a different but sometimes more natural form of manual dexterity for scar revisions. With the basic pencil grip scalpel position, almost all superficial skin lesions can be easily removed, and irregular facial scars can be improved by shaving the dermis followed by scraping the epidermal-dermal junction at the wound periphery (1).

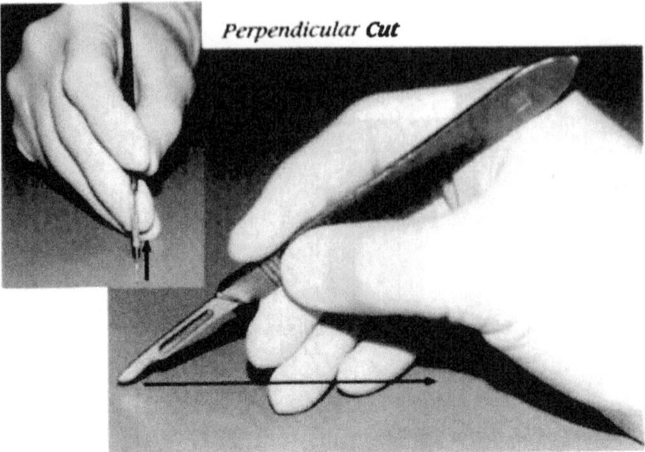

Figure 1 Traditional pencil grip position with scalpel held vertically for perpendicular incisions. Inset, vertical scalpel position (frontal view).

Three main scalpel techniques (Table 1) are used in skin surgery, depending on the how the scalpel is held between the fingers and the level of skin incision for which the particular scalpel-hand position is ideally suited (2). In addition, good skin traction is necessary to provide a relatively immobile surface while the skin is cut. To provide a greater degree of scalpel control, scalpel movement is preferably toward the surgeon.

A. Scraping Technique

Although the epidermis is normally tightly adherent to the papillary dermis, some of the superficial layers of the epidermis can be lightly deepithelialized at the edge of an open wound defect to a distance of 1 to 2 mm from the wound margin. In this technique (Fig. 2), the scalpel is held with a violin bow grip. The scalpel blade is placed perpendicular to the skin, with the blade handle about parallel to the skin surface. Generally, the scalpel handle is held between the thumb and three fingers as the scalpel is dragged across the skin with an acute blade angle toward the surgeon. Fragments of both the epidermis and dermis are scraped off together as the scalpel belly is brought across the skin in a repetitive broomlike

Table 1 Comparison of the Three Techniques of Excision and Their Application

Characteristic	Scraping	Reciprocating	Oblique
Microanatomy	Epidermis	Papillary dermis	Papillary-reticular dermis
Depth of excision	<0.1 mm	<0.5 mm	0.5–1.0 mm
Diameter of excision	1–2 mm	1–3 mm	3–10 mm
Lesion configuration	Pedunculated	Sessile	Intradermal
Examples	Whiskers	Hemangiomas	Freehand skin grafts
	Skin tags	Keloids	Micrographic surgical layers
	Seborrheic keratoses	Nevi	Perioral rhytids

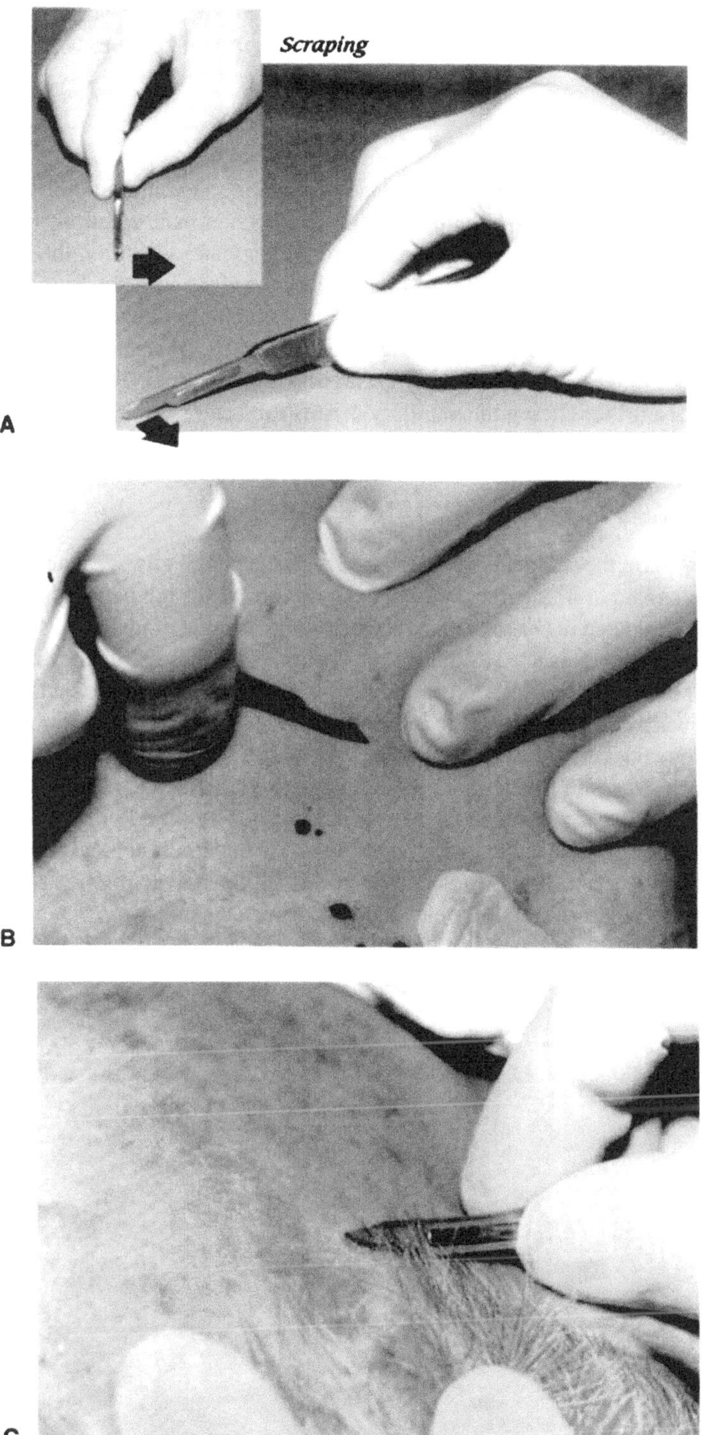

Figure 2 **(A)** Violin-bow grip position with scalpel held vertically for scraping the epidermal skin surface. Inset, vertical scalpel position (frontal view). **(B)** Scraping seborrheic keratoses with the violin-bow grip technique. **(C)** Scraping hair shafts with the violin-bow grip technique.

sweeping motion. On the flip side, scraping the skin with an obtuse blade angle works well to scrape off surface lesions such as hair shafts, skin tags, and seborrheic keratoses.

B. Reciprocating Technique

In the reciprocating technique (Fig. 3), the scalpel blade is positioned parallel to the skin surface while the scalpel is also held with a thumb-forceps grip or open-hand position. The cutting portion of the scalpel is the belly of the blade. To provide greater visibility, the direction of the cutting vector is generally to the side, rather than toward the surgeon. Surgery is easier and more stable when operating over a firm bony or cartilaginous convex skin site to allow clearance of the long surgical handle as it saws back and forth. Depending on surface convexity, from 1 to 3 mm of dermis is cut per oscillation of the scalpel. The reciprocating technique is very useful for slicing the papillary dermis for lesions on the forehead, scalp, or midline bridge and tip of nose.

C. Oblique Cutting Technique

In this technique (Figs. 4 to 6), the scalpel blade is grasped with the pencil grip. To start the surgery, the blade tip is angled at 45 degrees to pierce the dermis. After the dermis is incised, the hand is further supinated to permit a more acute 30-degree angle of incision while the wider belly portion of the blade is used as the cutting portion to increase efficiency and to maintain a more consistent level of incision in the dermis. The direction of the cutting vector is transversely toward the surgeon. As the incision proceeds, the blade is withdrawn and reinserted at the identical level of the dermis, advancing about 1 mm at a time with each stroke of the knife. The thickness of the dermal excision varies with the angle of the blade with the skin surface and the degree to which the dermis is expanded by intradermal injection of a local anesthetic. The oblique technique is a very versatile one to master and is frequently used to excise Mohs surgery layers for skin cancer evaluation, harvesting free skin grafts (3), and reducing the height of trap-door elevations, in selected cases.

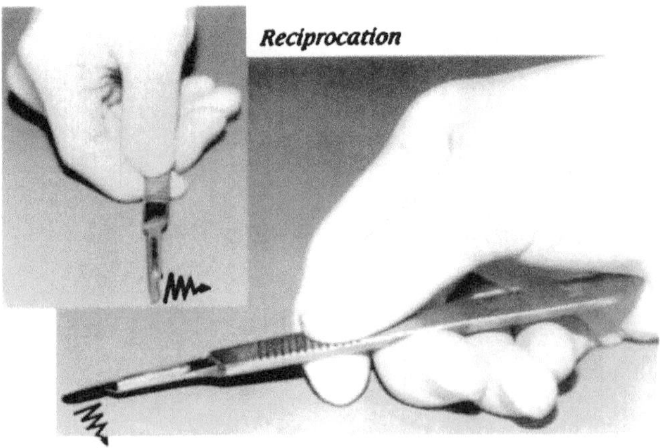

Figure 3 Violin-bow grip with scalpel held horizontal for cutting dermis parallel to the skin surface. Inset, horizontal scalpel position (frontal view).

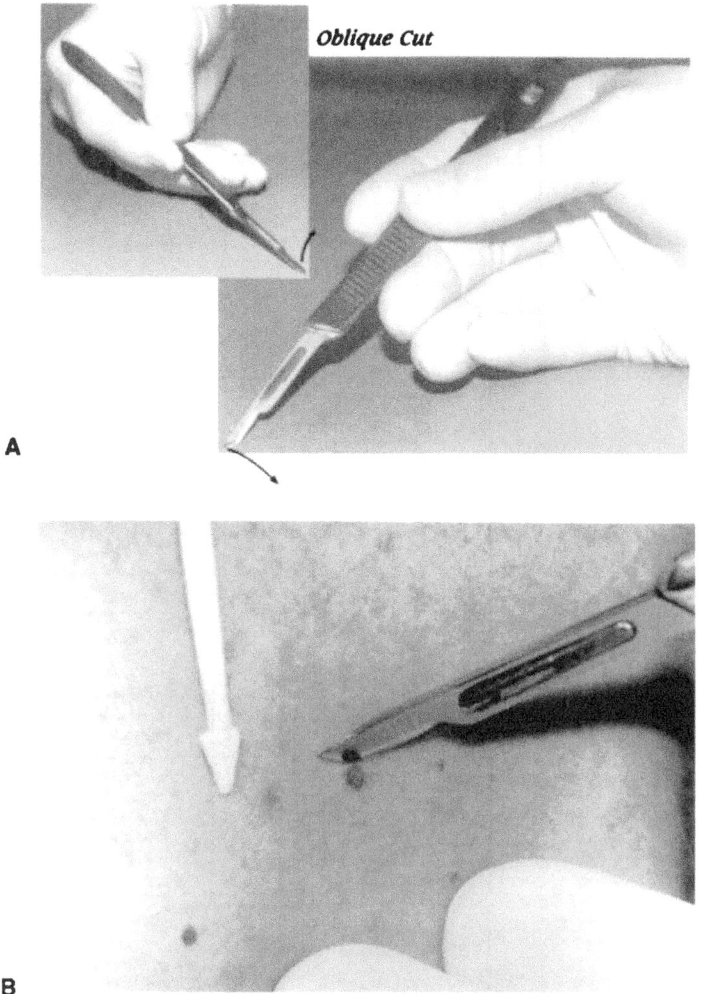

Figure 4 **(A)** Pencil grip position with scalpel held obliquely for transverse intradermal incision. Inset, oblique scalpel position (frontal view). **(B)** Scraping skin tags off the neck with the pencil grip technique.

III. PRACTICING THE TECHNIQUES

Fine skin surgery is an art that requires training, practice, and experience. At our institution, it often takes about 1 year of intensive daily hands-on cutaneous surgery to develop both the mechanical skill and the technical understanding to perform high-quality surgery on any facial site or from any position. There are several ways to practice sculpting, depending on the composition of the medium being cut and surgical technique used to slice it. The composition of an ordinary bar of soap closely mimics that of dermal tissue, an eggplant melon simulates fat, and the skin of a pig's foot resembles soft youthful human skin. Our preference is to practice on a bar of soap and a melon because they are readily available, can be hand held or taped for stability, and simulate opposite ends of human tissue composition. Your ability

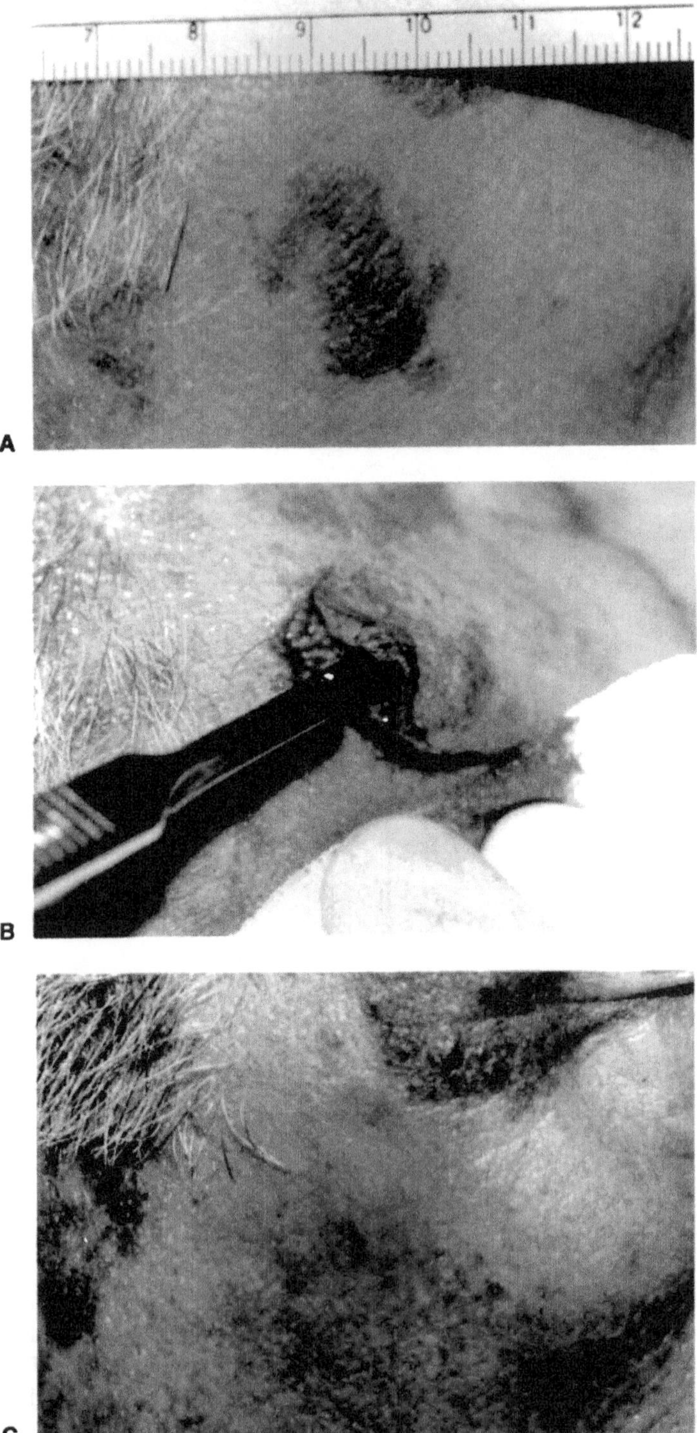

Figure 5 **(A)** Preoperative photograph of superficial hemangioma of the right cheek. **(B)** Intraoperative photograph showing intradermal excision by oblique technique. **(C)** Postoperative photograph after 1 month follow-up.

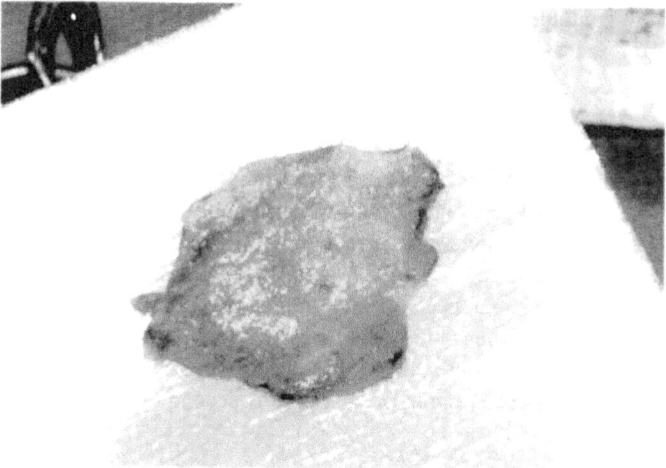

Figure 6 Freehand split-thickness skin graft harvested by oblique technique, size 2 cm, thickness less than 1.0 mm.

to control and finely sculpt these two different media equates with ability to cut any tissue (including skin) whose tissue composition lies in between these two extremes.

Practice whittling, scraping, and carving bits of soap using a relatively dull 1-inch-long blade such as found in a pocket knife or jackknife (Fig. 7). Safe handling techniques are learned by practicing whittling toward yourself, to understand not only blade distance but also force and direction of the sharp blade edge. When the flat scalpel handle is rotated, the fingertips and interosseous muscles finely control the scalpel tip to start the incision, while the wrist and forearm muscles control the scalpel belly and thickness of the intradermal excision. The reciprocating and oblique slicing techniques are practiced on an eggplant or cucumber. The body of these vegetables is soft and relatively inflexible, so that when scalpel sculpting is out of control, a series of unplanned cleavage planes and notches are

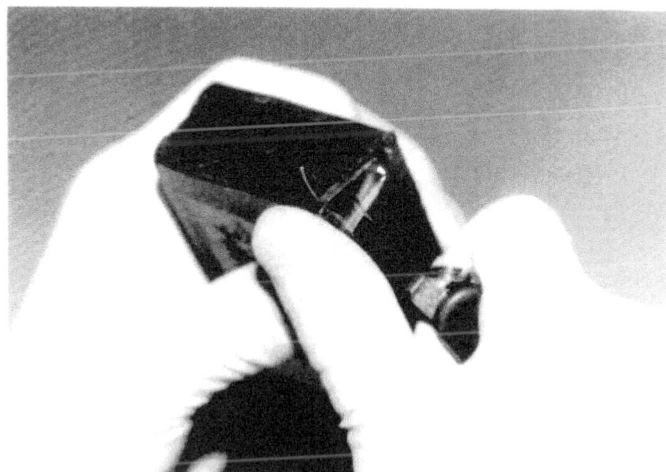

Figure 7 Shaving soap by whittling toward the operator increases dexterity and safety.

made instead of a smoothly cut contoured surface. As your dexterity improves, move on to pig's feet or a similar medium.

IV. APPLICATIONS

Performing scalpel sculpting well requires practice, experience, and understanding (Figs. 8 to 16). Each technique must be mastered separately and then harmoniously integrated into your surgical style to provide a systematic approach to managing the diversity of skin lesions that require skin sculpting surgery. Calibrating the surgery to reach the desired end point of aesthetic surgery is a difficult goal to achieve, because sculpting end points themselves are not hard fixed lines (like sutured closures) and the cosmetic results from second intention healing are 1 to 2 months in the future. In the end, the art of sculpting is the simplicity of the technique, and the end of simplicity is the beginning of sculpting by second nature.

A

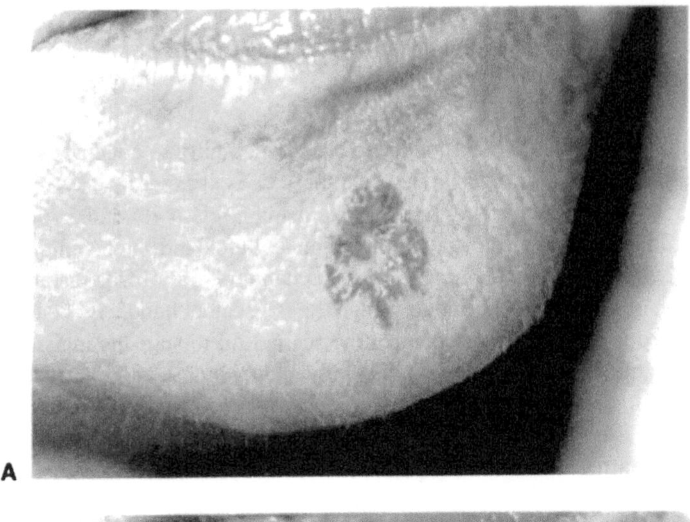

B

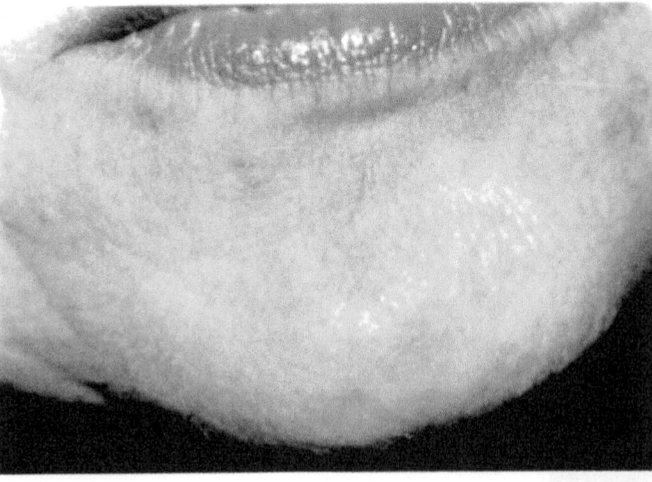

Figure 8 **(A)** Preoperative chin scar revised by reciprocation and scraping. **(B)** Postoperative result of scalpel sculpting.

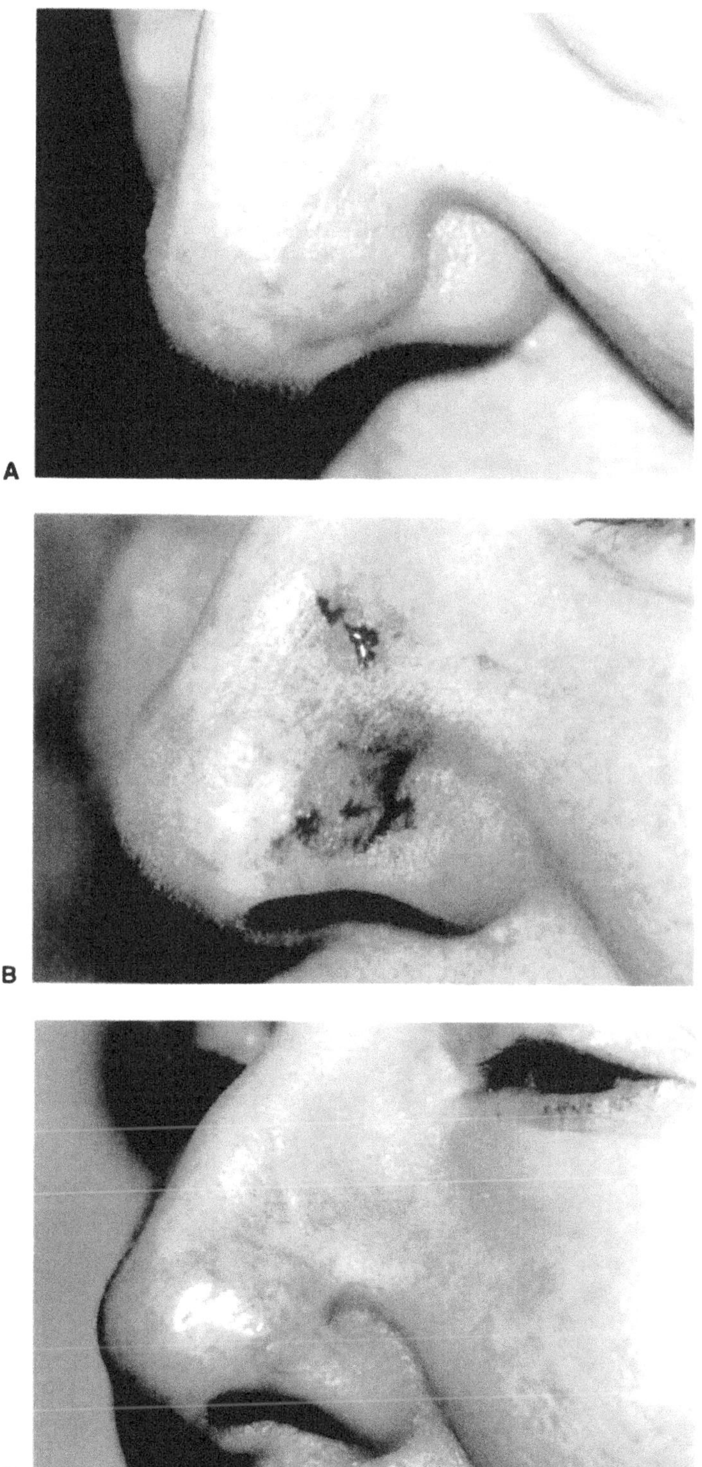

Figure 9 **(A)** Nasolabial transposition flap to left ala with subsequent development of trap-door deformity. **(B)** Revision of trap-door flap by scalpel sculpting. **(C)** Appearance of revision after 6 month follow-up.

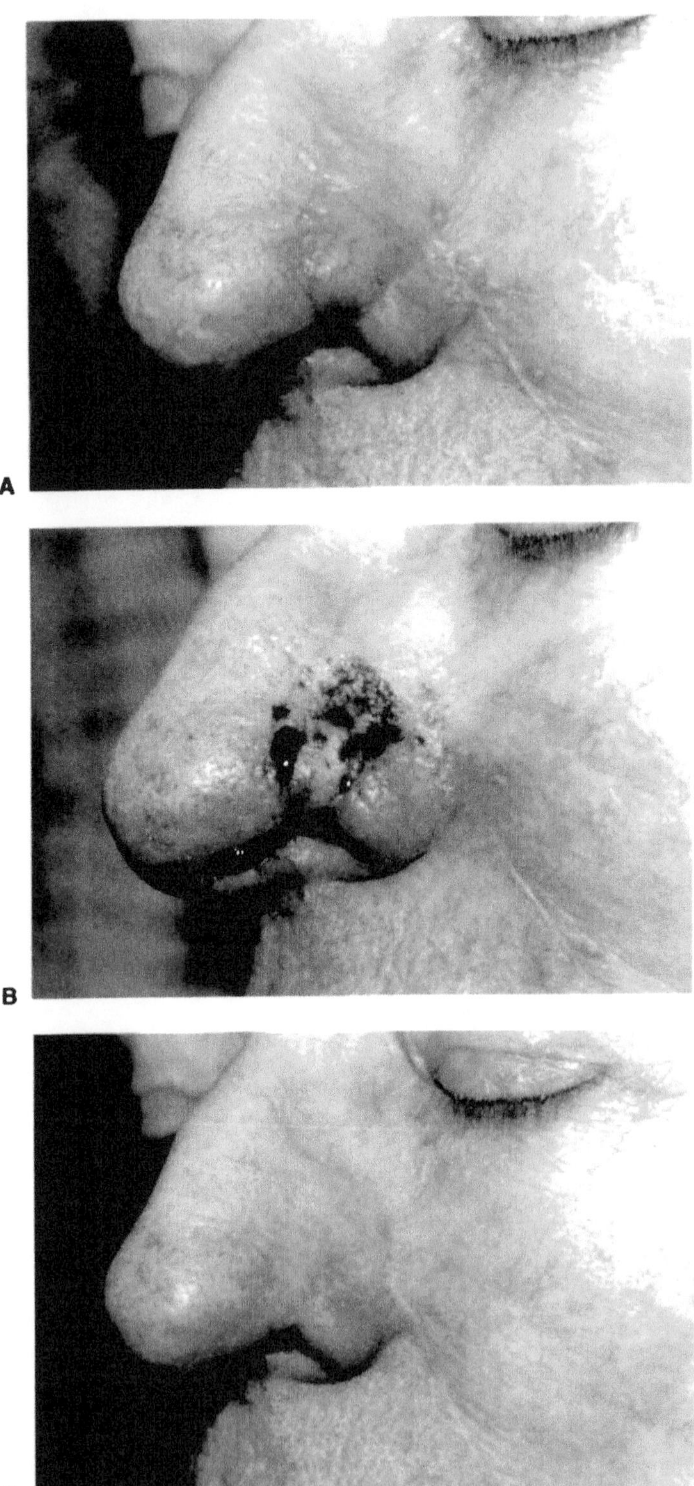

Figure 10 **(A)** Persistent trap-door deformity of nasolabial flap at 6 months follow-up. **(B)** Revision of trap-door flap by scalpel sculpting. **(C)** Appearance of flap revision at 7 month follow-up.

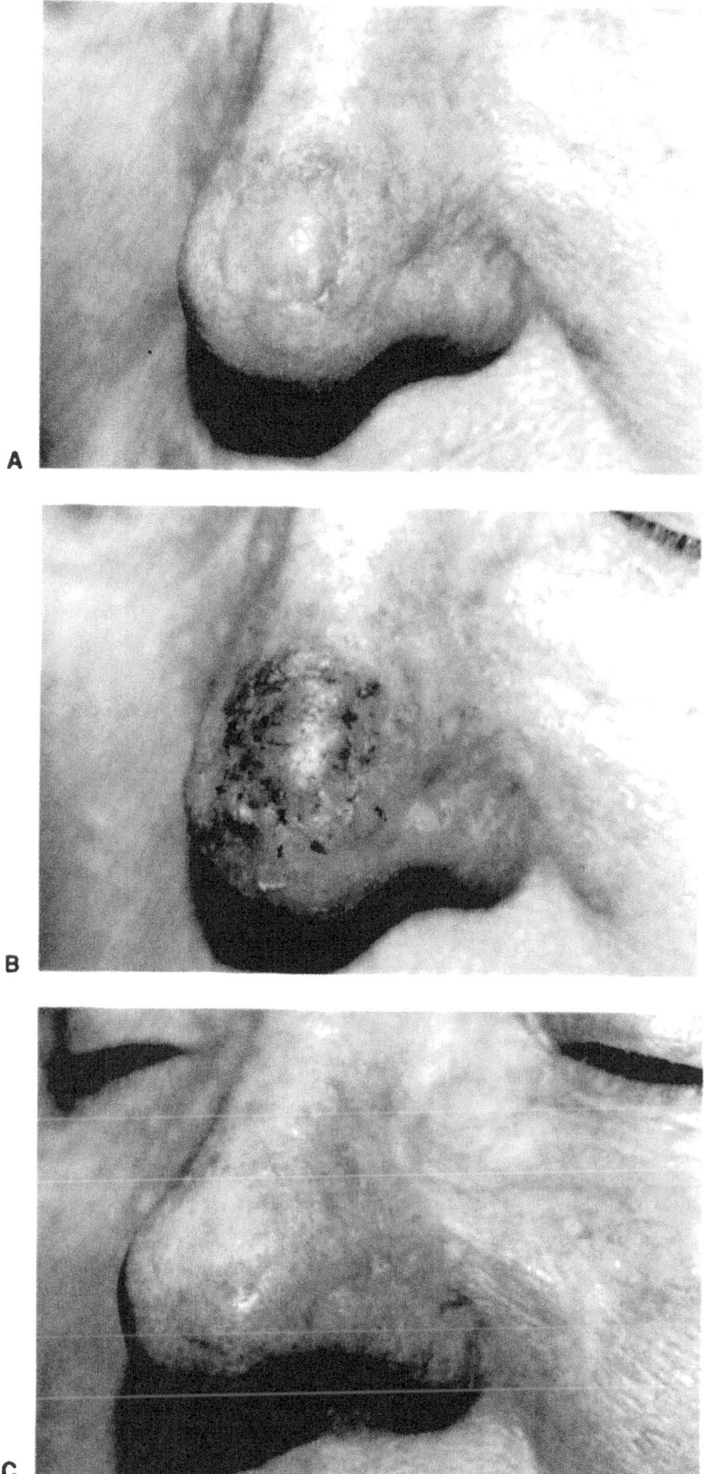

Figure 11 **(A)** Preoperative photograph of full-thickness skin graft of the left tip of nose. **(B)** Intraoperative photograph to show sculpting of the graft margin. **(C)** Postoperative photograph after 6 months of follow-up.

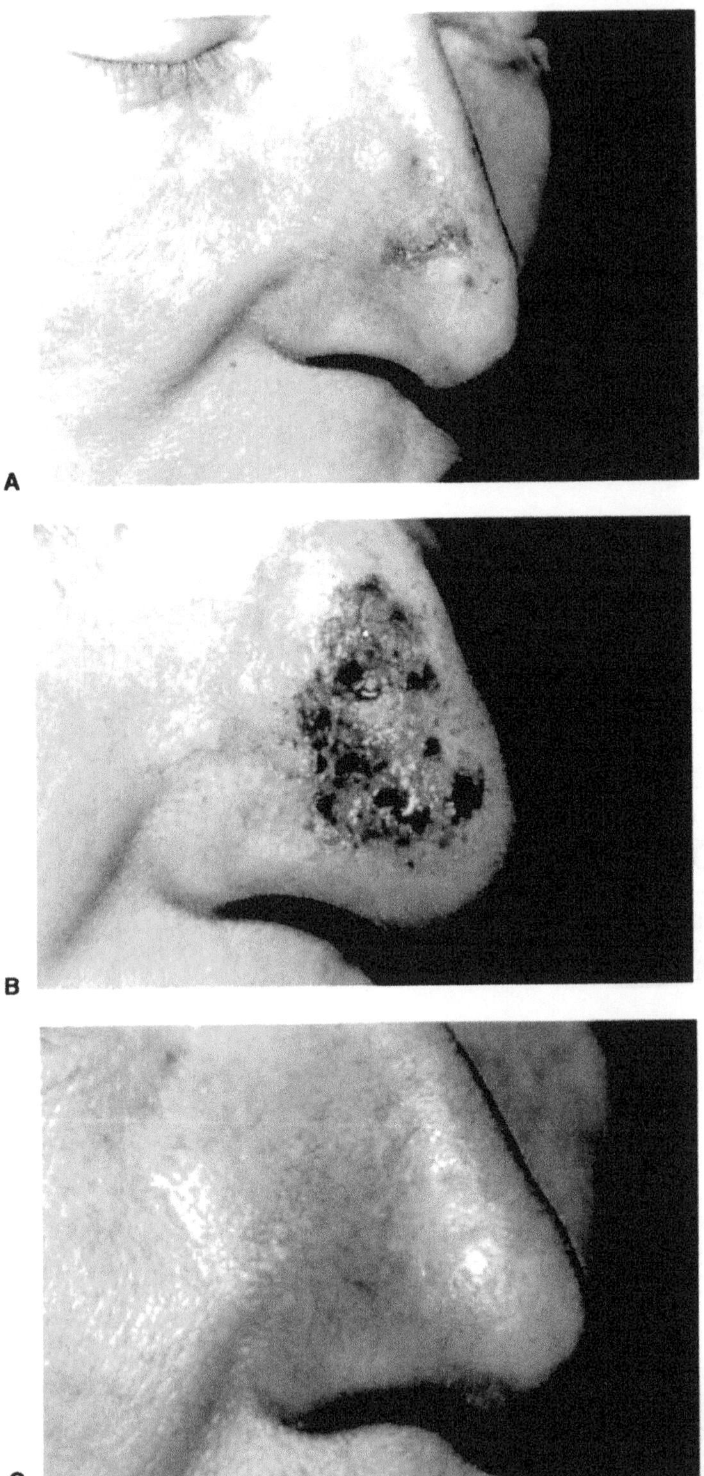

Figure 12 **(A)** Preoperative photograph of full-thickness skin graft of right bridge of nose. **(B)** Intraoperative photograph to show sculpting of entire graft. **(C)** Postoperative photograph after 6 months of follow-up showing smoother contour but slight hypopigmentation.

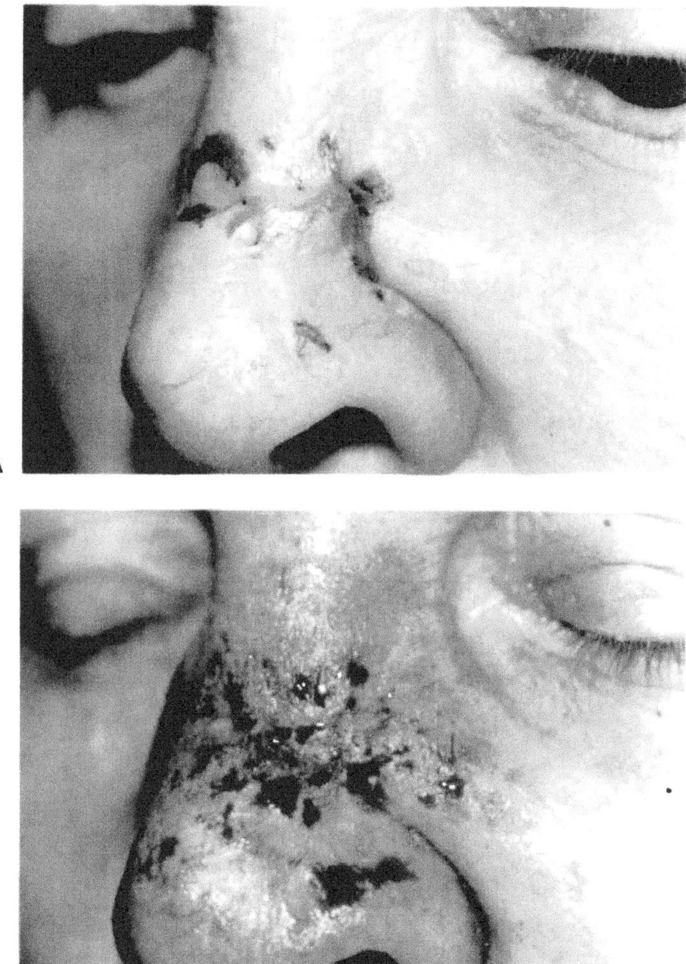

Figure 13 **(A)** Preoperative appearance of nasal bridge scar as a result of second intention healing. **(B)** Intraoperative appearance after hypertrophic stellate scar was sculpted followed by manual dermabrasion with sponge abrasive. **(C)** Postoperative result after 7 months of follow-up. **(D)** Close-up of sponge impregnated with coarse aluminum oxide abrasive. The sponge's right angle corner was cut to blunt its sharp edge. *(figure continues)*

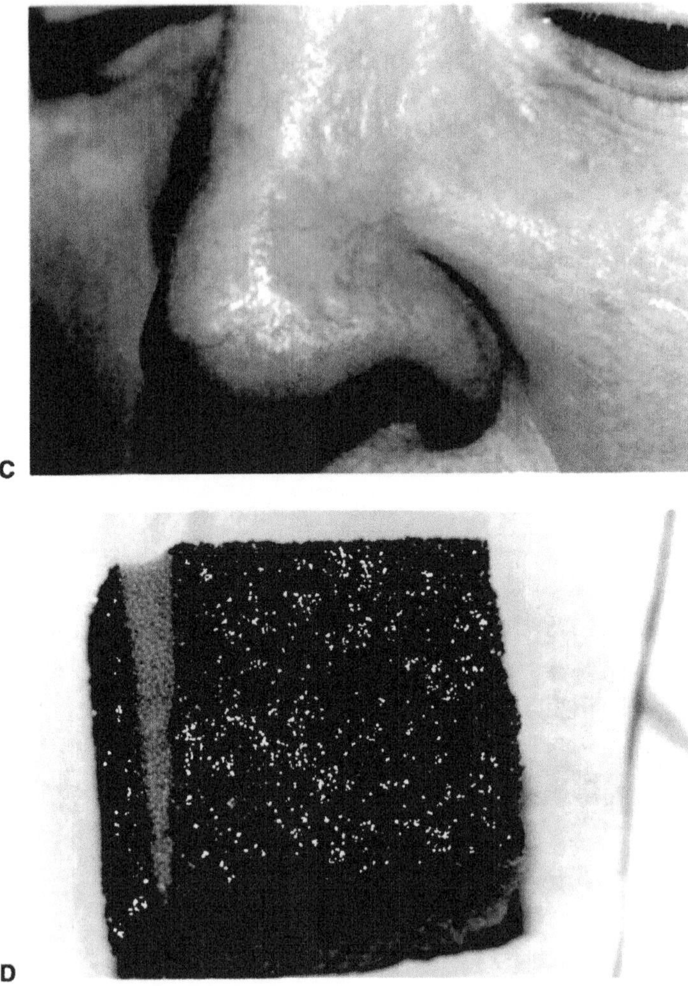

Figure 13 *(continued)*

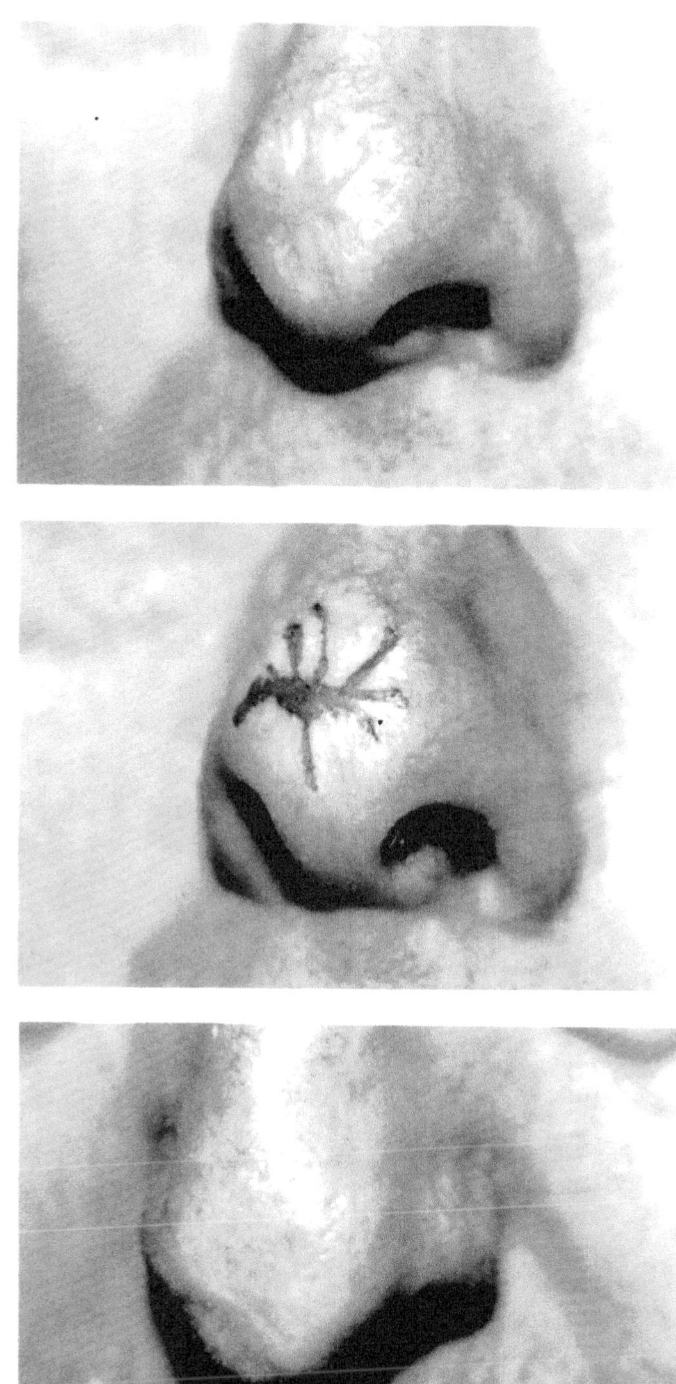

Figure 14 **(A)** Preoperative photograph to show nasal tip scar. **(B)** Photograph to show the stellate hypertrophic ridge pattern of the scar. **(C)** Postoperative photograph after sculpting and manual dermabrasion using sanding sponge.

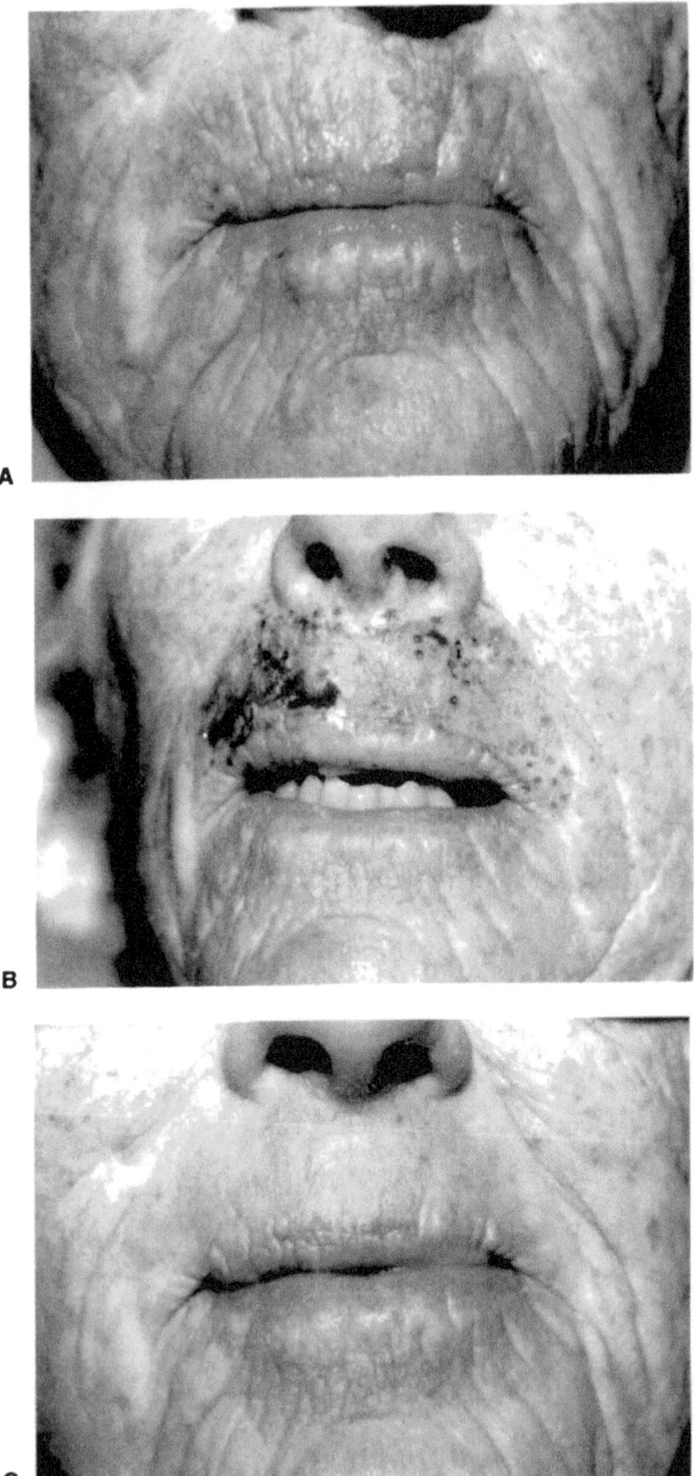

Figure 15 **(A)** Preoperative photograph showing extensive perioral rhytids of the upper lip. **(B)** Intraoperative photograph after sculpting left and then right upper lip. **(C)** Postoperative photograph of upper lip after 1 year of follow-up.

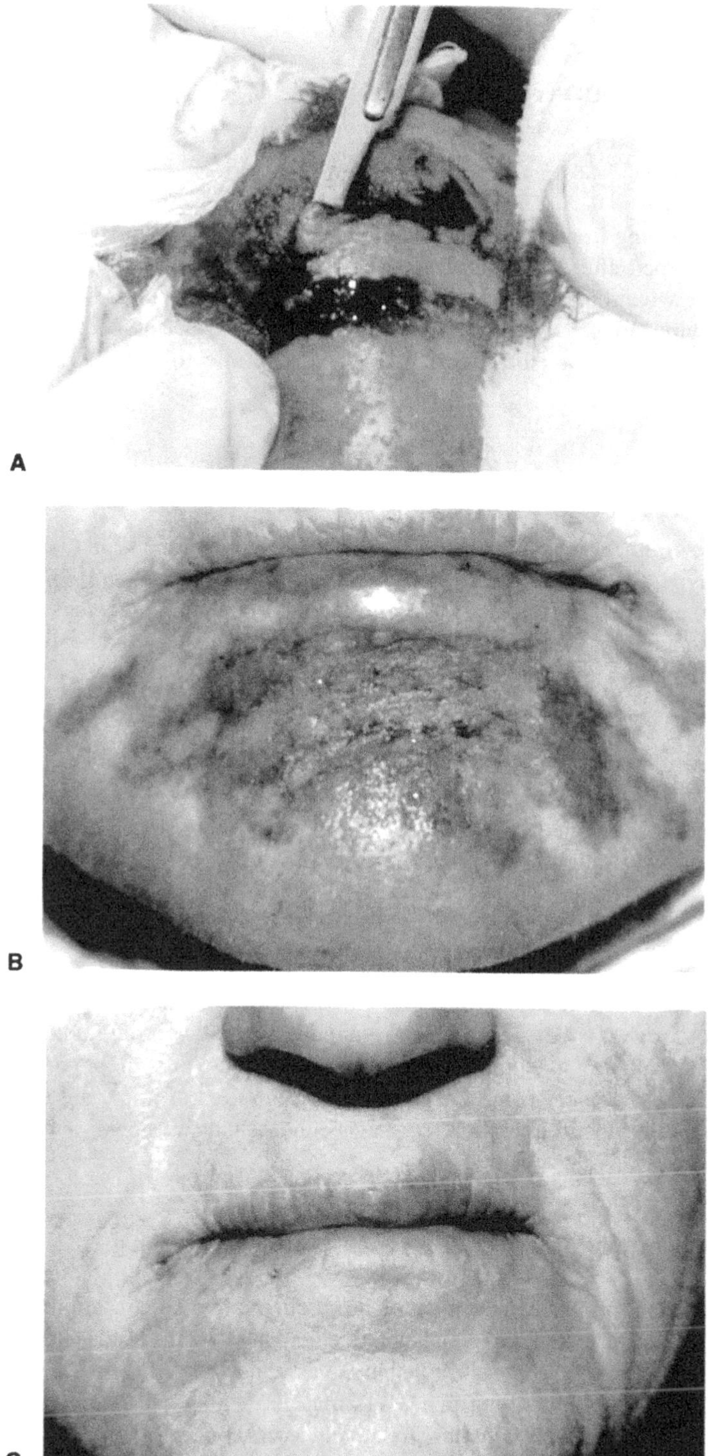

Figure 16 **(A)** Intraoperative photograph to show resculpting of skin of the lower lip and chin. **(B)** Immediate postoperative wound after sculpting. **(C)** Postoperative photograph after 6 months of follow-up. The upper lip was sculpted 1 year earlier, as reported in a previous publication (1).

V. DETERMINANTS OF GOOD WOUND HEALING

A. Timing

When smoothing scars resulting from healing by second intention, flaps, or grafts, scalpel sculpting is ideally performed after the perioperative edema and inflammation have resolved so that the uneven wound margins may be accurately assessed. Timing is not usually an issue when removing benign or malignant lesions of the skin surface unless the patient is taking an anticoagulant or isotretinoin (4), or susceptible to postoperative hyperpigmentation.

B. Skin Quality

There are three major determinants of rapid and uncomplicated healing of the skin: (a) the patient's intrinsic skin type, (b) the biologic age and composition of the skin, and (c) the condition of the underlying blood circulation. Successful surgical sculpting outcomes are predicated on an understanding of the basic microscopic events of human wound healing, balanced against the patient's own intrinsic healing nature.

C. Skin Type

Individuals with Fitzpatrick skin type I or II are particularly suited for surface skin work because they heal readily with minimum hypertrophic scars and dyspigmentation.

D. Biologic Age of the Skin

The chronologic age of the patient is usually known, but when dealing with open-wound healing, the skin's biologic age is a better predictor of wound healing. A youthful biologic skin results in quicker, high-quality wound healing. Excessive exposure to radiation or ultraviolet light ages the skin biologically, diminishing the concentration of important epidermal-adnexal cells and the blood circulation, so that wound healing is slower and of poorer quality.

E. Underlying Blood Circulation

The rate of skin regeneration is primarily dependent on its vascular circulation. Midline facial sites such as the forehead, nose, lips, and chin have excellent direct, collateral, and contralateral circulation. Also, in these midline sites the blood vessel network of the dermis is in direct communication with the underlying fascia and muscle without any intervening subcutaneous layer of fat which typically contains a relatively lower concentration of blood vessels per cubic millimeter of tissue. Skin flaps that are fed by a direct arterial blood supply can undergo more intrusive flap revision than flaps that have random blood. Because the circulation of skin grafts is marginal, scuplting should be performed delicately. Finally, patients who suffer from diabetes or smoke tobacco products incessantly are at risk of compromised tissue perfusion.

VI. WOUND CARE

The aim of open-wound management is to achieve the desired high-quality cosmetic result as easily, conveniently, inexpensively, and rapidly as possible. A successful outcome is based on developing a strategy that combines the current state of scientific art on wound healing tempered with the practical needs of your population of patients. For example, some patients prefer dry wounds, whereas others prefer moist wounds. The following is a brief focused description of how facial superficial wounds heal. These perspectives are honed after 15 years of observation and experience of wound healing by second intention of facial defects. The depth of the wound ranges from that of wounds made by laser ablation of the epidermis to deep subcutaneous wounds created by scalpel excision.

A. Horizontal Epidermal Wounds

True epidermal wounds clinically show scaling and exfoliation of epidermal cells without visible blood from capillaries in the dermal papilla. Wound healing is achieved by keratinocyte migration over a partially intact layer of basal cells. The application of a topical ointment or an occlusive dressing adds moisture and speeds the reepithelialization.

B. Horizontal Papillary-Dermal Wounds

Once the dermal envelope is breached, blood and extracellular fluids leak out to form a rudimentary fibrin lattice over the intact papillary dermis. Epidermal migration occurs under this lattice to reseal the wound. The duration of the reepithelialization varies from 1 to 2 days for direct closures to 7 to 10 days for punch biopsies. Immediately after surgery, the application of a thick layer of ointment and several minutes of pressure prevents evaporative water loss and creates an ideal wound-healing chamber. With carbon dioxide laser ablation surgery in older patients undergoing superficial epidermalectomy, the epidermis is reestablished in about 9 days after wounding. Because the papillary dermis is maintained, reepithelialization readily occurs, mainly from the centrifugal migration of epidermal cells originating from the periadnexal structures. The appearance of these superficial wounds is very good.

C. Horizontal Reticular Dermal Wounds

Wounds that expose the superficial reticular dermis heal more slowly and are of poorer cosmetic quality than papillary dermal wounds. Epidermal proliferation is reduced because the dermal section of ductal epithelium has less proliferative potential than the poral intraepidermal portion of the duct. Ideally, sculpting techniques should be above the midreticular dermis unless the blood circulation and adnexal concentration are of sufficient quality and magnitude to generate acceptable wound-healing cosmetic results, such as on the central regions of the face.

VII. COMPLICATIONS

Surgical sculpting recontours the topography of the skin. How the wound ultimately heals depends on the intrinsic quality of the host skin (skin type, age, degree of radiation damage, etc.) as well as the local care provided by the patient.

A. Pigment Alteration

Skin pigmentation is mainly a function of melanin synthesis and melanosome distribution within the melanocyte and epidermal cells. After sculpting, reepithelialization occurs by epidermal proliferation and migration. Repigmenation of the scar, however, is due to redistribution of pigment through a dendritic network maze within the scar. Hypothetically, postoperative hyperpigmentation may be due to the sudden unmasking of the protective epidermal umbrella, which exposes the underlying melanocytes to excessive sunlight, stimulating melanin synthesis and distribution of pigment throughout the partially fractured melanocytic network system. Irregular and prolonged pigmentation is aggravated when freed melanosomes and hemosiderin are captured in the papillary dermis, where pigment turnover is slow. For hemostasis we use light electrocautery and do not use aluminum chloride or ferric subsulfate. If the patient is taking aspirin, we use Oxycel cotton cellulose (Becton Dickinson, Franklin Lakes, NY 07417) and pressure for hemostasis. Use of sunscreens, steroids, and hydroquinone 2 weeks before surgery may prevent postoperative hyperpigmentation. A mixture of tretinoin (Retin-A), steroid, and hydroquinone often will diminish postoperative hyperpigmentation in patients with Fitzpatrick skin types III, IV, and V (5). Azelex (azeleic acid 20%) is also useful. Postoperative hypopigmentation can also result after sculpting fragile grafts (Fig. 11).

B. Hypertrophic Dermal Scars

Hypertrophic dermal scarring is best avoided by proper assessment of the site before surgery, matching proportionately the depth of dermal excision with the degree of local blood circulation, and avoiding postsurgical complications such as infection or bleeding. Hypertrophic scars are typically managed by intralesional injection of 0.2 mL of 0.1% triamcinolone per square centimeter of scar every 8 weeks until the desired result is achieved. There are some anecdotal reports that CO_2 laser excision may minimize hypertrophic scar formation.

C. Excessive Dilatation of Follicular Pores

Nasal tip wounds that heal by second intention sometimes have follicular poral openings that stretch toward the axis of contraction. When additional sculpting is performed to these sites, the diameter of these slits may be further enlarged because of either a more acute cutting angle through the poral cylinder or asymmetric contraction of the dermal collagen.

D. Infection

We usually prescribe cephalexin, erythromycin, or tetracycline when sculpting large scars or perioral rhytids. If the patient has a history of facial herpetic lesions, we also prescribe acyclovir before treatment (6). The risk of superinfection of facial sites less than 10 cm^2 in area is low.

VIII. CONCLUSION

Skin sculpting is a surgical art that requires a combination of experience and judgment to use a variety of treatment techniques applied in tandem or sequentially over time to achieve the desired cosmetic result for the patient. The experienced dermatologic surgeon will find some of these suggestions self-evident. Newly minted physicians may find them more helpful because there is no single scalpel technique that is appropriate for every blemish in all facial sites. Scalpel sculpting is about the intermixing of various hand and finger positions, and perhaps creating new positions unique to your own particular style, and wielding the scalpel in whatever manner is necessary to manipulate the skin to accomplish the desired outcome. One should always bear in mind that the competence of underlying blood circulation is critical to wound healing. Unlike skin grafts, well-vascularized perioral areas are more forgiving and can often be repeatedly sculpted. Having a good comprehensive and contemporary knowledge of the various simple and complex treatment options helps to bridge the gap between perfection and reality. Proper assessment of the skin and efficient surgical execution ensure quality wound-healing results and seamless surgical scars.

REFERENCES

1. Snow SN, Stiff MA, Lambert DR. Scalpel sculpturing. Techniques for graft revision and dermatologic surgery. J Dermatol Surg Oncol 1994; 20:120–126.
2. Anderson RM, Romfh RF. Technique in the Use of Surgical Tools. New York: Appleton-Century-Crofts, 1980.
3. Snow SN, Zweibel S. Freehand skin grafts using the shave technique. Arch Dermatol 1991; 127:633–635.
4. Rubenstein R, Roegnick HH Jr, Stegman SJ, Hanke CW. Atypical keloids after dermabrasion of patients taking isotretinoin. J Am Acad Dermatol 1986; 15:280–285.
5. Kligman AM, Willis I. A new formula for depigmenting human skin. Arch Dermatol 1975; 111:40–48.
6. Perkins SW, Sklarew EC. Prevention of facial herpetic infections after chemical peel and dermabrasion: new treatment strategies in the prophylaxis of patients undergoing procedures of the perioral area. Plast Reconstr Surg 1996; 3:427–433.

10

Laser Revision of Scars

Tina S. Alster

Washington Institute of Dermatologic Laser Surgery and Georgetown University Medical Center Washington, D.C.

I. INTRODUCTION

Laser irradiation of scars was first reported in the 1980s using a variety of available laser systems. Results were limited by scar recurrences, which were not unlike those observed after other surgical revision techniques. Since that time, refinements in laser technology as well as advances in laser techniques have enabled dermatologic surgeons to better define which lasers are best used for different types of scars without the adverse sequelae and recurrence rates noted with previous surgical treatments and laser systems.

II. SCAR CATEGORIZATION

A. History

The etiology and pathogenesis of excessive scar formation remain poorly understood despite the fact that the first documentation of an abnormal (keloid) scar was over a millennium ago in the 10th century writings of the Nigerian Yoruba tribe (1). The term "keloid" (Greek *chele* = crab claw), first introduced in 1817 by Alibert (2), is often used synonymously with the term "hypertrophic scar," although the two lesions are significantly different. Proper scar categorization is important in order to choose the appropriate laser for optimal scar treatment.

B. Clinical and Histologic Features

Because it is difficult to determine the quality and quantity of collagen on routine light microscopy, differentiation of scars solely on the basis of histologic differences is virtually impossible. Clinical differentiation may also be difficult, because several clinical features of hypertrophic scars and keloids overlap (Table 1).

C. Hypertrophic Scars

Hypertrophic scars usually develop within the first couple of months after surgery or trauma. They commonly present as erythematous, firm, and raised linear bands on the

Table 1 Scar Categorization

Characteristics	Atrophic scars	Hypertrophic scars	Keloids
Clinical	White or pink; indented below skin surface; usually asymptomatic	White, pink, or red; slightly raised, firm; follow wound borders; may be pruritic	Deep red or purple; very raised, firm; extend beyond wound borders; may burn or itch
Histologic	Dermal fibrosis without inflammation	Few thick collagen fibers, scant mucoid matrix	Thick hyalinized collagen bundles; mucoid matrix, disorganized arrangement of cells

presternal area, upper back, and deltoid region, but they can occur in any area (3). Hypertrophic scar tissue is typically confined within the inciting wound margins (4) and may be symptomatic, with pruritus and dysesthesia reported in upward of one third of patients (5). The increase in collagen synthesis and limited collagen lysis during the remodeling phase of wound repair are the likely explanations for the formation of hypertrophic scars.

D. Keloids

Unlike hypertrophic scars, keloids grow beyond the margins of the original sites of injury (3,4,6–8). The proliferation is evident clinically with extension of scar tissue into normal skin and histologically with thick bundles of hyalinized collagen in a nodular arrangement. The proliferative phase of wound repair is so prolonged that they have been described as being representative of incomplete tumors (9). They are most commonly seen on the earlobes, shoulders, chest, upper back, and nuchal region in patients with darker skin tones; however, any patient could potentially develop them.

E. Atrophic Scars

Atrophic scars manifest clinically as indented or pitted areas that are limited to previous areas of inflammation, trauma, or surgery. They are particularly common on the face, chest, upper back, and shoulders of individuals who have suffered repeated episodes of inflammatory or cystic acne. Early in their course, atrophic scars are typically erythematous, but become hypopigmented over time.

III. BACKGROUND OF LASER TREATMENT

A. Hypertrophic Scars and Keloids

1. Continuous-Wave (CW) Lasers

Initial reports on the use of lasers to treat hypertrophic scars and keloids appeared in the medical literature in the mid-1980s. The vaporizing systems used, such as the continuous-wave CO_2, argon, and neodymium:yttrium aluminum garnet (Nd:YAG) lasers, all led to early scar improvement followed by scar recurrence or worsening within 1 year after treatment (10–19).

The effect of CO_2 laser excision on keloids has been evaluated by several groups. In a retrospective study reported by Norris in 1991 (19), all but 1 of 23 patients with keloids were considered to have failed laser treatment, most requiring concomitant steroids to suppress recurrence. An earlier study by Apfelberg and colleagues (16) also found that CO_2 vaporization of keloids was not beneficial in the nine keloids studied, as merely a single patient with earlobe keloids showed significant improvement after laser irradiation and only with the concomitant use of compression earrings in the postoperative period. These reports were in contrast to a previous report by Henderson and colleagues (11), who obtained an improvement rate of 82% using the CO_2 and argon lasers, with 18% of patients rated as having excellent results.

Apfelberg and colleagues (10) also compared the argon and CO_2 lasers in the removal of keloids. They treated 13 patients with keloids, only 1 of whom experienced a long-lasting beneficial effect. In 1987, the same group reported their experience using an Nd:YAG laser with and without concomitant intralesional steroids on a variety of dermatologic lesions, including 22 keloids or hypertrophic scars (14). The scars treated with Nd:YAG laser irradiation alone uniformly recurred within 3 to 4 months, whereas combined laser and steroid treatment resulted in persistent flattening in five lesions.

2. *Pulsed Dye Laser*

In the early 1990s, the first reports on a series of experiments using a vascular-specific pulsed dye laser on hypertrophic scars and keloids were published (20–26). Early in its use, it was evident that the 585-nm pulsed dye laser could affect more than its intended microvascular target. Clinical improvement of hypertrophic scars and keloids has been reported without recurrences up to 10 years after pulsed dye laser irradiation (TSA, personal communication).

Alster and colleagues (20) first treated argon laser–induced scars in port-wine patients with five successive pulsed dye laser treatments, clearly demonstrating a significant improvement in scar texture (as measured by optical profilometry), histologic features, and clinical appearance after laser irradiation. Alster (21) later reported similar clinical and textural success in 14 patients with long-standing erythematous and hypertrophic scars. After one and two pulsed dye laser treatments, 57% and 83% improvements were observed, respectively. Dierickx and colleagues (25) later corroborated these favorable findings, reporting an average scar improvement of 77% after 1.8 pulsed dye laser treatments. Acne scars that were erythematous and hypertrophic were also found to be responsive to pulsed dye irradiation in a study reported by Alster and McMeekin (23).

Combination treatments may also enhance the clinical results obtained. Goldman and Fitzpatrick (26) used intralesional corticosteroids concomitantly with 585-nm pulsed dye laser irradiation in 11 of 37 patients with hypertrophic scars. Improvement was observed in all patients, without a clear distinction made between those who received laser treatment alone and those who also received steroid injections.

Keloids have also been improved with pulsed dye laser irradiation. Alster and Williams (22) irradiated median sternotomy scar halves and compared the clinical, textural, histologic, and symptomatic responses of treated scar halves with untreated control halves. The laser-treated scars became more pliable with significantly less hypertrophy, erythema, and pruritus. These clinical observations were substantiated by skin surface textural analyses, erythema reflectance spectrometry readings, scar height measurements, and pliability scores, all showing significant improvement after pulsed dye laser irradiation. Histopathologic examination of laser-irradiated scars revealed a finer and more fibrillar appearance of involved collagen. In addition, a possible etiologic explanation for the laser's effectiveness was indicated, with an increase in tissue mast cell numbers noted in the treated areas. As histamine has been shown to influence collagen synthesis both positively and negatively, its role in laser-induced scar improvement has yet to be determined. In addition, the fact that mast cells elaborate a wide variety of cytokines may account in some way for the clinical improvement seen—microvasculature destruction is effected, tissue factors are released, and collagen remodeling occurs. Other etiologic mechanisms include the possibility of collagen stimulation through dermal heat conduction from laser-targeted blood vessels or lack of tissue oxygenation leading to collagen catabolism and release of collagenase (25).

B. Atrophic Scars

1. *Carbon Dioxide Laser*

Continuous and superpulsed CO_2 lasers were initially used to resurface skin marred with atrophic scars (27). The older laser technology and limited scanning equipment were extremely operator dependent and often led to additional cutaneous depressions and/or scar worsening except in the most experienced operators' hands. Newer, high-energy, pulsed CO_2 laser systems are now widely available and have been shown to improve atrophic scars from acne, chickenpox, surgery, and trauma in a more controlled manner, with fewer significant side effects (28–32). In a study published by Alster and West (30), 50 patients with facial acne scars with a wide range of skin phototypes (I–V) were found to have an average clinical improvement of 81.4%. Skin texture analyses of the laser-irradiated scars demonstrated a return of normal skin surface markings, comparable to those seen in normal adjacent skin.

2. *Erbium:YAG Laser*

The most recent laser to become available for cutaneous laser resurfacing is the 2.94-μm erbium:YAG laser. There is considerable interest in this latest technology because of its high tissue ablation efficacy with minimal collateral thermal damage (which limits side effects such as scarring). As with the CO_2 laser, the long wavelength of the erbium laser (in the infrared range) allows specific absorption by water-containing tissue such as the epidermis and dermis. Early reports suggest that the erbium laser may prove useful in the treatment of mild atrophic scars (33,34). Deeper scars may still require resurfacing by the CO_2 laser to achieve deeper tissue vaporization, tissue tightening (from heat conduction), and subsequent collagen remodeling.

IV. PREOPERATIVE EVALUATION OF PATIENTS

Patients who desire laser treatment should receive an initial screening evaluation to ascertain whether their scars, skin types, and expectations are suitable for treatment. The appropriate laser system is determined on the basis of the scar type: hypertrophic, atrophic, or keloid (Table 2). Scar categorization also allows proper disclosure of information rele-

Table 2 Laser Treatment of Scars

Scar type	Laser	Treatment number
Hypertrophic	585-nm pulsed dye	2–4
Keloid	585-nm pulsed dye	2–6
Atrophic	High-energy, pulsed CO_2	1
	Erbium:YAG	1–2

vant to the laser being used, including the number of treatments anticipated to achieve the desired clinical effect.

The duration of the scar and its developmental history should also be ascertained. Younger scars (<1 year old) are typically more erythematous than older scars. Although younger scars are quite amenable to pulsed dye laser irradiation, they may not necessitate laser treatment, as some spontaneous improvement is expected over the first 12 months. In patients whose scars continue to worsen; however, it is best to advise laser intervention in order to prevent further abnormal scar growth and to effect speedier improvement.

Whether a patient has received prior treatment to the scar is also important, as additional fibrosis may be present within the scar as a result of failed attempts to remove it, making it even more difficult to treat. Atrophic scars that have been treated with prior dermabrasion may not be vaporized as readily with CO_2 laser resurfacing, possibly reducing the final clinical response. However, individuals who have simply received intralesional injections of corticosteroids (for hypertrophic scars and keloids, in particular) should not experience a significant reduction in response to subsequent pulsed dye laser treatment.

Patients with hypertrophic scars and keloids may report symptoms such as pruritus and dysesthesia within their scars, requiring the use of oral antihistamines. Pulsed dye laser irradiation of these scars may effect an improvement in symptoms within one or two treatment sessions (22).

Because patients with darker skin tones (phototypes IV and higher) have a greater amount of epidermal pigment and melanin can absorb 585-nm light, the amount of energy effectively delivered to dermal scar tissue is reduced. Thus, paler-skinned individuals would be expected to respond most favorably to pulsed dye laser irradiation.

A complete skin examination should be performed to assess for keloid tendencies. In patients who are known to be keloid prone, a laser test site should be considered prior to laser resurfacing of atrophic scars, as laser vaporization could lead to a hypertrophic tissue response. There does not appear to be an increased risk of scar worsening or new scar development using the pulsed dye laser to treat scars in individuals who are keloid prone; however, patients who have taken isotretinoin within the preceding 6 months are at an increased risk of developing hypertrophic scars. Thus, it is prudent to delay laser treatment for at least 6 months after a course of isotretinoin.

Patients who expect their scars to disappear after laser treatment will be uniformly disappointed with the clinical results effected, regardless of the amount of improvement actually achieved. If a patient continues to voice unrealistic expectations after adequate explanations regarding the laser procedure and its anticipated effect have been provided, laser treatment should not be performed.

V. LASER PROTOCOL

The number of laser treatments necessary to effect significant scar improvement is dependent not only on the type of scar present but also on each patient's tissue response and collagen remodeling capability. In general, two or more pulsed dye laser sessions are needed to improve hypertrophic scars and keloids, whereas a single laser resurfacing treatment is typically needed using either the carbon dioxide or erbium:YAG laser. Although atrophic scars can be effectively vaporized with the carbon dioxide or erbium:YAG laser without recurrence, hypertrophic scars and keloids universally recur with these resurfacing procedures.

A. 585-nm Pulsed Dye Laser

A 585-nm flashlamp-pumped pulsed dye laser is best used at average fluences of 6.0–7.0 J/cm^2 with a 5- or 7-nm spot size and at 4.5–5.0 J/cm^2 with a 10-mm spot size when treating hypertrophic scars and keloids (Table 3); Fig. 1A and B, 2A and B. Adjacent, nonoverlapping laser pulses are delivered to the entire scar. When laser spots are placed on top of one another, excessive heat (thermal damage) is produced in the treated skin, causing a significant increase in scarring risk.

Immediately after pulsed dye laser irradiation, a variable amount of tissue purpura is produced. The purpuric response is most evident (darker) in scars that are more erythematous (Fig. 3A–C). A reduced degree of purpura is seen when using the 10-mm spot size at the fluences indicated. The purpura typically resolve within 7 to 10 days, during which time the patient applies antibiotic ointment to the irradiated areas.

The patient is evaluated 4 to 8 weeks postoperatively. Depending on the clinical result obtained, another laser treatment at the same or slightly higher fluence is delivered. If the previously irradiated areas are hyperpigmented, it is advised to postpone evaluation and further evaluation for an additional 2 to 4 weeks in order to allow sufficient time for healing.

B. High-Energy, Pulsed or Scanned Carbon Dioxide Laser

The new pulsed or scanned CO_2 lasers can successfully ablate or vaporize thin layers of skin in a layer-by-layer fashion, enabling "sculpting" of atrophic scars. As described earlier, a much narrower zone of cutaneous thermal damage is produced by the new pulsed

Table 3 Laser Parameters

Laser type	Wavelength	Pulse width	Energy or power	Spot size	Scars treated
Pulsed dye	585 nm	450 μs–1.5 ms	5.0–7.0 J/cm^2	5–10 mm	Hypertrophic Keloid
Carbon dioxide	10,600 nm	<1 ms	300–500 mJ 5–7 W 60 W	 3-mm spot CPG scan	 Atrophic
Erbium:YAG	2940 nm	150–600 μs	500–1000 mJ	3–8 mm spot	Atrophic

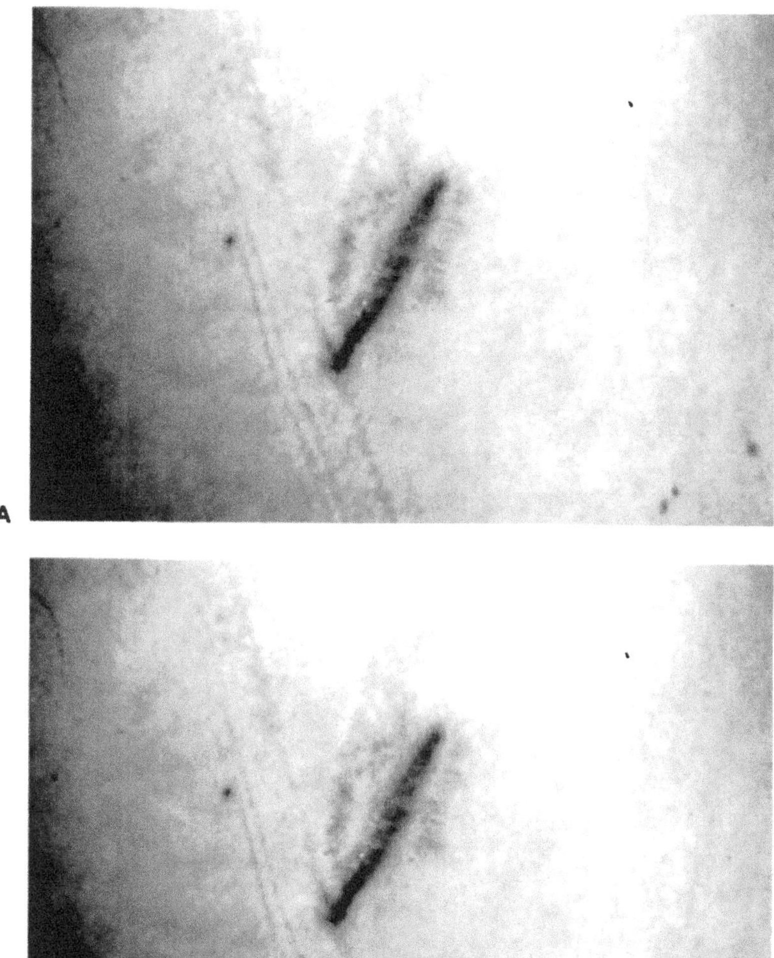

Figure 1 Hypertrophic and erythematous surgical scar of 5 years' duration before **(A)** and 8 weeks after **(B)** three 585-nm pulsed dye laser treatments (fluence 4.5 J/cm^2, pulse duration 1.5 ms, spot size 10 mm).

systems compared with the older continuous-wave systems. Several different pulsed and scanned CO_2 laser systems are currently available for cutaneous resurfacing, with separate guidelines for use. When used properly, these laser systems have been shown to yield clinically equivalent results despite differences in depth of vaporization and levels of residual thermal damage (Fig. 4A and B, 5A and B) (35).

In general, each laser system can be used at its maximum energy (up to 500 mJ) with short pulse widths (<1 millisecond) in order to effect tissue vaporization with minimal residual thermal damage to the surrounding skin. After each laser "pass," during which the

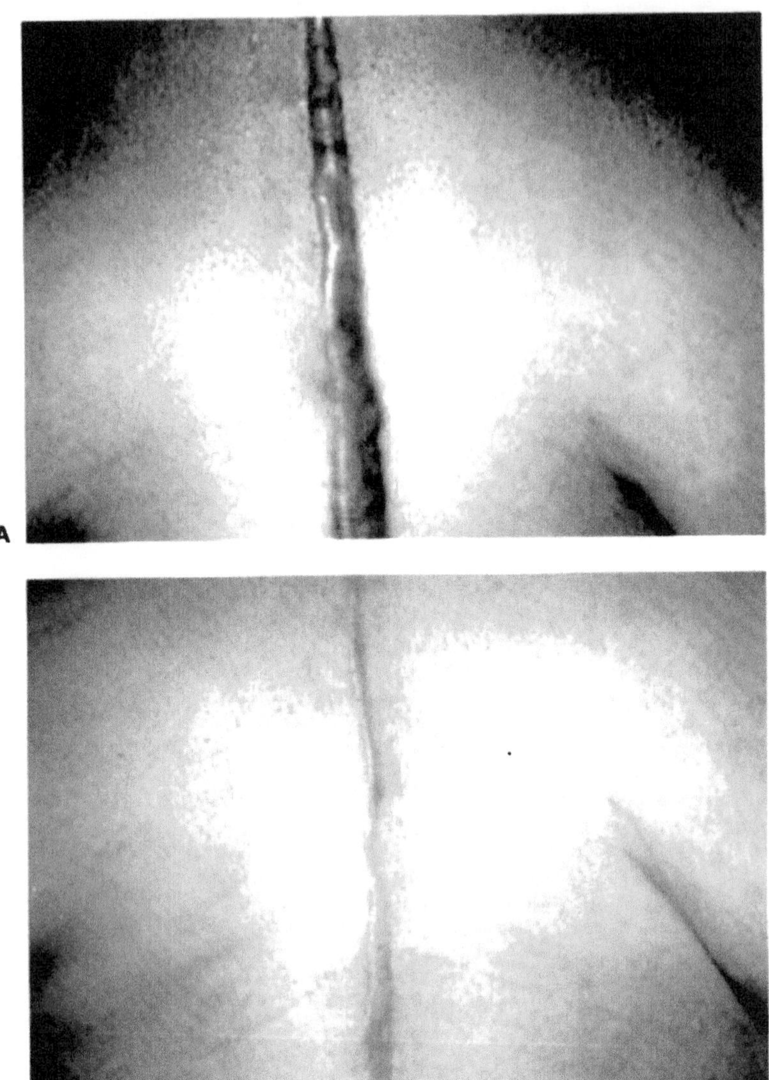

Figure 2 Keloid median sternotomy scar of 8 years' duration in a teenage girl before **(A)** and 1 year after **(B)** fourth pulsed dye laser treatment (average fluence 6.5 J/cm^2, pulse duration 450 μs, spot size 7 mm), showing marked improvement in scar color and height.

Figure 3 Hypertrophic burn scars induced by CO_2 laser resurfacing procedure before **(A)** and immediately after **(B)** 585-nm pulsed dye laser treatment, showing expected purpuric tissue response. Improvement of scars was noted 8 weeks after second laser treatment (fluences 4.5–5.0 J/cm^2, pulse duration 1.5 ms, spot size 10 mm) **(C)**.

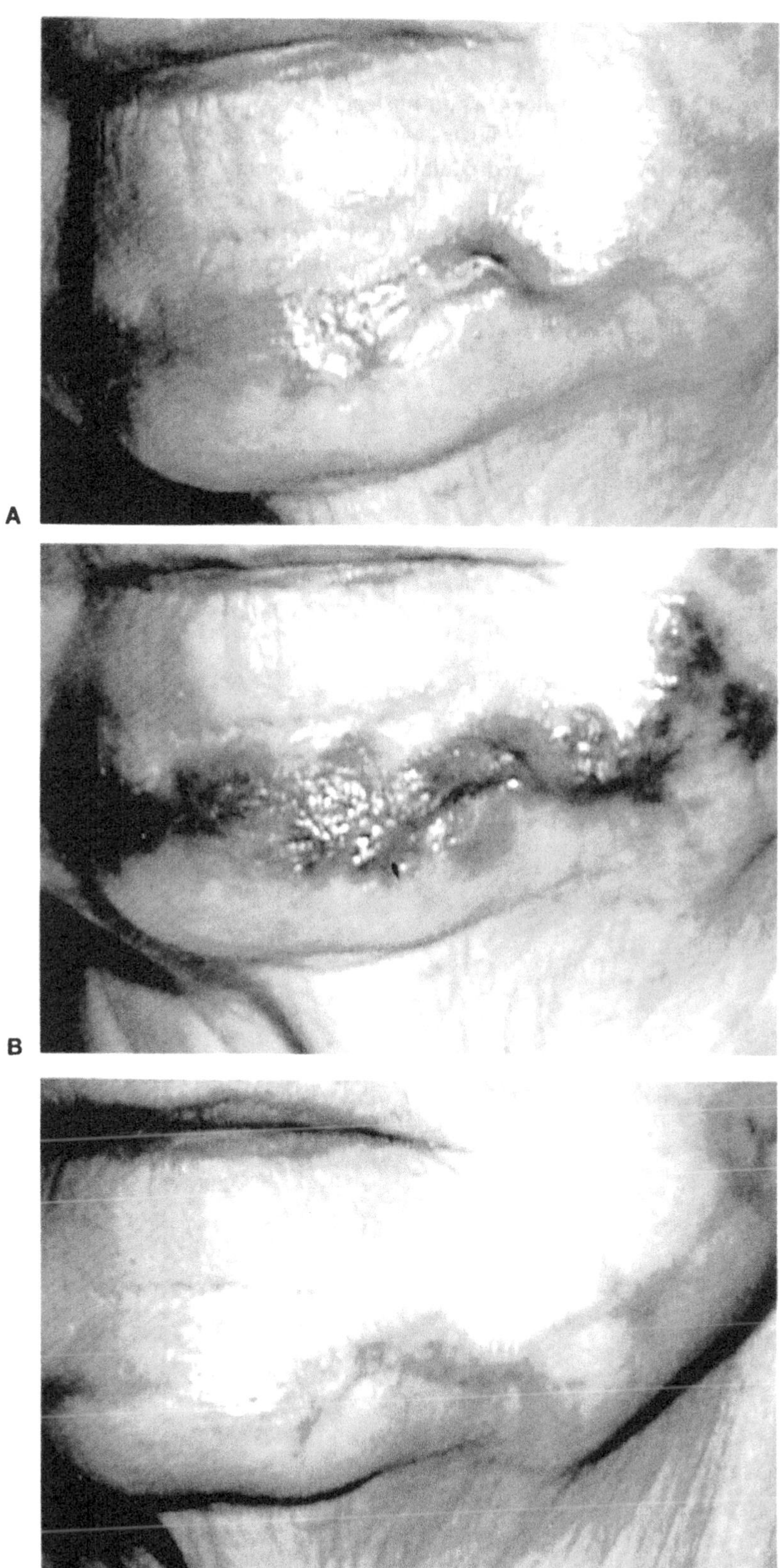
A
B
C

laser light interacts with the skin producing a puff of steam (vaporized tissue), the residual partially-desiccated tissue is manually removed with a saline-soaked gauze. Additional laser passes are delivered until the desired clinical result is obtained. In addition to the bloodless tissue vaporization observed, CO_2 laser resurfacing has been noted to produce an immediate skin-tightening effect due to the thermal denaturation of type I collagen. It is believed that it is the combination of tissue ablation and collagen shrinkage that accounts for the extensive collagen remodeling and improvement in surface irregularities seen after laser resurfacing.

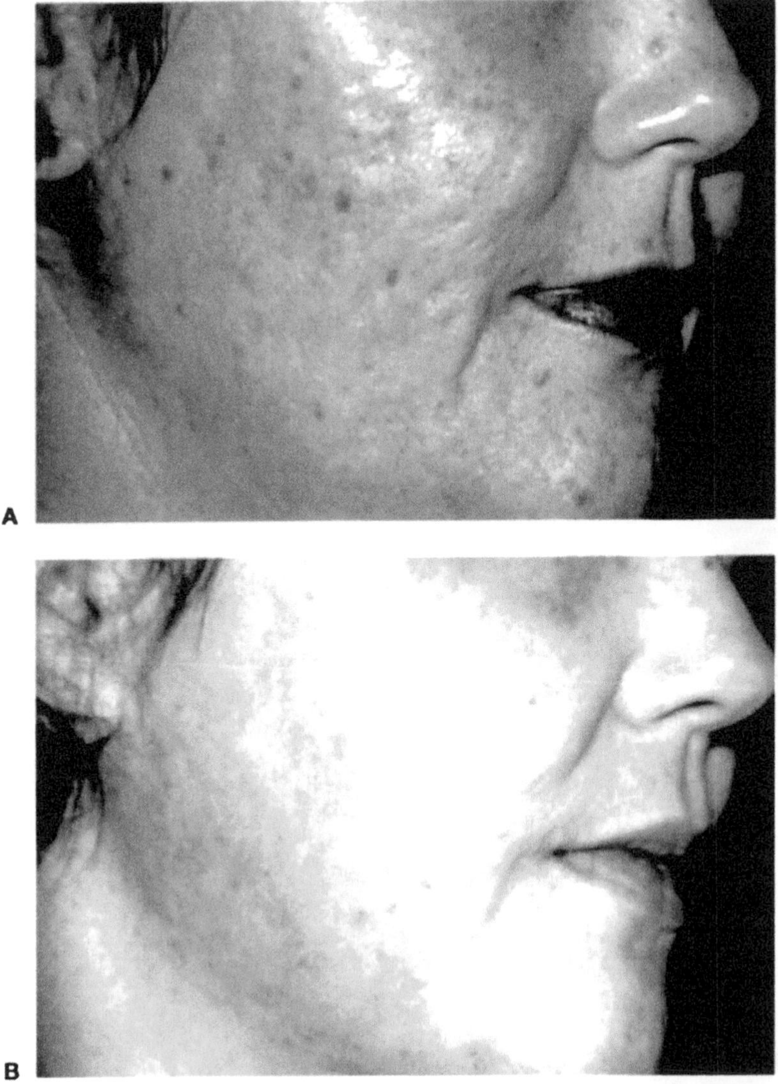

Figure 4 Atrophic facial acne scars in a 48-year-old woman before **(A)** and 6 months after **(B)** full-face high-energy, pulsed CO_2 laser resurfacing.

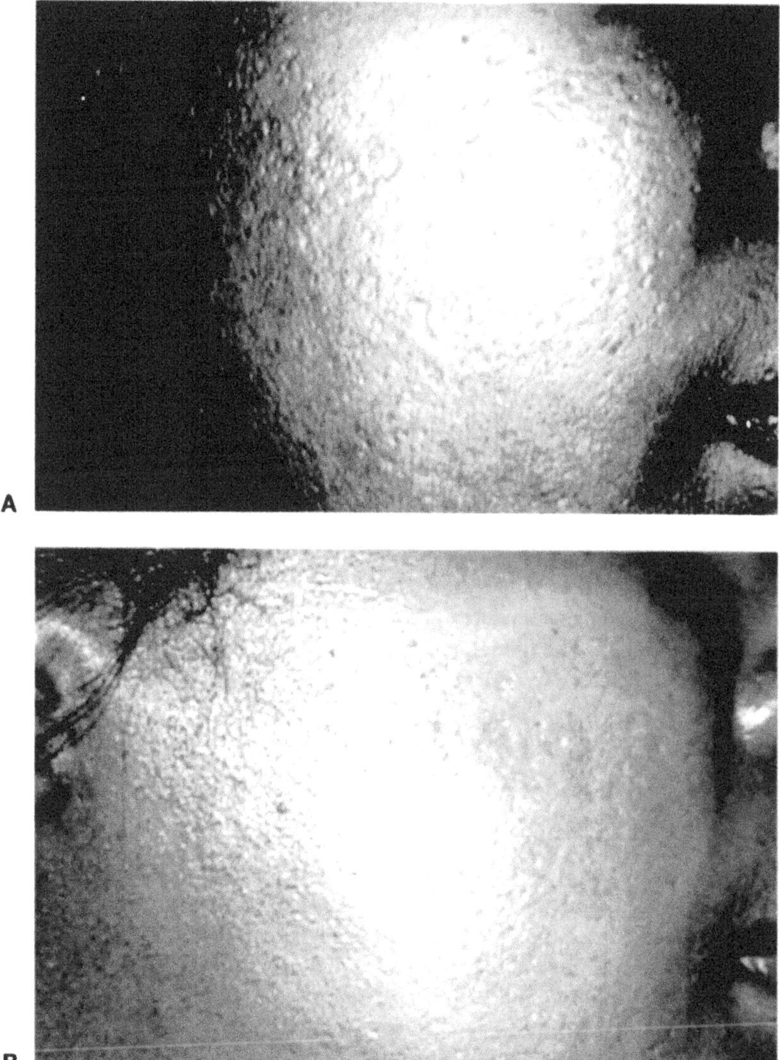

Figure 5 Atrophic acne scars in type V skin before **(A)** and 1 year after **(B)** CO_2 laser resurfacing.

The entire cosmetic unit should be treated to reduce the possibility of skin texture, color, or tonal irregularities. When an isolated atrophic scar is present, spot resurfacing can be performed. First, scars are deepithelialized across their entire breadth (including the atrophic portions), followed by "sculpting" of the scar edges with a smaller spot or scan size. When large skin areas require resurfacing, as is common with atrophic acne scars on the cheeks, it is best to use the largest scanning handpiece available in order to increase the speed of the procedure.

Immediately after the resurfacing procedure, the treated skin appears pale pink and slightly edematous. The erythema and edema intensify during the first 48 hours. Patients are encouraged to keep the laser-treated areas moist, either with continuous application of healing ointments or by covering with hydrogel wound dressings. Application of ice to the areas and administration of anti-inflammatories help to minimize swelling. After extensive resurfacing procedures, administration of oral antiherpetics and antibiotics is routinely prescribed.

Close follow-up of all patients is necessary during the first week after surgery in order to assess the skin for infection, poor wound healing, or irritation so that early treatment can be initiated when problems arise. After the first week, patients are instructed in the use of camouflage makeup and maintenance skin care, with subsequent follow-up visits scheduled on a regular basis (at least monthly) to assess further healing.

C. Erbium:YAG Laser

Atrophic scars are resurfaced with the erbium laser in the same manner as with the CO_2 laser (32, 36). However, wiping the skin between laser passes is not always necessary because there is minimal, if any, partially-desiccated tissue and a reduced residual thermal effect on the skin. The laser is typically used at energies of 500–1000 mJ, repetition rates of 7–15 Hz, and pulse durations of 200–300 microseconds using a 3–8-mm spot size.

Similar to CO_2 laser resurfacing, the erbium laser does not require the use of general anesthesia. Topical, local anesthesia with nerve blocks, and/or intravenous sedation is sufficient for even extensive resurfacing procedures. Postoperative recovery after erbium laser resurfacing is markedly shortened. The time to complete healing is reduced from months to weeks, and patients are able to return to their regular activities within a week after surgery with minimal erythema.

D. Combination Laser Treatment

A combined approach using a high-energy, pulsed CO_2 laser for scar deepithelialization followed by 585-nm pulsed dye laser irradiation has been shown to improve hypertrophic scars that are not clinically erythematous.(37) The pulsed CO_2 laser is not used to vaporize the scar flat (which would lead to scar recurrence) but is used to deepithelialize and provide collagen tightening or "shrinkage" of the scar. One or two passes of the CO_2 laser are delivered at an energy of 500 mJ/pulse and 5 W power using a 3-mm collimated handpiece. A 585-nm pulsed dye laser is then used at an energy density of 6.0–7.0 J/cm^2 and spot size of 5–7 mm in order to enhance the clinical effect achieved.

VI. SUMMARY

Lasers are being used successfully to treat a variety of scars. In order to optimize the treatment results obtained, scars need to be properly identified so that the correct laser technology can be employed. Hypertrophic scars and keloids respond best to a 585-nm pulsed dye laser, while atrophic scars can be ablated with high-energy, pulsed or scanned CO_2 laser systems. New erbium:YAG lasers may offer a viable alternative to CO_2 laser resurfacing with fewer postoperative side effects and complications; however, initial reports suggest decreased clinical effectiveness due to limited residual thermal damage and collagen remodeling.

When properly utilized, lasers can achieve significant clinical improvement of such recalcitrant lesions as hypertrophic scars and keloids. Future technologic advances as well as the addition of concomitant lasers or other therapies may enhance the clinical results obtained. It appears evident that by enhancing the remodeling phase of wound healing, abnormal scarring may be prevented or improved. Laser surgery may best be able to accomplish this goal through both direct (vaporization, collagen shrinkage) and indirect (microvascular destruction, tissue heating) means.

REFERENCES

1. Omo-Dare P. Yoruban contributions to the literature on keloids. J Natl Med Assoc 1973; 65:367–372.
2. Alibert JLM. Quelques recherches sur la cheloide. Mem Soc Med Emulation 1817; 744.
3. Rockwell WB, Cohen IK, Ehrlich HP. Keloids and hypertrophic scars: a comprehensive review. Plast Reconstr Surg 1989; 84:827–837.
4. Rudolph R. Wide spread scars, hypertrophic scars, and keloids. Clin Plast Surg 1987; 14:253–260.
5. Alster TS. Laser treatment of hypertrophic scars. Facial Plast Surg Clin North Am 1996; 4:267–274.
6. Datubo-Brown DD. Keloids: a review of the literature. Br J Plast Surg 1990; 43:70–77.
7. Muir IFK. On the nature of keloids and hypertrophic scars. Br J Plast Surg 1990; 43:61–69.
8. Murray JC, Pollack SV, Pinnell SR. Keloids and hypertrophic scars. Clin Dermatol 1984; 2:121–133.
9. Russell JD, Witt WS. Cell size and growth characteristics of cultured fibroblasts isolated from normal and keloid tissue. Plast Reconstr Surg 1976; 57:207–212.
10. Apfelberg DB, Maser MR, Lash H, et al. Preliminary results of argon and carbon dioxide laser treatment of keloid scars. Lasers Surg Med 1984; 4:283–290.
11. Henderson DL, Cromwell TA, Mes LG. Argon and carbon dioxide laser treatment of hypertrophic and keloid scars. Lasers Surg Med 1984; 3:271–277.
12. Kantor GR, Wheeland RG, Bailin PL, et al. Treatment of earlobe keloids with carbon dioxide laser excision: a report of 16 cases. J Dermatol Surg Oncol 1985; 11:1063–1067.
13. Hulsbergen-Henning JP, Roskam Y, van Gemert MJ. Treatment of keloids and hypertrophic scars with an argon laser. Lasers Surg Med 1986; 6:72–75.
14. Apfelberg DB, Smith T, Lash H, et al. Preliminary report on the use of the neodymium-YAG laser in plastic surgery. Lasers Surg Med 1987; 7:189.
15. Sherman R, Rosenfeld H. Experience with the Nd:YAG laser in the treatment of keloid scars. Ann Plast Surg 1988; 21:231–235.
16. Apfelberg DB, Maser MR, White DN, et al. Failure of carbon dioxide laser excision of keloids. Lasers Surg Med 1989; 9:382–388.
17. Stern JC, Lucente FE. Carbon dioxide laser excision of earlobe keloids: a prospective study and critical analysis of existing data. Arch Otolaryngol Head Neck Surg 1989; 115:1107–1111.
18. Lim TC, Tan WT. Carbon dioxide laser for keloids. Plast Reconstr Surg 1991; 88:111.
19. Norris JE. The effect of carbon dioxide laser surgery on the recurrence of keloids. Plast Reconstr Surg 1991; 87:44–49.
20. Alster TS, Kurban AK, Grove GL, et al. Alteration of argon laser–induced scars by the pulsed dye laser. Lasers Surg Med 1993; 13:368–373.
21. Alster TS. Improvement of erythematous and hypertrophic scars by the 585 nm pulsed dye laser. Ann Plast Surg 1994; 32:186–190.
22. Alster TS, Williams CM. Treatment of keloid sternotomy scars with 585 nm flashlamp-pumped pulsed dye laser. Lancet 1995; 345:1198–1200.
23. Alster TS, McMeekin TO. Improvement of facial acne scars by the 585 nm flashlamp-pumped pulsed dye laser. J Am Acad Dermatol 1996; 35:79–81.
24. Alster TS, Nanni CA. Laser treatment of hypertrophic burn scars. Plast Reconstr Surg 1998;102:2190–2195.

25. Dierickx C, Goldman MP, Fitzpatrick RE. Laser treatment of erythematous/hypertrophic and pigmented scars in 26 patients. Plast Reconstr Surg 1995; 95:84–90.
26. Goldman MP, Fitzpatrick RE. Laser treatment of scars. Dermatol Surg 1995; 21:685.
27. Garrett AB, Dufresne RG, Ratz JL, Berlin AJ. Carbon dioxide laser treatment of pitted acne scarring. J Dermatol Surg Oncol 1990; 16:737–740.
28. Fitzpatrick RE, Goldman MP, Ruiz-Esparza J. Clinical advantages of the CO_2 laser superpulsed mode. J Dermatol Surg Oncol 1994; 20:449–456.
29. Ho CH, Nguyen Q, Lowe NJ, et al. Laser resurfacing in pigmented skin. J Dermatol Surg Oncol 1995; 21:1035–1037.
30. Alster TS, West TB. Resurfacing of atrophic facial scars with a high-energy, pulsed carbon dioxide laser. Dermatol Surg 1996; 22:151–155.
31. Weinstein C, Alster TS. Skin resurfacing with high-energy, pulsed carbon dioxide lasers. In: Alster TS, Apfelberg DB, eds. Cosmetic Laser Surgery. New York: Wiley, 1996:9–28.
32. Alster TS. Cutaneous resurfacing with CO_2 and erbium:YAG lasers: Preoperative, intraoperative, and postoperative considerations. Plast Reconstr Surg 1999;10:619–632.
33. Kaufmann R, Hibst R. Pulsed erbium:YAG laser ablation in cutaneous surgery. Lasers Surg Med 1996; 19:324–330.
34. Nemeth AJ, Miller I, Glass LF, et al. Erbium:YAG laser for acne scarring/resurfacing. Lasers Surg Med 1997; 9(suppl):32.
35. Alster TS, Nanni CA, Williams CM. Comparison of four cutaneous resurfacing lasers: a clinical and histopathologic evaluation. Dermatol Surg 1999;25:153–159.
36. Alster TS. Clinical and histologic evaluation of six erbium:YAG lasers for cutaneous resurfacing. Lasers Surg Med 1999;24:87–92.
37. Alster TS, Lewis AB, Rosenbach A. Laser Scar Revision: Comparison of CO_2 laser vaporization with and without simultaneous pulsed dye laser treatment. Dermatol Surg 1998;24:1299–1302.

11
Cryosurgical Treatment

Christos C. Zouboulis and Constantin E. Orfanos
University Medical Center Benjamin Franklin, The Free University of Berlin
Berlin, Germany

I. INTRODUCTION

Cryosurgery—the well-aimed and controlled destruction of diseased tissue by application of cold—is an effective and efficient method for treating various skin diseases (1–4). The technique has several advantages (Table 1) and, especially, in the treatment of keloids and hypertrophic scars, it provides good therapeutic and cosmetic results with a few contraindications and a low incidence of complications (5–7). The therapeutic effects of freezing on tissues have also been used successfully in the treatment of superficial atrophic acne scars (8,9).

The first physician who used cold to treat a dermatological disease was Carl Gerhardt, a German dermatologist from Jena (10). In 1885, he published on the treatment of cutaneous tuberculosis with cold. Gerhardt had built a system in which the lesions were covered with ice bladders for 3 hours twice a day. Four patients improved considerably after a 2- to 4-week treatment (11). In 1899, A. Campell White, an American dermatologist from New York, used liquefied air for the first time to treat various skin disorders, such as verrucae vulgares, nevi, precancerous lesions, and tumors (12). In 1905 M. Juliusberg, a Berliner dermatologist, introduced the term "cryotherapy" for the treatment of skin lesions with cold. He applied the first cryospray, a small balloon filled with carbon dioxide released in spurts (13). Modern cryosurgery was born at the 1960s after liquid nitrogen became available (14) and closed-circuit devices working with liquid nitrogen, freon gas, and nitrogen protoxide were developed by the American neurosurgeons Irving S. Cooper and A. S. Lee and their Italian colleagues V. A. Fasano et al. (15–17). Since then, numerous sophisticated devices have been developed and commercialized, not only to preserve and deliver cryogens but also to monitor the temperatures in and underneath the treated lesions, allowing controlled and reliable cryosurgery of the diseased skin.

II. CRYOBIOLOGY

The biological changes that occur in cryosurgery have been studied in vitro and in vivo and are caused by reduction of tissue temperature and consequent freezing (18–21). Tissue in-

Table 1 Advantages of Cryosurgery

Safe and relatively simple technique	Low rates of complications
Outpatient procedure	Few contraindications
Short duration of treatment	High healing rates, also in "difficult" areas
Low cost	No general anesthesia required—local anesthesia optional
Repeatable as often as needed	Protects important tissue structures
Excellent cosmetic results	Applicable in old, nonoperable patients and in pregnancy

jury is induced by the direct physical effects of cell freezing and by the vascular stasis that develops in the tissue after thawing. The cryoreaction is, therefore, characterized by physical and vascular phases. A postulated third phase of cryoreaction, the immunologic phase, is still under investigation. The factors that influence the effects of freezing on tissue and the optimal parameters for the treatment of keloids and hypertrophic scars are shown in Table 2.

A. Physical Phase of Cryoreaction*

1. *Tissue Freezing: Homogeneous and Heterogeneous Nucleation*

Very rapid freezing (100–260°C/min) leads to intracellular ice formation and gives rise to cellular death through an irreversible destruction of the cells known as homogeneous nucleation. Damage to cell organelles, such as mitochondria and endoplasmic reticulum, has been postulated to be caused by intracellular ice formation. Ice crystal size is important: the larger the crystals, the greater the induced damage. Very high freezing speeds are required in the treatment of malignant skin tumors, where cryosurgery has to be lethal. In the treatment of benign skin tumors, such as keloids and hypertrophic scars, moderate freezing speeds (up to 100°C/min) can also be applied. Moderate freezing speeds lead to differential freezing in the different parts of the tissue, resulting in extracellular ice formation and hypertonic and sensitization damage. These phenomena, which can also induce irreversible destruction of the cells, are known as heterogeneous nucleation. Extracellular ice formation alone is not sufficient to kill cells, because disruption of cell membranes barely occurs de-

* Reviewed in Refs. 19 and 22.

Table 2 Factors Influencing the Effects of Freezing in Tissue

Factor	Optimal parameters for the treatment of keloids and hypertrophic scars
Speed of tissue freezing	Moderate speed (up to 100°C/min)
Speed of thawing	Slow speed (10°C/min, spontaneous rewarming)
Intra- or extracellular osmotic phenomena	Heterogeneous and homogeneous nucleation
Probe tip temperature	−85 to −190°C
Tissue temperature	−20 to −25°C
Duration of freezing	30 seconds
Repetition of freeze-thaw cycles	No
Vascular reaction	Yes
Immunologic reaction	Probable

spite the volume changes in the extra- and intracellular compartments. However, the temperature changes occurring in tissue with moderate freezing speeds are rapid enough to induce additional intracellular ice formation. When extracellular ice is formed, changing osmotic gradients between cells and extracellular fluid are produced, which lead to passage of electrolytes out of the cells and a decrease in cell volume. When a certain concentration of essential intracellular molecules is reached, they also pass out of the cell, causing irreversible cell damage (hypertonic damage). However, gross cell damage can be observed even if the necessary hypertonic conditions are not achieved. This leads to the assumption that this "sensitization" damage is the result of phospholipid disruption in cell membranes.

Slow freezing leads only to extracellular ice formation and, together with the addition of cryoprotective agents, such as dimethyl sulfoxide, in order to prevent hypertonic damage, is used in cryoconservation of cells and tissues.

2. *Tissue Thawing*

Slow thawing (10°C/min) induces volume changes in the extra- and intracellular compartments, leading to an increase of the intracellular water content. Rapid electrolyte transfer has been incriminated as the cause of damage to cell proteins and enzyme systems. Reverse osmotic gradients during thawing may give rise to sensitization damage. In addition, intracellular recrystallization of ice is responsible for tissue destruction. The latter process is as important as the initial freezing in causing cell death. Adequate freezing has been achieved when the thawing time is 1.5 times the freezing time or longer.

3. *Tissue Temperature*

Freezing takes place in the tissue at −0.6°C, but this is not the lethal temperature. Various cell populations have different abilities to tolerate cold (23–25). Melanocytes are the skin cells most sensitive to low temperatures; they die at −4°C to −7°C. Sebaceous glands and hair follicles are also rather sensitive to cold; temperatures lower than −20°C are lethal for them. Keratinocytes die at about −20°C to −30°C. Fibroblasts are rather resistant to cold, dying at −30°C to −35°C. Therefore, it is difficult to achieve optimal cooling rates capable of killing all cells during cryosurery. Theoretically, the formation of ice crystals in tissue, and therefore tissue freezing, starts from temperatures lower than −21.8°C, which is the eutectic temperature of sodium chloride solutions (19). The water content of rapidly dividing cells is directly proportional to the mitotic index, hense they are more likely to be damaged. A probe tip temperature lower than −180°C and a tissue temperature at least as low as −50°C have been shown to be essential for killing all target cells (24,26,27). These parameters are required in cryosurgery of malignant skin tumors; optimal cryosurgery of benign skin lesions, such as keloids and hypertrophic scars, requires only tissue temperatures of −20°C to −25°C (2).

4. *Duration of Freezing*

Cell death rates in vitro have been shown to increase not only with lower temperatures but also with longer freezing times (18). However, the effect of freezing on cell viability reaches a maximum at about 100 seconds, followed by a plateau in cell death rates with time.

5. *Repetition of Freeze-Thaw Cycles*

The importance of more than one freeze-thaw cycle in causing increased rates of cell death has been demonstrated in several in vitro and animal studies (18). Electron microscopic studies of normal skin showed damage to all cell structures after a second freeze-thaw cycle (28). Repeated freeze-thaw cycles are essential in the treatment of cutaneous tumors (27,29) but are not required in the treatment of keloids and hypertrophic scars (5).

B. Vascular Phase of Cryoreaction

Cryogenic injury leads to vascular stasis and inevitable tissue anoxemia resulting in ischemic necrosis. Ischemia produces cell damage in addition to that due to intra- and extracellular ice formation (22,30). Microscopic examination of injured tissue in animals has shown that edema, focal capillary damage, hemorrhages, and isolated microthrombi begin to occur after 2 hours and that by 5–8 hours focal or segmental necrosis of blood vessels is present. Thrombosis of terminal arteries leading to gangrene appears between 1 and 7 days, but only when injury is severe. Even after mild cold injuries, the initial circulatory impairment is irreversible, which implicates delayed progressive thrombosis as the main factor producing tissue loss (31,32). Thrombosis in 65% of the capillaries and 35–40% of the arterioles and venoles occurs at tissue temperatures of 11°C to 3°C, and thrombosis of all vessels is detectable at −15°C to −20°C in tissue (33,34).

In an attempt to explain the exudation that occurs after cryosurgery, ultrastructural studies of endothelial cells were performed. These studies have shown that cell damage in the first hour after freezing and thawing includes rupture of cell membranes, thinning and later condensation of ground substance, and swelling of rough endoplasmic reticulum and mitochondria (35).

C. Immunologic Phase of Cryoreaction

The possibility of an immunologic response after cryosurgical treatment was first raised when circulating antibodies directed against prostatic or adrenal tissue that had been treated by cryosurgery in the rabbit were observed (36,37). Clinically, regression of tumor masses beyond the region treated by cryosurgery or even in distant metastases has been observed (38,39). It has been demonstrated in both the rabbit and human that antigens are released by cell lysis after freezing. The antibody response is directed against tissue antigens rather than tumor antigens (40). Further confirmation of an immunologic response after cryosurgery has been provided. Natural killer cell cytotoxicity was found to be enhanced after cryosurgery of normal liver and liver tumors in animals (41). A parallel study of patients with benign tumors in the lungs and bronchial or pulmonary cancer treated with combined operative intervention and cryosurgery showed a stimulating effect of cryodestruction of malignant tumors and their subsequent spontaneous thawing on the content of large granule–containing lymphocytes and natural killer activity (42). An interesting study was performed in rats with liver carcinoma that was incompletely or completely frozen. In the incompletely frozen group, the survival days were significantly prolonged compared with controls. Phytohemagglutinin blast formation and CD4 positivity exhibited high levels at 8 weeks after cryosurgery. In the completely frozen group, survival time was not prolonged and three cases of early death were observed. Moreover, CD4 positivity significantly decreased at 3 days and CD8 positivity significantly increased at 2 weeks after cryosurgery. These results led to the conclusion that the immunologic response after cryosurgery for liver carcinoma may be induced by changes in tumor cell immunity (43). Langerhans cell activity after cutaneous cryosurgery was found to be enhanced in another study (44). Finally, in an experimental study, the concentration of ascites fibrosarcoma tumor cell membrane proteins increased in frozen tumor cells compared with the native cells. In addition, they increased further with the number of freeze-thaw cycles applied. The cell surface protein pattern, which was heterogeneous before freezing, became more homogeneous after freezing because of depolymerization and breaking of higher molecular weight components (45).

III. CRYOSURGERY IN THE TREATMENT OF KELOIDS AND HYPERTROPHIC SCARS

Keloids and hypertrophic scars are benign cutaneous lesions produced by uncontrolled synthesis and deposition of dermal collagen as a result of abnormal wound healing. They usually follow injury to the skin of predisposed individuals but can also occur spontaneously. The chest, shoulders, head-neck area, and upper back are the most susceptible regions of the body (46,47). Whereas keloids have a strong tendency to grow beyond the confines of the previous wound, hypertrophic scars remain within the borders of the original dermal trauma (48,49). In contrast to hypertrophic scars, keloids do not regress with time and do not provoke scar contractures. Keloids contain large, thick collagen fibers composed of numerous fibrils closely packed together. In contrast, hypertrophic scars exhibit modular structures in which fibroblastic cells, small vessels, and fine, randomly organized collagen fibers are present (49).

The primary cell in keloids has shown to be the myofibroblast with prominent rough endoplasmic reticulum and bundles of myofilaments with focal densities in the cytoplasm (49–52). Enhanced secretory activity was reflected in the prominence of the Golgi apparatus and the frequent presence of intracellular collagen within the tubular membranes (52). Proliferating dermal fibroblasts in the periphery of the keloid tissue have been shown; their numbers were increased in comparison with hypertrophic scars and normal skin (53,54). In contrast, no proliferating cells were found in the central region of the keloid (54). Northern blot analysis of total RNA obtained from keloids with a high growth tendency in vivo and immunohistochemistry of keloids and hypertrophic scars showed a marked induction of the small proteoglycan biglycan and collagen-$\alpha 1$ (I) expression in comparison with normal skin (55,56). In another study, increased levels of $\alpha 1$ (I) and $\alpha 1$ (III) collagen messenger RNA (mRNA) were observed in fibroblasts from the edge and outside of hypertrophic scar tissue, whereas normal levels were noted in fibroblasts from the center of this tissue. In addition, decreased levels of collagenase mRNA were found in the hypertrophic scar fibroblasts, suggesting that decreased expression of collagenase in hypertrophic scar fibroblasts may be one possible cause for the excessive accumulation of collagen in the skin lesions of hypertrophic scars (57). On the other hand, increased collagen synthesis by normal collagen degradation has been found in keloid fibroblasts in vitro (58). Tenascin, a large extracellular matrix glycoprotein, was shown to be strongly expressed in keloids, demarcating their borders in tissue (59,60). Significantly increased levels of tenascin expression were also found in keloidal fibroblasts in comparison with normal cells in vitro. As in vivo, normal and keloidal fibroblasts have been shown to exhibit similar basal rates of fibrin matrix gel contraction in vitro, and fibroblasts from hypertrophic scars exhibited a consistently higher basal rate of fibrin matrix gel contraction than other fibroblasts (61). Furthermore, only nodules of hypertrophic scars contained α-smooth muscle actin–expressing myofibroblasts when compared with keloid and normal skin tissue (49). The presence in hypertrophic scar myofibroblasts of α-smooth muscle actin, the actin isoform typical of vascular smooth muscle cells, may represent an important element in the pathogenesis of increased contraction in hypertrophic scars.

Patients wish treatment mainly for cosmetic reasons; pruritus, pain, and restriction of movement by lesions close to joints are often additional ones. A variety of therapeutic regimens has been used with unsatisfactory final results, because these lesions, especially keloids, are notoriously recurrent (47,48,62–65). Cryosurgery was found effective and safe for keloids and hypertrophic scars in several studies during the past years. Because of its major advantage of rarely involving recurrences the technique, as monotherapy or in combinations, has been established as the treatment of choice for keloids and hypertrophic scars.

A. Effects of Freezing on the Connective Tissue

An advantage of cryosurgery often cited is that of minimum scarring. The collagen fiber network of the dermis has been shown to remain largely undamaged by the standard cryosurgical procedures performed by clinicians (25). With the young domestic pig as a model and two 1-minute freeze-thaw cycles, no alteration in the periodicity of fibrillar cross-banding and no fracturing or distortion of collagen fibrils were found. In another study on rats, wound contraction after freeze injury was minimal, whereas with burn damage contracture was the rule (66).

B. Effects of Freezing on Keloidal Fibroblasts

Fibroblasts are rather resistant to freezing (25,60) and cryosurgery was shown to increase their proliferation in vivo (21) and in vitro (60,67). Suspended fibroblast cultures established from keloids and normal skin samples incubated in sterile cryotubes were frozen in precooled ethanol (−75°C) and consequently seeded on culture dishes. The proliferation of keloidal fibroblasts significantly increased immediately after cryotherapy in vitro in four of six cultures tested. After subcultivation, persistence of significantly increased proliferation was determined in three of four cultures. On the other hand, the proliferation of normal fibroblasts decreased in three of six cultures immediately after cryotherapy but returned to higher rates after subcultivation. These data correspond to the increase in the number of dermal fibroblasts observed 3 weeks after cryosurgery of the young domestic pig skin (21). Furthermore, cryosurgery induced a significant reduction of collagen I synthesis in two of four cultures examined after freezing in comparison with nonfrozen cultures, whereas increased synthesis of collagen IV was found in two of four cultures (60,67). No uniform changes of collagen III and fibronectin synthesis were detected. After subcultivation, increased collagen IV synthesis of keloidal fibroblasts persisted in two of two cultures, and the synthesis of collagen I was no longer suppressed. Collagens I and III represented more than 90% of the total amount of collagen produced by keloidal fibroblasts in vitro. Normal fibroblasts showed no uniform changes of collagen and fibronectin synthesis either immediately after cryotherapy or after subcultivation. It is likely that cryotherapy has a temporary inhibitory effect on the synthetic activity of keloidal fibroblasts, while it does not affect the activity of normal cells.

C. Structural Changes in Keloids and Hypertrophic Scars After Cryosurgery

Significant skin thickening was found to occur 3 weeks after cryosurgery of pig skin, which was compatible with an increase in the number of fibroblasts, followed by significant thinning at 6 months, probably due to the chronic ischemia induced by cryosurgery (21). In humans, neovascularization, a regular linear arrangement of collagen bundles, increased fibroblasts in a stroma running parallel to the skin surface, and mononuclear cells mostly arranged at the perivascular area were found in clinically responding lesions after cryosurgery (5). In a prospective, randomized study of 40 patients with keloids comparing the clinical and histological effects of cryosurgery as a single regimen or combined with intralesional steroids, an increased vessel number and lumen dilatation in both groups and a reduction of the number and length of rete ridges in the monotherapy group were the major structural changes observed (68). Immunhistologically, enhancement and diffusion of tenascin expression in the whole treated dermal region and depletion of interferon-γ expression, indicating immune regulation, were found (69). These histological and immunohistological studies indicate that cryosurgery can induce changes in keloids that are compatible with rejuvenation of the scars.

D. Clinical Results

Cryosurgery was initially applied in the treatment of keloids and hypertrophic scars as a weak cryotherapy regimen prior to intralesional corticosteroids in order to induce tissue edema and to facilitate intralesional injections (70). Cryosurgery as a monotherapy regimen was first used by Shepherd and Dawber in 1982 (71). They treated 17 patients with keloids with a single cryosurgical session and achieved 80% improvement of the lesions; however, they observed a high recurrence rate of 33%. With the exception of case or technical reports (72–74), further monotherapy studies were probably delayed by the rather disappointing recurrence rate, until Mende (1987) (75) and Zouboulis and Orfanos (1990) (76) showed that repeated cryosurgical sessions can have a beneficial effect on keloids and hypertrophic scars and also prevent relapses.

Cryosurgery was shown to yield significantly better results than intralesional triamcinolone (5 mg per lesion) in a randomized study with 11 patients with multiple acne keloids, especially in early, vascular lesions (77). It is now regarded as an established treatment for keloids and hypertrophic scars (78), possibly the treatment of choice (4,5). The following techniques are established or currently under evaluation.

1. *Cryosurgery as Monotherapy*

In 241 of 356 patients with keloids (68%) and 72 of 89 patients with hypertrophic scars (81%) a higher than 50% improvement or complete regression has been observed (five studies; Table 3) (5–7,68,75). Acne keloids also showed 73% improvement or complete regression in 16 patients treated (79). To achieve these results, 1 to more than 20 sessions of an average of 30 seconds each applied once monthly using the contact method of treatment were required. Progression or recurrence was rare (2%). The number of sessions, the diagnosis, and the duration of lesions were significantly correlated with the result of the treatment. The age and the sex of the patient, the size and the localization of lesions, and pretreatment with another method did not influence the outcome of cryosurgical treatments (5)

Table 3 Cryosurgery of Keloids and Hypertrophic Scars: Clinical Results

Study	Number of patients	Significant to complete remission	%	Recurrences	
Cryosurgery as monotherapy		Keloids			
Mende (1987)	7	5	71	—	
Zouboulis et al. (1993)	55	28	51	—	
Rusciani et al. (1993)	40	34	85	—	
Ernst and Hundeiker (1994)	234	158	68	9	
Zouridaki et al. (1996)	20	16	80	—	
Total	356	241	68%	9	2%
		Hypertrophic scars			
Zouboulis et al. (1993)	38	29	76	—	
Ernst and Hundeiker (1994)	51	43	84	2	
Total	89	72	81%	2	2%
Cryosurgery combined with intralesional corticosteroids		Keloids			
Hirshowitz et al. (1982)	58	41	71	9	
Ernst and Hundeiker (1994)	56	38	68	2	
Zouridaki et al. (1996)	20	19	95	—	
Banfalvi et al. (1996)	25	21	84	—	
Total	159	119	75%	11	7%

(Table 4). The cryosurgical treatment was generally well tolerated and only minor complications occurred. About one third of the patients treated complained of mild local pain, which was easily managed, if necessary. From 12 to 100% of the subjects experienced lesional hypopigmentation and 1–8% skin atrophy. The complications were dependent on the duration of freezing and the number of freeze-thaw cycles applied (5,6,75).

2. *Cryosurgery Combined with Intralesional Corticosteroids*

Initially performed in 1982 by Hirshowitz et al. (80) with the impressive result of 71% complete remission in 58 patients with keloids, the combination of cryosurgery prior or fol-

Table 4 Variables Affecting the Outcome of Cryosurgery in Keloids and Hypertrophic Scars

Factors that influence the outcome of cryosurgery in keloids and hypertrophic scars	
Diagnosis	Hypertrophic scars respond significantly better than keloids.
Number of sessions	Improved responses were detected in subjects treated with three or more sessions compared to subjects treated once or twice.
Age of the lesion	Lesions younger than 2 years responded better than older ones.
Factors that do not influence the outcome of cryosurgery in keloids and hypertrophic scars	
Age of the patient	
Sex of the patient	
Size of the lesion	
Localization of the lesion	
Pretreatment	

lowing intralesional corticosteroids resulted in significant regression of keloids in 78 of 101 patients (77%) treated in three further studies (Table 3) (7,68,81). Cryosurgery performed before corticosteroid treatment induces tissue edema and facilitates intralesional injections. However, the combined therapy was not superior (90% with more than 50% reduction of lesional volume) to monotherapy (83% with more than 50% reduction of lesional volume) in a randomized trial with 40 patients with keloids (68).

3. *Surgical Debulkment Prior to Cryosurgery With or Without Intralesional Corticosteroids*

Lesions refractory to cryosurgery or cryosurgery combined with intralesional corticosteroids can be surgically removed, and postsurgical cryoprevention with or without intralesional corticosteroids can be applied in order to avoid recurrences. This regimen is unavoidable with large keloids, although recurrences are not rare despite the promising initial result (82–85). Intramarginal excision is advisable because it is followed by a lower recurrence rate than extramarginal excision (86). Removal of lesions by surgery or carbon dioxide laser involves similar recurrence rates (87); however, a carbon dioxide laser provides a high degree of hemostasis and avoidance of sutures.

4. *Intralesional Cryosurgery*

A method of intralesional cryosurgery for keloids and hypertrophic scars developed by modification of the technique of Weshahy (88) is under evaluation in our department.

5. *Cryopeeling*

The freezing peel (cryopeeling) is a full-face, superficial cryosurgical treatment for atrophic acne scarring that is especially useful for patients with mild to moderate circinate scars. Results are similar to those obtained with chemical peeling but not as good as those obtained with dermabrasion. Repeated sessions, sometimes over 2 to 3 years, are required to obtain optimal results (9).

IV. CRYOSURGICAL EQUIPMENT AND TREATMENT TECHNIQUES

A. Simple Cryosurgical Units: The Cotton-Tipped Applicator and the "Hard Tail" Dipstick

The simplest cryosurgical modality, still in current use, is the cotton-tipped applicator method using small or large swabs soaked in liquid nitrogen (14) (Fig. 1). Both instruments lack the capacity of active freezing and, therefore, can induce only slow freezing, which limits their application in the treatment of keloids and hypertrophic scars. In addition, large swabs create large frozen surfaces, generally exceeding the limits of the area intended for treatment in small lesions, and small swabs have a limited liquid nitrogen reservoir capacity. A modification of the classic cotton-tipped applicator is the "hard tail" dipstick, which has been devised in an attempt to avoid these disadvantages (89). The hard tail dipstick is made of a standard large cotton-tipped applicator (Fig. 1). At its end, a tiny amount of cotton is pinched between the index finger and thumb and strongly twisted in order to obtain the so-called hard tail. The distal part of the tail is cut down so that the total tail does not exceed 5 mm. This dipstick is soaked in liquid nitogen. Because a large swab is used, a large amount of liquid nitrogen is absorbed by the cotton reservoir. Only the tail of the swab is put in contact with the lesion. Liquid nitrogen is slowly released at the pointed end of the

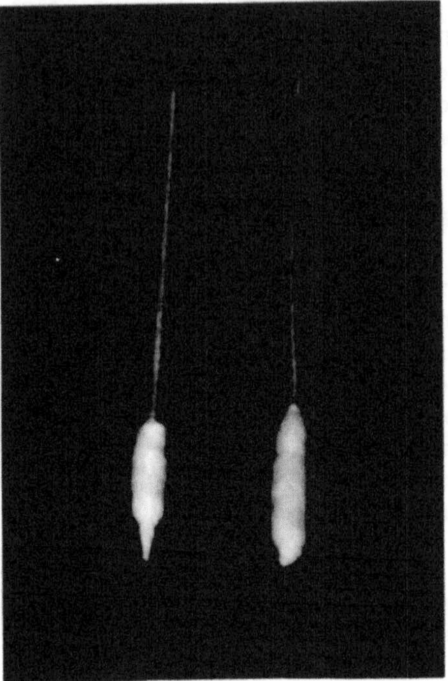

Figure 1 Cotton-tipped applicator using a large swab (right) and hard tail dipstick (left) before cutting the distal part of the tail.

swab, producing an accurate freezing effect. The degree of hardness of the tail is a factor that must be stressed. If it is not hard enough, the tail cannot easily remain in contact with the lesion and is useless. Therefore, one should not pull a tiny amount of cotton but only pinch it before twisting it strongly. When application with the hard tail begins, some drops of liquid nitrogen may run. This can be avoided by shaking the swab once or twice in the air before the application. The method is sufficient to treat epithelial benign lesions but does not induce temperatures low enough for sufficient cryosurgery of dermal benign lesions, such as keloids and hypertrophic scars. However, it can be used as an alternative technique when other cryosurgical devices are not available or for very small scar lesions (smaller than 5 mm).

B. The Modern Cryosurgical Unit

Today, there many commercially available, well-functioning cryosurgical units with variable design, function, and performance characteristics (90,91). Sufficient cold for cryosurgery can be produced by direct or indirect application of a solid or liquid cryogen stored at low temperatures, by lowering the pressure of a gas (Joule-Thompson effect), electromechanically, or simply by refrigeration. The devices are mainly characterized by the applied cryogen and the means of cryogen application to the skin (Table 5). A cryosurgical unit consists of five main components: a liquid Dewar or gas cylinder, the cryogen, a pressure gauge, a cryogun with tubing, and assorted cryoprobe or spray tips.

Table 5 Classification of Cryosurgical Devices

According to the cryogen used
Liquid nitrogen units (probe tip temperature −170 to −190°C)
Nitrous oxide units (probe tip temperature −65 to −85°C)
Units using a Peltier thermoelectric element (probe tip temperature −32 to −40°C)
According to the means of cryogen application
Devices using the contact technique
Devices using the spray technique
Devices for intralesional cryosurgery

1. The Liquid Dewar or Gas Cylinder

Liquid Dewars and gas cylinders are of widely varying size (Fig. 2). The efficiency of cryosurgery using nitrous oxide is dependent on maintaining adequate gas pressure in the cylinder. Internal gas pressure decreases during freezing and must be regenerated at room temperature between freezes to maintain adequate pressure. In contrast, most units using liquid nitrogen are not pressurized until the unit becomes activated. Most units incorporate regulators to reduce or control tip pressures for economy and safety. The regulators provide constant performance at various cylinder pressure levels.

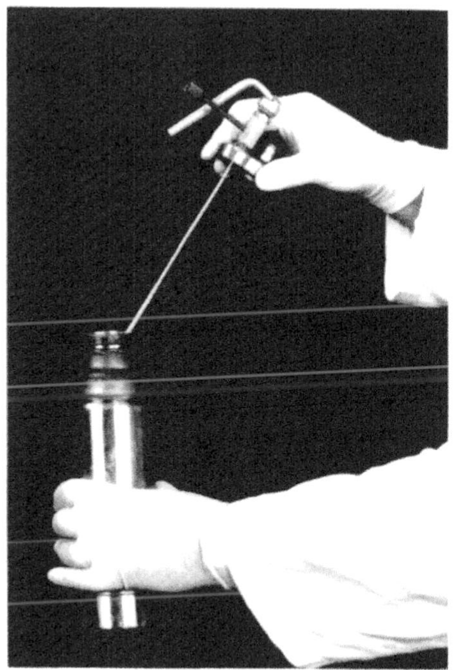

Figure 2 Liquid Dewar (lower part) of a cryosurgery unit using liquid nitrogen as the cryogen. The upper part of the device includes the activation trigger, which must be pressed during the freezing, the regulator vent, the cryoprobe stem, and the cryogun stem.

2. *The Cryogen*

The most common cryogen today is liquid nitrogen, which can generate low target tissue temperatures because of its boiling point of −195.8°C. It is considered to be the cryogen of choice for dermatological cryosurgery and the only cryogen advocated for treatment of malignant skin lesions. Nitrous oxide, a nonflammable gas with a boiling point of −89.5°C, is a sufficient cryogen for the treatment of benign skin lesions.

3. *The Gas Pressure Gauge*

Nitrous oxide cryosurgical units feature a gas pressure gauge located between the cylinder and the cryogun (Fig. 3). The gauge indicates the pressure within the cylinder and is divided

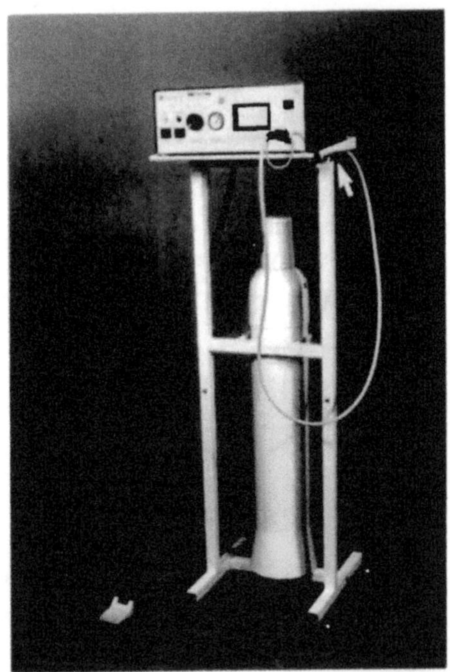

a

Figure 3 **(a)** Nitrous oxide cryosurgery unit with a 10-L gas cylinder, the on-off switch (pedal), and the cryogun (arrow) supplied with a pyrometer recording the actual temperature of the cryoprobe tip. In **(b)** a gas pressure gauge (closed arrowhead), a pressure indicator (cross), and an incorporated chronometer (star) can be seen. The temperature is registered on an indicator (open arrowhead).

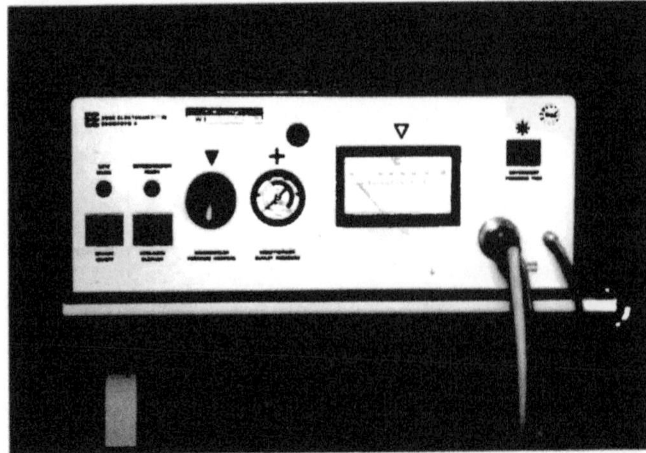

b

into three pressure zones. The high zone of the gauge reflects excessive cylinder pressure (a safety hazard) and the low gas pressure results in inefficient and probably inadequate freezing. The middle zone indicates adequate freezing.

4. The Cryogun

The cryogun consists of a hand grip, activation trigger, cryogun stem, and cryoprobe stem. In some units, the on-off switch for the gas valve is located on the cryogun (Fig. 2); in others it consists of a pedal (Figs. 3 and 4). Activation triggers vary in function. In the majority of the units, depression of the trigger initiates the freeze (Figs. 3, 4, and 13); in a few others it defrosts the probe tip. Some triggers feature a locked position setting so that the trigger need not be depressed during the freeze (Fig. 4).

5. Cryoprobe and Spray Tips

Cryoprobe tips must be made of a good thermal conducting metal, such as silver, gold, or copper. The interchangeable tips are available in various shapes and sizes to enable maximum contact of the tip with the tissue and avoid freezing of healthy areas (Figs. 5–7). The majority of cryosurgical units feature pyrometers, which indicate the actual temperature of the cryoprobe tip. By applying the spray technique, spray tips with different aperture sizes are used (Fig. 8). Intralesional cryosurgery involves single-use, 20-gauge or larger needles instead of tips (Fig. 9).

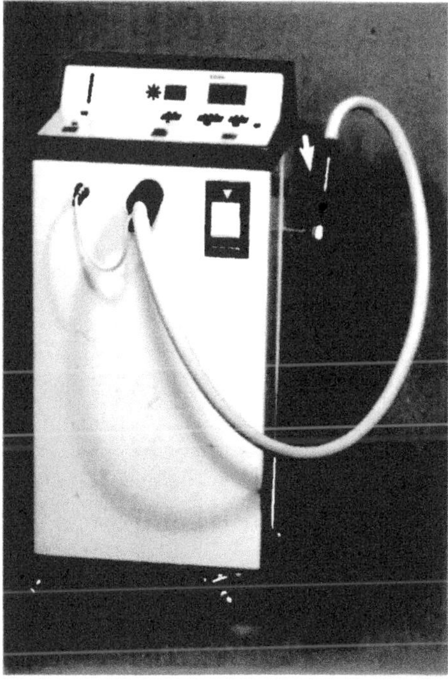

Figure 4 Large liquid nitrogen hospital cryosurgery unit with a 10-L liquid Dewar (inside the body of the device), the on-off switch (pedal) with a locked position setting, the cryogun (arrow) supplied with a pyrometer recording the actual temperature of the cryoprobe tip (closed arrowhead), and an incorporated chronometer (star). The unit includes a rapid rewarming device (for quick detachment of the cryoprobe) with a heating option (for tissue coagulation or hemostasis).

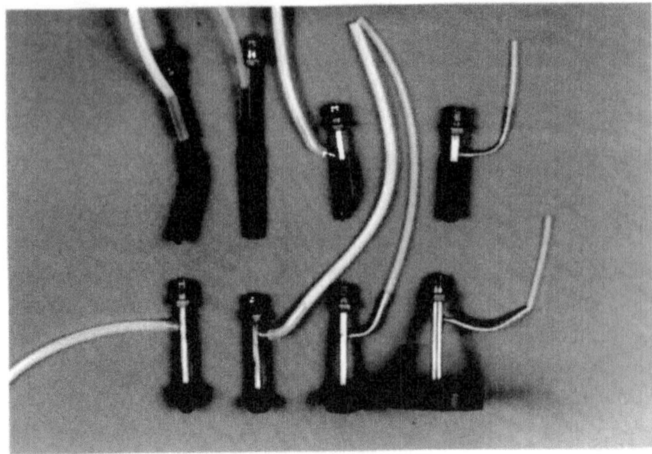

Figure 5 Cryoprobe tips in different shapes for a liquid nitrogen device. All cryoprobes have exhaust valves with exhaust silicone tubings.

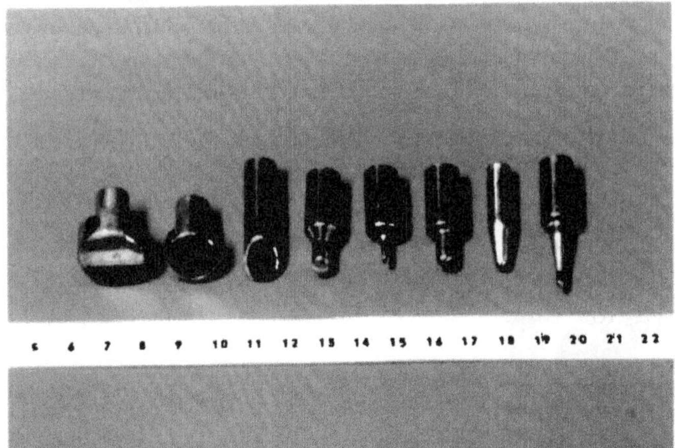

Figure 6 Cryoprobe tips in different shapes for a nitrous oxide device.

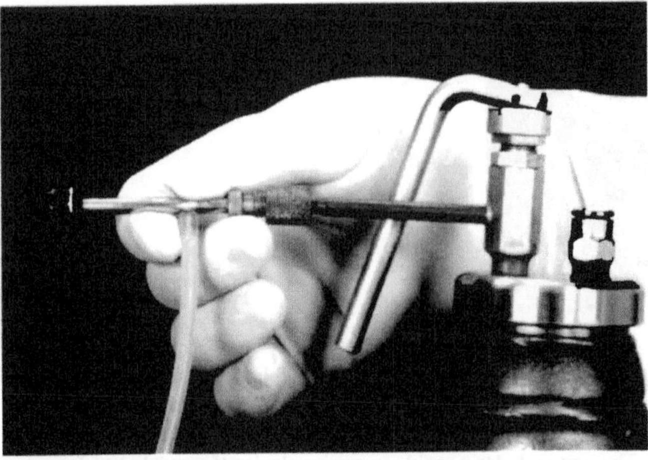

Figure 7 A cryoprobe tip for a liquid nitrogen device is going to be fixed in the cryoprobe stem.

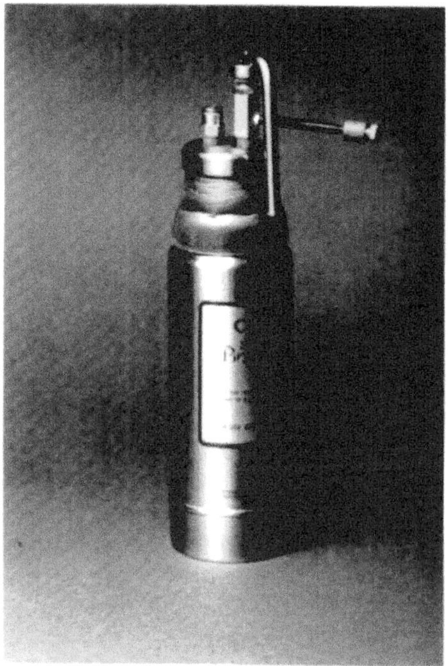

Figure 8 Small liquid nitrogen cryosurgery unit with a spray tip instead of cryosurgery probe.

C. Classification of Cryosurgical Devices According to the Cryogen Used

1. Liquid Nitrogen Units

Liquid nitrogen units are open systems that can be used for both cryoprobe and spray applications. They develop a probe tip temperature of −170 to −190°C and, therefore, rapid freezing of over 100°C/min. Handheld simple units with a liquid Dewar capacity of 250 mL to 1 L (Figs. 7 and 8) as well as large instruments with sophisticated temperature controls and a liquid nitrogen Dewar capacity of up to 10 L (Fig. 4) are available. Most units are not pressurized until the spray is desired. Liquid nitrogen requires a storage container (91).

2. Nitrous Oxide Units

Nitrous oxide units are closed systems that operate by the Joule-Thomson effect (92). They can be only used for cryoprobe applications. The refrigeration results from the expansion of the gas through a small opening (adiabatic principle). Pressurized nitrous oxide advances down the narrow cryogun stem [high-pressure cryoprobe (19)]. When it reaches the hollow cryoprobe tip, the gas rapidly expands, lowering the tip temperature below freezing. The temperature of the nitrous oxide cryoprobe drops to −65 to −85°C and, therefore, a moderate freezing speed of less than 100°C/min is developed. High-pressure devices have several advantages over liquid nitrogen probes (19) (Table 6).

3. Units Using a Peltier Thermoelectric Element

Units using a Peltier effect cooler (19) are closed systems used only for cryoprobe applications. They develop a probe tip temperature of −32 to −40°C by a thermoelectric proce-

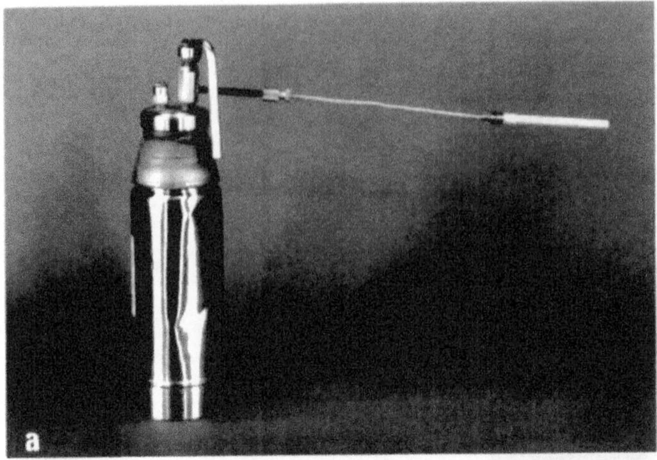

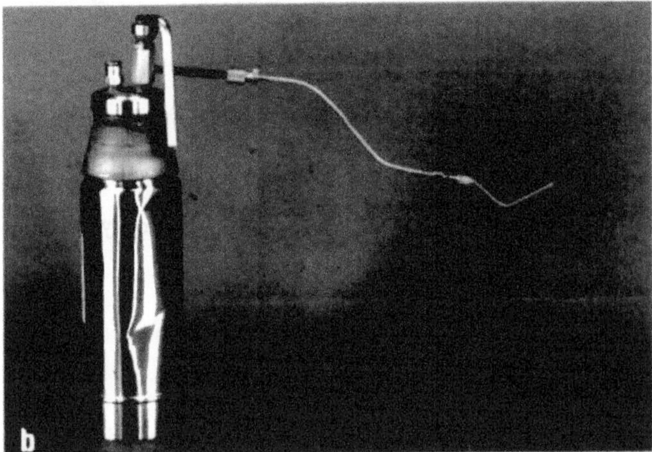

Figure 9 Small liquid nitrogen cryosurgery unit for intralesional cryosurgery with a single-use 20-gauge needle **(a)** and a flexible, long metallic cryoprobe stem Luer locked to the needle **(b)**.

dure, and therefore they do not involve the use of a cryogen. The low freezing speed makes these devices sufficient only in the treatment of superficial benign epithelial lesions and in cosmetic dermatology; they are insufficient in the treatment of keloids and hypertrophic scars.

D. Classification of Therapeutic Techniques According to the Means of Cryogen Application

The methodology of cryosurgery has now become sophisticated and the techniques standardized. There are three different techniques that may be used for the treatment of keloids and hypertrophic scars.

Table 6 Advantages and Disadvantages of High-Pressure and Liquid Nitrogen Devices

High-pressure devices (nitrous oxide)	Liquid nitrogen devices
Advantages	Disadvantages
Relatively inexpensive and robust	More expensive because of the quick evaporation of liquid nitrogen and the requirement for a storage Dewar
The working fluid is supplied at room temperature; highly insulated supply lines are not required.	Insulated supply lines are required.
They operate efficiently without pre-cooling; the cooling expansion occurs within the tip itself.	The cooling expansion occurs within the whole device.
Disadvantages	Advantages
Freezing at moderate speed only	Freezing at high speed
Moderately low temperature at cryo-probe tip	Very low temperature at cryoprobe tip
Available for contact technique only	Available for both contact and spray techniques

1. The Contact Technique

The contact method uses metallic probes that function according to the principle of temperature exchange (Fig. 10). These probes are circulated by a gas cryogen. As the tip removes heat from the tissue, the tissue gradually cools. The size, material, composition, and temperature of the probe tip determine its tissue-cooling capacity. Other factors, such as tissue moistness, extent of tissue contact, duration of freezing, and pressure exerted on the probe, affect heat diffusion. When the cryosurgical unit is activated and the probe is placed

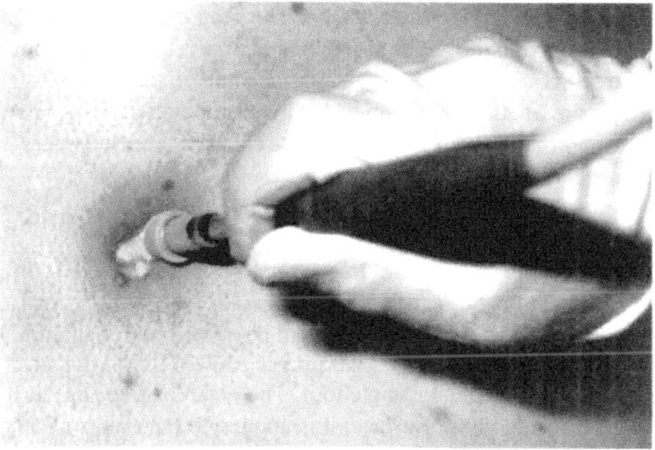

Figure 10 The contact method uses metallic probes with a circulating gas refrigerant that function after the principle of temperature exchange. The size, material, composition, and temperature of the probe tip determine its tissue cooling capacity. (From Ref. 4, copyrighted 1995, Kassenarzt-Verlag.)

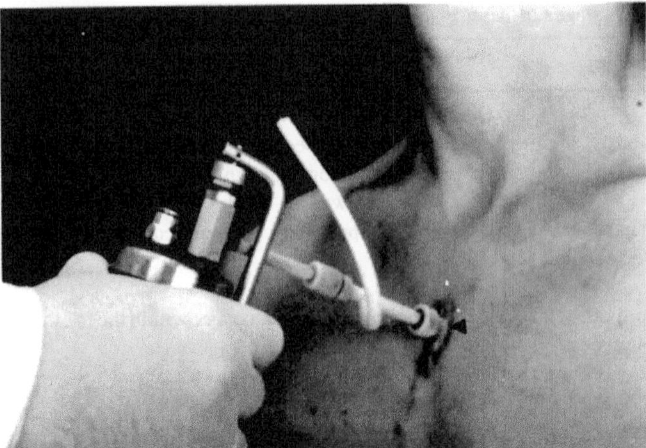

Figure 11 Contact freezing technique: when the cryosurgical unit is activated and the probe is placed in firm contact with the tissue, an area of frozen tissue or ice ball may be observed extending radially from the cryoprobe tip (arrowhead).

in firm contact with the tissue, an area of frozen tissue or ice ball may be observed extending radially from the cryoprobe tip (Fig. 11). The interface between the ice ball and unfrozen tissue represents the 0°C isotherm, which is the line of connection points representing 0°C at the given time. The greater the duration of freezing, the farther the iceball radiates from the cryoprobe tip margin (18). The distance between the tip margin and the 0°C isotherm represents the lateral spread of freezing. The depth of the 0°C isotherm from the tip indicates the depth of freezing. Although variable, the lateral spread of freezing approximates the depth of freezing by a ratio of 1:1.3 (93). The volume of tissue located between the −22°C isotherm and the probe tip is called the lethal zone. Cells within this zone undergo cryonecrosis (19). The cells situated in the warmer region between the −22°C isotherm and the 0°C isotherm generally survive the freezing. This important zone represents the recovery zone (Fig. 12). Although the depth of freezing is time related, as the duration of freezing extends toward 100 seconds the lethal zone becomes flat. The contact method is the method of choice for the treatment of keloids and hypertrophic scars, because it provides controllable as well as reproducible results. The results can be modulated as cryoprobe pressure can induce vessel contraction.

2. *The Spray Technique*

The spray technique uses an open freezing system with freeze secure vents (Fig. 13). It directly emits a fine spray of a cryogen at the target area. It is particularly useful for irregular lesions and lesions with a curved surface. For large lesions to be treated in one session, a paintbrush or spiral pattern of spray can be used (94). The spray is emitted from a distance of 1 to 2 cm from the target site and at a 90-degree angle to it. The depth of freezing may be judged by the lateral spread of freezing on the surface; it is about half the radius of the surface area (95) (Fig. 14). Intermittent spraying of liquid nitrogen is desirable, because it results in a more uniform temperature in the ice ball and greater depth, while it limits lateral spread. The depth of freezing can reach only 10 mm (95), so this is not the appropriate technique for voluminous keloids and hypertrophic scars. There are two variants of the

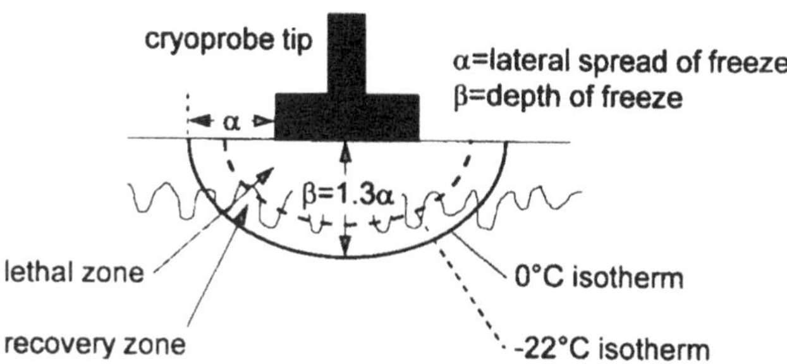

Figure 12 Ice ball induced by a cryoprobe tip. The interface between the ice ball and unfrozen tissue represents the 0°C isotherm. The longer the duration of the freeze, the farther the iceball radiates from the cryoprobe tip margin. The distance between the tip margin and the 0°C isotherm represents the lateral spread of freezing. The depth of the 0°C isotherm from the tip indicates the depth of freezing. Although variable, the lateral spread of freezing approximates the depth of freezing by a ratio of 1:1.3. The volume of tissue located between the −22°C isotherm and the probe tip is called the lethal zone. Cells within this zone undergo cryonecrosis. The sells cituated in the warmer region between the −22°C isotherm and the 0°C isotherm generally survive the freeze. This area represents the recovery zone.

spraying procedure, the described open-spray technique and the confined-spray technique. The latter directs the spray into cones (91), individually prepared plastic moulages (4), or other materials that are open at both ends with one end placed on the skin. The confined-spray technique restricts the spray to the lesion and avoids wide freezing of the healthy peripheral tissue; however, it makes impossible clinical evaluation of the depth of freezing (Fig. 13).

3. *Intralesional Cryosurgery*

The inability of skin surface cryosurgery to freeze more than 20 mm in depth (96) led Weshahy (88) to develop a method for applying cryosurgery in depth. One or more needles are introduced into the skin from one point, run through the deeper tissues of the lesion, and appear at the surface on the opposite border. A sprayed cryogen is then passed through the needle by inserting the spray tip of the cryosurgical device into the headpiece of the needle. The cryogen is passed through the lumen and exits to the atmosphere from the other end of the needle. An ice cylinder is formed around the embedded part of the needle within the deeper tissues. The distance of extension of freezing can be clinically estimated from the degree of extension of the whitish ice balls formed around the points of contact between the skin surface and the visible portions of the needle. The needles can be angled, curved, and hook shaped. Compression of the lesions is accomplished by pooling the visible parts of the needle up. We currently evaluate intralesional cryosurgery in the treatment of keloids and hypertrophic scars. We have developed a device consisting of a small liquid nitrogen Dewar with a single-use, 20-gauge needle instead of a tip to spray liquid nitrogen through connected by a flexible, long metallic cryoprobe stem (Fig. 9). The cryoprobe stem is Luer locked to the needle. The shape of the cryoprobe stem is variable so that the Dewar can stay upright during freezing. The shape of the needle can also be changed in order to form a hook. The main advantage of intralesional cryosurgery compared with the contact and

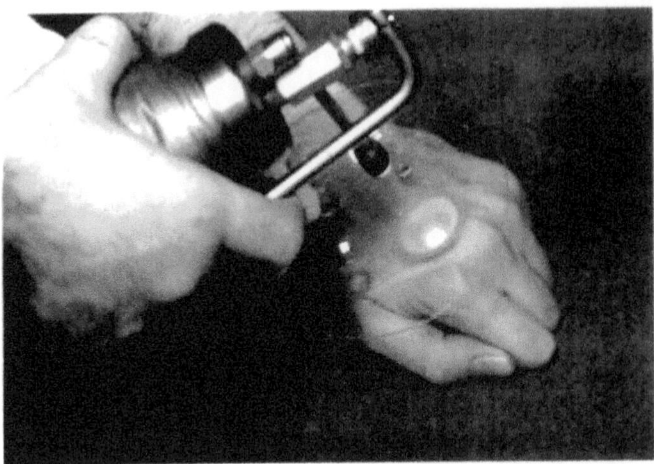

Figure 13 The confined-spray technique. The liquid nitrogen spray is directed into a plastic moulage with an opening size fitting the size of the lesion to be treated. The confined-spray technique restricts the spray to the lesion and avoids wide freezing of the healthy peripheral tissue. (From Ref. 4, copyrighted 1995, Kassenarzt-Verlag.)

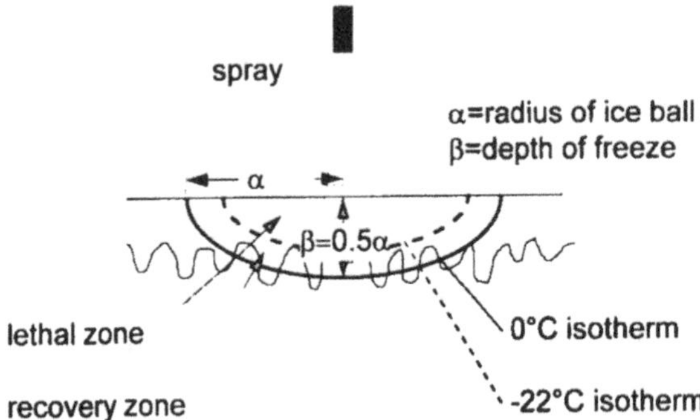

Figure 14 Ice ball induced by a cryogen spray. The interface between the ice ball and unfrozen tissue represents the 0°C isotherm. The longer the duration of the freeze, the larger the radius of the ice ball becomes. The maximum depth of the 0°C isotherm from the skin surface indicates the depth of freezing. Although variable, the lateral spread of freezing approximates half the radius of the ice ball. The volume of tissue located between the −22°C isotherm and the skin surface is called the lethal zone. Cells within this zone undergo cryonecrosis. Those cells situated in the warmer region between the −22°C isotherm and the 0°C isotherm generally survive the freezing. This area represents the recovery zone.

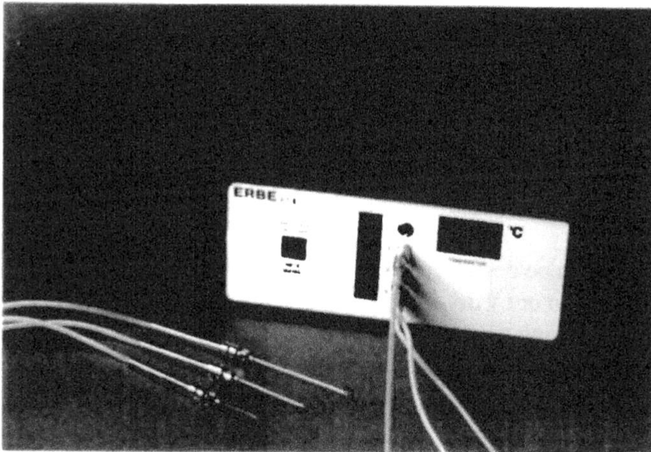

Figure 15 Pyrometer-thermocouple apparatus with three thermocouples mounted in needles of different width and length.

spray techniques is minimal surface destruction, which can be further reduced by using peripherally insulated needles.

E. Methods of Monitoring Tissue Temperature

Although the depth of tissue to be frozen should be exactly monitored in cryosurgery of malignant skin tumors (91), in the treatment of keloids and hypertrophic scars monitoring of freeze depth is optional. The progress of freezing can be clinically judged from the duration of freezing, the thawing of the lesion, and the measurement of the lateral spread of freezing (contact technique) or radius of the ice ball. To supplement clinical estimation, the tissue temperature can be monitored with a pyrometer-thermocouple apparatus using thermocouples mounted in 25- to 30-gauge needles (97) (Fig. 15). The thermocouples are inserted into the skin so that the tip lies beneath or lateral to the lesion. Other monitoring techniques are measurement of the electrical impedance in frozen tissue (98) and ultrasonography (99,100). Further improvement could provide a device combining a 27-mm nitrous oxide cryoprobe and an ultrasound microtransducer (20 MHz, 3.6 mm) at the center of the probe tip, permitting ultrasonographic monitoring of the tissue during freezing (101).

V. PRACTICAL PROCEDURES

In the following, practical procedures for the cryosurgical treatment of keloids and hypertrophic scars are described step by step. Although the techniques seem rather simple, the physician using cryosurgery has to be a certified dermatologist in order to diagnose the disease and have knowledge of the skin and subcutaneous tissues. In addition, the physician should have had training in cryosurgery. Prior to treatment the following general measures have to be taken:

1. The patient has to be informed about the procedure, the reported results of the technique, and the personal experience of the cryosurgeon as well as the complications that may occur. For sensitive patients, lidocaine-prilocaine 1:1 creme (102) has to be prescribed and be occlusively applied by the patient to the lesion(s) to be treated 1 hour prior cryosurgery. Instead of long explanations of the technique, which may confuse patients simplified information or a letter about cryosurgery can be prepared and distributed to the patients while awaiting their treatment (Fig. 16).
2. The cryoprobe tips have to be desinfected after every treatment either by soaking them in ethanol solution or by dry sterilization.
3. Gloves have to be worn during the procedures.
4. The lesion to be treated has to be disinfected using a sterile gauze soaked in ethanol solution (Fig. 17).

A. Contact Technique

1. The cryoprobe tip has to be chosen so that it fits to the size of the lesion in order to avoid freezing of the peripheral healthy tissue (Fig. 18). The sizes of the probe tips have to be similar to or, even better, a little smaller than the size of the lesion, taking into consideration that an ice ball is formed during freezing that spreads laterally to the lesion.
2. When using a liquid nitrogen hand unit with silicone exhaust tubing, the tubing has to be frozen at a position away from the patient and the physician, otherwise the tubing will flail and finally freeze to a position that may interfere with the treatment (Fig. 19).
3. The time of freezing for each lesion or a part of it has to be controlled. For keloids and hypertrophic scars a single freeze-thaw session of 20 to 60 seconds has to be used, depending on the volume of the lesion (Fig. 20).
4. Large scars can be treated with specially formed cryoprobes, such as a flat linear probe for a linear scar (72) (Fig. 5), or classical small probes in order to induce significant pressure and vasocontraction on fragments of the lesion (Fig. 21).
5. As mentioned earlier, optimal use of the technique allows exact freezing of the lesion without any freezing of the peripheral healthy tissue (Fig. 22).
6. If there is no intervention after cryosurgery, the physical course of the cryoreaction is as follows:
   (a) Peripheral erythema, occurring immediately to 30 minutes after cryosurgery (Fig. 23).
   (b) Edema of the lesion, occurring between a few minutes and some hours after treatment (Fig. 24).
   (c) Bulla formation, usually presenting between 1 and 3 days after treatment (Fig. 25).
   (d) Exudation, lasting between a few to 14 days after cryosurgery.
   (e) Mummification, wherein a serum crust is formed between the second and the fourth posttreatment week.
   (f) Healing, with a flat, slightly atrophic scar.
7. In order to minimize erythema and edema after cryosurgery, a mild, nonatrophogenic steroid cream (e.g., hydrocortisone aceponate, hydrocortisone

University Medical Center Benjamin Franklin
The Free University of Berlin
Department of Dermatology
Director: Prof. Dr. Prof. h.c. C.E. Orfanos

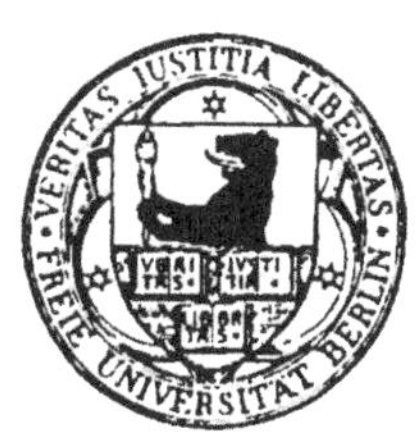

University Medical Center Benjamin Franklin
Hindenburgdamm 30, D-12200 Berlin, Germany

Secretariat:	(030) 8445 - 2292
Direct call:	(030) 8445 - 2284
Telephone center:	(030) 8445 - 0
Fax:	(030) 8445 - 4262
e-mail:	zoubbere@zedat.fu-berlin.de

For Your Information

Cryosurgery and Post-Operative Skin Care

Dear patient:

Your dermatologist has proposed you a treatment by "cryosurgery". How does this technique work?

"Cryosurgery" is a surgical treatment administering low temperatures to the skin by which diseased tissue is removed and substituted by new-formed healthy one.

What happens during the treatment session?

Skin is a living tissue. It is constituted by numerous cells which have to fulfill several functions. The reduction of environmental temperature, like in winter, leads to decreased skin and body temperature. In extreme cases, skin can cool down until it freezes, skin blisters can occur.

During treatment with cryosurgery the diseased skin will be frozen in a similar, but controlled, manner for a few seconds. The tissue water freezes, the cells dye. Consequently, the tissue thaws. This cold shock leads to a controlled destruction of the diseased tissue, only. Local swelling results after the treatment due to local water collection in the tissue.

How does the dermatologist make diseased tissue freeze?

Diseased tissue freezes through the contact and slight pressure of a cold metal probe on the skin. This probe is already cold enough to freeze together with the skin for a short time. After thawing the probe can be removed from the skin surface. Skin can also be frozen by spraying nitrous oxide on it through a spray tip of a liquid dewar vessel.

Is cryosurgical treatment painful?

The small nerve endings in skin can perceive the acute tissue freezing as painful. However, an injection with local anesthetic solution is rarely required. The application of an anesthetic ointment 1 to 2 hours before the cryosurgical session could sufficiently minimize local pain in the most of the cases.

What happens after the cryosurgical treatment?

Immediately after treatment the skin reacts with irritation and swelling. Both reactions are signs that a sufficiently low temperature could be achieved in the tissue. In the next hours to days small or large skin blisters can occur with or without liquid loss. All these skin reactions are normal and expected, they indicate that destruction of the diseased tissue had taken place.

Figure 16 A simplified information letter about cryosurgery used in the Department of Dermatology, University Medical Center Benjamin Franklin, The Free University of Berlin, which informs the patient about the technique, its advantages, possible complications, and what the patient has to do to help the physician give optimal care. The letter is distributed to the patient either when he decides to have cryosurgery and books an appointment or while waiting for treatment. *(figure continues)*

You do not need to do anything else except of protecting the skin blister until it breaks up spontaneously or visit your dermatologist so that he can puncture the blister and aspirate its content with a sterile fine needle 2 days after the treatment.

Therefore, you do not have to be anxious because of the presence of the skin reaction mentioned above; if you have any questions call or visit your dermatologist.

What happens after the blister is broken up?

After the skin blister is broken up the wound has to be treated with an antibacterial solution once daily until it dries and develops a crust. In that time the healing procedure has begun. Healthy skin tissue grows up from the wound borders and continuously makes the wound smaller. At that phase of skin reaction it is important to keep the wound dry in order to avoid infections, your dermatologist is going to provide you the required advice and topical medication.

When is wound healing completed?

Wound healing is completed in average three weeks after the cryosurgical treatment. During this period of time your dermatologist or your general medicine physician has to regularly control the procedure of wound healing.

Are scars to be expected after cryosurgery?

Scar formation after cryosurgery is usually not visible. The patient can often recognize the treated area only by the occurring thinner skin and its whitish color. Later, skin can pigment again to the normal color so that the treated area cannot be recognized any longer.

What is further important to know?

In individual cases wound healing can proceed with formation of a small scar at the center of the treated area raised over the skin surface and persisting over 2 to 4 weeks. This is not a hint that the treatment was insufficient but indicates that the skin overreacted to the treatment. Such skin changes usually heal spontaneously.

Can cryosurgical treatment take place on an outpatient basis?

Cryosurgery can take place on an outpatient basis presupposed that (a) the skin lesion is not very large, (b) it is located in areas being prone to wound infections and (c) the post-operative care is guarantied. "Difficult" lesions and patients with severe systemic diseases have to be treated on an inpatient basis in order to be optimally controlled. Your dermatologist is going to evaluate your individual case and discuss with you the adequate procedure.

Can cryosurgery be performed in very old patients?

Cryosurgery is often the surgical treatment of choice in very old patients who are unable to stand other operative procedures. With only exception the long-term wound healing period, cryosurgery is usually an easy-to-perform surgical procedure.

Please always ask! Your dermatologist is happy to answer your questions!

With best regards

Constantin E. Orfanos, M.D.
Professor and Chairman

Christos C. Zouboulis, M.D.
Responsible for Cryosurgery

Figure 16 *(continued)*

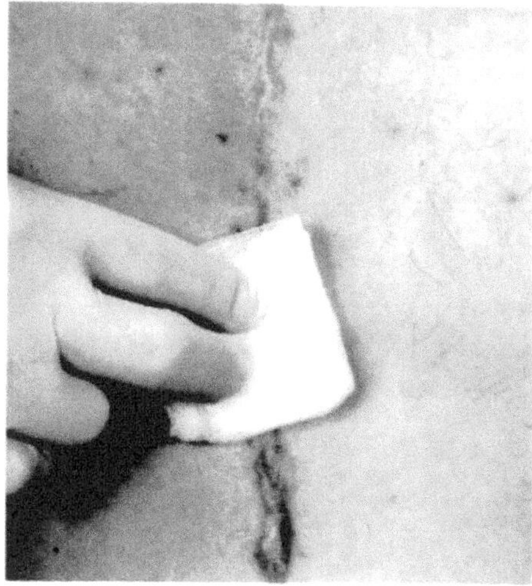

Figure 17 Disinfection of the lesion to be treated using a sterile gauze soaked in ethanol solution.

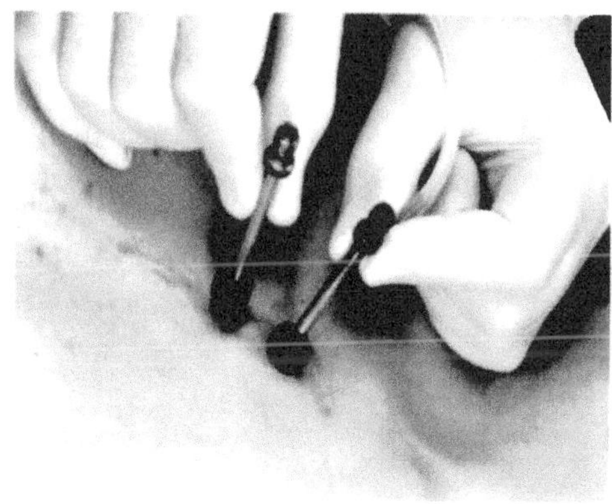

a

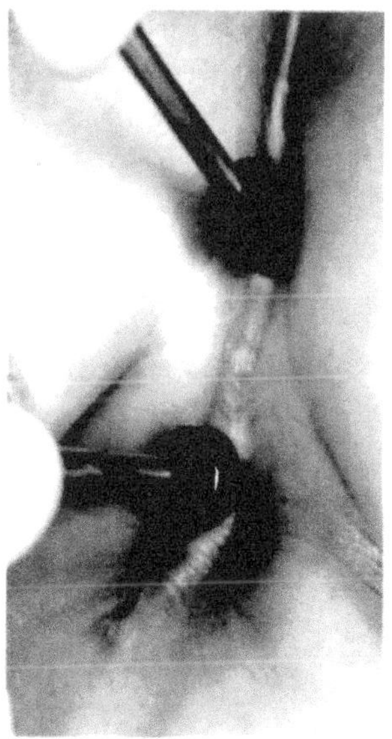

b

Figure 18 Choice of adequate cryoprobe tip for the different areas of the lesion to be treated **(a)** so that it fits the size of the lesion or, even better, is a little smaller than the size of the lesion **(b)**.

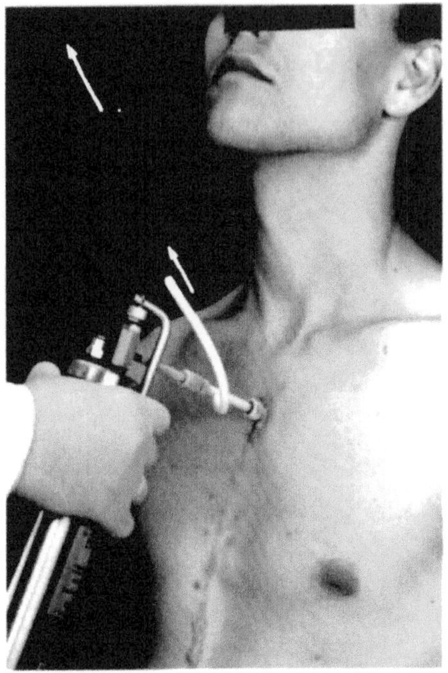

Figure 19 Direction of the silicone exhaust tubing and the liquid nitrogen (arrows) away from the patient and the physician during treatment in order to avoid unwanted freezing.

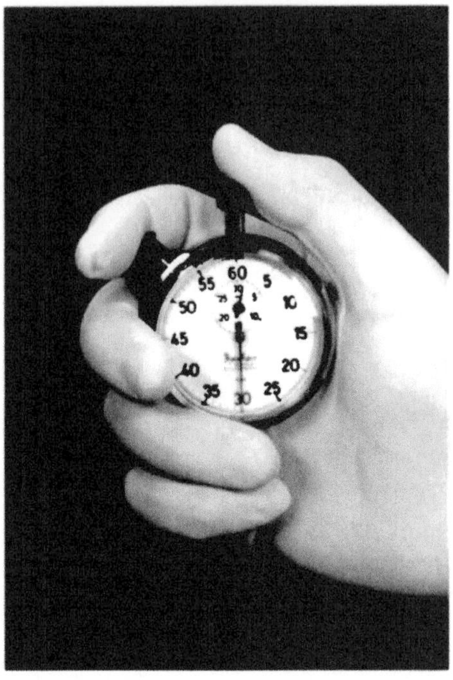

Figure 20 Control of freezing time is performed by a chronometer incorporated in the device or by a hand-operated chronometer.

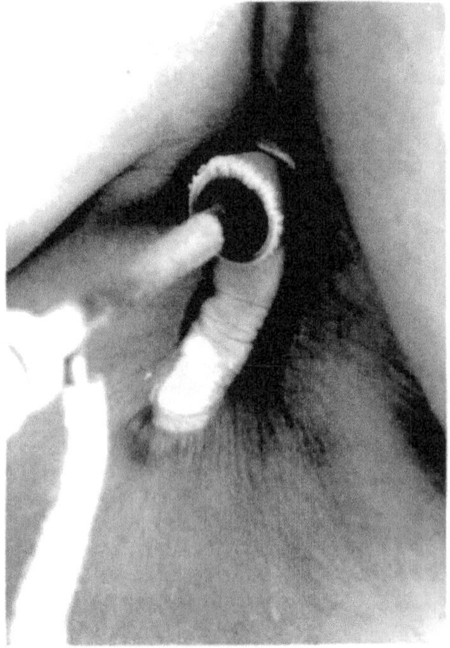

Figure 21 Treatment of large keloid by a small cryoprobe tip in order to induce significant pressure and vasocontraction on the lesion. Treatment is performed by repeated freezes on consecutive fragments of the lesion.

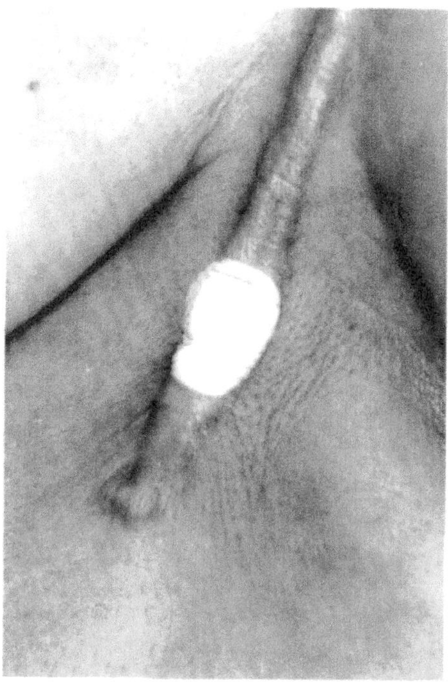

Figure 22 An example of optimal cryosurgery: exact freezing of the lesion without any freezing of the peripheral healthy tissue.

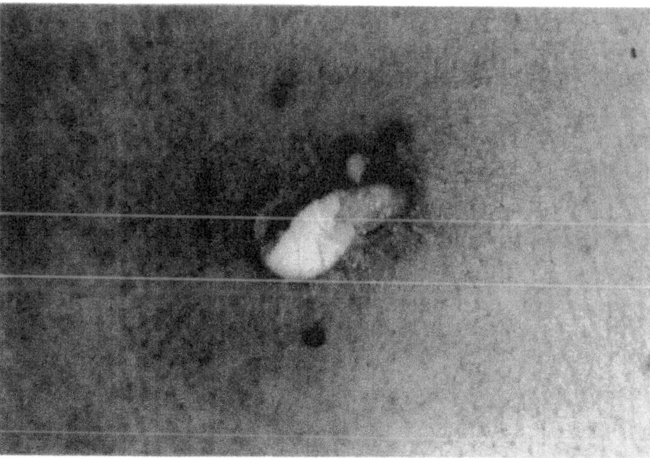

Figure 23 Peripheral erythema immediately after cryosurgery. Erythema is already present during thawing of the lesion.

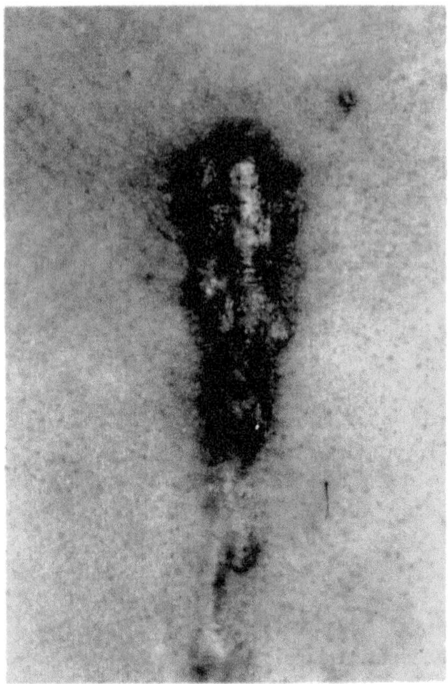

Figure 24 Lesional edema presenting a few minutes after cryosurgical treatment.

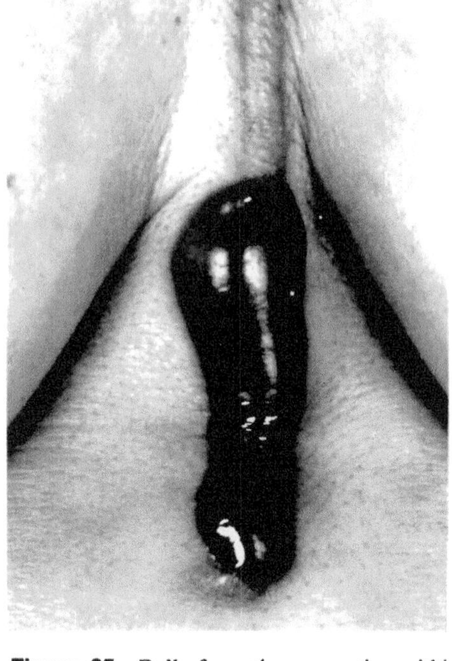

Figure 25 Bulla formation presenting within 3 days after cryosurgical treatment.

buteprate, hydrocortisone-17-butyrate, methylprednisolone aceponate, prednicarbate) has to be applied on the lesion immediately after treatment, especially in areas that are prone to react with strong edema (e.g., facial area).

8. The patient is requested to visit the physician again when a bulla is formed so that the physician or assistant can aspirate the serum content with a sterile fine needle (e.g., 26 gauge). The bulla roof must be left on the lesion as a natural protective film (Fig. 26). The bulla has to be disinfected using a sterile gauze soaked in ethanol solution before being aspirated.

a

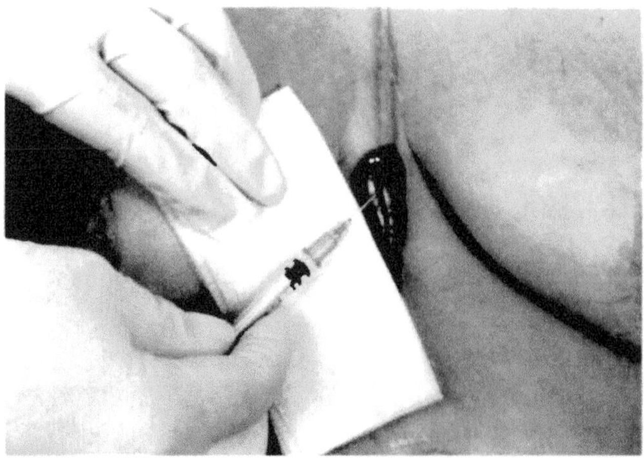

Figure 26 After disinfecting the lesion, the serum content is aspirated with a sterile 26-gauge needle **(a, b)**. The procedure is completed without destroying the bulla roof **(c)**, which is left on the lesion as a natural protective film **(d)**. (*figure continues*)

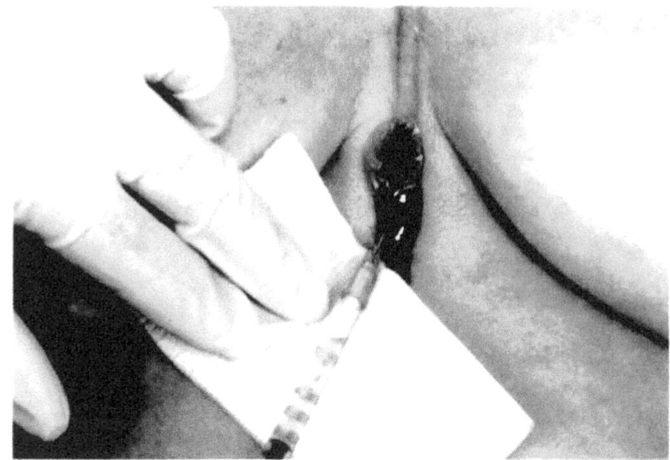

b

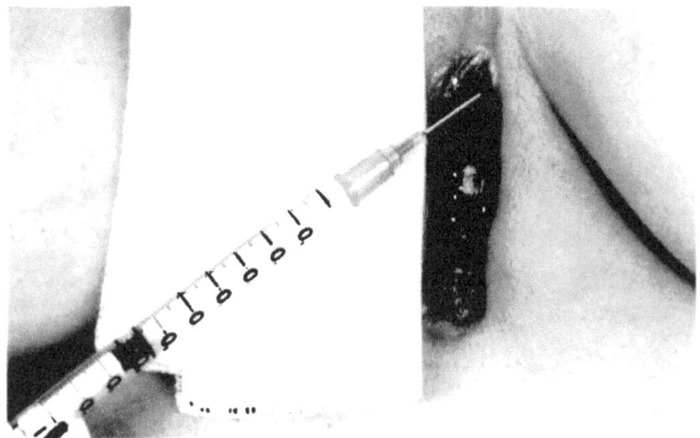

c

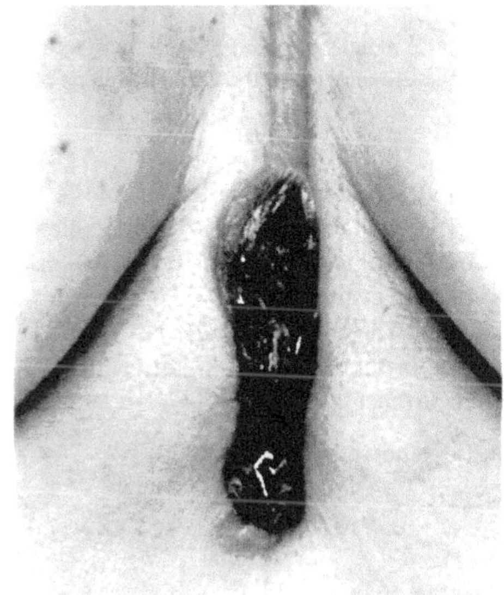

d

Figure 26 *(continued)*

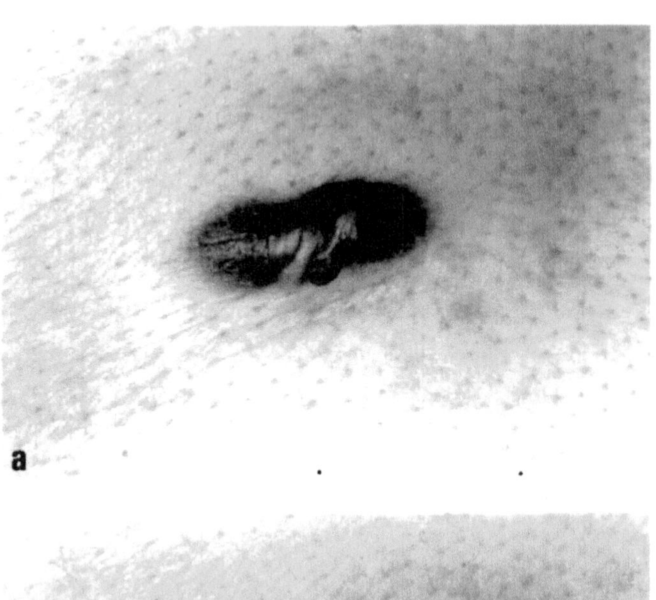

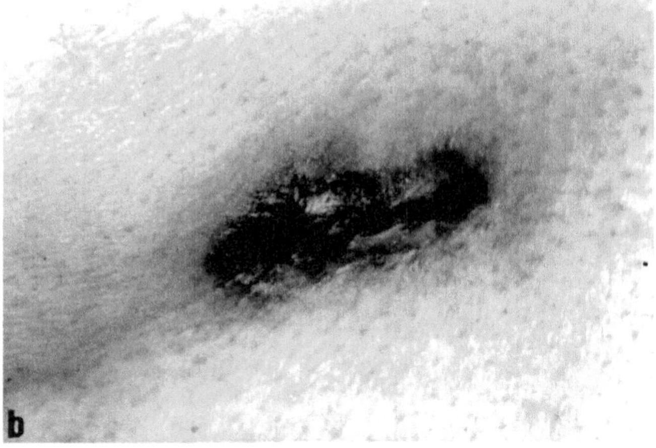

Figure 27 Keloid on the chest of a patient before **(a)** and 2 months after **(b)** a single session of cryosurgery with nitrous oxide, 30 seconds, contact technique. A reduction of the lesional volume of more than 50% can be observed.

9. The patient is prescribed a disinfection-drying solution (e.g., Castellani colorless solution, chlorhexidine 1%, merbromin 2%, polyvidone-iodine 10%) or a lotion (e.g., chlorhexidine 1% in lotio alba aquosa) to be used once daily on the lesion.
10. A new appointment with the patient is made to evaluate the result and perform the next session of treatment 4 weeks later. The treatment must be repeated once monthly, if required. A total of three or more sessions significantly increase the response rates and minimize recurrences.

The clinical results obtained by the technique are shown in Figs. 27 to 38.

B. Spray Technique

The spray technique is not advisable for the treatment of keloids and hypertrophic scars. However, physicians who prefer to apply this technique because of their overall experience should use the confined-spray technique (Fig. 13) following a procedure similar to the one described for the contact technique. The following additional measures have to be taken:

1. The spray has to be emitted from a distance of 1 to 2 cm from the target site and at a 90-degree angle to it.
2. A single freeze-thaw session of 20 to 60 seconds should be used, depending on the volume of the lesion. If the open-spray technique is applied, two freeze-thaw sessions of 20 to 30 seconds are required in order to limit the ice ball radius and to obtain results similar to those obtained by the contact method.
3. Point spraying yields better results for keloids and hypertrophic scars than a paintbrush or spiral pattern of spray.

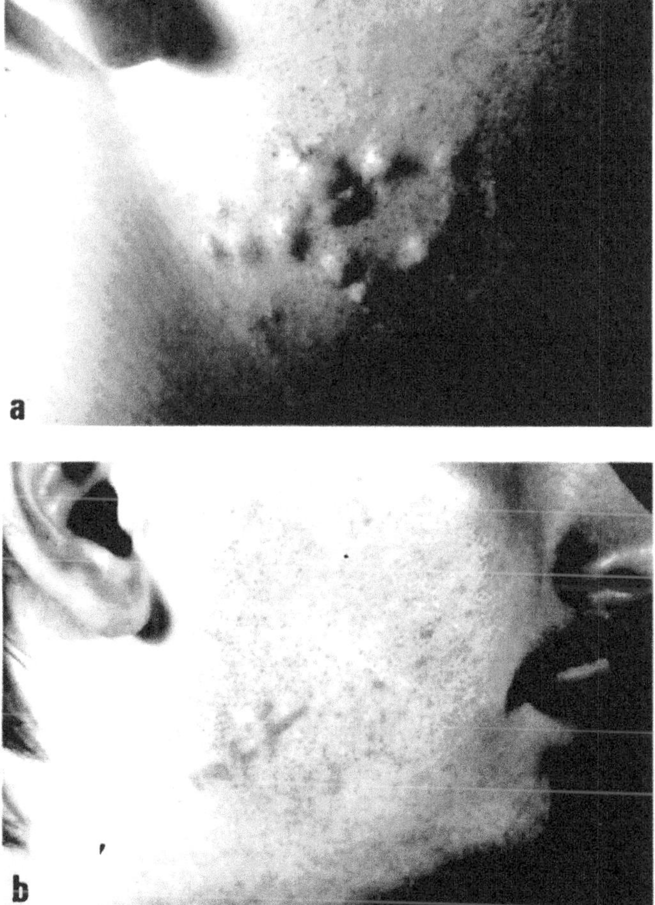

Figure 28 Two-year-old postacne keloids on the right cheek of a patient before **(a)** and 8 months after **(b)** the last of seven sessions with liquid nitrogen, 30 seconds per lesion, contact technique. (From Ref. 5, copyrighted 1993, American Medical Association.)

a

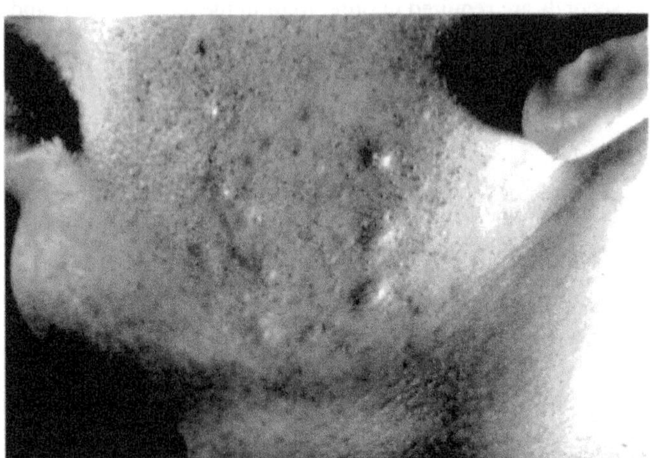

b

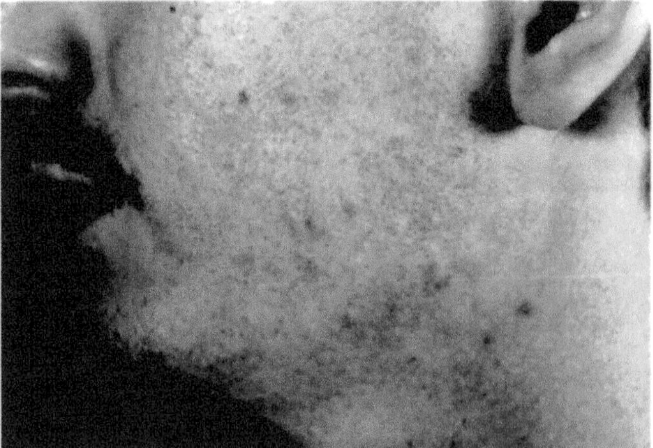

Figure 29 The left cheek of the same patient before **(a)** and 8 months after **(b)** the last of seven sessions with liquid nitrogen, 30 seconds per lesion, contact technique.

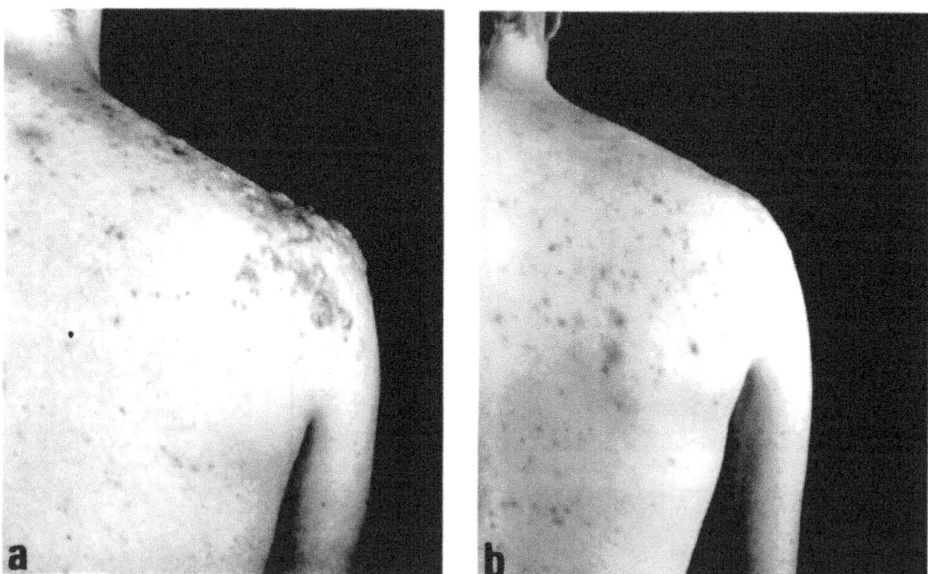

Figure 30 Large acne keloids on the right shoulder of an 18-year-old male patient before **(a)** and 2 months after **(b)** 12 sessions with nitrous oxide, 40–60 seconds per lesion, contact technique.

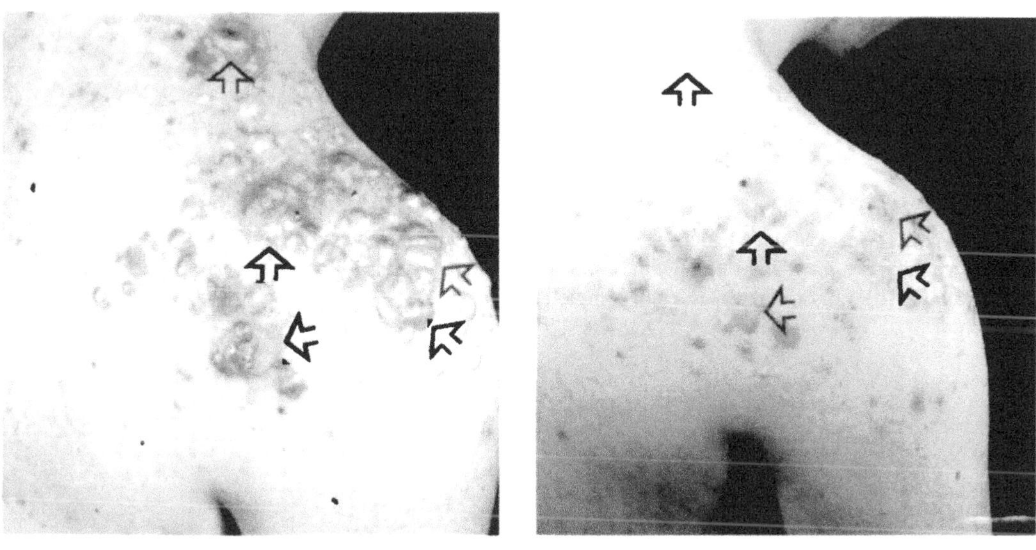

Figure 31 Detail from Fig. 30. Impressive improvement of the keloids registered by arrows **(a)** 2 months after 12 sessions with nitrous oxide, 40–60 seconds per lesion, contact technique **(b)**. (From Ref. 76, copyrighted 1990, Springer-Verlag.)

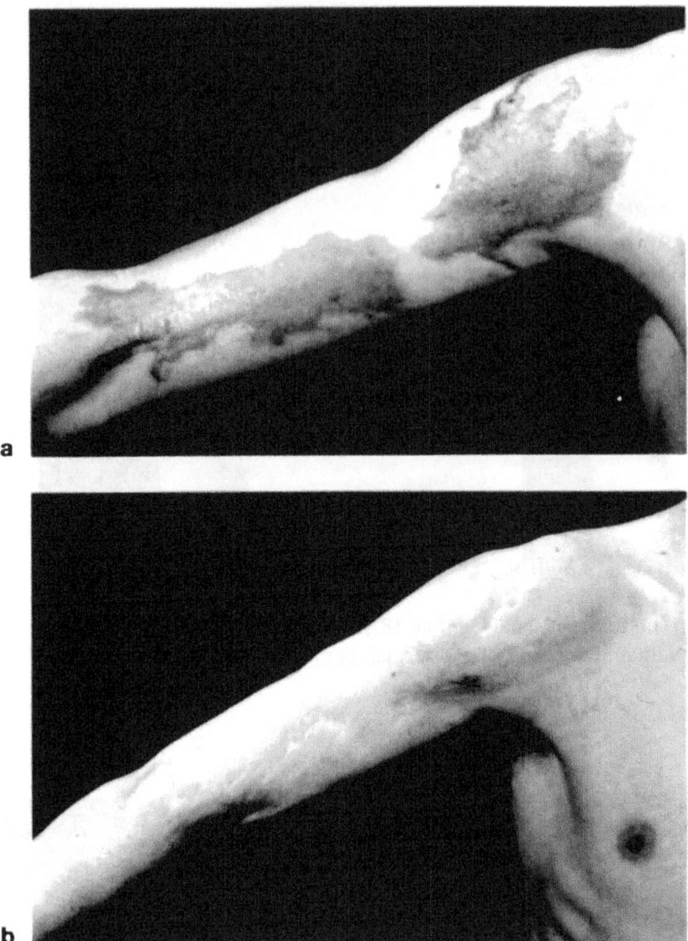

Figure 32 Huge keloids after chemical burn with sulfuric acid and contraction of the right elbow joint in a 21-year-old male patient before **(a)** and 1 year after nine sessions initially with liquid nitrogen (four sessions) and finally with nitrous oxide (five sessions), 30 seconds per lesion, contact technique **(b)**. Elbow mobility is again complete.

Figure 34 Two-year-old hypertrophic scar before **(a)** and 2 months after the last of four sessions with liquid nitrogen **(b)**, 30 seconds per lesion, contact technique. (From Ref. 5, copyrighted 1993, American Medical Association.)

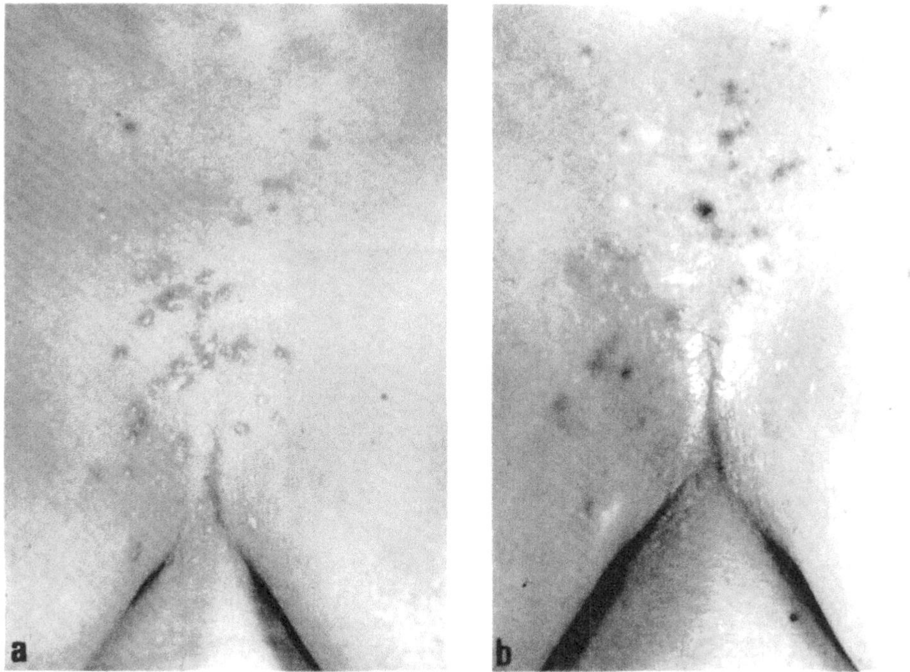

Figure 33 Acne scars on the chest of a 22-year-old female patient before **(a)** and 1 month after the last of nine sessions with nitrous oxide, 30 seconds per lesion, contact technique **(b)**.

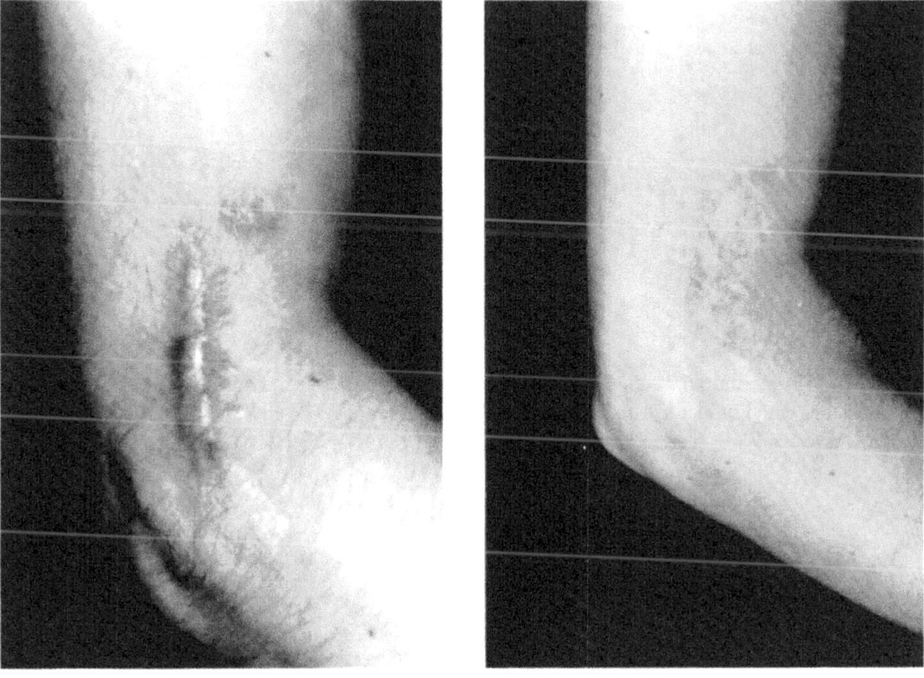

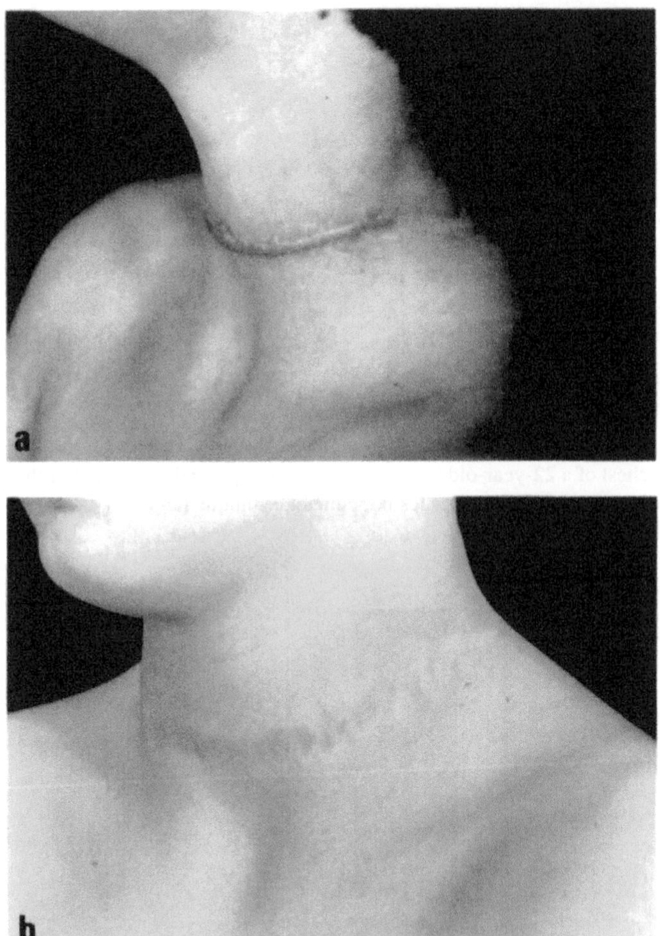

Figure 35 Six-month-old 22-cm-long hypertrophic scar before **(a)** and 6 months after **(b)** the last of five sessions with liquid nitrogen, 30 seconds, contact technique. (From Ref. 85, copyrighted 1993, Johann Ambrosius Barth-Verlag.)

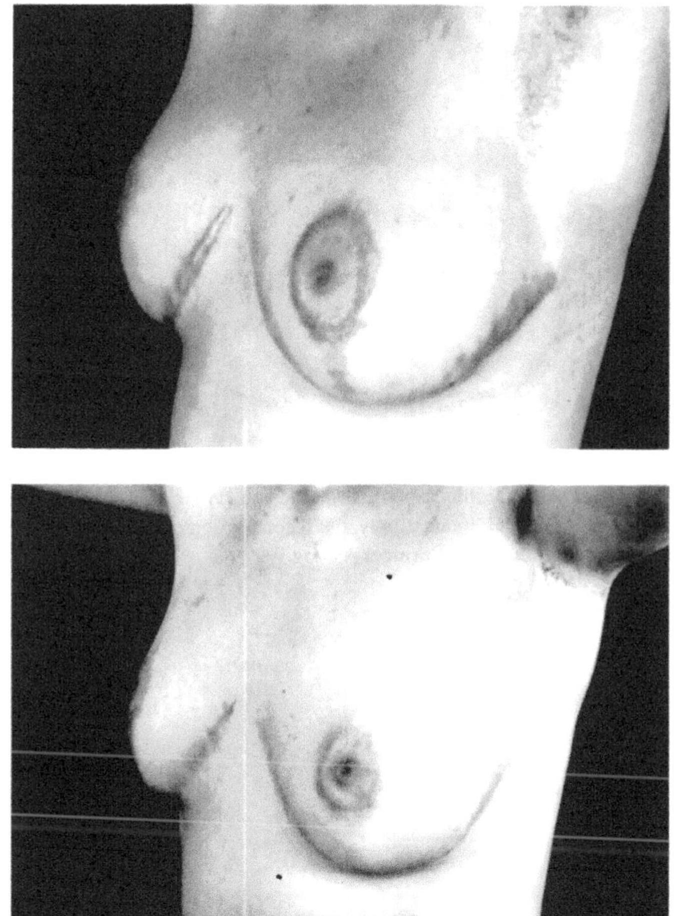

Figure 36 Two-year-old hypertrophic scars before **(a)** and 10 months after the last of six sessions initially with liquid nitrogen (two sessions) and finally with nitrous oxide (four sessions), 30 seconds per lesion, contact technique **(b)**.

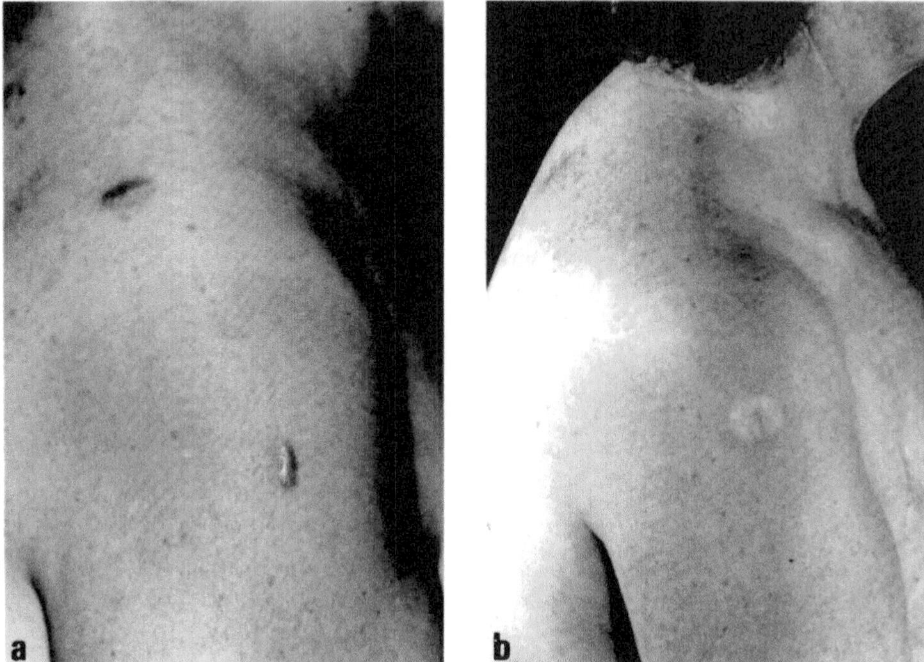

Figure 37 Five-month-old hypertrophic scars before **(a)** and 1 year after three sessions with nitrous oxide, 30 seconds per lesion, contact technique **(b)**. In the lesion on the arm long-term hypopigmentation due to cryosurgery is observed; interestingly, the second lesion on the shoulder is not hypopigmented. (From Ref. 76, copyrighted 1990, Springer-Verlag.)

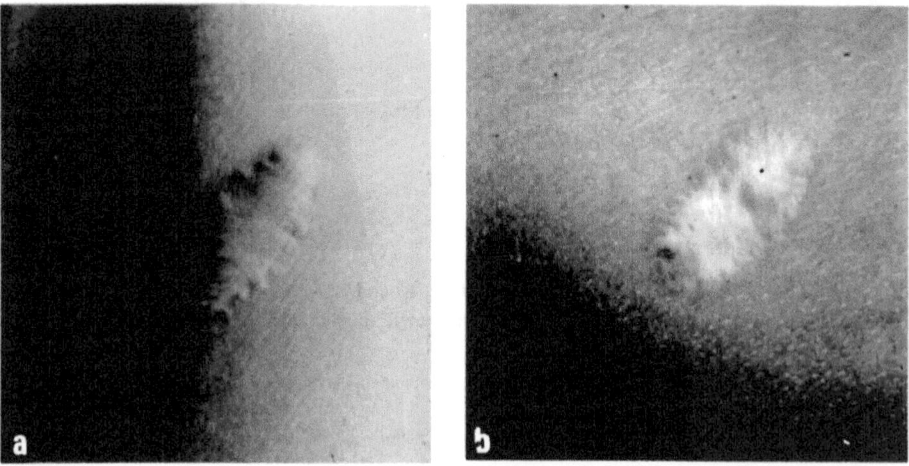

Figure 38 Hypertrophic scar on the upper arm of a 22-year-old female patient before **(a)** and 3 months after the last of seven sessions with liquid nitrogen, 30 seconds, contact technique **(b)**. An excellent clinical result, but lesional hypopigmentation and slight peripheral hyperpigmentation can also be seen.

C. Cryosurgery Combined with Intralesional Corticosteroids

Lesions, mostly keloids, that are refractory or minimally responsive to cryosurgery performed as monotherapy after at least six sessions may improve with a combination of cryosurgery and intralesional steroids. Intralesional betamethasone or triamcinolone injections (up to 2 mg/cm^2 lesional surface) are applied with a Luer-locked 26-gauge needle 30 to 60 minutes after cryosurgical treatment, performed as described earlier. This delay is required in order to allow the lesions to enter the edematous phase of cryoreaction, making intralesional injections easier and leading the fluid to the area of minor resistance, which is the lesion because of the edema.

a

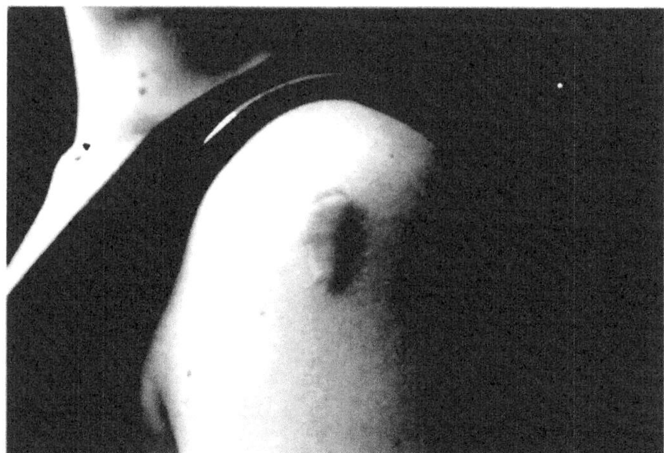

b

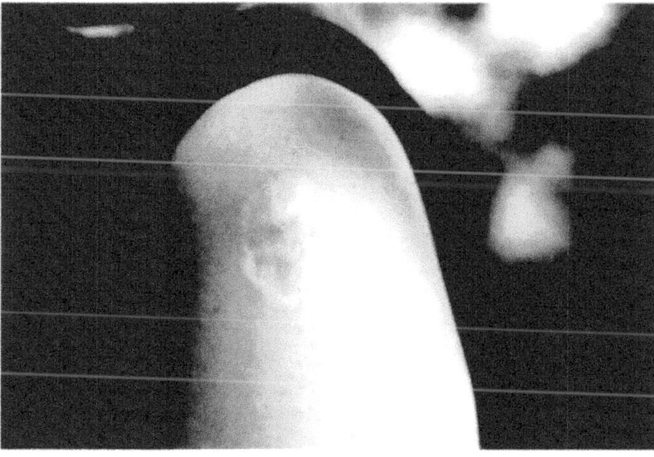

Figure 39 Hypertrophic scar **(a)** treated with three sessions of combined cryosurgery (liquid nitrogen, 30 seconds, contact technique) and intralesional corticosteroid injections (betamethasone, 2 mg/cm^2 lesional surface). A good clinical result, but a characteristic skin atrophy expanding over the borders of the initial scar is seen as a side effect of the applied corticosteroid **(b)**. (Courtesy of E. Zouridaki, M.D.)

If intralesional injections were performed prior to cryosurgery or as monotherapy, the lesion would show resistance to accepting the fluid volume, leading to a concentration of the fluid at the healthy periphery of the lesion and finally to the well-known perilesional atrophy after intralesional corticosteroid injections in keloids. In addition, corticosteroid concentrations of up to 2 mg/cm^2 lesional surface have been defined in order to avoid perilesional atrophy. On the other hand, corticosteroid injections in keloids are painful, and a better acceptance is obtained if the injections are performed in edematous tissue. In patients who, despite this improved procedure, continue to feel pain during the corticosteroid injection, a mixture of corticosteroid and lidocaine (1%) 1:1 can be injected. Results of the technique are shown in Fig. 39.

D. Surgical Debulking Prior to Cryosurgery

Cryosurgery of large voluminous keloids is a difficult task. It is better to remove these lesions surgically and apply postsurgical cryoprevention with or without intralesional corti-

a

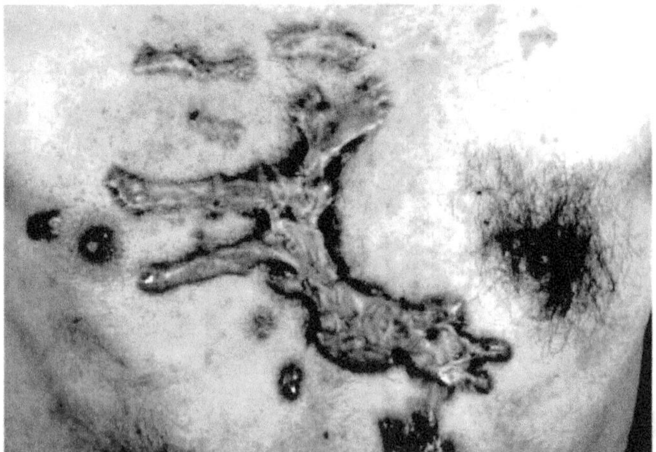

b

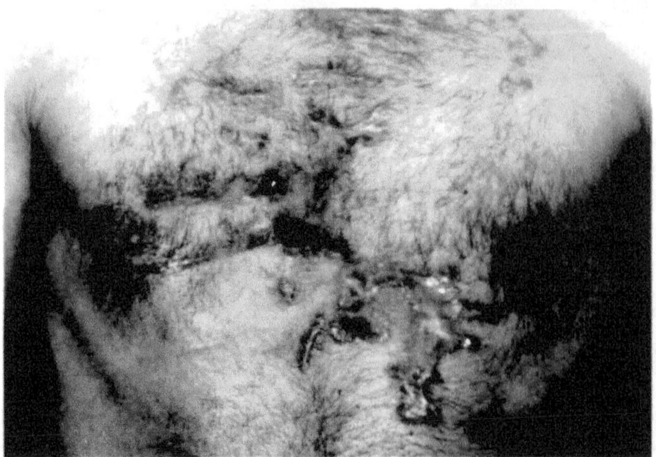

Figure 40 Intramarginal removal of huge keloids **(a)** with the carbon dioxide laser and intraoperative application of intralesional corticosteroid injections into the scars followed by three sessions of cryoprevention (liquid nitrogen, 30 seconds per lesion, contact technique) **(b)**.

costeroids in order to decrease the recurrence rate. However, recurrences are unavoidable. Before surgery is performed, the following facts have to be taken into consideration.

1. Intramarginal excision is advisable because it is followed by a lower recurrence rate than extramarginal excision (Fig. 40).
2. Removal of the lesion with a carbon dioxide laser provides a high degree of hemostasis and avoids sutures.

The carbon dioxide laser setting is 11 W, 2 mm beam diameter, continuous discharge, and energy 350 W/cm^2.

Cryoprevention (20 to 30 seconds at −86°C or −196°C) has to be performed on the resulting fresh scar after healing and repeated every 4 weeks for at least 6 months. If intralesional corticosteroids are also applied, the first injection has to be made intraoperatively, followed by injections once monthly combined with cryosurgery according to the procedure described above. Results can be seen in Fig. 41 and 42.

E. Intralesional Cryosurgery

1. The lesion is disinfected and perilesional anesthesia is performed with 1% lidocaine solution (Fig. 43a).
2. The lesion is grasped between the fingers and a single-use 20-gauge needle is introduced into the skin at one border of the lesion and exits on the surface at a point on the other border of the lesion (Fig. 43b).

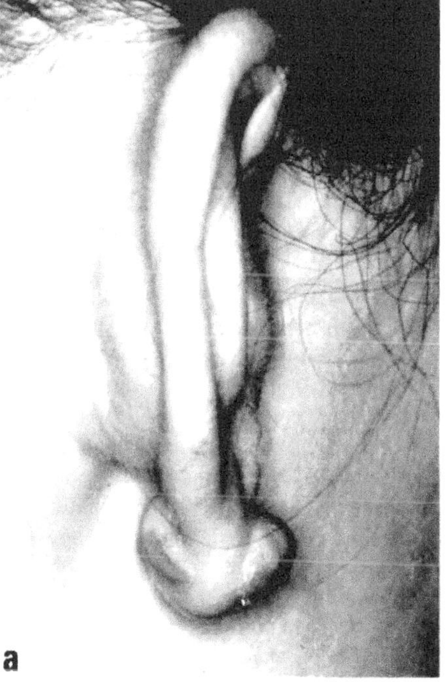

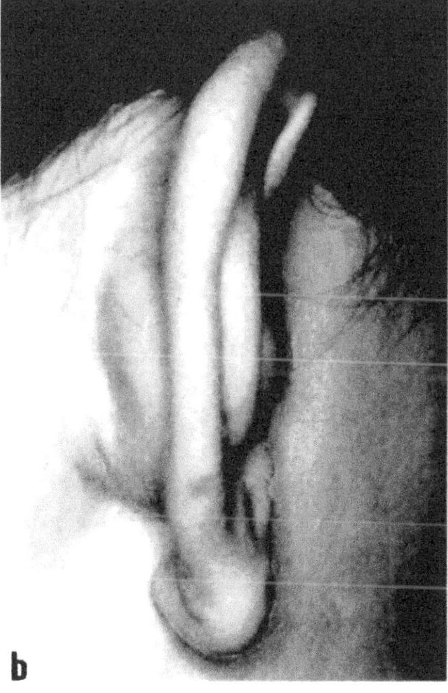

Figure 41 Earlobe keloid before **(a)** and 2 months after intramarginal excision with the carbon dioxide laser followed by four sessions for cryoprevention initially with liquid nitrogen (one session) and finally with nitrous oxide (three sessions), 30 seconds per lesion, contact technique **(b)**. (From Ref. 85, copyrighted 1993, Johann Ambrosius Barth-Verlag.)

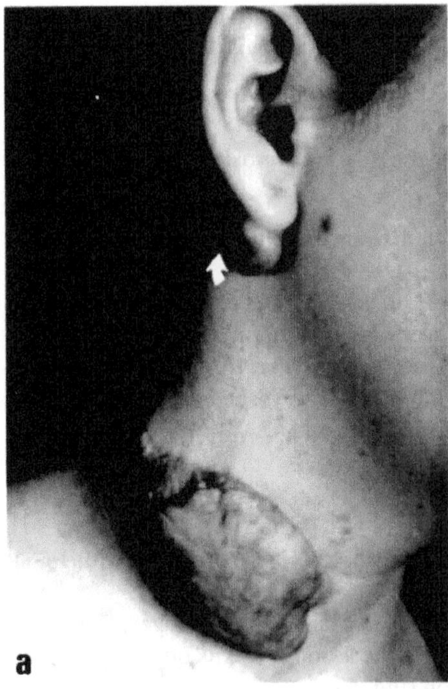

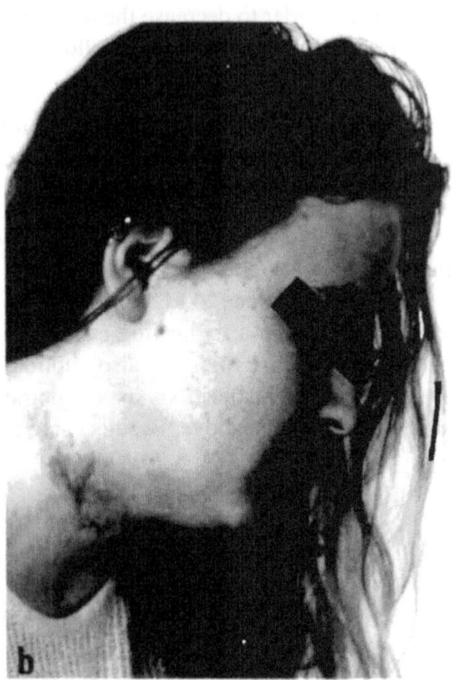

Figure 42 Huge keloids on the neck and the earlobe (arrow) before **(a)** and after intramarginal excision with the carbon dioxide laser with general anesthesia and intraoperative intralesional corticosteroid injections followed by 12 sessions of cryoprevention (liquid nitrogen, 30 seconds per lesion, contact technique) and intralesional corticosteroids (triamcinolone, 2 mg/cm^2 lesional surface) **(b)**.

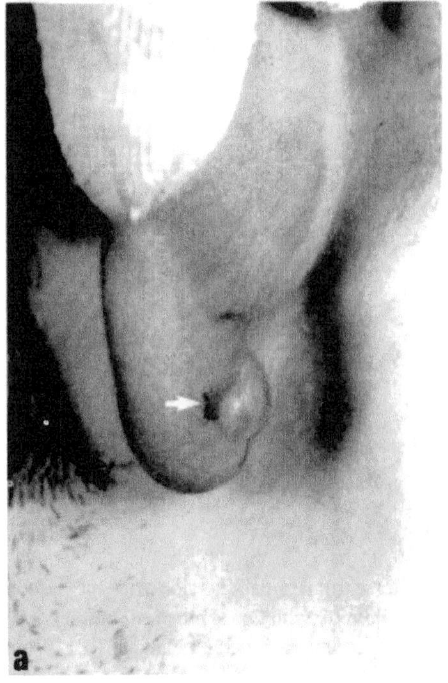

Figure 43 Intralesional cryosurgery: after lesional disinfection, perilesional anesthesia is performed (arrow) with lidocaine, 1% solution **(a)**. A single-use 20-gauge needle is introduced into the skin at one border of the lesion to exit on the surface at a point on the other border of the lesion **(b)**. The needle is connected to the cryoprobe, the cryogun is activated, and liquid nitrogen is passed through the needle lumen, exiting to the atmosphere from the other end of the needle. Two ice balls are formed at the sites of contact between the visible portions of the needle and the skin. In addition, an ice cylinder is formed around the embedded part of the needle in the deeper tissue. This is visible through the skin **(c)** and gradually spreads toward the surface **(d)**. Cryosurgery ends when the whole lesion is frozen **(e)**. *(figure continues)*

3. The needle has to be directed in such a way that the cryogen spray will not come in contact with the patient's healthy skin during treatment.
4. The needle is connected to the cryoprobe stem, and this is connected to the liquid nitrogen Dewar (Fig. 9).
5. Compression of the lesion is accomplished by pulling the visible parts of the needle up with the help of the connected cryosurgical device.

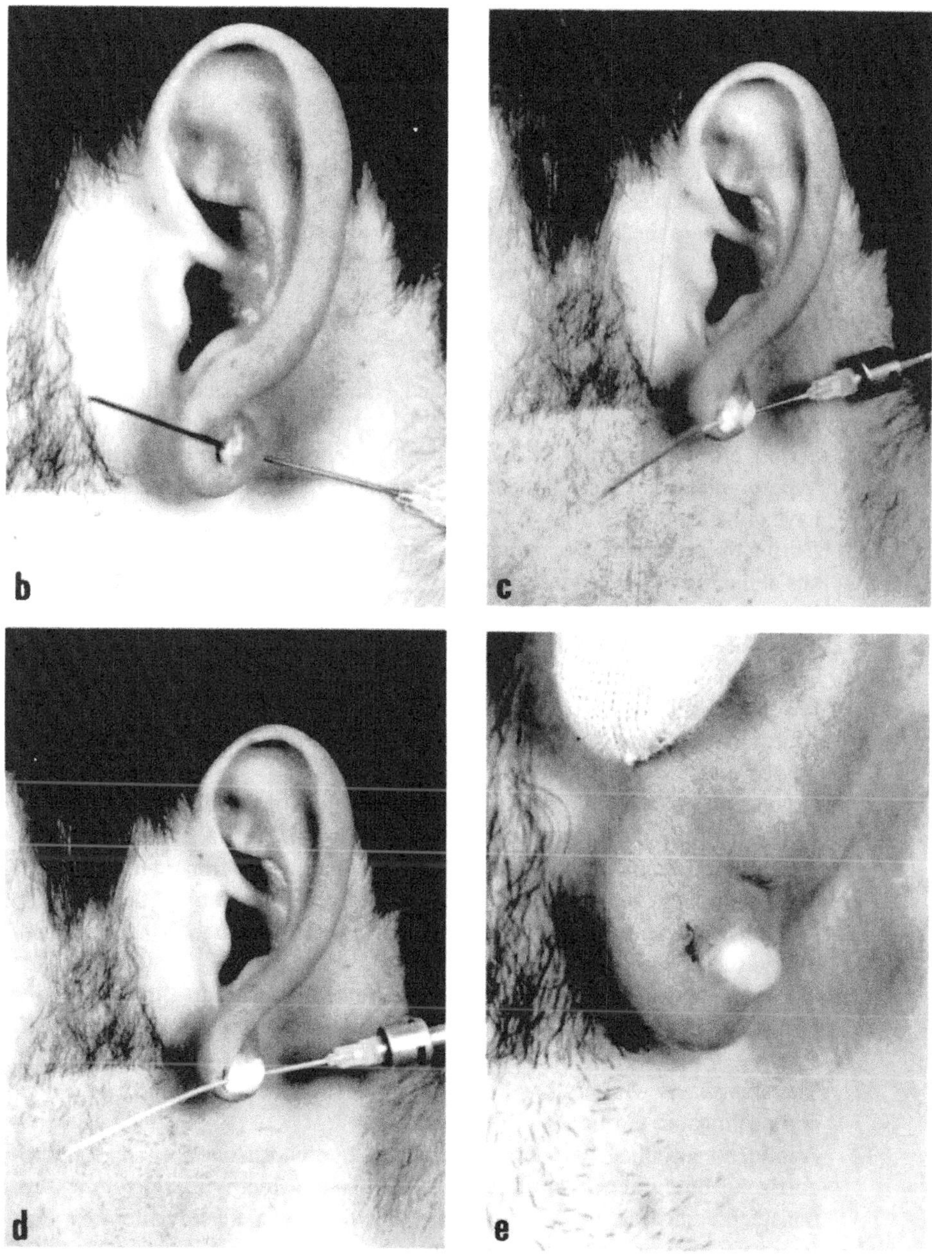

Figure 43 *(continued)*

6. The cryogun is activated and liquid nitrogen is passed through the needle lumen, exiting to the atmosphere from the other end of the needle. At the beginning of freezing two ice balls are formed at the sites of contact between the visible portions of the needle and the skin (Fig. 43c).
7. These circles increase in diameter with continued freezing (Fig. 43d). In addition, an ice cylinder is formed around the embedded part of the needle in the deeper tissue. This is visible through the skin and gradually spreads toward the surface.
8. The procedure ends when the whole lesion is frozen, regardless of the duration of freezing. The needle is left to thaw and is pulled out of the lesion (Fig. 43e).
9. Because some bleeding may occur after thawing, a sterile, firm dressing has to be applied.
10. Postsurgical care is similar to that described earlier.
11. The treatment has to be repeated every 3 weeks. The optimal number of sessions to obtain the best results is still under investigation.

F. Cryopeeling

1. Selection of patients has to be performed. Dark white-skinned patients; patients who do not avoid sunbathing for 1 month before treatment, during the treatment period, and for 2 months after treatment; patients who take drugs that induce hyperpigmentation; and patients who want to experience immediate results have to be excluded.
2. During the treatment, the patient lies in a reclining armchair and the physician sits at the top of the patient's head.
3. No sedation or premedication is required.
4. The patient's eyes can be covered by a pair of goggles.
5. The facial skin is cleaned with a gauze soaked in ethanol solution. Ethanol is allowed to evaporate before starting the treatment.
6. A nitrous oxide cryosurgical device (contact method) with a round cryoprobe tip of 2 cm diameter is used for cryopeeling.
7. Cryopeeling is started horizontally from the middle of the forehead in either direction and continues according to the plan shown in Fig. 44. The cryoprobe tip is slowly moved over the skin in order to leave a fine ice film on it.
8. The skin is stretched and held tight to ensure even application of the ice film.
9. Individual deeper scars are treated for a longer period of time to increase depth of cryosurgery.
10. The whole facial skin surface has to be treated in order to limit borderline postinflammatory hyperpigmentation, which is one of the disquieting side effects.
11. The skin reacts with erythema and light edema presenting immediately after cryopeeling and lasting up to 24 hours.
12. A mild, nonatrophogenic steroid cream (e.g., hydrocortisone aceponate, hydrocortisone buteprate, hydrocortisone-17-butyrate, methylprednisolone aceponate, prednicarbate) can be applied on the lesion immediately after treatment in order to reduce the erythematous reaction.
13. After 2 to 3 days, fine scaling of the superficial epidermis is observed.

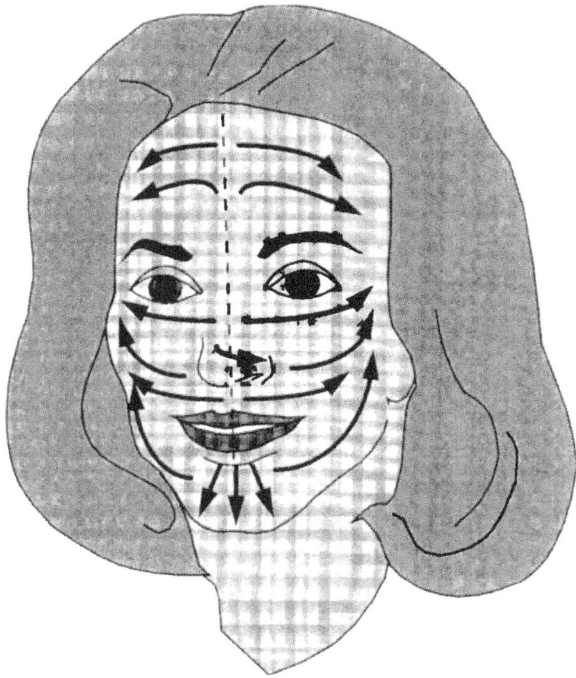

Figure 44 Cryopeeling starts from the forehead and ends at the chin. The cryoprobe tip is slowly moved from the middle of the face toward the periphery in either direction in order to leave a fine ice film on the skin. The skin is stretched and held tight to ensure even application of the ice film. The treatment is applied to the whole facial area.

14. Treatment has to be repeated once monthly during the winter (October to April in the northern hemisphere, six sessions per year) and can last 2 to 3 years.
15. A sunscreen has to be worn during the intermissions between treatment sessions.

The results of the treatment are shown in Fig. 45. A more aggressive cryopeeling procedure has been described by Graham (8) and Chiarello (103) using liquid nitrogen spray for 5 to 30 seconds on 8-cm^2 facial skin fragments by the paintbrush technique. This technique leads to long-lasting erythema. In our opinion, cryopeeling should be a mild technique, as dermabrasion with or without punch excision and punch elevation is more adequate and better controlled in the treatment of deeper atrophic scars.

VI. COMPLICATIONS AND CONTRAINDICATIONS

Among the various temporary or permanent complications described after cryosurgery (2,8,78) local pain during and/or shortly after treatment and lesional hypopigmentation and/or peripheral hyperpigmentation (Figs. 37 and 38) are the major side effects in the treatment of keloids and hypertrophic scars. Large local edema, wound infection, local hypoesthesia, local necrosis, and formation of milia have been reported in single patients (5).

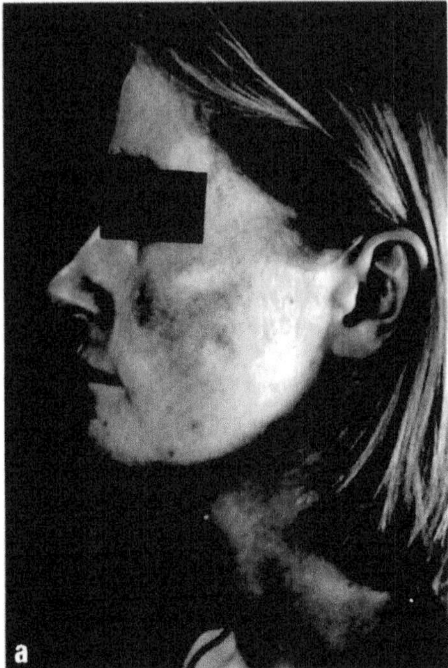

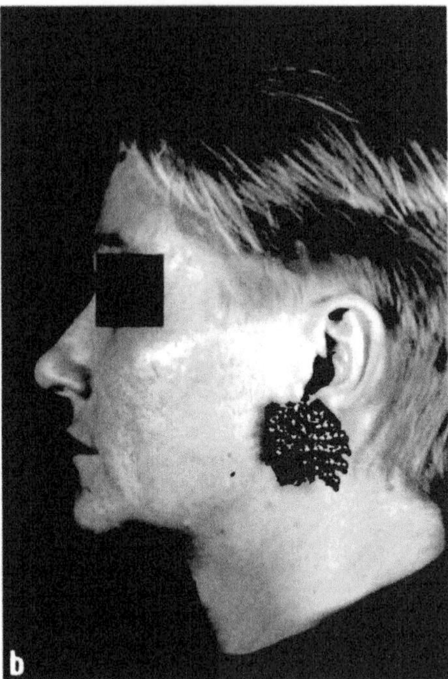

Figure 45 Atrophic acne scars before **(a)** and 6 months after cryopeeling (12 sessions in 2 years) **(b)**.

Delayed wound healing is an additional side effect, mostly occurring after combined cryosurgery with intralesional corticosteroids (68). There are a few absolute contraindications, including cold-inducible urticaria, cryoglobulinemia, cryofibrinogenemia, and Raynaud's disease (4). Relative contraindications are collagen diseases, lesions at the extremities of old patients, and black skin because of the long-term depigmentation occurring with melanocyte death.

REFERENCES

1. Graham GF. Cryosurgery. Clin Plast Surg 1993; 20:131–147.
2. Kuflik EG. Cryosurgery updated. J Am Acad Dermatol 1994; 31:925–944.
3. Zacarian SA. Cryosurgery in the management of cutaneous disorders and malignant tumors of the skin. Compr Ther 1994; 20:379–401.
4. Zouboulis ChC, Blume-Peytavi U. Kryotherapeutische Verfahren in der Dermatologie. Kassenarzt 1995; 7:38–50.
5. Zouboulis ChC, Blume U, Büttner P, Orfanos CE. Outcomes of cryosurgery in keloids and hypertrophic scars. A prospective consecutive trial of case series. Arch Dermatol 1993; 129:1146–1151.
6. Rusciani L, Rossi G, Bono R. Use of cryotherapy in the treatment of keloids. J Dermatol Surg Oncol 1993; 19:529–534.
7. Ernst K, Hundeiker M. Ergebnisse der Kryochirurgie bei 394 Patienten mit hypertrophen Narben und Keloiden. Hautarzt 1995; 46:462–466.

8. Graham G. Cryosurgery for acne. In: Zacarian SA, ed. Cryosurgery for Skin Cancer and Cutaneous Disorders. St. Louis: Mosby, 1985:59–76.
9. Röhrs H. Dokumentation therapeutischer und kosmetischer Ergebnisse bei der kryochirurgischen Behandlung von Hauterkrankungen. Dissertation, The Free University of Berlin, Berlin, Germany, 1997.
10. Thulliez M, Geerts M, Zouboulis ChC. History of cryosurgery. Dermatol Monatschr 1993; 179:234–236.
11. Gerhardt C. Lupus-Behandlung durch Kälte. Dtsch Med Wochenschr 1885; 11:38–43.
12. White AC. Liquid air, its application in medicine and surgery. Med Rec 1899; 56:109–112.
13. Juliusberg M. Gefrierbehandlung bei Hautkrankheiten. Berl Klin Wochenschr 1905; 42:260–263.
14. Allington H. Liquid nitrogen in the treatment of skin diseases. Calif Med 1950; 72:153–155.
15. Cooper IS, Lee AS. Cryostatic congelation: a system for producing a limited controlled region of cooling or freezing of biologic tissues. J Nerv Ment Dis 1961; 133:259–263.
16. Cooper IS. Cryogenic surgery: new method of destruction or extirpation of benign or malignant tissues. N Engl J Med 1963; 268:734–749.
17. Fasano VA, Broggi G, De Nunno T, Baggiore P. Cryothérapie et neurochirurgie. Neurochirurgie 1964; 10:172–179.
18. Farrant J, Walter CA. The cryobiological basis of cryosurgery. J Dermatol Surg Oncol 1977; 3:403–407.
19. Orpwood RD. Biophysical and engineering aspects of cryosurgery. Phys Med Biol 1981; 26:555–575.
20. Mazur P. Freezing of living cells: mechanisms and implications. Am J Physiol 1984; 247:125–142.
21. Dawber R. Cold kills! Clin Exp Dermatol 1988; 13:137–150.
22. Shepherd J, Dawber RPR. The historical and scientific basis of cryosurgery. Clin Exp Dermatol 1982; 7:321–328.
23. Gage A, Meenaghan M, Natiella J, Greene G. Sensitivity of pigmented mucosa and skin to freezing injury. Cryobiology 1979; 16:348-361.
24. Gage AA, Caruana JA Jr, Montes M. Critical temperature for skin necrosis in experimental cryosurgery. Cryobiology 1982; 19:273–282.
25. Shepherd JP. The effects of low temperature on dermal connective tissue components. Dissertation, University of Oxford, Oxford, United Kingdom, 1979.
26. Torre D. Depth dose in cryosurgery. J Dermatol Surg Oncol 1983; 9:219–225.
27. Zouboulis ChC, Blume U, Pineda Fernandez MS, Mielitz H, Orfanos CE. Outcomes of cryosurgery in patients with basal cell carcinoma. Skin Cancer 1994; 9:7–22.
28. Breitbart EW, Schaeg G. Electron microscopic investigation of the cryolesion. In: Breitbart EW, Dachow-Siwiec E, eds. Clinics in Dermatology: Advances in Cryosurgery. New York: Elsevier, 1990:30–38.
29. Gage AA. Experimental cryogenic injury of the palate; observations pertinent to cryosurgical destruction of tumors. Cryobiology 1978; 15:415–425.
30. Zacarian SA. Cryogenics: the cryolesion and the pathogenesis of cryonecrosis. In: Zacarian SA, ed. Cryosurgery of Skin Cancer and Cutaneous Disorders. St. Louis: Mosby, 1985:1–30.
31. Kulka JP. Cold injury of the skin. The pathogenic rate of microcirculatory impairment. Arch Environ Health 1965; 11:484–497.
32. Sebastian G, Scholz A. Histopathology of the cryolesion. Dermatol Monatsschr 1993; 179:237–241.
33. Rinfret AP. Cryobiology. In: Vance RW, ed. Cryogenic Technology. New York: Wiley, 1962.
34. Zacarian SA, Stone D, Clater M. Effect of cryogenic temperature on the microcirculation of the golden Syrian hamster cheek pouch. Cryobiology 1970; 7:22–29.
35. Rabb JM, Renaud ML, Bradt PA, Witt CW. Effect of freezing and thawing on microcirculation and capillary endothelium of the hamster cheek pouch. Cryobiology 1974; 11:508–518.

36. Yantorno C, Soanes WA, Gonder MJ, Shulman S. Studies in cryoimmunology. I. The production of antibodies to urogenital tissue in consequence of freezing treatment. Immunology 1967; 12:395–410.
37. Ablin RJ, Witebsky E, Jagodzinski RV, Soanes WA. Secondary immunologic response as a consequence of the in situ freezing of rabbit male adnexal gland tissues of reproduction. Exp Med Surg 1971; 29:72–88.
38. Ablin RJ, Soanes WA, Gonder MJ. Prospects for cryoimmunotherapy in cases of metastasizing carcinoma of the prostate. Cryobiology 1971; 8:271–279.
39. Gursel E, Roberts M, Veenema RJ. Regression of prostatic cancer following sequential cryotherapy to the prostate. J Urol 1972; 108:928–932.
40. Ablin RJ, Gonder MJ, Soanes WA. Elution of cell-bound antiprostatic epithelial antibodies after multiple cryotherapy of carcinoma of the prostate. Cryobiology 1974; 11:218–221.
41. Bayjoo P, Rees RC, Goepel JR, Jacob G. Natural killer cell activity following cryosurgery of normal and tumour bearing liver in an animal model. J Clin Lab Immunol 1991; 35:129–132.
42. Kindzel'skii LP, Zlochevskaia LL, Zakharychev VD, Tsyganok TV. Changes in cytotoxicity of natural killer cells and level of large granule–containing lymphocytes in patients with lung cancer under the effects of cryosurgery. Klin Khir 1991; (5):3–5.
43. Hanawa S. An experimental study on the induction of anti-tumor immunological activity after cryosurgery for liver carcinoma, and the effect of concomitant immunotherapy with OK432. Nippon Geka Gakkai Zasshi 1993; 94:57–65.
44. Horio T, Miyauchi H, Kim YK, Asada Y. The effect of cryo-treatment on epidermal Langerhans cells and immune function in mice. Arch Dermatol Res 1994; 286:69–71.
45. Roy A, Ghosh S, Lahiri S, Lahiri P, Santra A, Roy B. Some aspects of the causes of enhanced immune response of in vitro frozen ascites fibrosarcoma tumor cells in mice. Cryobiology 1995; 23:306–313.
46. Muir IFK. On the nature of keloid and hypertrophic scars. Br J Plast Surg 1990; 43:61–69.
47. Datubo-Brown DD. Keloids: a review of the literature. Br J Plast Surg 1990; 43:70–77.
48. Peacock EE Jr, Madden JM, Trier WC. Some studies on the treatment of keloids and hypertrophic scars. South Med J 1970; 63:755–760.
49. Ehrlich HP, Desmouliere A, Diegelmann RF, Cohen IK, Compton CC, Garner WL, Kapanci Y, Gabbiani G. Morphological and immunochemical differences between keloid and hypertrophic scar. Am J Pathol 1994; 145:105–113.
50. James WD, Besaucenaey CD, Odom RB. The ultrastructure of a keloid. J Am Acad Dermatol 1980; 3:50–57.
51. Matsuoka LY, Uitto J, Wortsman J, Abergel P, Dietrich J. Ultrastructural characteristics of keloid fibroblasts. Am J Dermatopathol 1988; 10:505–508.
52. Lee YS, Vijayasingam S. Mast cells and myofibroblasts in keloid: a light microscopic, immunohistochemical and ultrastructural study. Ann Acad Med Singapore 1995; 24:902–905.
53. Nakaoka H, Miyauchi S, Miki Y. Proliferating activity of dermal fibroblasts in keloids and hypertrophic scars. Acta Derm Venereol 1995; 75:102–104.
54. Appleton I, Brown NJ, Willoughby DA. Apoptosis, necrosis, and proliferation: possible implications in the etiology of keloids. Am J Pathol 1996; 149:1441–1447.
55. Hunzelmann N, Anders S, Sollberg S, Schonherr E, Krieg T. Coordinate induction of collagen type I and biglycan expression in keloids. Br J Dermatol 1996; 135:394–399.
56. Scott PG, Dodd CM, Tredget EE, Ghahary A, Rahemtulla F. Immunohistochemical localization of the proteoglycans decorin, biglycan and versican and transforming growth factor-beta in human post-burn hypertrophic and mature scars. Histopathology 1995; 26:423–431.
57. Arakawa M, Hatamochi A, Mori Y, Mori K, Ueki H, Moriguchi T. Reduced collagenase gene expression in fibroblasts from hypertrophic scar tissue. Br J Dermatol 1996; 134:863–868.
58. Diegelmann RF, Cohen IK, McCoy BJ. Growth kinetics and collagen synthesis of normal skin, normal scar and keloid fibroblasts in vitro. J Cell Physiol 1979; 98:341–346.
59. Dalkowski A, Schuppan D, Orfanos CE, Zouboulis ChC. Increased expression of tenascin-C by keloids in vivo and in vitro. Br J Dermatol 1999, in press.

60. Dalkowski A. Immunhistochemische Untersuchungen an Keloiden und keloidalen Fibroblasten und der Einfluβ der Kryotherapie auf Proliferation, synthetische Aktivität und Immunphänotyp humaner keloidaler und normaler Fibroblasten in vitro. Dissertation, The Free University of Berlin, Berlin, Germany, 1997.
61. Younai S, Venters G, Vu S, Nichter L, Nimni ME, Tuan TL. Role of growth factors in scar contraction: an in vitro analysis. Ann Plast Surg 1996; 36:495–501.
62. Brown LA Jr, Pierce HE. Keloids: scar revision. J Dermatol Surg Oncol 1986; 12:51–56.
63. Rudolph R. Wide spread scars, hypertrophic scars, and keloids. Clin Plast Surg 1987; 14:253–260.
64. Kelly AP. Keloids. Dermatol Clin 1988; 6:413–424.
65. Berman B, Bieley HC. Keloids. J Am Acad Dermatol 1995; 33:117–123.
66. Ehrlich HP, Hembry RM. A comparative study of fibroblasts in healing, freeze and burn injuries in rats. Am J Pathol 1984; 117:218–224.
67. Wulff A, Zouboulis ChC, Blume-Peytavi U, Sommer Ch, Schuppan D, Orfanos CE. Cryotherapy modifies proliferation and collagen synthesis of keloidal fibroblasts. Arch Dermatol Res 1996; 288:303.
68. Zouridaki E, Trautmann Ch, Alvertis H, Katsambas A, Orfanos CE, Zouboulis ChC. Cryosurgery alone and cryosurgery combined with intralesional steroids are equally effective on keloids but induce different histological changes: results of a prospective randomised study. J Eur Acad Dermatol Venereol 1996; 7(suppl 2):87.
69. Zouboulis ChC, Zouridaki E, Wulff A. The treatment of keloids, hypertrophic and atrophic scars. J Eur Acad Dermatol Venereol 1996; 7(suppl 2):22.
70. Ceilley RI, Babin RW. The combined use of cryosurgery and intralesional injections of suspensions of fluorinated adrenocorticosteroids for reducing keloids and hypertrophic scars. J Dermatol Surg Oncol 1979; 5:54–56.
71. Shepherd JP, Dawber RPR. The response of keloid scars to cryosurgery. Plast Reconstr Surg 1982; 70:677–681.
72. Meltzer L. A cryoprobe for the therapy of linear keloid. J Dermatol Surg Oncol 1983; 9:111–112.
73. Muti E, Ponzio E. Cryotherapy in the treatment of keloids. Ann Plast Surg 1983; 11:227–232.
74. Cirne de Castro JL, Pereira dos Santos A, Morais Cardoso LP, Ribeiro R. Cryosurgical treatment of a large keloid. J Dermatol Surg Oncol 1986; 12:740–742.
75. Mende B. Keloidbehandlung mittels Kryotherapie. Z Hautkr 1987; 62:1348–1355.
76. Zouboulis ChC, Orfanos CE. Kryochirurgische Behandlung von hypertrophen Narben und Keloiden. Hautarzt 1990; 41:683–688.
77. Layton AM, Yip J, Cunliffe WJ. A comparison of intralesional triamcinolone and cryosurgery in the treatment of acne keloids. Br J Dermatol 1994; 130:498–501.
78. Drake LA, Ceilley RI, Cornelison RL, Dobes WL, Dorner W, Goltz RW, Lewis CW, Salasche SJ, Chanco Turner ML, Lowery BJ, Graham GF, Detlefs RL, Garrett AB, Kuflik EG, Lubritz RR. Guidelines of care for cryosurgery. J Am Acad Dermatol 1994; 31:648–653.
79. Röhrs H, Orfanos CE, Zouboulis ChC. Cryosurgical treatment of acne keloids. J Invest Dermatol 1997; 108:396.
80. Hirshowitz B, Lerner D, Moscona AR. Treatment of keloid scars by combined cryosurgery and intralesional corticosteroids. Aesthetic Plast Surg 1982; 6:153–158.
81. Banfalvi T, Boer A, Remenar E, Oberna F. Treatment of keloids (review of the literature, therapeutic suggestions). Orv Hetil 1996; 137:1861–1864.
82. Lubritz RR. Cryosurgical approach to benign and precancerous tumors of the skin. In: Zacarian SA, ed. Cryosurgery for Skin Cancer and Cutaneous Disorders. St. Louis: Mosby, 1985:41–58.
83. Glazer SF, Sher AM. Adjunctive cryosurgery in the surgical approach to keloids. In: Zacarian SA, ed. Cryosurgery for Skin Cancer and Cutaneous Disorders. St. Louis: Mosby, 1985:91–95.

84. Sebastian G, Scholz A. Unsere Erfahrungen mit konservativen Therapiemethoden bei hypertrophen Narben und Keloiden. Dt Derm 1990; 38:872–877.
85. Zouboulis ChC, Blume U, Orfanos CE. Keloids and hypertrophic scars: cryosurgical treatment and postsurgical cryoprevention. Dermatol Monatsschr 1993; 179:278–284.
86. Engrav LH, Gottlieb JR, Millard SP, Walkinshaw MD, Heimbach DM, Marvin JA. A comparison of intramarginal and extramarginal excision of hypertrophic burn scars. Plast Reconstr Surg 1988; 81:40–45.
87. Stern JC, Lucente FE. Carbon dioxide laser excision of earlobe keloids. A prospective study and critical analysis of existing data. Arch Otolaryngol Head Neck Surg 1989; 115:1107–1111.
88. Weshahy AH. Intralesional cryosurgery. A new technique using cryoneedles. J Dermatol Surg Oncol 1993; 19:123–126.
89. Simon CA. A simple and accurate cryosurgical tool for the treatment of benign skin lesions: the "hard tail" dip-stick. J Dermatol Surg Oncol 1986; 12:680–682.
90. Ferris DG, Ho JJ. Cryosurgical equipment: a critical review. J Fam Prac 1992; 35:185–193.
91. Torre D. Instrumentation and monitoring devices in cryosurgery. In: Zacarian SA, ed. Cryosurgery for Skin Cancer and Cutaneous Disorders. St. Louis: Mosby, 1985:31–40.
92. Garamy G. Engineering aspects of cryosurgery. In: Rand RW, Rinfret AP, von Leden H, eds. Cryosurgery. Springfield, IL: Charles C Thomas, 1968:92–132.
93. Torre D. Understanding the relationship between lateral spread of freeze and depth of freeze. J Dermatol Surg Oncol 1979; 5:1–3.
94. Lubritz RR. Cryosurgical spray patterns. J Dermatol Surg Oncol 1978; 4:138–139.
95. Elton RF. Epilogue. In: Zacarian SA, ed. Cryosurgery for Skin Cancer and Cutaneous Disorders. St. Louis: Mosby, 1985:313–322.
96. Gage AA. Deep cryosurgery. In: Epstein E, Epstein E, eds. Skin Surgery. Springfield, IL: Charles C Thomas, 1982:857–877.
97. Gage AA. Correlation of electrical impedance and temperature in tissue during freezing. Cryobiology 1979; 16:56–62.
98. LePivert P, Binder P, Oughier T. Measurement of intratissue bioelectrical low frequency impedance: a new method to detect preoperatively the destructive effect of cryosurgery. Cryobiology 1977; 14:245–250.
99. Kimmig W, Hicks R, Breitbart EW. Ultrasound in cryosurgery. In: Breitbart EW, Dachow-Siwiec E, eds. Clinics in Dermatology: Advances in Cryosurgery. New York: Elsevier, 1990:65–68.
100. Hoffmann K, Dirschka Th, Stücker M, Rippert G, Hoffmann A, el-Gammal S, Altmeyer P. Ultrasound and cryosurgery. Dermatol Monatsschr 1993; 179:270–277.
101. Laugier P, Laplace E, Berger G. Cryosurgery in dermatology monitored by ultrasonography: in vitro results with a new prototype. In: Homasson JP, ed. Abstracts of the 9th World Congress of Cryosurgery, Paris, 1995:13.
102. Juhlin L, Evers H, Broberg F. A lidocaine-prilocaine cream for superficial skin surgery and painful lesions. Acta Derm Venereol (Stockh) 1980; 60:544–546.
103. Chiarello SE. Full-face cryo- (liquid nitrogen) peel. J Dermatol Surg Oncol 1992; 18:329–332.

12
Implant

Larry E. Millikan
Tulane University Medical Center
New Orleans, Louisiana

I. INTRODUCTION

A recent approach to cosmetic resurfacing and correction of defects is the use of safe and reasonably long-lasting and effective implants that can be injected. This provides an easy solution for many patients who have scars, depressions, etc. that result from trauma, infections, chickenpox, acne, or other conditions and under certain circumstances can also be used effectively for the treatment of wrinkling.

There is a long history of products available for this use, and over the years various products' side effects, availability, and longevity, and lack thereof, have stimulated the concept and development of an ideal implant (Table 1). Ease of use of the product is perhaps the most important aspect. Ease in shipping, ease in handling in the doctor's office, and acceptance by patients are all important in this area. Some of these products require refrigeration, which complicates the delivery and storage. Many of the products have a shelf life that can create a problem for dermatologists who do not do a large volume of dermal implants.

The permanence of the correction can be a two-edged sword. If the clinician is less skilled and the correction is less than optimal, a permanent solution will mean a permanent overcorrection or miscorrection. Most of the products today require more than one injection, which does provide some user-friendly characteristics. The ideal product has to be enough like the host that there is a minimal reaction, and it seems that in the most successful types of implants, the permanent correction is related more to turnover of the collagen implant and replacement with neonative collagen.

II. HISTORY

The correction of deep-pitted scars has been attempted with a variety of products, and the difficulties with products that created a significant host reaction are documented in the literature. Early on, the use of paraffin gave initial satisfactory correction but resulted in the formation of paraffinomas and very significant host reactions with inflammation, draining sinuses, and scarring. This and some other similar products all resulted in a host reaction that was totally unacceptable, and the use of these products fell out of favor.

Silicone has been around since the early 1950s. The silicone molecule appears to be one of the most nonreactive products (inspite of popular news to the contrary) and was met

Table 1 Ideal Implant

Easily obtained by usual shipping mechanism
Stable, shelf life
Ease of use
Minimal host reaction
Inert or replaced by natural collagen
Permanent correction

with a great deal of enthusiasm early on. Skill in using silicone is essential for an ideal result with the implant. Recent concerns about host reactions to silicone implants, associated arthritis-like syndromes, and other illnesses have certainly tempered the enthusiasm for these products. In addition, the adjuvant syndrome seen with silicones and some other oils tended to underscore concerns about the safety of these products, culminating in the Food and Drug Administration (FDA) decisions with regard to the silicone implant situation. There is no doubt that under certain circumstances, the adjuvant syndrome can occur with some oils and some silicones (often products of questionable preparation). The exact pathways involved are not entirely clear but seem to be partially related to host susceptibility, and in many of these cases the patients have had a family history of collagen-vascular disease and increased susceptibility to agents promoting this problem. Some of this can be avoided by a careful and complete history and skin testing, but there remain some patients who have a severe debilitating syndrome who defy medical association and good therapy. One of the last major discussions of silicone at the ASDS Regional Dermatologic Surgery Update (1984) (1) involving Drs. Orentreich, Yarborough, and Rathkin (Dow-Corning) was of note, in that Dow Corning at that time was still very interested in making the product available if they could provide the appropriate intermediary to oversee distribution, injection technique, and appropriate evaluation of patients (and potential liability!). It is understandable that pharmaceutical firms have concerns about making a product available that can have variable success and variable reaction rates related to the skills of the treating physicians. At the time of that discussion, silicone still had a reasonable reputation, and it would seem now that other circumstances have made silicone a historical item and no longer a clinically useful agent. It is a fact that a large number of silicone implants are without problems, and this is related to the skill of the treating physician. Perhaps the key is in-depth evaluation of the patient in regard to avoiding problems, and the availability and legal status of silicone in the future seem unlikely.

III. COLLAGEN PREPARATIONS

In the 1970s, Collagen Corporation began working on studying bovine collagen as a suitable implant for correction of wrinkles, depressed scars, and other cosmetic defects. The early acceptance was broad and enthusiastic, but the biggest problem with the first product made available was the short duration of the correction. Zyderm I had a few months' correction life at the maximum, and after the first round of enthusiastic usage, the need for a longer lasting correction became obvious, and Zyderm II was made available and a slightly different injection technique was used for this product. Zyderm I is a suspension of 3.5% collagen of bovine origin, and it is essentially type I (with only 5% type III) collagen in a physiologic saline solution with lidocaine added. Some of the antigenicity of this product was removed by pepsin digestion of the peptide ends, and this provided a reasonably satisfactory safety profile, although reactions may occur with any and all implants.

Because of the short-lived response with Zyderm I, the product Zyderm II became available, and it is characterized by a higher concentration of the collagen (6.5%), but the physiologic saline lidocaine base is essentially the same. Ultimately, one other product, Zyplast, became available; it has 3.5% lidocaine and physiologic saline but differs from the other products by formaldehyde cross-linking of the molecules to form a lattice that is thicker and slightly more difficult to inject, but it seems to have greater permanence. These are biologic products with a potential for immunogenicity, which can largely be circumvented by the use of skin testing.

Early skin testing was straightforward using a single test followed by the injections. Reactions to the implant led to the concept of double testing (2,3).

Double skin testing has been the obvious answer for any physician who has had the problem of caring for a patient who has reacted to the collagen injection. Elson (4) did perhaps the best review of this in 1989, in the Journal of Dermatologic Surgery and Oncology (now Dermatologic Surgery), where he described his experience with 200 patients with single testing and 200 patients with double testing. Of the single-tested patients, five had an adverse reaction and therefore were not considered candidates. The remaining patients, who had implants had a 3% adverse reaction rate in spite of a negative skin test. In the second group, with double skin testing, there were five positive first skin tests and seven positive second skin tests, and the patients who were negative on double testing had no adverse reactions to the implants.

IV. ZYDERM TECHNIQUES

Skin testing is done in a similar manner to a tuberculin test, on the volar aspect of the arm using 0.1 mL. The skin test is then read, and repeated skin testing is done. Several approaches to skin testing can be used. One is to skin test in one arm and then, 2 to 4 weeks later, skin test in the contralateral arm. Elson in his review also pointed out another approach, which is skin testing the arm and then skin testing the face. Reading the skin test at 48–72 hours, as one would a tuberculin test, we feel is important, with a final reading in 4 weeks. The author has preferred a skin testing reading at 4 weeks, retesting and reading 2 to 3 weeks after that, allowing a minimum of 6 weeks after the initial skin test to pick up any delayed and slow responding reactions to the implant.

A. Treating with the Implants

The technique of injection has become easier with the greater availability of finer needles (5) (Fig. 1). Currently, a 30-gauge needle is standard, but a 32- or 33-gauge needle may also be used. These have the advantage of decreasing the patient's discomfort and allowing easier depth placement of the implant. With Zyderm I, one uses the needle bevel up and superficial, so that one can actually see the implant placement. Overcorrection, because of the low concentration of collagen, is routine, and one can see over the subsequent days rapid

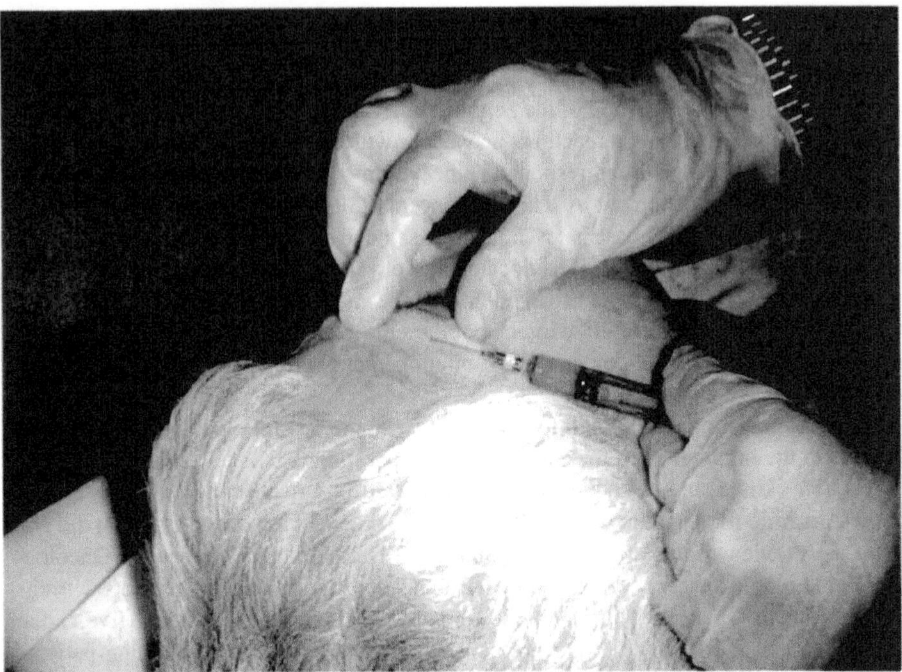

Figure 1 Injection technique. Injection techniques for most of the filler substances are identical. Slight variations depend on the viscosity and particular preparation in relation to the depth of placement of the implant. The usual technique is illustrated here in a treatment of a patient for a scar.

resolution of the overcorrection. With Zyderm II the technique is the same as with Zyderm I, but usually the overcorrection is somewhat less. Zyplast is different because the product is thicker: the overcorrection is minimal, and the placement is deeper than with Zyderm. The results of these implant injections correlate very directly with the experience and skill of the treating physician. Training in use and technique is essential, and the company has made available small Petri dish size practice units that we have found very useful for one who does this technique infrequently to keep his or her skills at a high level.

B. Clinical Usefulness

In the treatment of depressed scars secondary to acne, varicella, and trauma, the results are very good (Figs. 2 and 3). Implants are generally considered less useful in the treatment of wrinkles, because there is a dynamic or gravitational process that results in reinstitution of the abnormality in short order after the correction.

The principal promise of these implants to correct the wrinkling effects of aging is yet to be fully realized, but the public has accepted the need for occasional reinjection to correct the problem. Also, current usage of Zyplast and Zyderm is often coordinated, with the base for the correction being applied with Zyplast and fine touching up done more superficially with Zyderm I or II. In many people's hands this provides a significant amount of flexibility. Newer products are in the process of development.

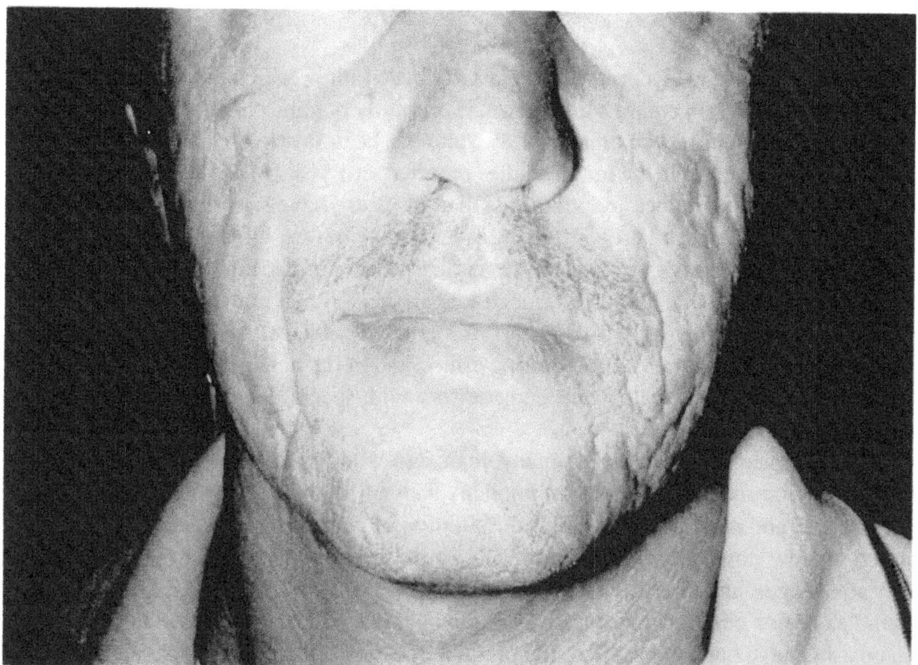

Figure 2 Patient with very severe postacne scarring.

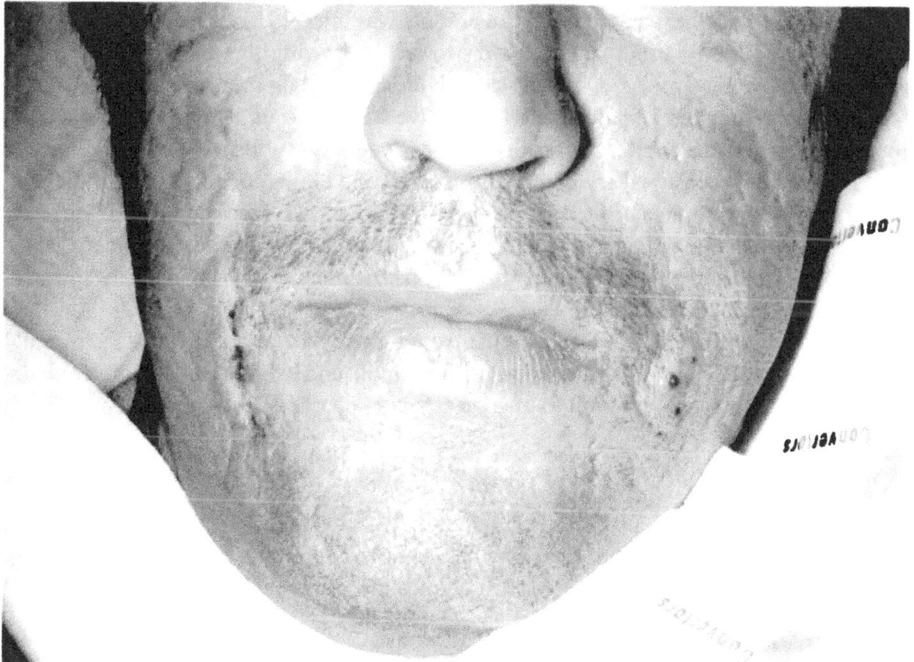

Figure 3 The same patient several months later with a number of the areas filled in, showing good improvement.

V. FIBREL

The major alternative to Zyderm and Zyplast has been Fibrel, which has been available for nearly a decade. This, in contrast to Zyderm, is primarily porcine collagen. It has a reported lower rate of reactions, approximately 1.8%, and has been favored by some because of its longer lasting correction in the initial studies reported, at 1 year (6), 2 years (7), and 5 years (8). Again, with this product, individuals skilled in its use have significant success in correction for the patients, and proper training is key to the best results.

Fibrel has differences from Zyderm that are worth noting. First of all, it comes as a lyophilized product, which gives it a much longer shelf life and obviates the need for refrigerated shipping. This is perhaps one of its stellar advantages. An additional difference is that the product has a much more lasting effect, and in the author's hands complete correction of some ice-pick scars has been necessary with special techniques using a custom needle (see later).

The premise for Fibrel began many years ago with Spangler (9), Gottleib (10), and others, who first used gel foam as an implant. The gel foam was augmented with the patient's serum, and another key aspect is the addition of ϵ-aminocaproic acid, which was instituted to slow down fibrinolysis at the site of the implant injection. In theory, this has many advantages, and in reality most of those seem to be true. However, the use of patient's serum has been a complicating factor from the beginning for many physicians, and variations on this have been done. Also, the product does not come with a local anesthetic incorporated in it; it has just the saline and the lyophilized preparation, to which the patient's serum is added. For many busy dermatologic surgery offices this is not a major problem. Many dermatologists early on began adding xylocaine to the mixture, feeling that it would provide some anesthetic benefit. In the original studies on wrinkles, regional or field blocks were done with xylocaine, and then the pure product was injected to correct the wrinkle defect. Others have tried various modifications to avoid drawing the patient's serum, and some reports show nearly as good results as with the traditional product, although the data are for only small numbers of patients. Retrospective studies are under way to compare traditional with nonplasma Fibrel, but results have not yet been published. An intriguing aspect of Fibrel is the occasional erythematous response and dramatic remodeling of the scar site with total disappearance of the scar, suggesting that growth factors or other cytokines are activated with the injection, and this has been explored by some to look at other uses of Fibrel in skin grafts and other tissue repair situations. At present, this is primarily speculation and scientific data are lacking.

The growth of the use of Fibrel was hampered in the past by some setbacks in availability of the product, but availability now seems assured, and exploration of simpler methods of application may allow Fibrel to assume a greater percentage of the implant usage.

A. Skin Tests

The skin test is available as a separate preparation, just as is the case of Zyderm. The skin test application is essentially the same as with Zyderm, and at present double testing has not become the usual pattern, and there still seems to be a low incidence of reactions.

B. Techniques and Exceptions

The technique of Fibrel injection begins with or without the patient's serum being used in preparation of the product. This is mixed with the saline, and then the lyophilized gelatin powder is thoroughly mixed and stored until ready for injection. It is usual to prepare the product freshly with each implant injection. However, some physicians reportedly store some patients' plasma for varying periods of time, introducing some variability in the process. One who uses Fibrel frequently will notice variations in the viscosity of the implant in different patients and at different times; this is not entirely predictable but has been thought to be related to blood lipid levels in the patient. When plasma is not used, the implant product is fairly standard in viscosity.

VI. ALTERNATIVE PREPARATIONS

Alternative preparations include using smaller amounts of the patient's serum or none. When no serum is used, the saline is used as the primary diluent, and in most instances some xylocaine is added prior to the implant injection. An excellent video is available showing the technique of mixing and injection; this is recommended to familiarize the staff with the product, and it has also been used on occasion for education of patients. The injection technique is very similar to that with Zyderm. The injection plane is usually somewhere between the planes for Zyplast and Zyderm, and a very superficial implant with Zyderm I is difficult to do except in some patients in whom the final reconstituted product has a great deal of fluidity. The original studies that we reported showed excellent results and excellent correction, but these were done with just one injection, and one can surpass these results routinely with touch-up injections at 6- to 8-week intervals as needed. One additional injection is usually all that is necessary to achieve the desirable correction. The correction of traumatic, varicella, or acne scars is essentially 100%. In the case of wrinkles, as with Zyderm, the fluid nature of gravity stress and muscle stress that causes wrinkling predisposes individual patients to recurrence of the wrinkles. Deep ice-pick scars resist implant elevation and special techniques are necessary for optimal results. Our approach is covered in the next section. The use of botulinum toxin in some patients seems to be an important additional approach to maximize the benefit but will not be dealt with in this chapter.

The most reliable and reproducible implant usage is in the correction of depressed scars. Shallow dome-shaped scars respond best, especially when they are distensible. So-called ice-pick scars always represent a challenge. Several approaches have been used to deal with these. In the punch-and-float technique, the depressed area of the scar is punched out with an appropriate size dermal punch, the epidermis then is freed from the deep dermis and allowed to float up, and a clot forms under the scar tissue. This elevates the scar and sometimes by itself provides satisfactory cosmetic results. However, many dermatologists augment the resurfacing with dermabrasion, allowing areas too deep for the wire brush or fraise to be corrected. We have found that it is possible to utilize the Fibrel kit with the custom needle as an instrument to free up the bound-down part of these deep ice-pick scars and then place the implant to elevate the depressed area. This generally mandates a two-stage procedure, because the large hole that is created by the large custom needle will not allow much of the implant to stay in the tissue and so a touch-up injection is usually done 2 to 7 days later. This has been a successful approach in our hands.

An alternative with any of the implants is to use a no. 11 blade in the same manner to free up the bound-down scar and then use the implant of choice to fill in. The problem with wrinkles has been mentioned several times previously, and the increasing use of Botox is of interest. Other defects that are often a challenge are furrows in the glabella, which for many patients are more of a cosmetic concern than fine wrinkles or simple expression lines.

This is an area in which injection has to be done with caution, because of the necrosis that sometimes occurs with improper injection techniques in the glabella.

The future of these implants has some intriguing twists. The author and other colleagues, including Dr. Gary Monheit, have on occasion noticed very remarkable reactions after implants that result in erythema (Fig. 4), but no obvious infection, and the outcome has been a significant cosmetic result. The mechanism of what happens under these circumstances is still unclear but is under investigation in some laboratories. The use of these collagen-like products as a lattice in wound healing has been considered before, and they have sometimes been used for preparing surgical sites to enhance healing and/or enhance coverage of a defect that is being repaired.

Another form of collagen is the Japanese form of a telocollagen under the Koken brand name, which is available outside the United States. It is a clear solution of calf collagen without the telopeptide. The author has no experience with the use of this product but has seen it demonstrated at international meetings. It comes in an easy-to-use dental syringe.

The use of autologous collagen has had some advocacy, and research into this has been done by our department and others. This is a follow-on from the initial use of autologous fat from liposuction as a filler. It appears that in most of the instances in which this lipoinjection seemed to provide some benefit, much of the long-lasting effect was related to the collagen present in the liposuction material rather than the fat. Subsequently, we and others have looked at separation of the fat from the septa and other collagenous materials

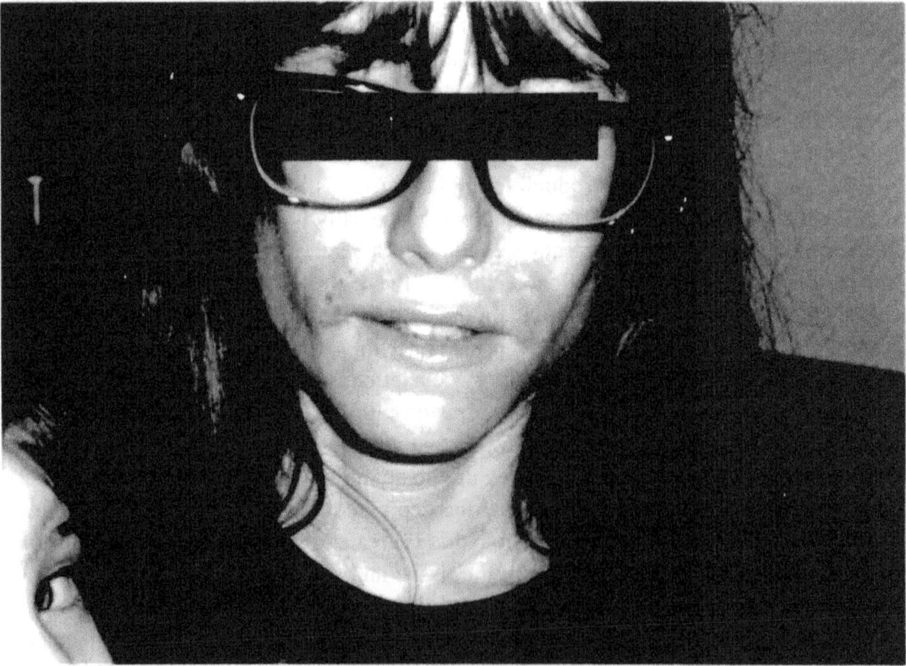

Figure 4 The erythematous response sometimes seen with a significant reaction. This, in our experience, attends inflammation, neocollagen formation, and very good cosmetic results. A reaction such as this must be carefully monitored to be absolutely certain there is no infection.

in the autologous liposuction material and then with minimal preparation use of that as an implant (12). This is a very labor-intensive procedure but it seems to work in many instances; however, at present it has not gained widespread acceptance.

VII. OTHER PRODUCTS

Investigation of other collagen sources is under way, including catfish collagen (13) and new studies of a form of collagen from China (14). Most collagen is derived from other species, and the immunogenicity has yet to be determined in most of these cases. However, it is clear that the enthusiasm for implants has declined somewhat.

Gortex threads have been used in Europe to fill in the areas of wrinkles, and the reaction around the threads causes collagen deposition and filling of the fold. This is perhaps too new for us to judge the long-term results, reactivity, and side effects. Here again, one needs to have a skilled surgeon, very familiar with the technique, to achieve the optimal results (15).

VIII. DISCUSSION

Implants are currently available around the world in a variety of preparations, the primary ones being those from bovine collagen. Other sources of collagen, including porcine and other species, are available or under study. All of these products seem to offer satisfactory correction, albeit temporary, and the cosmetic results seem to have a very direct relationship to the experience and skills of the surgeon. They represent a very useful additional procedure for patients and their margin of safety seems quite high. They are a recommended procedure for dermatologic surgeons to utilize in their practice. The availability of products and approval vary from country to country, but some product is available to the clinician, to the best of the author's knowledge, around the world.

REFERENCES

1. Personal communications, Tulane/ASDS Conference on Dermatologic Surgery, New Orleans, LA, July 4–8, 1984.
2. Clark DP, Hanke CW, Swanson NA. Dermal implants: safety of products injected for soft tissue augmentation. J Am Acad Dermatol 1989; 21:992–1998.
3. Cooperman LS, Mackinnon V, Bechler G, et al. Injectable collagen: a six-year clinical investigation. Aesthet Plast Surg 1985; 9:145–151.
4. Elson ML. The role of skin testing in the use of collagen injectable materials. J Dermatol Surg Oncol 1989; 15:301–303.
5. Klein AW. Indications and implantation techniques for the various formulations of injectable collagen. J Dermatol Surg Oncol 1988; 14:27–30.
6. Millikan L. Long-term safety and efficacy with Fibrel in the treatment of cutaneous scars: results of a multicenter study. J Dermatol Surg Oncol 1989; 15:837–842.
7. Millikan L, Rosen T, Monheit G, et al. Treatment of depressed cutaneous scars with gelatin matrix implant: a multicenter study. J Am Acad Dermatol 1987; 16:115–162.
8. Millikan L, Banks K, Purkait B, et al. A 5-year safety and efficacy evaluation with Fibrel in the correction of cutaneous scars following one or two treatments. J Dermatol Surg Oncol 1991; 17:223–229.

9. Spangler AS. New treatment for pitted scars. Arch Dermatol 1957; 76:708–711.
10. Spangler AS. Treatment of depressed scars with fibrin foam: seventeen years of experience. J Dermatol Surg 1975; 1:65–69.
11. Gold MH. Fibrel. Dermatol Clin 1995; 13:353–361.
12. Coleman WP III, Lawrence N, Sherman RN, et al. Autologous collagen? Lipocytic dermal augmentation: a histopathologic study. J Dermatol Surg Oncol 1993; 19:1032–1040.
13. Rose C, Mandal AB. The interaction of sodium dodecyl sulfate and urea with cat-fish collagen solutions in acetate buffer: hydrodynamic and thermodynamic studies. Int J Biol Macromol 1996; 18(1–2):41–53.
14. Liu B, Xu Z, Yu R. Experimental and clinical observation on wrinkle correction by medical cosmetic collagen injection. Chung Kuo I Hsueh Ko Hsueh Yuan Hsueh Pao 1994; 16:197–200.
15. Elson ML. Soft tissue augmentation. A review. Dermatol Surg 1995; 21:491–500.

13

Subcutaneous Incisionless (Subcision) Surgery for the Correction of Depressed Scars and Wrinkles*

David Scott Orentreich and Norman Orentreich
Orentreich Medical Group, LLP
New York, New York

A complex problem confronts the skin surgeon who attempts to correct depressed scars and wrinkles. In light of the various causes, anatomy of depressed areas, type of patient, and response of patient to past or current trauma and/or surgery, it is unlikely that one treatment modality will successfully improve all depressions. Therefore, the greater the number of treatment options available, the more likely the surgeon is to obtain successful correction.

The use of injectable soft tissue–augmenting implants has grown in both frequency and type. However, there is no ideal injectable augmentation agent. Existing materials have one or more disadvantages, including lack of persistence, risk of allergic reactions (1,2), localized tissue necrosis (1), and amaurosis (3,4). Other procedures, such as lipoinjection and autologous collagen injection, require additional surgery at the harvesting sites.

The shortcomings of currently available materials have spurred the ongoing development of techniques to correct depressed scars, wrinkles, and contours. The term Subcision (5) describes a unique form of incisionless local subcuticular undermining. The word Subcision is a contraction of "subcutaneous incisionless" surgery, and the method involves cutting under a depressed scar, wrinkle, or contour using a tribeveled hypodermic needle (now standard on most disposable needles) inserted under the skin through a needle puncture. The procedure attempts to raise the base of the defect to the level of the surrounding skin surface. The integrity of the skin surface is minimally compromised as with a routine needle puncture.

The effectiveness of Subcision for correcting various types of skin depressions depends on two distinct phenomena. First, the act of surgically releasing the skin from its attachment to deeper tissues results in skin elevation. Second, the introduction of a controlled

---

* Reprinted with permission from Dermatologic Surgery, Vol. 21, No. 6, David S. Orentreich, M.D. and Norman Orentreich, M.D., F.A.C.P. Subcutaneous Incisionless (Subcision) Surgery for the Correction of Depressed Scars and Wrinkles. pp 543–549, June 1995. Elsevier Science, Inc. 655 Avenue of the Americas, New York, NY 10010-5107.

trauma initiates wound healing with consequent formation of connective tissue, resulting in augmentation of the depressed site.

To the best of our knowledge, the use of subcuticular undermining to improve scars and wrinkles without the additional benefit of injectable augmenting agents was first reported by the authors in 1995 in the Journal of Dermatologic Surgery (6). In 1957, Spangler (7) reported using a Bowman iris needle to cut the fibrous strands beneath deeply depressed facial scars prior to injecting fibrin foam into the resulting cavity. In 1977, Gottlieb (8) pursued this approach, eventually leading to the development of Fibrel (9). The Fibrel kit is equipped with a 20-gauge needle that is used to undermine fibrotic depressed scars. This undermining creates a pocket in the dermis into which the Fibrel is injected (10). However, the studies evaluating Fibrel's efficacy did not include positive controls, i.e., fibrotic scars treated by undermining alone (2,9). In 1989, Koranda (11) reported the treatment of bound-down acne "crater" scars by inserting a no. 69 Beaver blade through a stab incision in the skin, sweeping through the scar tissue under the crater and allowing clot formation followed by fibrosis to maintain the elevation. In 1992, Hambley and Carruthers (12) used an 18-gauge needle inserted through the skin to release depressed, bound-down, full-thickness skin grafts on the nose prior to microlipoinjection. Again, no positive controls were reported.

It is possible that a majority of the long-term benefit derived from fibrin foam (13), Fibrel (2), or lipoinjection (1) after undermining may occur not primarily as a result of the implant substance, which is eventually absorbed, but rather as a consequence of connective tissue formation resulting from the preinjection undermining intended to create a pocket for the implant.

Subcision corrects depressed defects through two mechanisms. The first is the surgical act of cutting under and releasing the tethered bound-down site; the second is the formation of new connective tissue.

The first mechanism is exemplified by cutting through the scar tissue under depressed, bound-down scars. In comparison, subcising facial wrinkles releases the skin from its fibromuscular attachments to deeper tissue. These attachments include the muscles of facial expression that insert into the overlying skin (14), unlike skeletal muscles, which have no such attachments. In addition, numerous fibrous septa connect the superficial musculoaponeurotic system (SMAS), a broad, fibrous fascia enveloping and linking the muscles of facial expression, to the overlying dermis (14). The SMAS transmits the mimetic muscular contractions that create facial expressions and, with repetition, result in facial wrinkles that form at right angles to the direction of muscle contraction.

The second corrective mechanism is the creation of controlled trauma to promote new connective tissue formation under the defect in the course of wound healing. After a Subcision procedure, wound healing begins with a vascular response, then subsequent phases of inflammation, granulation tissue formation, and fibroplasia. Surface reepithelialization is essentially absent, because Subcision only minimally involves the epidermis. Ground substance is produced, and collagen synthesis (peaking at 6–7 days) continues for 2–4 weeks (15). Finally, long-term collagen remodeling occurs. Collagen production is possibly influenced by physical factors such as location and tension (16). This, in part, may explain the occasional appearance of a localized hypertrophic reaction following Subcision (see sequelae in Sect. II). The degree of response to Subcision varies with each patient's response to wounding.

The physiologic consequences of Subcision demonstrate that the releasing action and the associated wound healing process can, in many instances, be harnessed to correct distensile and bound-down skin depressions without need of injectable augmentation agents.

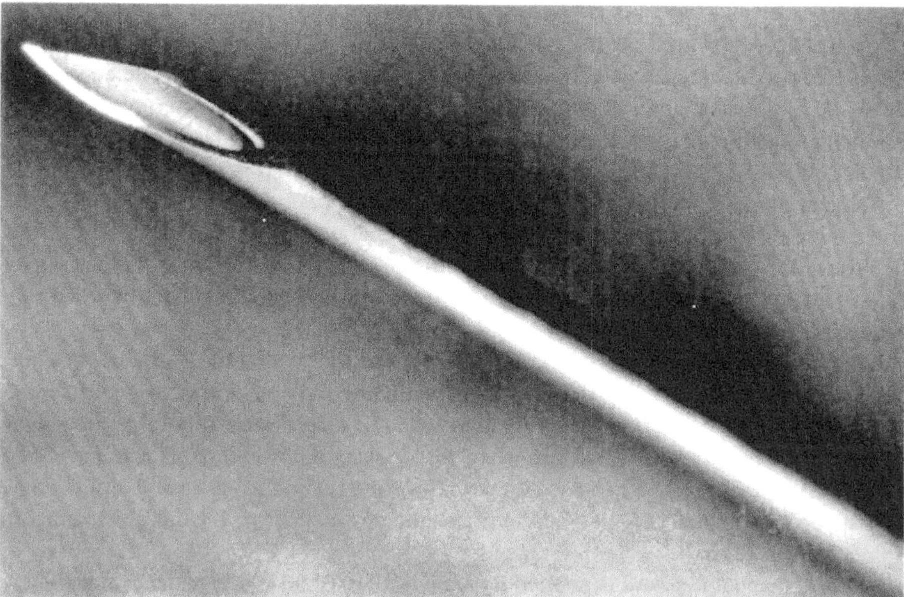

Figure 1 Tribeveled hypodermic needle. Note its sharp edges.

I. TECHNIQUE

Subcision surgery uses standard, readily available, and inexpensive materials. A sterile, disposable, 1-inch, 22- or 27-gauge, hypodermic B-D® needle suffices for most cases; however, needles of different lengths and gauges are also useful. Close inspection reveals that these needles are tribeveled to enhance their ability to puncture skin with minimal resistance (Fig. 1). During Subcision, the sharp edges are manipulated while under the skin to cut subsurface tissue. Needles as large as 16 gauge may be used to treat cellulite and large, bound-down scars such as healed surgical drain sites. Needles of 25–27 gauge (and even 30 gauge) can be used on particularly small, superficial facial scars and wrinkles, although care must be taken not to bend the finer caliber needles.

Areas to be subcised are first cleansed to remove dirt and makeup. Overhead lighting is adjusted to delineate fully and precisely the depressions, which are then outlined with a marking pen and subsequently anesthetized, typically with a 2% lidocaine with 1:100,000 epinephrine solution. Epinephrine is not used when contraindicated. A eutectic mixture of local anesthetic (EMLA)® cream may be used to produce topical analgesia prior to anesthetic injection. Local anesthesia should extend for several millimeters beyond the border of a marked area to ensure pain-free entry of the Subcision needle.

How one holds the Subcision needle is a matter of personal preference, influenced by the needle size and the treatment site. Generally, one either grasps the needle by its hub or clamps the needle in a needle holder.

® The B-D needle is a registered trademark of Becton-Dickinson and Co.

® EMLA is a registered trademark of Astra USA, Inc.

After sufficient time has elapsed for maximal vasoconstriction, a needle of chosen gauge is inserted a few millimeters from the depressed site and advanced underneath it. The bevel is oriented upward on insertion, and the angle of insertion is acute. The entry point into the skin acts as a pivot about which the needle is moved. The sharp edges of the tribeveled needle tip are maneuvered to cut under the skin surface. The free hand acts as a guide to Subcision and is used as needed to pinch, stretch, or stabilize the treatment site. If the needle is shorter than the full length of the wrinkle or scar, multiple puncture sites are chosen, depending on the size and shape of the depression.

The term "lancing" Subcision describes a simple linear inserting-withdrawing movement of the needle; this technique may be used under "crow's feet" wrinkles or when subcising very fibrotic scars (Fig. 2A).

"Fanning horizontal" Subcision describes moving the needle, bevel side up, in a horizontal plane, from side to side, back and forth, while inserting and withdrawing it in a fan-like motion (Fig. 2B). After insertion, the bevel may be turned vertically to cut in a plane that is perpendicular to the skin surface when withdrawing the needle. This is termed "vertical" Subcision (Fig. 2C). When used on wrinkles, vertical Subcision cuts at a right angle across superficially situated facial muscle fibers, thereby hampering the muscle's ability to wrinkle the skin.

Direct, manual pressure is applied by a medical assistant or the patient immediately after a site is treated, and pressure is maintained for several minutes to obtain hemostasis.

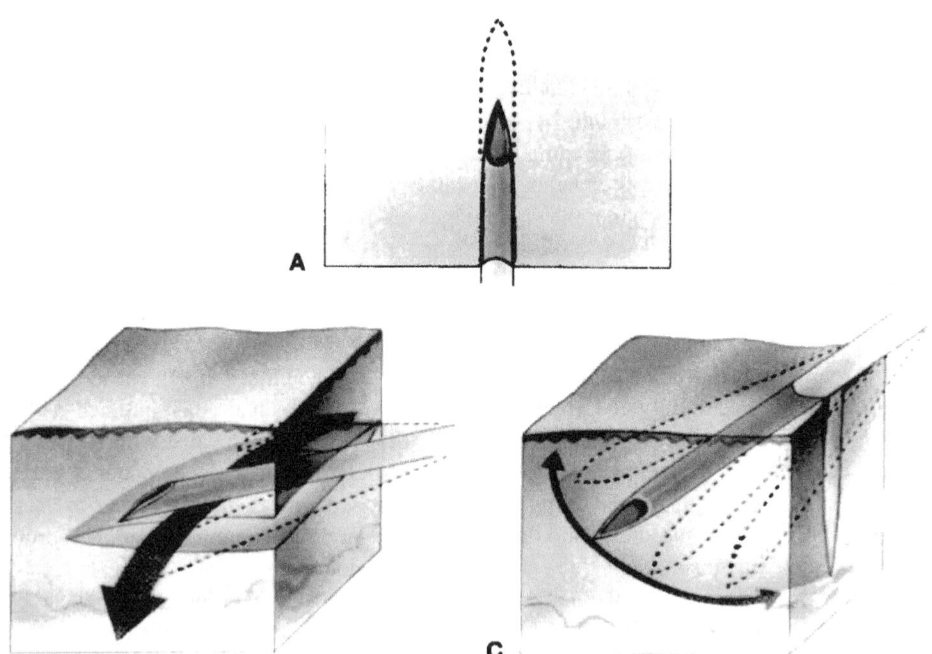

Figure 2 Nomenclature. **(A)** Lancing Subcision denotes inserting and withdrawing movements. **(B)** Horizontal fanning Subcision denotes side-to-side movements. Note that bevel is facing upward. **(C)** Vertical Subcision denotes cutting in a plane that is perpendicular to the skin surface. Note the bevel is oriented vertically.

Antibiotics are not usually prescribed unless there is a particular indication. Patients may apply makeup or Micropore tape to camouflage bruised areas.

Subcision is performed at precise, predetermined depths to ensure optimal results. The depth chosen depends on the indication, location of tethering structures, and the local microanatomy.

When treating depressed, bound-down scars, Subcision is usually performed in the mid- to deep dermis. Cutting through the fibrous bands of scar tissue permits the skin surface to elevate (Fig. 3). To correct distensile, depressed scars, Subcision is usually performed in the deep dermis or subdermally.

When treating facial expression lines, Subcision is subdermal in order to release facial muscle fiber and SMAS insertions into the dermis (Fig. 4). Small, superficial wrinkles (such as those radiating from the lateral canthus or from the vermilion border) may be treated with upper dermal, middermal, or subdermal Subcision, depending on wrinkle morphology and on the patient's response to previous Subcision.

The dimpled appearance of skin on the upper legs and buttocks, commonly known as "cellulite," is partially caused by fibrous septa arising from the deep fascia investing skeletal muscles, traversing the adipose layer, and inserting into skin, thereby tethering it. These fibrous septa can be divided by Subcision in the adipose layer.

Because the ability of individuals to form collagen varies, it is not possible to predict precisely how many Subcision treatments will be needed for any given defect. In general, Subcision is not a single treatment. The approximate number of Subcisions required to correct a specific depression depends on such variables as the type of depression (Table 1), its location, the patient's wound healing response, and the intensity of each treatment. Three to six visits suffice for the majority of cases of moderate wrinkling or scarring. Additional visits to treat other depressed sites and to retreat partially elevated sites (or treat a hypertrophic site) are scheduled at intervals of about 1 month. Usually, 1 month between Subcisions allows sufficient time for bruising and swelling to resolve and for connective tissue formation to plateau. Longer intervals delay but do not diminish the quality of the end result.

During the first session, it is prudent to limit the number and intensity of Subcisions until the patient's response is established. On subsequent visits, more or less intensive Subcision may be performed, depending on the patient's previous response. Generally, deeply depressed sites require more intensive Subcision carried out over more treatment sessions.

Certain anatomical locations including areas of increased skin tension may have a greater propensity for fibroplasia (16); therefore, these areas are treated less intensively, particularly during initial sessions. The periorbital, glabellar, labial commissure, and upper

Table 1 Indications for Subcision

Depressed distensile scars	Depressed, bound-down scars
Acne	Acne (excluding deep ice-pick scars)
Traumatic	Varicella
Surgical	Traumatic
Anetoderma	Surgical (e.g., healed drain site)
	Wrinkles
	Depressed contours (e.g., malar groove)
	Cellulite dimples

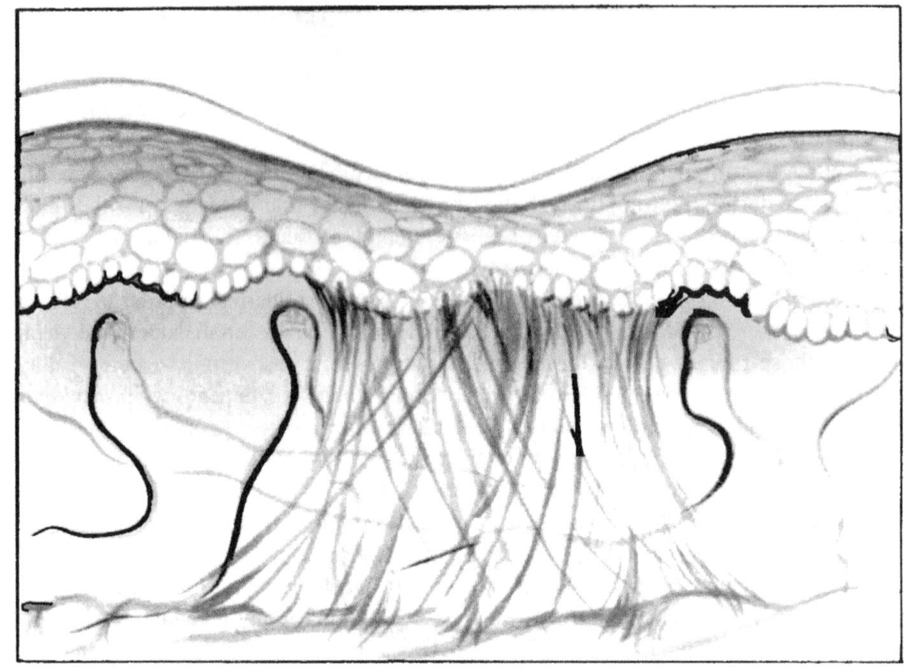

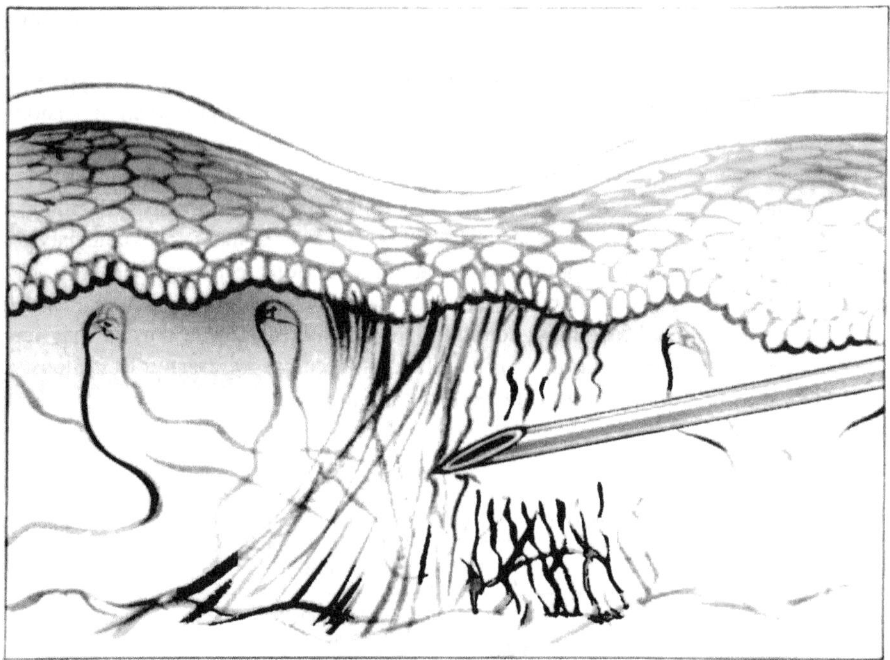

Figure 3 Treatment of bound-down scars. **(A)** Fibrous bands tether scar surface down. **(B)** Subcision of tethered scar releases depressed area. **(C)** Extravasated blood collects in Subcision wound. **(D)** Wound heals with formation of new connective tissue, which further augments depressed areas.

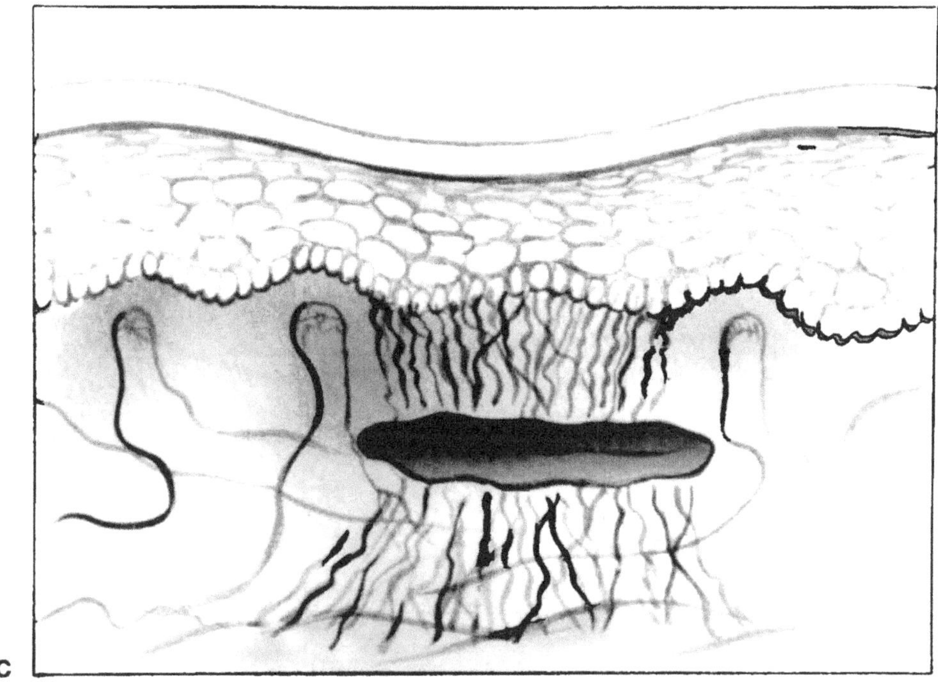

C

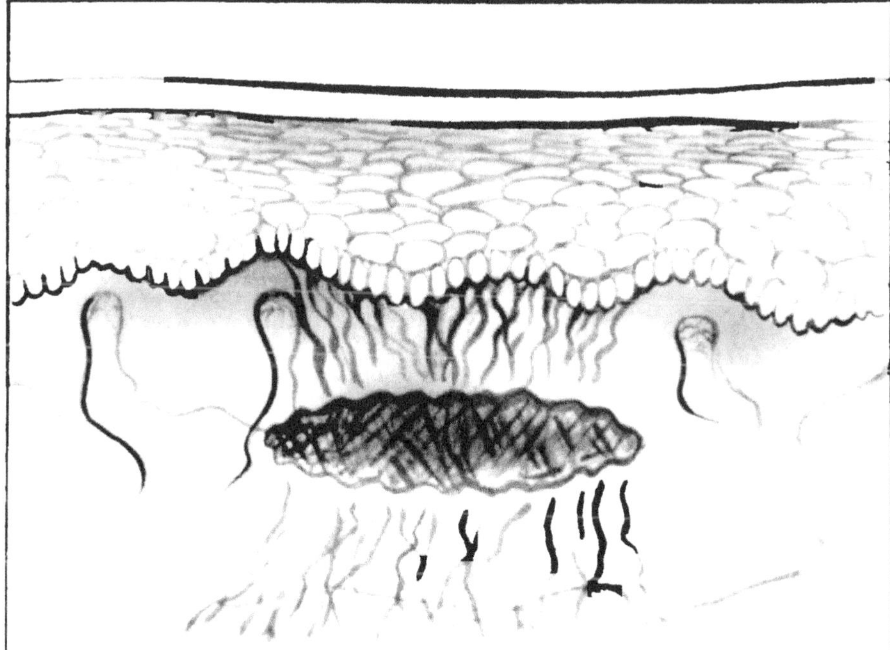

D

Figure 3 *(continued)*

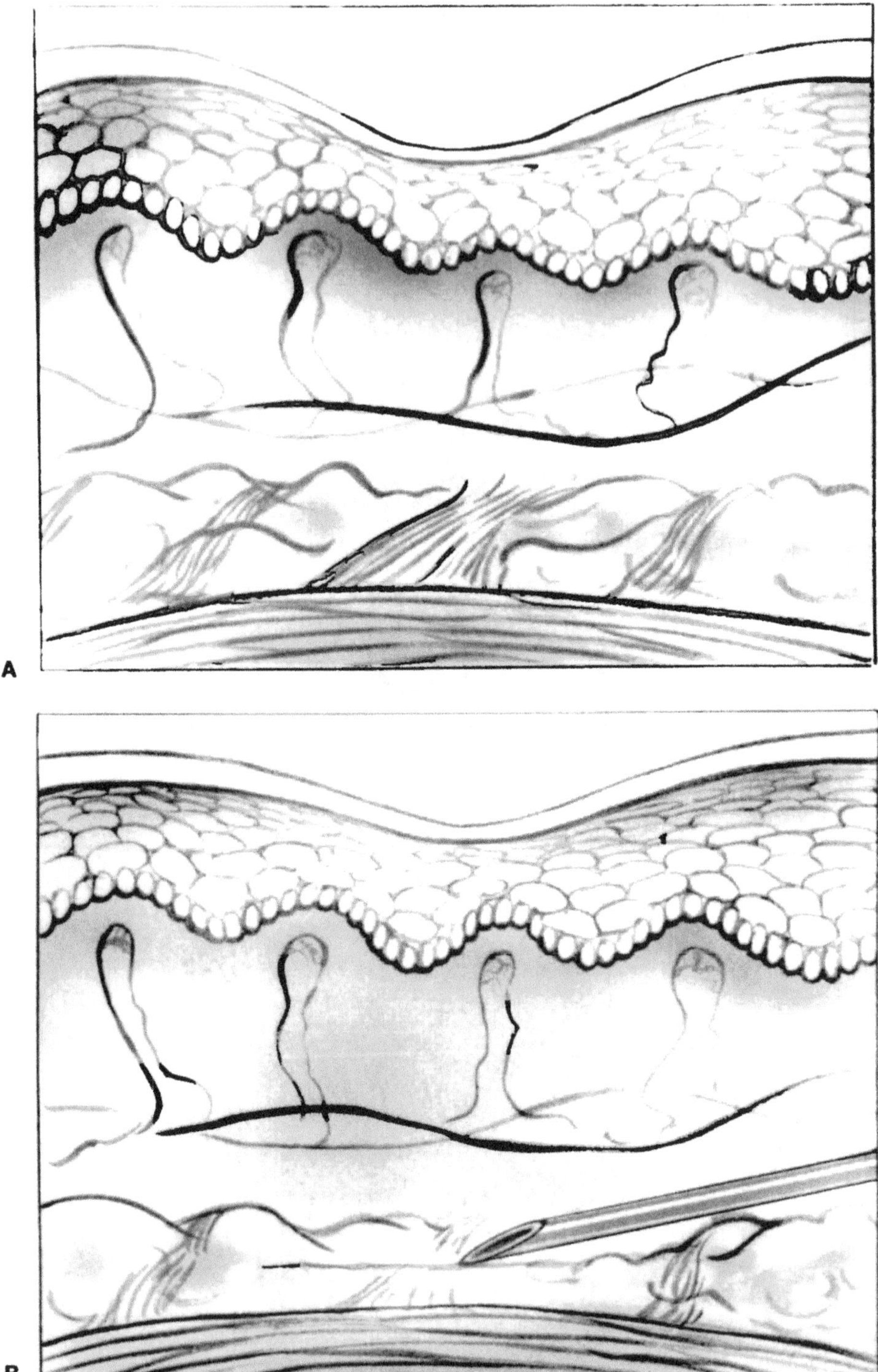

Figure 4 Treatment of wrinkles. **(A)** Mimetic muscle fibers and fibrous septa from the SMAS insert directly into the dermis. **(B)** Needle maneuvered to release insertions from facial muscles and SMAS. **(C)** Extravasated blood collects in Subcision wound. **(D)** Wound heals with formation of new connective tissue, which further augments depressed areas.

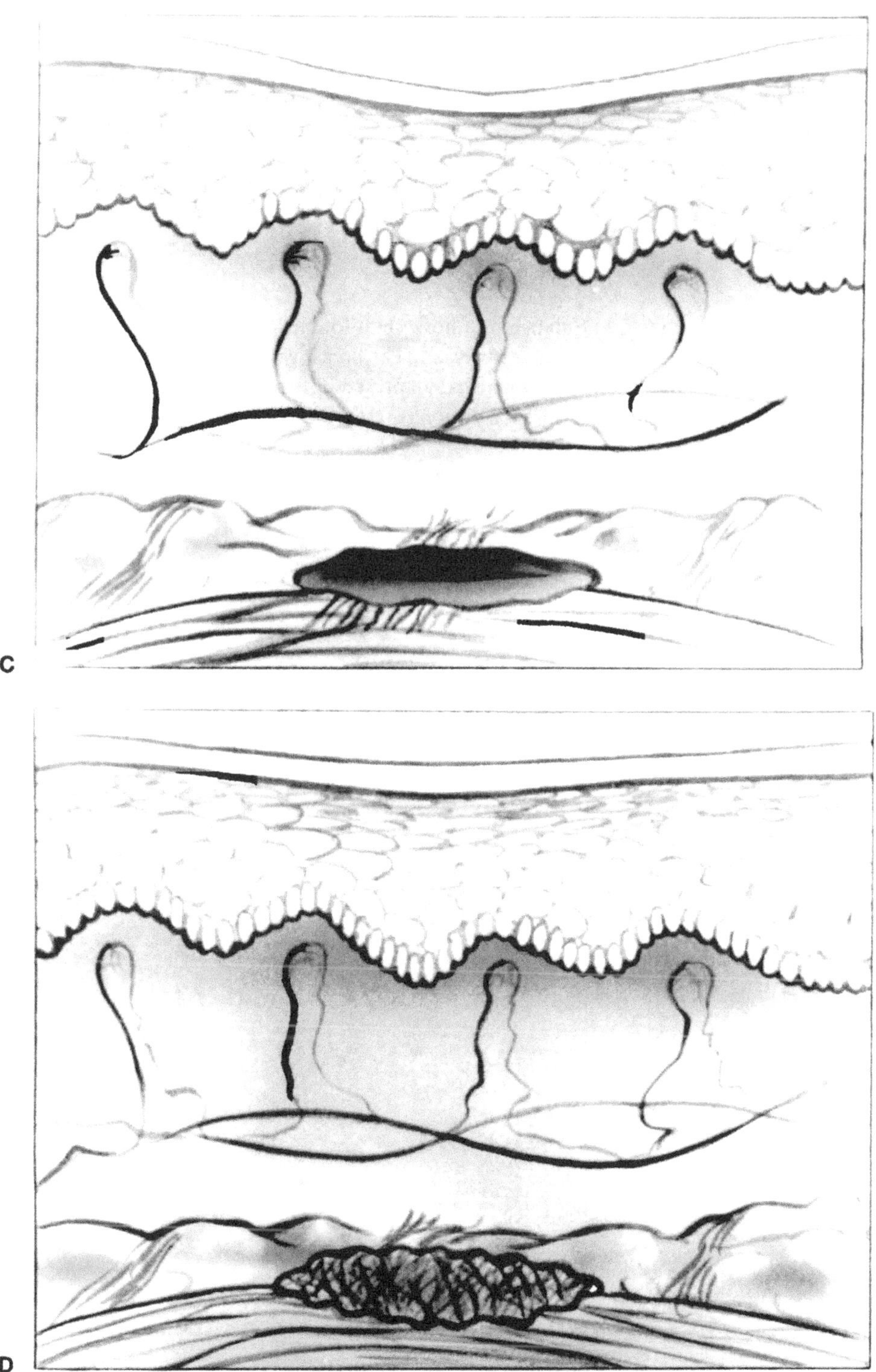

Figure 4 *(continued)*

lip areas are among those that appear to have a greater propensity to hypertrophic reactions in response to Subcision.

Although scar correction is generally permanent, wrinkles may deepen or re-form with time. Patients are advised that follow-up treatments at 6 to 12-month intervals may be needed to correct either new or recurring areas of wrinkling.

The following cases show the results of Subcision for wrinkles and depressed bound-down scars.

A. Case 1

A 43-year-old man underwent Subcision of horizontal forehead wrinkles (Fig. 5A). Three sessions were performed over a 3-month period. The areas were prepared as described. A 22-gauge, 1-inch needle was used. Other than expected bruising, there were no sequelae. Follow-up examination and photographs 4 months after the last session revealed satisfactory improvement (Fig. 5B).

B. Case 2

A 21-year-old woman presented with a depressed, bound-down, varicella scar, approximately 4 mm in diameter, on the left tip of her nose (Fig. 6A). The area was prepared as de-

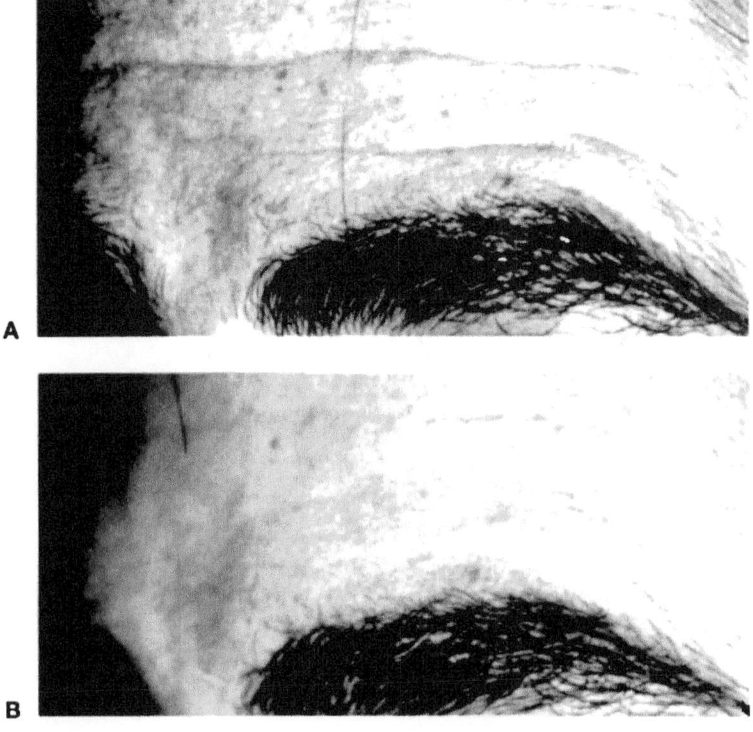

Figure 5 Case 1. **(A)** A 43-year-old man with forehead wrinkles before treatment. **(B)** Follow-up examination 4 months after the last of three sessions of Subcision reveals satisfactory improvement.

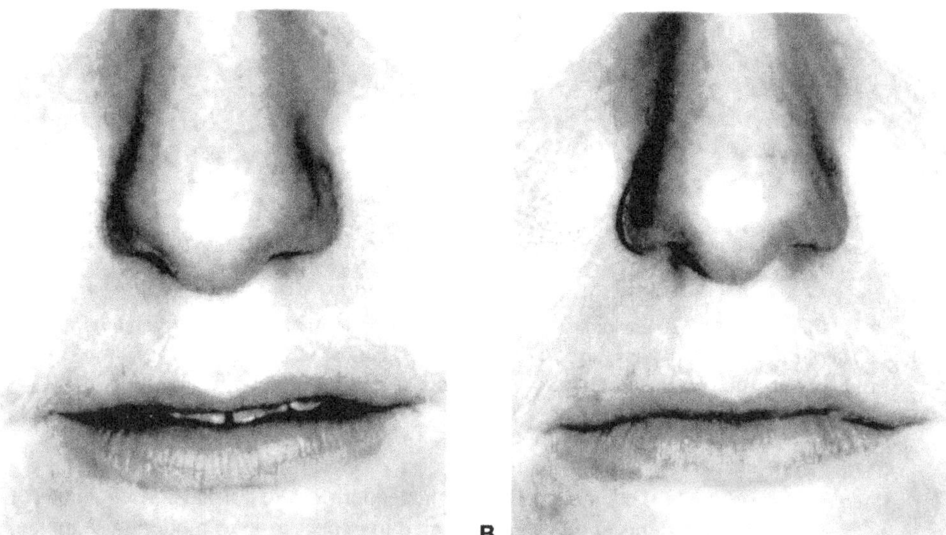

Figure 6 Case 2. **(A)** A 21-year-old woman before Subcision to correct a varicella scar on left tip of nose. **(B)** One month after Subcision, with nearly complete correction.

scribed, and a 22-gauge needle was used to perform Subcision. Follow-up at 10 days showed one small comedo, which was expressed, and one incipient acneiform lesion, which was incised and drained. The photograph at 1 month after Subcision shows nearly complete correction (Fig. 6B).

C. Case 3

A 42-year-old woman presented with three bound-down scars, between 10 and 15 mm in length, on the lower abdomen (Fig. 7A). The scars resulted from drains inserted during abdominal surgery 5 years previously. The areas were treated with one session of Subcision using a 22-gauge, 1-inch needle. Follow-up at 10 weeks showed substantial correction (Fig. 7B).

II. CONTRAINDICATION AND SEQUELAE

The only known contraindication to Subcision is active infection, at or immediately adjacent to the site to be treated. Deep ice-pick scars will not respond well to Subcision; punch grafting is usually preferred (16).

There are three relative contraindications. Although depressed, atrophic scars may be successfully raised to normal skin level, the appearance of the surface will remain atrophic. Nevertheless, correction by Subcision may be preferable to excision or grafting.

Patients with bleeding diathesis should be treated conservatively.

Any history of keloid scarring after trauma or surgery should prompt the physician to consider the possibility of keloid formation, and a carefully chosen test site may be subcised.

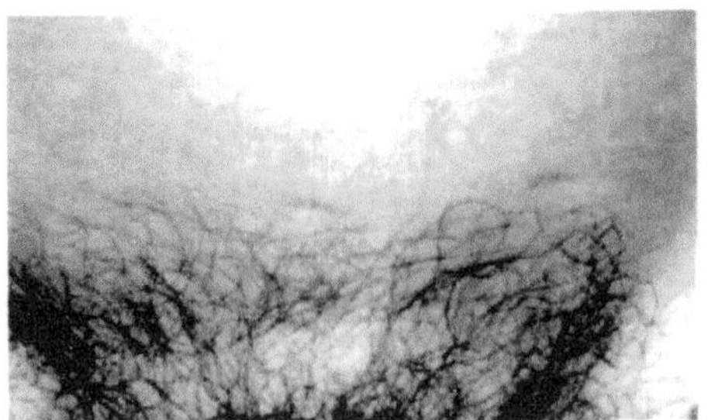
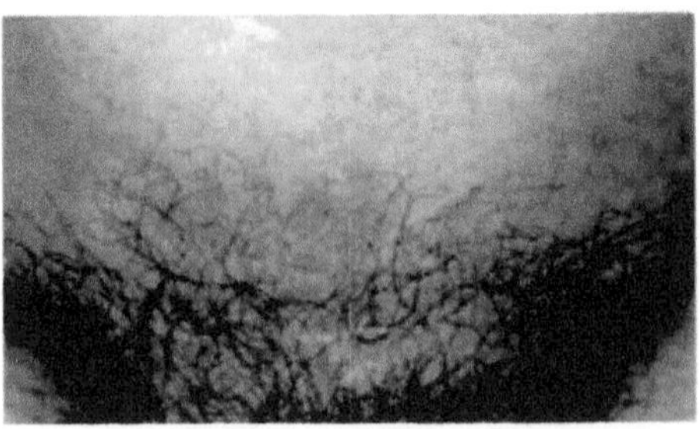

A B

Figure 7 Case 3. **(A)** A 42-year-old woman with three bound-down scars of 5 years duration, developed after healing of abdominal surgical drain sites. **(B)** Follow-up examination at 10 weeks after one session of Subcision revealed satisfactory correction.

Sequelae: Ecchymosis, edema, erythema, and tenderness are normal consequences of wounding. Patients should be counseled to expect mild to moderate sequelae, depending on the intensity and amount of treatment.

Infection: Occasionally, localized acneiform, cystlike lesions are observed. It is likely that subcutaneous disruption of the pilosebaceous apparatus is responsible for these lesions. These lesions respond to incision and drainage, intralesional corticosteroid injections (0.05–0.10 mL of triamcinolone acetonide, 1 mg/mL), and oral antibiotics, if needed.

Altered physical consistency of treated sites: The new connective tissue produced occasionally imparts a somewhat firmer skin texture. However, the improved overall appearance of the defect usually outweighs any change in physical consistency.

Discoloration: Temporary postinflammatory hyperpigmentation may appear in predisposed individuals. Patients are instructed to avoid sun exposure for at least 1 month after Subcision.

Suboptimal response: Partial elevation of the defect is a common occurrence after a single Subcision. Prior to treatment, patients are advised that multiple sessions are usually required to correct a specific defect.

Excess response: In approximately 5–10% of cases, excess fibroplasia develops, and an elevated or hypertrophic response results about 2–4 weeks postoperatively. These elevations usually have normal skin surface markings, in contrast to hypertrophic scars that appear after scalpel surgery. They respond favorably to intralesional corticosteroid injections (0.05–0.10 mL of triamcinolone acetonide, 1–5 mg/mL).

Keloid scarring: See relative contraindications earlier.

The advantages of Subcision are long-lasting scar correction and reasonably persistent correction of wrinkles. The materials required to perform Subcision are readily available and inexpensive. Furthermore, Subcision is not associated with a risk of allergic reactions (1,2) or amaurosis (3,4). Disadvantages of Subcision are bruising and occasionally hypertrophic reactions and acneform lesions.

In our experience, the combination of surgical release and spontaneous fibroplasia induced by Subcision is effective in treating cutaneous depressions such as scars, wrinkles, and cellulite. We find Subcision a valuable addition to the cutaneous surgeon's armamentarium of rehabilitative techniques.

REFERENCES

1. Hanke CW, Higley HR, Jolivette DM, Swanson NA, Stegman SJ. Abscess formation and local necrosis after treatment with Zyder m(R) or Zyplast(R) collagen implant. J Am Acad Dermatol 1991; 25:319–326.
2. Millikan L, Banks K, Purkait B, Chungi V. A 5-year safety and efficacy evaluation with Fibrel in the correction of cutaneous scars following one or two treatments. J Dermatol Surg Oncol 1991; 17:223–229.
3. Teimourian B. Blindness following fat injections (Letter). Plast Reconstr Surg 1988; 82:361.
4. Zyplast(R) Implant Physician Package Insert. Collagen Corporation, Palo Alto, CA.© 1985, 1987.
5. U.S. trademark for Subcision(R). Registration no. 1,841,017. Date granted: June 21, 1994.
6. Orentreich D. Punch grafting. In: Moy RL, Lask G, eds. Principles and Techniques of Cutaneous Surgery. New York: McGraw-Hill, 1996.
7. Spangler AS. New treatment for pitted scars. Arch Dermatol 1957; 76:708–711.
8. Gottlieb S. GAP repair technique (Poster Exhibit). Annual Meeting of the American Academy of Dermatology, Dallas, TX, December 1977.
9. Multicenter Study. Treatment of depressed cutaneous scars with gelatin matrix implant. J Am Acad Dermatol 1987; 16:1155–1162.
10. Cohen IS. Fibrel(R). Semin Dermatol 1987; 6:228–237. Fibrel(R) is a registered trademark of the Mentor Corporation.
11. Koranda FC. Treatment modalities in facial acne scars. In: Thomas JR, Holt GR, eds. Facial Scars: Incision, Revision & Camouflage. St. Louis: Mosby, 1989:285.
12. Hambley RM, Carruthers JA. Microlipoinjection for the elevation of depressed, full-thickness skin grafts on the nose. J Dermatol Surg Oncol 1992; 18:963–968.
13. Spangler AS. Treatment of depressed scars with fibrin foam: seventeen years of experience. J Dermatol Surg Oncol 1975; 1:65–69.
14. Salasche I, Bernstein G, Senkarik M. Surgical Anatomy of the Skin. Norwalk, CT: Appleton & Lange, 1988:70, 90.
15. Zitelli SA. Wound healing and wound dressings in dermatologic surgery. In: Roenigk RK, Roenigk HH Jr, eds. Dermatologic Surgery: Principles and Practice. New York: Marcel Dekker, 1989:98–101.
16. Ketchum LD, Kelman Cohen I, Masters FW. Hypertrophic scars and keloids: a collective review. Plast Reconstr Surg 1974; 53:140–154.

14
Punch Transplant Technique for Pitted Scars

Edmond I. Griffin
Dermatology Associates of Atlanta, P.C.
Atlanta, Georgia

I. INTRODUCTION

Acne patients with scarring rarely have just one type of scar. The scars vary in type, number, and extent. Acne scars are characterized most commonly as papules, nodules, depressions, and pits (ice-pick scars or craters). They are further described as deep, shallow, narrow, broad, hypertrophic, hypotrophic, keloidal, hyperpigmented, hypopigmented, mottled, white, pink, brown, or purple. It is most important to match the scar type to the technique that produces the best cosmetic result. In the past, deep pitted scars were treated with simple surgical excision with closure resulting in a white linear scar. The purpose of this chapter is to isolate the pitted scars and describe the techniques of punch grafting or punch elevation used for reconstruction (Fig. 1a and b).

II. BACKGROUND OF ACNE

Although much is understood about acne and its "cure" (Accutane-Roche Laboratories), why a person with relatively minor acne develops scars is a mystery. The genetic code for the poor-healing gene has not been identified, although a genetic predisposition is suggested by a familial tendency. The pilosebaceous unit is central to the cause of acne. When this follicular unit is plugged with sebum, the walls become necrotic, break down, and become inflamed, resulting in a scar. Scarring, superficial and deep, occurs around the follicular structure, resulting in an enlarged pore or an ice-pick scar.

III. ANATOMY OF THE PITTED SCAR

The ice-pick scar is a depressed epithelium-lined tract with fibrotic attachments to the subcutaneous layer. It collects sebum, makeup, and cellular and bacterial debris. Whereas the acne scar called a crater or shallow pit is only about 1 mm or less in depth, the deeply reaching ice-pick scar extends down to 2 mm or more. Neither laser resurfacing, chemical peeling, nor dermabrasion will erase the ice-pick scar. The pitted crater can be improved by

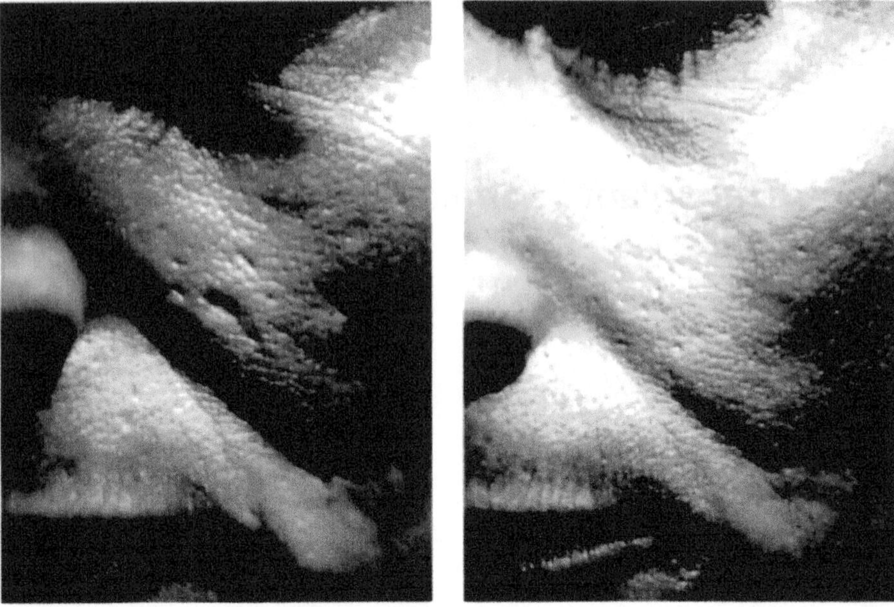

Figure 1 **(A)** Before photograph of female patient with acne pits; **(B)** photograph of the same patient 6 months after the last procedure (history of multiple procedures): Punch grafting, punch elevation, simple excisions, subcisions, dermabrasion, and dermal grafting.

both dermabrasion and laser resurfacing, which smooth the edges, decreasing shadows. Subcisions (undermining) will improve craters but not ice-pick scars. Whereas acne depressions and broad craters are oriented in the horizontal plane, ice-pick scars are oriented more vertically (Fig. 2). Punch grafting (with excision) is needed when the base of the pit or crater has a scar or abnormal pigmentation. This scarred area needs to be discarded and replaced with a normally pigmented smooth-surfaced graft (full thickness) from a distant site behind the ear (Fig. 3a and b).

IV. SUPPLIES AND EQUIPMENT

1. Well-sharpened Orentreich-type cylindrical punches: 1.5, 1.75, 2.00, 2.25, 2.5, 2.75, 3.0, 3.5, 4.0, and 5.0 mm
2. Hand engine with steam autoclavable chuck
3. Iris scissors
4. Fine forceps with teeth, fine forceps without teeth
5. Needle holder
6. Liquid adhesive (Mastisol by Ferndale Labs) and adhesive remover (Detachol by Ferndale Labs)
7. 4 × 4 gauze sponges; cotton Q-tips; alcohol swabs
8. Marking pen—gentian violet
9. Anesthetics: lidocaine without epinephrine and with epinephrine, bupivacaine (Marcaine)
10. 30-gauge needles

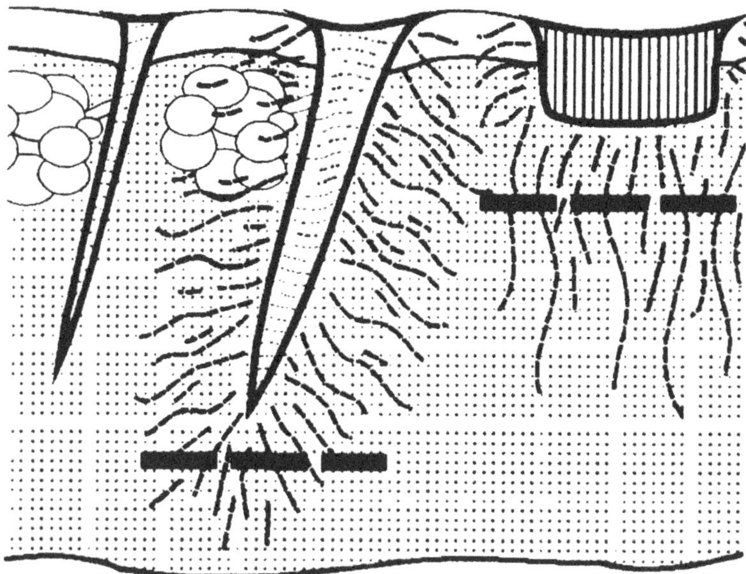

Figure 2 (Left) Normal pilosebaceous unit with normal-sized pore and sebaceous gland; (Middle) ice-pick pitted scar with radial fibrotic bands; (Right) crater pitted scar with downward fibrotic bands. Dark dotted lines at bases in the middle and at the right represent Subcisions, showing minimal effect on the ice-pick scar and a greater effect on the crater.

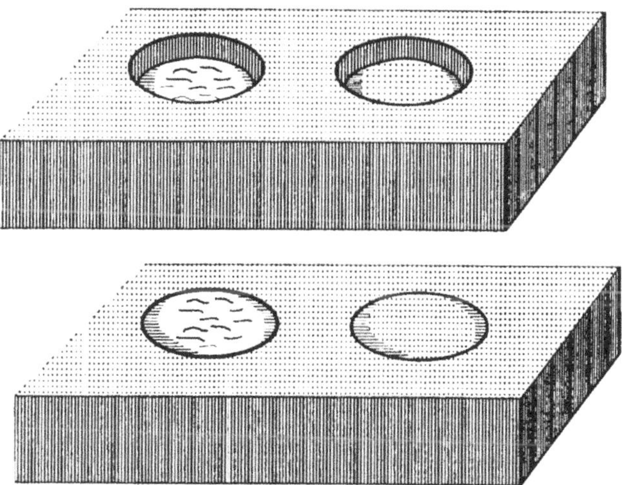

Figure 3 (Top) Shallow craters: the crater at the left shows a hypopigmented scarred base ideal for punch graft replacement by donor graft; the crater at the right shows normal epidermis in the base ideal for punch elevation. (Bottom) Both craters at the top treated only by punch elevation; note good match on right but now raised, hypopigmented scar on left.

11. Petri dishes with smooth filter paper
12. Normal saline, ice
13. Tegaderm (3M) or Omiderm dressings (ITG Laboratories)

V. MAGNIFICATION AND STAFFING

The details of the operation will go unnoticed unless magnification is required and used for all operating surgeons and staff. In addition to the surgeon, at least one assistant (sterile gloved) is needed to perform this procedure efficiently. An additional circulating assistant also speeds the process, especially if multiple elevations are being performed.

VI. PATIENTS' WRITTEN INSTRUCTIONS

Before Your Surgery

1. Avoid acetylsalicylic acid (ASA) or ASA-containing drugs 1 week prior to and after surgery.
2. Discontinue smoking 2 weeks prior to and 2 weeks after surgery. Continuation of smoking has resulted in loss of grafts and poor healing.
3. Start Retin-A (Ortho) at least 2 weeks prior to surgery. If you have olive or darker skin coloring, also start your bleaching creams at the same time. A cortisone cream will stop any itching and redness produced by these medications. Stop all toners, masques, scrubbing sponges, and detergent cleansers: Use Cetaphil (Galderma) cleanser daily.
4. Take the prescribed antibiotic the day before and the morning of surgery.

After Your Surgery

1. Take the prescribed antibiotic for 5 days after surgery.
2. On the night of surgery do not disturb your dressings in any way. Do not touch or press the sites.
3. Avoid unnecessary facial contortions, excessive talking, and bulky food, especially on the night of surgery and for 3 days.
4. Pain is usually minor. Take the analgesic every 4 hours if needed.
5. On the morning after your surgery, you may remove any gauze dressing that was applied on your surgery day. Do not disturb the clear plastic-like dressing or the skin-colored Steri-strips (3M) that are covering your grafts.
6. If the clear plastic dressing with the strips comes off, use warm water compresses for 20 minutes four times a day. Apply an antibiotic ointment.
7. If a graft comes out, place it on a moistened gauze, place in a sandwich bag, put it into the refrigerator; and notify the office.
8. If regrafting a site is necessary, this will be done in 2–6 weeks. If the grafts need to be smoothed, this is best done after 6 weeks. Some swelling and hardening of the elevated skin or transferred graft occur and peak at 6 weeks. Too early removal may result in a depression that will be difficult to repair.

VII. PUNCH RELEASE FOR ICE-PICK SCARS OR SMALL PITS

Before deciding on the best treatment, a careful examination under unidirectional spotlighting helps identify the exact defect to be reconstructed. Although bound-down craters and depressions may be helped by the usual undermining referred to as Subcision, the usual deep ice-pick scar will not respond to this technique. The fibrotic bands of the ice-pick scar pull radially away and downward from the sides, whereas the fibrotic bands of the larger crater pull downward. When a cylindrical punch is placed around the ice-pick scar it severs these radial bands in the same manner that the Subcision releases the downward bands of the craters. The released cylinder is now free to contract because it has been released from the fibrotic bands. The dilated pore or ice-pick scar shrinks in diameter and becomes smaller with time (2–6 months). In like manner, the small pit also contracts. Surprisingly, no ring scar or dilated pore remains among the normal pores (Fig. 4a–c).

Punch elevation is the term also applied to the release of a crater with a normal (nonscarred, normally pigmented) base. For these craters with normal bases the punch elevation can be performed without adjunctive procedures. For craters with hypopigmented and scarred bases, punch grafting is necessary. The cicatricial base is punch excised, discarded, and replaced. If a depressed crater is small enough, it can be surrounded and elevated by a punch. For large craters tissue augmentation may be necessary to elevate the center of the crater.

A. Technique of Punch Release and Punch Elevation for Small Pits and Ice-Pick Scars

The ultrasharp cylindrical punch (Orentreich) is rotated at medium speed by a hand engine. A thick conical biopsy punch cannot be used. Manually rotating the Orentreich punch does not produce consistent results. Select the smallest (1.5-mm) punch and incise all pits that fit easily within the bounds of that size. Increase next to the 1.75-mm punch and incise the scars that fit that size. Repeat at each size of punch upward until all pits and craters have been incised but not severed from their base. This is especially true of the larger grafts above 3.5 mm. When the punch enters fat (about 3 mm or less), stop the spin or withdraw the punch. If the incision is too deep in the fat, there is a greater chance that the graft will become detached, lost, or lodge inside the punch. Although the detached graft is still viable, it delays surgery and generally does not heal as well. The punched tissue is elevated just above the surface of the surrounding skin. With forceps, this elevation is maintained for 1–2 minutes for a coagulum to form beneath the tissue. When doing the punch elevations, the angle of the punch should be at 90 degrees unless the angle of the pit is different. The deep ice-pick scar may follow the original angle of the pilosebeceous unit. The punch must completely surround the entire length of the ice-pick scar and not transect it at any point. If the cylindrical punch is not large enough or is not angled along the axis of the ice-pick scar, it will cut off part of the epithelialized track and produce an epidermal inclusion cyst (Fig. 5a–c). If the graft has been spun around in the cutting process, it will need to be rotated to match the original cutting angle.

Mastisol (Ferndale Labs) skin adhesive is applied thinly with the cotton Q-tips around all punch elevations, followed by Tegiderm (3M) dressing. This dressing is sized to cover one or more of the sites. It is preferable, because of skin movement, to have multiple

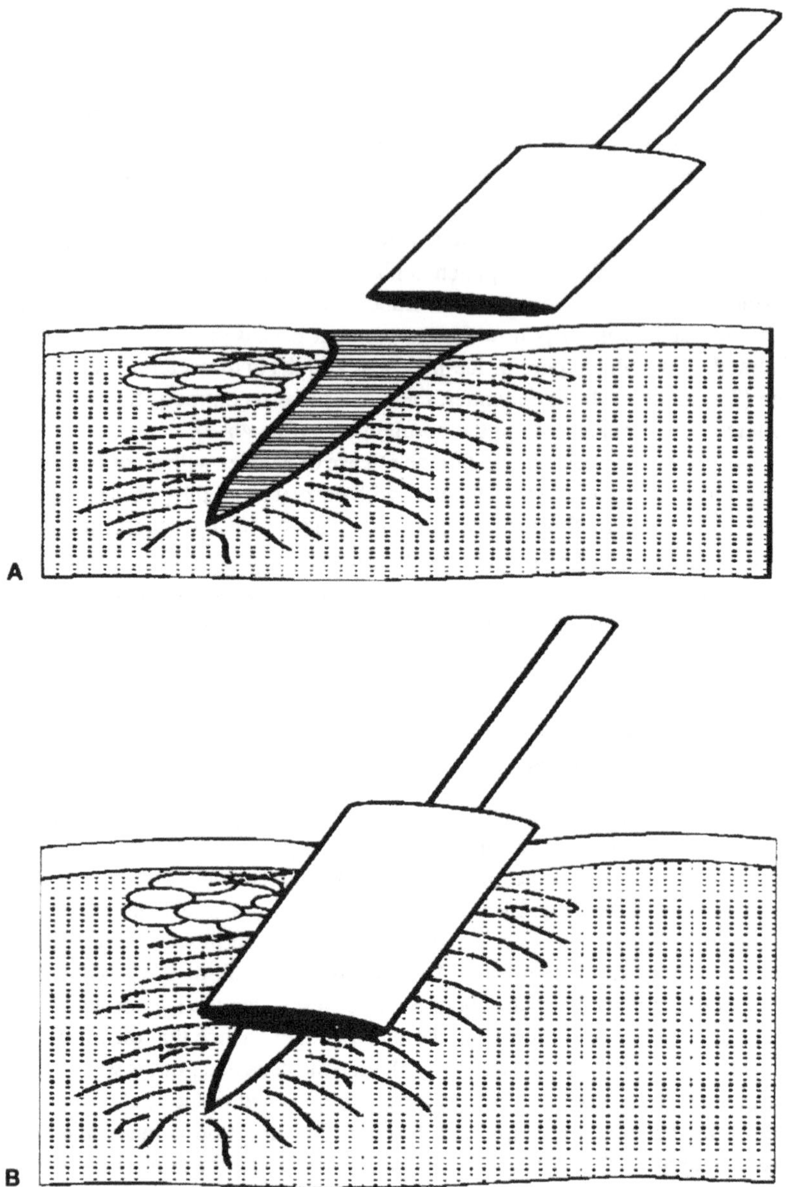

Figure 4 **(A)** Ice-pick scar (angled) with punch also angled along axis of scar; **(B)** punch completely surrounds ice-pick scar while releasing fibrotic bands; **(C)** healed and released scar shrinks to form normal pore opening.

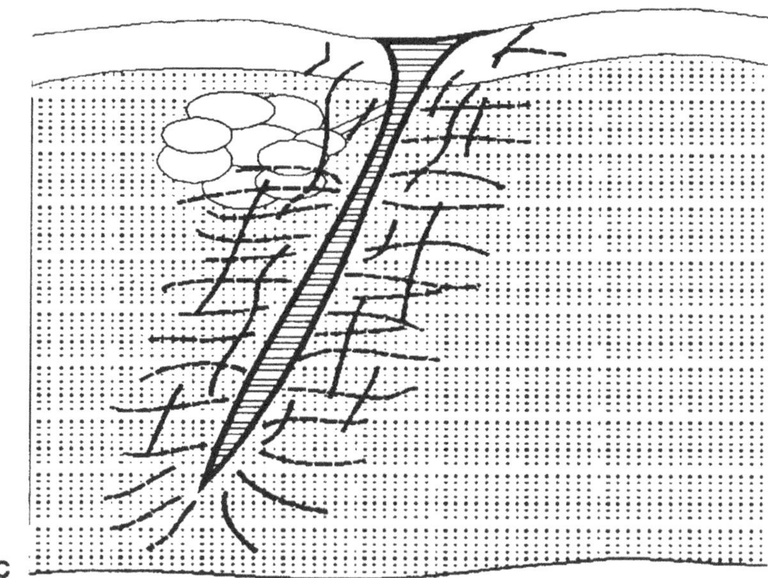

Figure 4 *(continued)*

small pieces rather than one large one. This clear occlusive dressing has the advantage of minimally adhering to the skin and releasing easily in a few days without dislodging the graft. The graft position and condition can be inspected through this clear dressing. Steri-strips (skin colored) can then be applied. No glue, sutures, or steel pins are used. For areas that continue to bleed, a pressure (gauze) dressing can be applied, to be removed the next day.

On return to the office at 2–3 days, the dressings can be left in place if the inspection reveals that all is well. The patient can remove the dressings at 5–7 days or return to the office. The patient returns to the office at 6 weeks. If a slight elevation is noted, the patient is reassured and encouraged to allow at least several weeks for it to flatten. Intradermal injections of triamcinolone, 1 mg/mL, can be used for more rapid flattening. For significant elevation, the area is flattened with a double-edge Personna blade (Fig. 6). The patient is examined again in 3–4 weeks. Laser resurfacing or dermabrasion may be considered if necessary after the sixth postoperative week. Many patients are not further benefited by additional procedures. Others, according to severity of their scarring, may need further grafting, dermal grafting, or soft tissue augmentation by fat transfers (lipofilling), Alloderm (dermal allografts by Lifecell Corporation), Gortex (W. L. Gore and Associates), Fibrel (Mentor H/S, Inc.), collagen (Collagen Corporation of America), or others (Fig. 7a and b).

B. Summary of the Punch Elevation

1. Photograph the patient with and without his or her makeup.
2. Cleanse the skin with povidone-iodine (Betadine) and wipe with alcohol. Allow to dry.

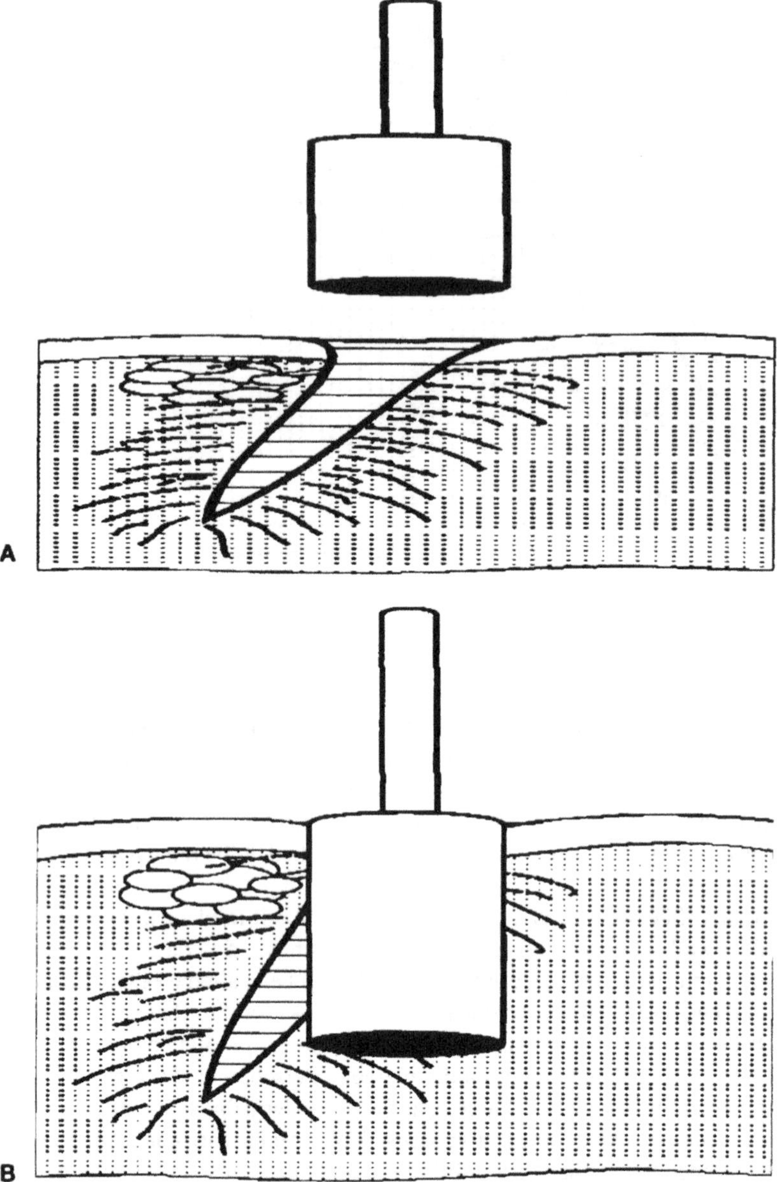

Figure 5 **(A)** Ice-pick scar (angled) punch at 90 degrees; **(B)** punch misses part of epithelium-lined pit while releasing the fibrotic bands; **(C)** healed punch leads to epidermal cyst formation.

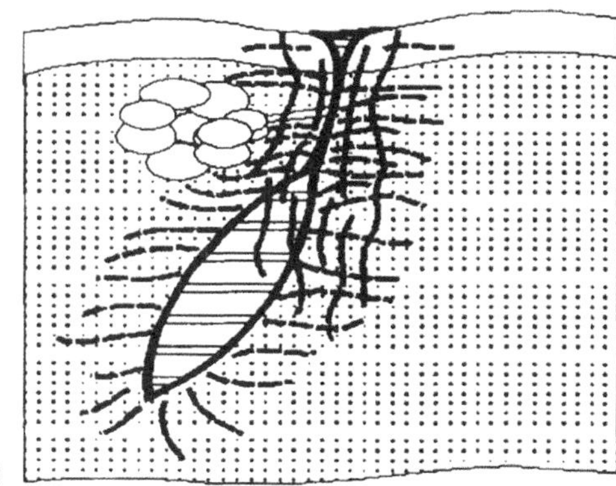

Figure 5 *(continued)*

3. With a mirror in the patient's hand and a spotlight angled across the skin, mark with gentian violet all the areas to be punch elevated. Identify the elevations and the transfers.
4. Lidocaine with epinephrine is used, followed by Marcaine (for the longer procedures).
5. Use proper punch size for scar.
6. When incising deeply pitted scars at less than a 90-degree angle, note adjacent fine hairs. All other pits should be incised at 90 degrees.
7. The punch should just enter the subcutaneous fat and go no deeper.
8. Rotate graft in opening for the best fit. The graft should be freely floating, not detached and not twisted.
9. Cover with moistened gauze. The final desired position of the punch elevation is slightly elevated, never depressed. If depressed, raise the graft to the desired level for 1–2 minutes.
10. Apply Mastisol around the incision sites (not on the incisions).
11. Apply Tegaderm dressings; Secure Tegaderm with Steri-strips. Use overlying gauze dressing for drainage.
12. Review written postoperative instructions with the patient.
13. Follow-up in office in 2–3 days, then about 5–7 days and again at 6 weeks and 3 months.

C. Punch Graft Transplant

In the past, deep pitted scars and craters were treated with simple surgical excision, resulting in a linear scar. For the punch graft technique, the best hairless donor site that is easily accessible is the postauricular region of the scalp. If this site has acne or cysts, another site is chosen. Although the preauricular skin is a possibility, it too is usually ravaged by acne scarring and/or cysts, so look above the clavicles, the back of the arms, or the back of the ears. If replacing an area of the nose where the sebaceous glands and pores are largest, look for a similar type of skin (the hairline of the forehead may have large pores and a similar amount of actinic damage).

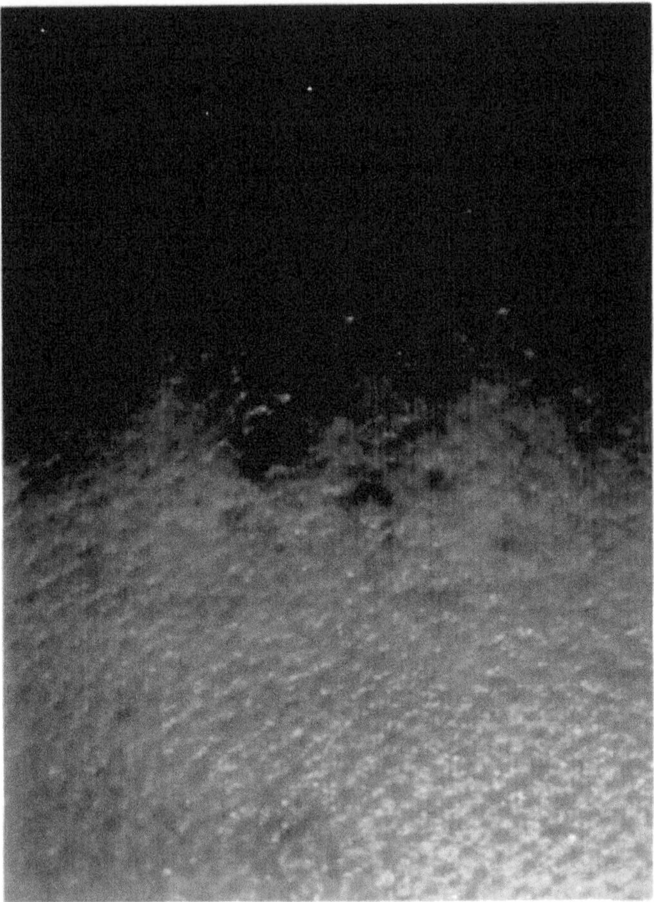

Figure 6 Photograph of male patient at 6 weeks after operation. Grafts are slightly raised; most will resolve spontaneously by 3–6 months.

Select a punch size for each defect. If the punch is too small, epidermis will be left extending into the pit and leave a groove or cyst. Punch and discard the scarred area; note the size and location of each. Cover the openings with cool normal saline gauze to aid hemostasis. Because of the natural elastic nature of the skin, the recipient openings dilate while the donor grafts contract. The smaller the grafts, the less the effect. This should be individualized for every patient. Usually, for the smaller graft sizes, 1.5 to 2.25 mm, the donor graft should be 0.25–0.5 mm larger than the recipient opening; for the larger grafts it will tend to be larger and may extend to 1.5 mm larger than the openings. Because of multiple factors, grafts larger than 4.0 mm and grafts smaller than 1.5 mm do not take well. Keep the donor site unsutured and available. Additional grafts may be necessary to replace grafts with a poor fit. All donor grafts should be inspected. Trailing fat is removed; the prepared grafts are placed on well-moistened normal saline filter paper in cold Petri dishes according to size. If large numbers are performed, the sizes of the grafts are written on the filter paper with the gentian violet marker.

The angle of the punch to the skin should be 90 degrees both for the opening and for the donor graft. Any variation of this will lessen the chances for a perfect fit. Placing a

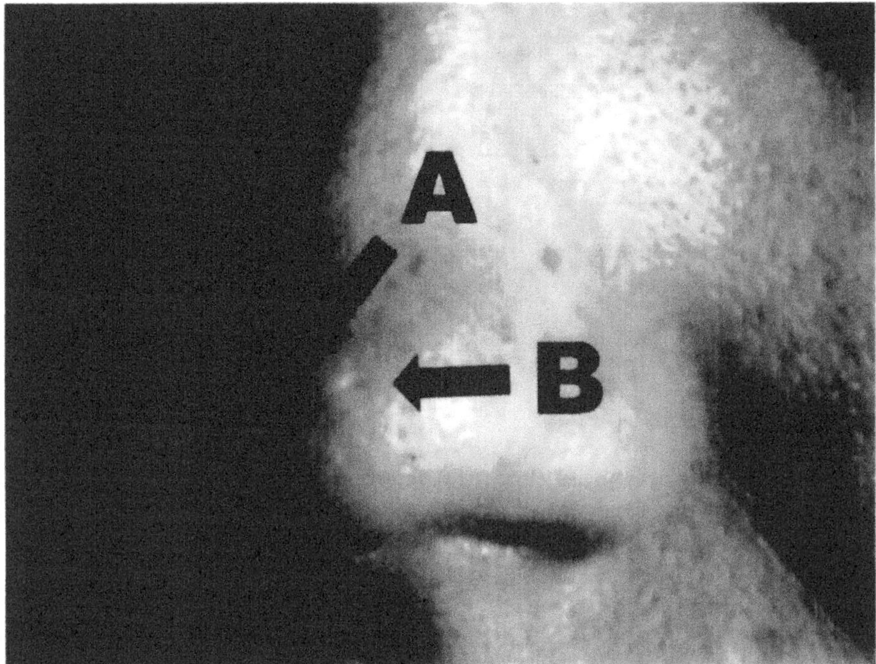

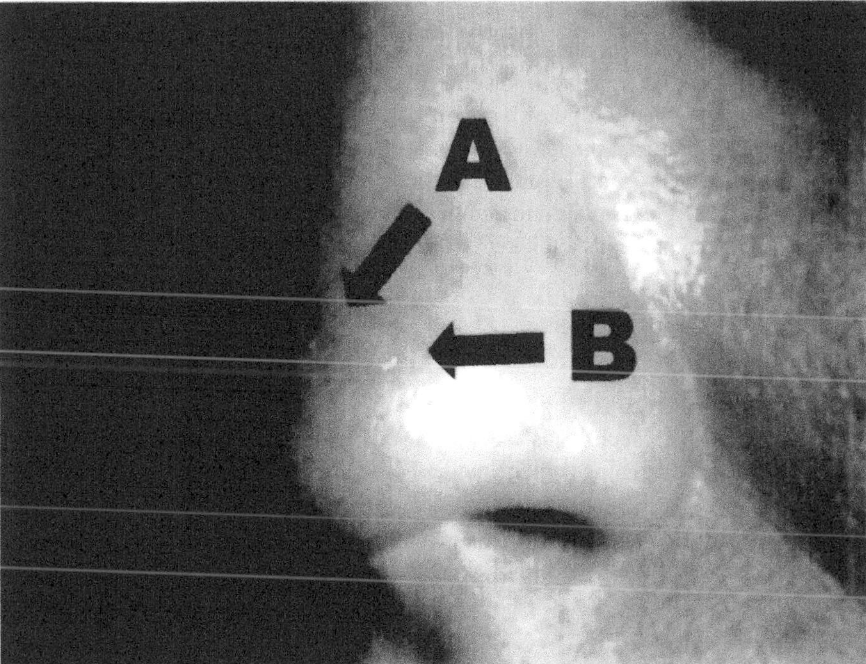

Figure 7 Photograph of female patient's nose before and 3 months after operation; **(A)** and **(B)** treated with punch elevation showing decreased size of pore with slight persistent ring scar.

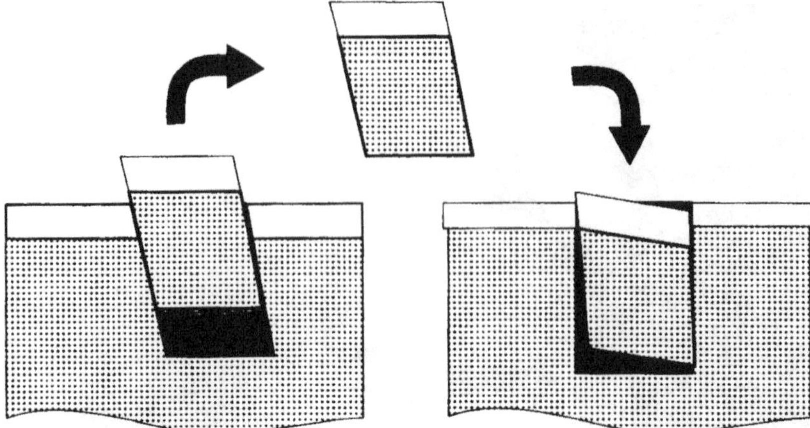

Figure 8 Donor graft taken at an angle (left to right), then placed into a recipient opening that is cut at 90 degrees. Note tendency to lip on the left edge and to groove on the right edge.

beveled graft into a nonbeveled opening will lead to a poor fit with a groove and a lip (Fig. 8). These missed details will lead to poor results and the possibility of a visual scar. Above 2.25 mm, the possibility of a visible round scar is greater. Above 4.0 mm, the chance for a failed graft is greater.

Some areas on the face produce oval openings because of the resting skin tension lines (RSTLs). Age, degree of scarring, and actinic damage are all factors that influence the elasticity of the skin and, therefore, the sizing of these openings and grafts. An oversized graft may later elevate and even pincushion upward. If a graft is too small, the edges will retract and create a groove or "moat" around a portion of the graft, resulting in a curved depression (Fig. 9a and b). An oval graft into a round opening may produce grooves with central elevation. If the opening needs a thicker or thinner piece of skin, another donor site is selected and cut.

D. Summary of Punch Graft Transfer

1. Photograph, cleanse, and mark as described.
2. Lidocaine with epinephrine is used, followed by Marcaine (for the longer procedures) where all openings will be made. For the donor site(s) behind the ear, use lidocaine without epinephrine. Lidocaine with epinephrine can be injected into the donor area(s) for hemostasis as soon as all grafts are removed. At that point, when numbers of grafts and fit of all grafts are proper, the donor site is sutured.
3. Use proper punch size for scar (pit or pick) removal; note the size and number of openings.
4. Incise at a 90-degree angle unless the pit is deep and angled. The full-thickness scar is discarded. If angled, a similarly angled donor graft must be made.
5. Place the properly sized graft into the opening and rotate the graft to confirm a snug fit. Adjust the graft so that it is slightly above skin level, never depressed.
6. As described for punch elevation, use the same dressings and follow-up care.

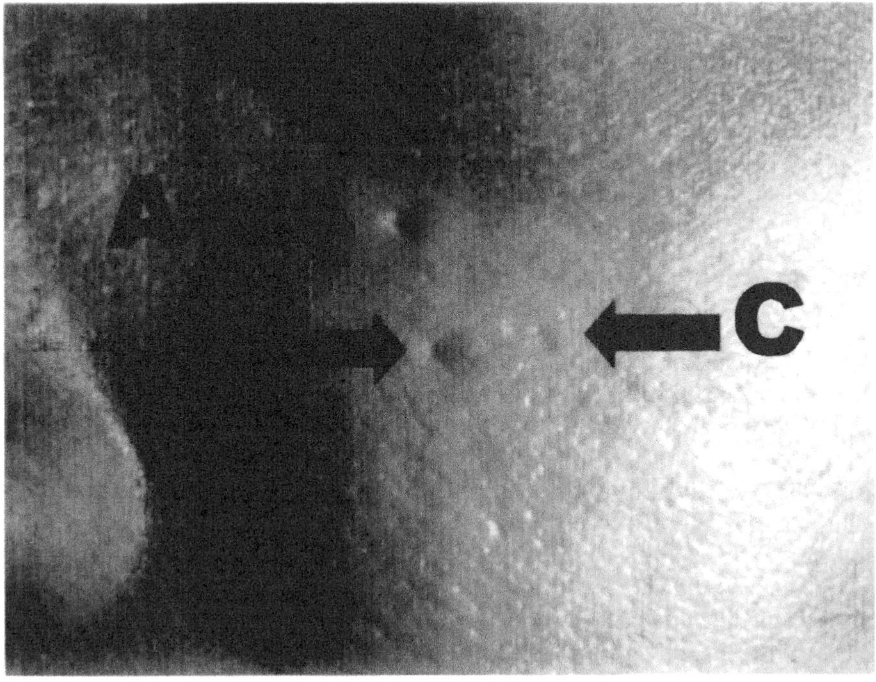

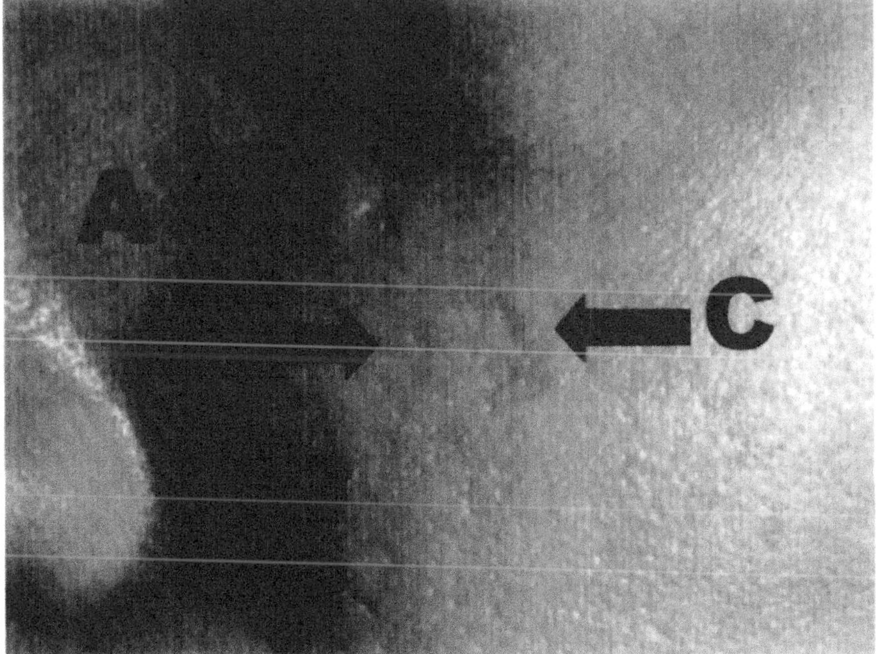

Figure 9 Photograph of female patient at 6 months after operation (before and after). **(A)** Punch graft too small, resulting in grooves around the edge; **(B)** punch graft properly sized; **(C)** control, no treatment.

E. Complications

Complications include failure of the graft to take, a depressed groove at the junction with normal skin, a depressed or elevated graft, a cyst, and a hypertrophic or hypotrophic scar. Some of the transplants have to be redone. Causes of these complications include excessive bleeding, lack of bleeding to seal the wound, poorly angled punches, poorly sized grafts, and trauma to the grafts. Infections are rare.

F. Problem Areas

Special problem areas are the nose with its large dilated pores, the bearded areas of men and the areas surrounding the mouth because of movement of this area after surgery. The thicker skin with larger pores may not be replaced by thin, small-pored skin from behind the ear, where minimal sun damage occurs. Another location for donor grafts must be identified and used as the source for nose grafts for a better match. In the bearded area of men, because of the possibility of trauma to normal hair shafts, the initial punch excision must parallel the hair follicles. Especially in dark-haired men, it is most important to use grafts with follicles. These can be taken from the occipital region.

Mouth movement makes it difficult for the graft to take. If multiple grafts are taken in this area, a modified dressing is needed in which the Tegaderm is separated from other pieces; the steri-strips are shorter and placed at right angles to the opening of the mouth and the patient is given extra warnings about facial movements, especially when talking and eating.

VIII. OBSERVATIONS ON ADJUNCTIVE PROCEDURES

1. Dermal grafting can be used as a soft tissue autologous filler that is placed subdermally. Alloderm (Lifecell Corp.) is an excellent and convenient dermal filler.
2. Scars that are bound down by subcutaneous fibrotic bands must be released at least 6 weeks before resurfacing by laser or dermabrasion. An 18-gauge NoKor (B-D) needle is ideal for severing these bands of scar tissue, which allows release and formation of a clot or coagulum beneath them that maintains elevation.
3. For deep ice-pick scars with a cicatrix at the base for which punch grafting is not indicated, excision with direct suture closure is used before or at the time of dermabrasion or laser resurfacing.
4. Chemical peel as a single procedure rarely results in significant improvement of scars.
5. A flashlamp-pumped pulsed dye laser improves both hypertrophic and erythematous facial acne scars.
6. It is possible for openings less than 2 mm to heal by second intention with little scarring.
7. When cutting openings, have the skin stretch at right angles to the skin lines. This will allow better closure as an ellipse.
8. Dermabrasion and laser resurfacing may actually worsen a deep ice-pick scar if the infundibulum (deeper portion) of the scar is wider than the surface opening (pore).

BIBLIOGRAPHY

Arouete J. Correction of depressed scars on the face by a method of elevation. J Dermatol Surg Oncol 1976; 2:337–339.

Griffin EI. Dermal filling of acne scars with Alloderm. Second Annual Advances in Cosmetic Dermatology and Surgery of the Face, Head and Neck, London, Sept 1997.

Johnson WC. Treatment of pitted scars: punch transplant techniques. J Dermatol Surg Oncol 1986; 12:260–265.

Koranda FC, Thomas JR. Treatment and modalities in facial acne scars. In: Facial Scars. St. Louis: Mosby, 1989:278–289.

Orentreich N, Durr NP. Rehabilitation of acne scarring. Dermatol Clin 1983; 1:405–413.

Solotoff SA. Treatment for pitted acne scarring: postauricular punch grafts followed by dermabrasion. J Dermatol Surg Oncol. 1986; 12:1079–1084.

Yarborough JM Jr, Pitard EF. Punch float technique for "ice-pick" scars. In: Robins P, ed. Surgical Gems in Dermatology. New York: Journal Publishing Group, 1988:47–50.

15
Recollagenation of Acne Scars

Steven Burres
University of California, Los Angeles
Los Angeles, California

I. INTRODUCTION

Once severe acne inflammation destroys the full thickness of dermis, the familiar wound healing process is triggered, in which a thin, glossy scar bed is created to span the area of dehiscence. Although the fibrous sheet of collagen seals off the deeper tissues from external contamination, the normal elasticity, volume, texture, and color that are needed to match the neighboring skin are lost. A primary goal of aesthetic restoration is to eliminate the dents and crevices whose shadows make the acne scars so disfiguring.

As an alternative or supplement to existing forms of acne scar management, the author introduced the process of recollagenation in 1994 (1,2). Recollagenation is defined simply as the generation of native collagen at a site of prior collagen destruction (1,2). With regard to acne scars, recollagenation is a means of smoothing out the unsightly depressions by augmenting the thickness of the collagen layer of the previously healed scar.

II. BACKGROUND

Preserved fascia lata has been adapted to repair a wide variety of defects since its original presentation by Koontz in 1926 (3). Historically, diverse surgical subspecialties have employed some form of preserved fascia to help solve problems of tissue deficiency (2–6). These clinical trials indicated that functional restitution often occurred on a long-term basis (4–6). Based on these reports from its earlier proponents, fascia lata was developed for the purpose of intradermal reconstruction as reported in 1994 (1,2).

The histologic fate of preserved, irradiated, cadaver fascia has been established by many investigators (3–9). In both animal and clinical studies, an acute inflammatory response surrounds and permeates the graft immediately after implantation. Once this response subsides, the material provides a framework for the invading fibroblasts that eventually deposit an indigenous, vascularized collagen bed to bridge the tissue gap (3–9).

III. MATERIAL

While searching for the optimal stimulator materials for recollagenation, the author tested an assortment of banked allografts, e.g., dura and dermis (Alloderm), and fresh autografts, e.g., temporalis fascia, scar. The extent to which the choice of material or details of the tissue preparation influence the outcome of grafting is unknown (2,9,10). Varying success was achieved with different substances, but banked fascia lata combined the positive features of the many materials available to choose from (3–10).

Banked fascia lata stimulates the proliferation of collagen, which is the specific tissue desired. Biocompatibility or migration problems of the sort that might occur with silicone or Teflon (Gortex) are unreported to date with banked fascia lata (3–11). Histologic studies demonstrate that banked fascia lata is completely reabsorbed, eliminating the concern about long-term rejection (4–10).

Sterility is a vital issue with any foreign implant. Besides the careful screening of donors, banked fascia lata supplied by the American Red Cross (Tissue Services, Washington, DC; released by region no. 006) has been freeze dried, irradiated, and vacuum sealed (Fig. 1). In addition, we store the material for 60 days before use. Banked fascia lata has an unblemished contamination record in a large number of clinical applications (2–6).

Banked material preserved in this fashion is easy to handle, cut, and implant compared with the more slippery, fresh preparations. In our experience, the thickness of banked fascia lata matches the depth of most of the defects created by acne. Refrigeration or tissue activation is not required.

As compared with the retail prices charged by the manufacturers of materials such as bovine collagen or Fibrel, the material cost for treating equivalent numbers of lesions with banked fascia lata is small. The donor stock supplied by the tissue bank may be divided into lots, as long as multiple donors are not used for the same recipient. Likewise, the inconvenience and potential morbidity of harvesting from a donor site are avoided by using banked

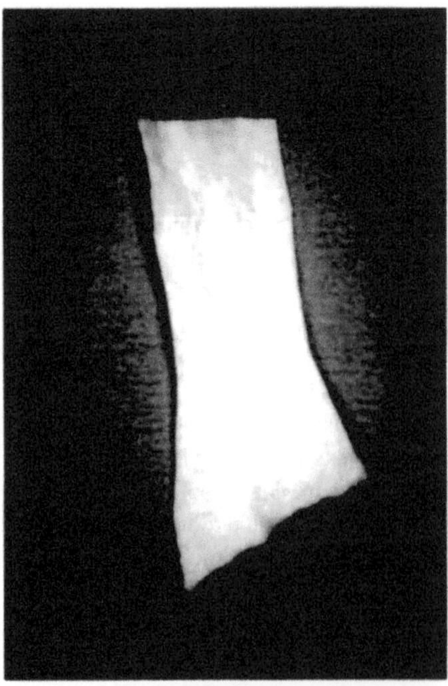

Figure 1 Freeze-dried, irradiated, human cadaver fascia lata.

material. At some donor sites, the quantity of tissue available for autografting may be so limited as to preclude retreatment.

Unlike materials whose approval by the Food and Drug Administration (FDA) is limited to specific purposes only, present federal guidelines permit physicians to implant banked, cadaver tissues at their own discretion (12).

IV. SELECTION OF PATIENTS

Careful selection of patients is critical to achieving a satisfactory outcome. To date, age, gender, race, and skin type do not appear to influence the results in terms of contour restoration. Local hyperpigmentation may be a significant concern in some ethnic groups or in people with dark hair and eye colors. We have never implanted known keloid formers.

Although recollagenation was not performed during a significant flare-up of acne, a few, small circumscribed areas of acne inflammation on the patient's face do not prohibit the recollagenation of more distant areas. In general, grafts were placed only in healed scars with healthy surrounding skin.

Prior or ongoing isotretinoin (Accutane) treatment is not a contraindication to recollagenation and, by virtue of ability to inhibiting collagenase and possibly other inflammatory mediators, offers theoretical advantages (13). In fact, antecedent treatment by any modality, including dermabrasion, laser abrasion, or chemical peels, appeared to be irrelevant as long as the inflammatory reaction in the skin was completely resolved. Associated systemic medical conditions, e.g., diabetes mellitus, have not been considered factors that precluded treatment.

An equally important aspect of the selection process for patients is preoperative education of the patient, which can eliminate misconceptions or inappropriate expectations and allow patients to choose recollagenation on an informed basis. Patients should understand that recollagenation is distinct from other types of intervention and that, for instance, a more extensive healing process is required to generate a native collagen reaction when compared with bovine collagen injections. Patients must also realize that the treatment goal is to repair skin depressions rather than discoloration, and they must anticipate that their improvement may be limited to this aspect of their problem. Although many surgeons cite high improvement percentages to prospective acne scar patients and show comparison photographs of their best cases, this practice can be very misleading.

Test areas are occasionally offered to reassure patients further and demonstrate to them the systematic results that can be obtained by recollagenation.

V. METHOD

Good technique and experience are vital to obtaining a successful result by recollagenation. The details of this art are protected under U.S. Patent 5, 397, 352, issued March 14, 1995, although some modification has been made subsequent to patent approval.

Excellent photography with appropriate lighting is critical for measuring the surgical results. As the photographs of acne scars are essentially a record of shadows, each slight alteration in the lighting and camera angle may deceptively alter the perceived improvements. Photographic cheating, which is easy, common, and tempting, must be eliminated if the integrity of the investigator is to be maintained.

Before the procedure is begun, the skin is prepared and draped sterilely. Next, with the patient seated, the individual depressions to be treated are marked with gentian violet in accordance with a schema agreed upon by the doctor and patient. Because the depressions are actually elevated by the anesthetic injections, the marks will become the only record of the intended treatment sites and so they must be accurate.

Through a 30-gauge needle, the scars are anesthetized with 1% lidocaine with 1:100,000 epinephrine in a 1:25 solution of hyaluronidase (Wydase). The entry stab is made 4 to 5 mm peripheral to the margin of the defect with a disposable 20-gauge hypodermic needle, and the pockets are incised. While the anesthetic is taking effect, the banked fascia lata is fashioned into grafts of varying size and thickness, according to the surgeon's estimate of the defects' dimensions. Grafts are then inserted into the appropriate pockets (Fig. 2). The graft must fit completely in the pocket, otherwise extrusion is certain. Typically, 2 to 3 cm^2 of graft material can fill 40 to 50 scars.

After graft insertion, the skin surface is again cleansed, first with alcohol to remove the overlying gentian violet and then with hydrogen peroxide to dissolve dried blood. Grafts that fit tightly into their pockets will not extrude with the agitation of vigorous skin cleaning. Any grafts that are exposed should be removed and exchanged with fresh ones.

Preferably, all of the patient's defects are treated in the initial session in order to avoid piecemeal restoration, which can be confusing and haphazard after several sessions. As many as 80 to 100 scars can be filled in 1 or 2 hours with practice. Recovery is generally painless and uneventful, and postoperative analgesia is unnecessary.

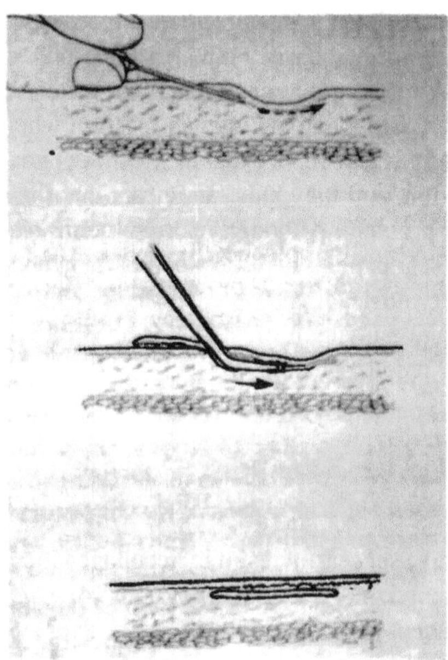

Figure 2 The intradermal insertion of the fascia lata graft. (Elsevier Science Inc. 655 Ave. of the Americas, New York, NY 10010)

VI. RESULTS

The author has filled approximately 8000 scars in 300 patients over the past 6 years with a high degree of success in contour restoration. Demographic factors, such as age, race, or gender, do not seem to influence the outcome in an adverse or positive manner.

The time course of graft healing is predictable. As described, the implanted graft produces an elevated papule for 4 to 10 weeks (2). As the graft material is decomposed, the site flattens and gradually blends into the neighboring skin. Premature flattening of the area indicates faulty graft insertion. Local blood products in the graft pocket that cause ecchymosis are typically reabsorbed over the first 2 to 3 weeks. Likewise, the needle insertion site invariably heals without scarring.

In the author's estimation, 30% to 40% of defects are filled completely and another 30% to 40% are grossly improved in a typical first session (Figs. 3–5). Almost all of the remaining spots demonstrate some measure of improvement. Routinely, patients are advised to have a second, touch-up session 6 weeks later, in which any residual defects, usually 10% of the initial treatment, are retreated. Individual spots can be retreated as many as four or five times to reach the desired height.

The exact details of the skin surface after recollagenation may show some variation from spot to spot. If the scar is elevated flush with the level of the skin surface, the epidermis can overgrow the lesion and produce an undetectable result. In other cases, a fine, residual surface irregularity may remain after treatment. Other potential outcomes include either a persistent indentation or a flat area of normal skin that has residual erythema or hyperpigmentation.

Satisfaction of patients is generally very high as long as information about the healing process is made clear and the patients' expectations are appropriate. The decision to undergo retreatment usually depends on the patient's motivation, and about 10% of them return at some later date for further touch-up procedures. There is no time limit on the later treatment sessions.

VII. COMPLICATIONS

A. Persistent Defects

Grafts fail for many reasons. Some defects are thicker than the standard graft, and a graft 1 or 2 mm thick will not repair defects 3 or 4 mm thick, unless it provokes an exceptional collagen response. Furthermore, although the widening of the tissue by the graft in the external direction alone is desired, half of the graft's expansive effect is directed internally and does not contribute to the visible change. If the graft extends subcutaneously, the dermal effect will be reduced accordingly, if not completely lost. Likewise, if the graft travels into neighboring tissues and does not settle directly and completely under the defect, because of poor pocket formation or graft placement, results will be diminished.

No patient has ever returned with a treated defect that was appreciably deeper.

B. Discoloration

Discoloration results from two independent events—ecchymosis resulting from the persistent blood products that mix with the graft immediately after insertion and hyperpigmentation resulting from later melanocyte invasion. Patients are warned that the lesions will typ-

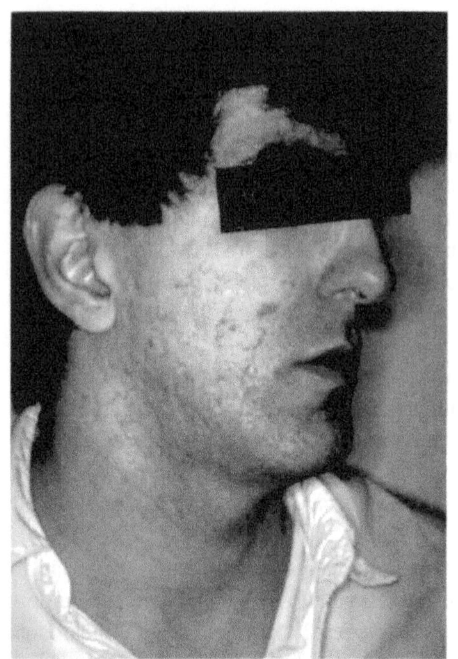

A

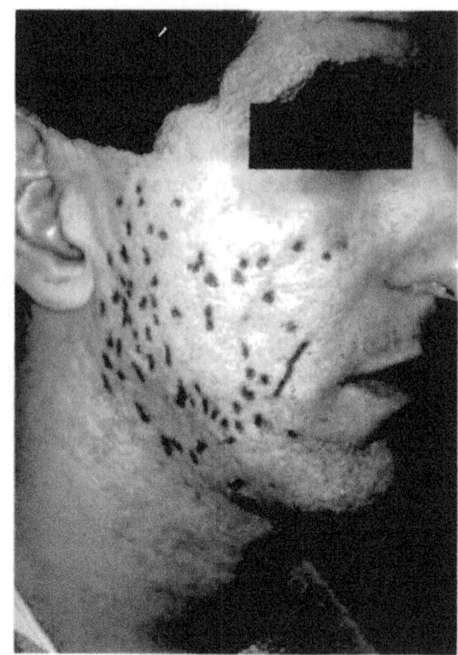

B

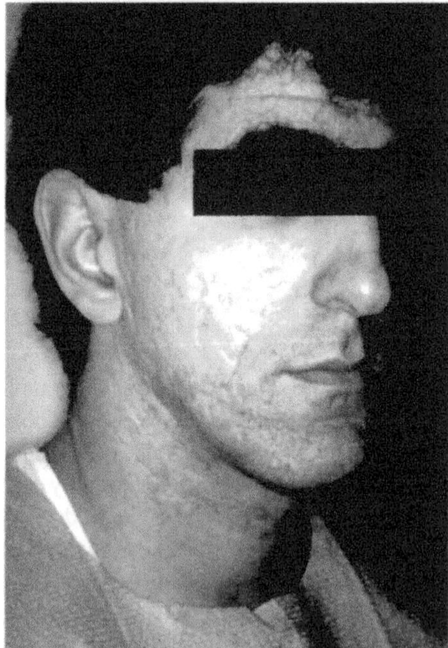

C

Figure 3 **(A)** A 30-year-old male with severe acne scars of the face and neck. **(B)** Scars marked with gentian violet immediately prior to implantation. **(C)** After three courses of recollagenation.

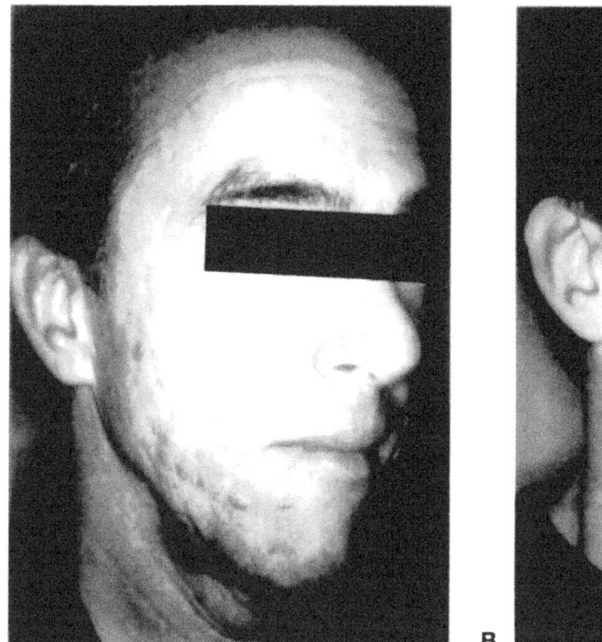
A

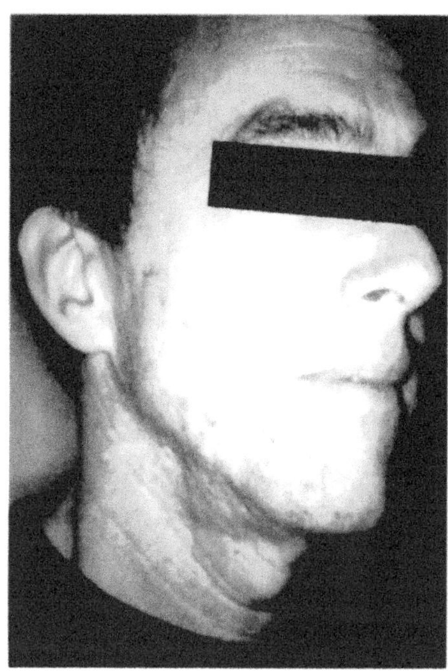
B

Figure 4 **(A)** A 37-year-old male with severe acne scarring before recollagenation therapy. **(B)** After two courses of recollagenation. (Elsevier Science Inc. 655 Ave. of the Americas, New York, NY 10010)

ically be discolored during the healing process and that whatever coloration was present at the bottom of the scar prior to treatment should be expected after healing is complete. Dark skin types are especially prone to localized hyperpigmentation, but because the spots are relatively isolated defects, they do not create a comprehensive cosmetic disability that interferes with most people's routine activities. Local hyperpigmentation generally resolves completely or subsides acceptably.

In fact, the overgrowth of surrounding skin may eliminate the discoloration present in the scar from before treatment, but patients are advised not to expect this fortuitous outcome.

C. Graft Extrusion

Graft extrusion may be 10% to 30% with poor technique but can be reduced to 1% or 2% with experience. Extrusion begins when the graft's tip appears through the needle hole after 2 or 3 days and may continue for a week or more.

If the graft extrudes, recurrence of the defect is the rule.

D. Infection

Local infection occurs infrequently. Over the past 5 years, approximately five or six furuncles or seromas with less than 0.5 mL of fluid inside have occurred. Although they all responded well to needle puncture and a short course of antibiotics, they may leave a tissue

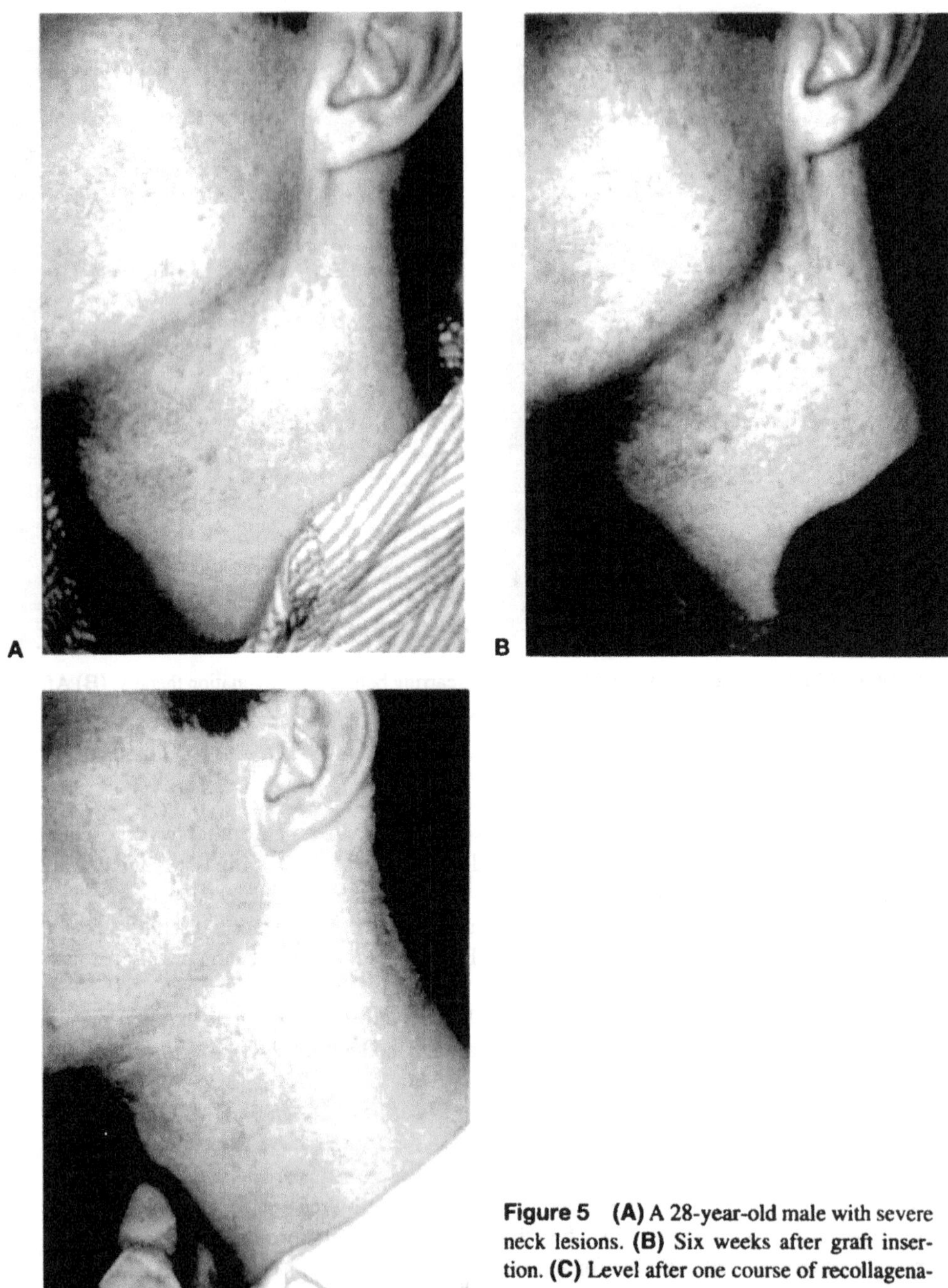

Figure 5 **(A)** A 28-year-old male with severe neck lesions. **(B)** Six weeks after graft insertion. **(C)** Level after one course of recollagenation. (Elsevier Science Inc, 655 Ave. of the Americas, New York, NY 10010)

defect that requires treatment later. Neither a generalized facial infection, e.g., erysipelas, nor a herpes outbreak occurred during the treatment of any subjects prior to the time of this report.

E. Scarring

Patients are advised that the goal of treatment is to generate scar, so they realize that the graft is not generating new skin. Hypertrophic scarring has not occurred.

F. Allergic Reaction

True allergic reactions have not been observed to date with either single or repeated applications.

VIII. DISCUSSION

Recollagenation is a new method for repairing the topographic irregularities created by acne's inflammatory assaults (1,2). Introducing a graft of collagen intradermally can evoke native collagen production and in some instances stimulate the overgrowth of neighboring skin. Recollagenation does not damage adjacent tissue, employs convenient banked graft material, involves a low risk of significant side effects, and has an overall recovery and improvement that are reliable (1,2). To date, there has not been a single episode of a true hypersensitivity reaction reported after deep implantation of banked fascia lata (2–6).

Many procedures may enhance skin contour. Filling techniques typically include the injection of liquid silicone, fat, Fibrel, or bovine collagen to replace defects (11). Because these materials are not incorporated in the host's collagen matrix, they are either digested locally or dispersed into neighboring tissues as scar integrity resumes. Likewise, treatment with liquid injectables alone does not divide the mature vertical scar bands that restrict elevation and epidermal realignment.

Resurfacing techniques, e.g., dermabrasion, laser abrasion, and chemical peels, rely on both the destruction of the edges of the normal skin and the inflammation in the underlying tissues to even out surface irregularities and evoke a fresh collagen response (14–17). A long recovery can be anticipated when resurfacing is performed to the level intended to remove deep scars, and still the elimination of full-thickness scars cannot be anticipated. Likewise, complications such as persistent erythema, hyper- or hypopigmentation, loss of skin elasticity, bridging of deep scars, and hypertrophic scarring must be addressed when deep resurfacing is performed with any agent (13–15). Our experience with laser resurfacing parallels that of Ho et al. (18), who found only a marginal improvement in the treatment of deep scars, perhaps 25% over a long term.

On occasion, punch grafting may return all of the lost skin elements to the desired spot (19,20). However, grafts are often poor matches for the defects in terms of shape, color, texture, and depth. Punch elevation can help restore the contour if the defect tissue is compatible with regrowth in the new plane. Scars may also be surgically recut and sutured when their configuration is appropriate.

Subcision is the division of the intradermal scar bands with a hypodermic needle (21). Orentreich and Orentreich introduced this procedure with the expectation that the fibrin clot generated by the local extravasation of blood into the dermis will separate tissue layers and instigate some fibroblast activity. However, dissolution of this clot occurs expeditiously, followed by abrupt readherence of the prior cellular bridges and return of the preexisting intradermal environment and anatomy. Our experience has shown that successful graft insertion is vital to ultimately achieving an optimal, enduring result.

Laboratory and clinical reports concur that the fascia graft interstices are highly conducive to collagen deposition (3–6,22,23). A collagen matrix appears to be valuable as a nest for fibroblast ingrowth (22,23). During the weeks of healing, the graft prevents the cellular bridges from reattaching to the normally adjacent cells. The local intradermal graft environment, with its altered temperature, pH, tissue tension, and relative hypoxia, provides an ongoing stimulus to scar formation (22,23).

Unfortunately, there is no "gold standard" by which to quantify objectively the results of acne scar correction, so most studies rely on observers, who are notoriously inaccurate and biased (18,24,25). The distinct problems of depressed scars and skin discoloration probably deserve independent consideration, among many other issues, e.g., scar shape, in the entire problem of acne scar grading. Therefore, reported improvement figures from different studies may show either wide discrepancies or close concurrence, both without any scientific basis.

Surgeons should be discouraged from applying a single treatment method to acne scars. Each patient's treatment plan must be developed according to the patient's own needs and desires by a surgeon experienced in all of the available techniques of correction. Frequently, small, superficial scars may respond to resurfacing techniques that freshen the epidermal edges and stimulate the ingrowth of new skin. Deeper scars require some form of tissue implantation to replace lost volume, in which case we recommend recollagenation as the preferred method.

REFERENCES

1. Burres SA. Recollagenation: a new technique for the restoration of pitted acne scars. Min Inv Ther 1994; 3:231–232.
2. Burres SA. Recollagenation of acne scars. Dermatol Surg 1996; 22:364–367.
3. Koontz AR. Experimental results in the use of dead fascia grafts for hernia repair. Ann Surg 1926; 83:523–536.
4. Crawford JS. Nature of fascia lata and its fate after implantation. Am J Ophthamol 1968; 67:900–906.
5. Bedrossian EH. Banked fascia, lata as an orbital floor implant. Ophthalmol Plast Reconstr Surg 1993; 9:66–70.
6. Bright RW, Green WT. Freeze-dried fascia lata allografts: a review of 47 cases. J Pediatr Orthop 1981; 1:13–22.
7. McGregor JC, Lindop GB. The behavior of Cialit-stored and freeze-dried human fascia lata in rats. Br J Plast Surg 1974; 27:155–164.
8. Klen R. Biological Principles of Tissue Banking. Oxford: Pergmon, 1982:207.
9. Hinton R, Jinnah RH, Johnson C, Warden K, Clarke HJ. A biomechanical analysis of solvent dehydrated and freeze-dried human fascia lata allografts. Am J Sports Med 1992; 20:607–612.
10. Thomas ED, Gresham RB. Comparative tensile strength study of fresh, frozen, and freeze-dried human fascia lata. Surg Forum 1963; 14:442–443.
11. Duffy D. Silicone: a critical review. Adv Dermatol 1990; 5:93–110.
12. American Red Cross Tissue Services, verbal communication.
13. Brinckerhoff CE, McMillan RM, Dayer JM, Harris MD. Inhibition by retinoic acid of collagenase production in rheumatoid synovial cells. N Engl J Med 1980; 432–436.

14. Fulton JE. Dermabrasion. In: Harahap M, ed. Complications of Dermatologic Surgery. New York: Springer-Verlag, 1993:31–39.
15. Moritz D, McGillis ST, Vidimos AT, Bailin PL. Cutaneous Laser Surgery, ibid., pp 51–67.
16. Collins PS. Chemical face peeling. ibid., pp 68–83.
17. Elson ML. Collagen implantation. ibid., pp 92–100.
18. Ho C, Ngueyn Q, Lowe NJ, Griffin ME, Lask G. Laser resurfacing in pigmented skin. Dermatol Surg 1995; 21:1035–1037.
19. Sotoloff SA. Treatment for pitted acne scarring: postauricular punch grafts followed by dermabrasion. J Dermatol Surg Oncol 1986; 12:1079–1084.
20. Johnson WC. Treatment of pitted acne scars: punch transplant technique. J Dermatol Surg Oncol 1986; 12:260–264.
21. Orentreich DS, Orentreich N. Subcutaneous incisionless (Subcision) surgery for the correction of depressed scars and wrinkles. Dermatol Surg 1995; 21:543–549.
22. Germain L, Jean A, Auger FA, Garrel DR. Human wound healing fibroblasts have greater contractile properties than dermal fibroblasts. J Surg Res 1994; 57:268–273.
23. Philips TJ. Biological skin substitutes. J Dermatol Surg Oncol 1993; 19:794–800.
24. Burres SA, Fisch U. The comparison of facial grading systems. Arch Otolaryngol Head Neck Surg 1986; 112:755–758.
25. Alster TS, Lewis AB. Dermatologic laser surgery: a review. Dermatol Surg 1996; 22:797–805.

16

Dermal Overgrafting

Abdel-Fattah M. A. Abdel-Fattah
University of Alexandria
Alexandria, Egypt

I. DEFINITION

"Dermal overgrafting" means the application of a split-thickness skin graft to a recipient bed of dermis or scar tissue denuded of surface epithelium. The depth of excision and the thickness of the graft are determined by the lesion, the location being treated, and the desired outcome. The technique is sometimes called "shaving and skin grafting."

II. ORIGINS OF DERMAL OVERGRAFTING

Webster (1) first developed overgrafting in 1954 as a convenient and rapid substitute for pedicle flap repair for unstable scars over bone prominences of the lower extremities and other areas that lack normal skin and subcutaneous tissue. Webster et al. (2) employed the dermabrasion technique described by Iverson (3) to remove the scar surface epithelium and to prepare the deep normal layer to receive a split-thickness skin graft. After healing, the graft was abraded and a second split-thickness graft was placed over it, thus building a layered repair. In one patient, as many as three separate grafts were piled up on top of one another at three separate operations; each graft took successfully and completely on the bleeding, abraded surface of the graft or scar beneath it.

Hynes (4), in 1956, independently described overgrafting to resurface shaved large pigmented moles. Hynes (5,6) widened the spectrum of application of dermal overgrafting, under the designation "shaving and skin graft," to include scars and chronic radiodermatitis.

III. INDICATIONS OF DERMAL OVERGRAFTING

Dermal overgrafting is a simple and useful technique that is well established in the treatment of a variety of surface lesions.

A. Scars

1. Unstable Scars

Unstable scars have been treated as described by Webster (1) and Hynes (5).

2. Depressed or Atrophic Scars

Hynes (5) and Rees and Casson (7) reported the successful use of the technique on depressed scars to build up the area to a level with the surrounding skin. Trimble (8) used the technique successfully for depressed, linear acne scar of the cheek. The present author has been using dermal overgrafting to improve the aesthetic look of atrophic burn scars with great success, as will be shown in the following.

3. Hypertrophic and Keloidal Scars

Moustafa and Abdel-Fattah (9) reported excellent results of shaving and skin grafting, i.e., dermal overgrafting, for matured, pale, nonsymptomatic hypertrophic burn scars. Variable degrees of recurrence were almost inevitable in active, florid, telengiectatic, itchy hypertrophic scars. In the present author's experience, the same applies to keloids of various etiologic origin. The active lesion (Fig. 1) should be left untouched until activity has completely subsided and the telengiectasia disappeared. When the lesion becomes pale and quiet, success with dermal overgrafting is more probable. The symptom-free period should be no less than 3 months before embarking on the technique.

Moustafa and Abdel-Fattah (9) modified Hynes' original technique in three ways:

1. Shaving went slightly deeper in the center of the scar than the periphery, i.e., "saucerization" of the scar rather than shaving it flush with the surrounding skin as in the original Hynes technique.
2. A narrow peripheral edge of scar tissue was left to hold the stitches and avoid puncturing the skin, with possible development of unsightly hypertrophic stitch marks. Hynes, in contradistinction, thinly shaved a narrow rim of the adjacent skin, which was grafted together with the scar to reduce the peripheral scar line.
3. The authors used intermediate-thickness skin grafts instead of the thin grafts used by Hynes.

4. Scars Difficult or Dangerous to Excise

Some scars that are difficult or dangerous to excise because of their contiguity to important structures may need to be strengthened. This can be done safely without scar excision by light shaving of the surface of the scar followed by the application of a thick skin graft (5).

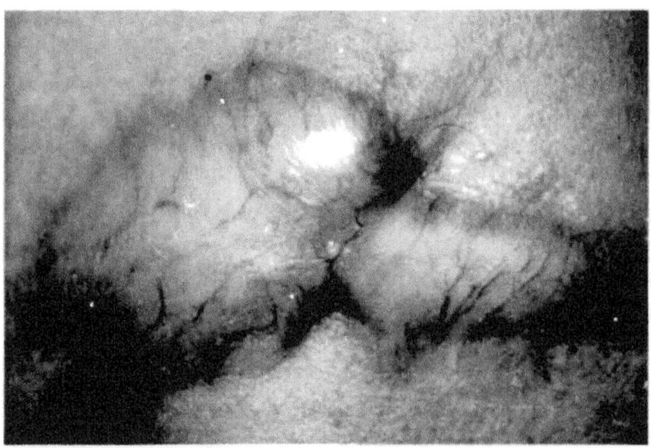

Figure 1 An active keloidal scar showing wide spread telengiectasia.

5. *Contracted and Tight Scars*

There are some scars in the region of a joint that either produce a mild contracture of the joint or, if no actual contracture is present, cause a feeling of tightness when the joint is moved in certain directions. A scar of this type can be strengthened, improved in appearance, and elongated by shaving it and then dividing the whole thickness of the residual scar tissue by a number of parallel cuts at right angles to the direction of the contracture. The shaved surface is then covered with a thick skin graft (5).

6. *Colored Scars*

Many burn scars, particularly those on the face, are reasonably flat but are conspicuous because of their permanent red color. Other scars, resulting from deep burns, may show patches of dark brown pigmentation. Hynes (5) reported very promising results with shaving and skin grafting such scars.

B. Chronic Radiodermatitis

Hynes (6) used the technique successfully in the treatment of skin damage caused by irradiation on the same lines mentioned above. Rees and Casson (7) suggested that partial-thickness excision and overgrafting were the techniques of choice for treating skin damage caused by irradiation in the absence of ulceration or deep necrosis. It need not be feared that potential nests of cells prone to malignancy are being masked if the split-thickness removal of the diseased area extends below the dermal-epidermal junction. Skin appendages are rare or absent in irradiated skin, yet the vascularity of the dermis is usually sufficient to support a split-thickness graft unless the dosage of ionizing radiation was excessive. Trimble (8) confirmed the usefulness of the technique for x-ray scars.

C. Chronic Traumatic Ulcers of the Extremities and Venous Stasis Ulcers of the Lower Limb

Thompson and Ell (10) reported 10 years of experience with dermal overgrafting in such cases. The surface to be treated usually consisted of a wound that had been grafted with split skin or a healed ulcer. A protective pad of dermis was built up at the site by thinly removing the surface epithelium and then applying a thick split-skin graft. The graft was similarly treated 3 weeks later, virtually doubling the thickness of the dermal tissue present. By applying two, three, or even more skin grafts as successively superimposed laminae at intervals, the protective dermal pad could be thickened sufficiently to produce stable healing even on pressure areas of the distal parts of the extremities. Thompson and Ell (10) believed that this pad was sufficient to withstand functional pressure and had the quality of firm mobility, resilience, and protective sensation to a greater degree than cross-leg flap skin. It also avoided the "loose glove-slipper" effect so often found following a flap repair. The postoperative complications of dermal overgrafting were minimal because failure of a skin graft to "take" was almost unknown. Advanced age was not a contraindication because prolonged immobilization was not entailed in the procedure. Hospitalization was decreased compared with that involved in distant flap repair.

D. Large Pigmented Nevi

Hynes (4), Rees and Casson (7), and Trimble (8) reported the adequate use of dermal overgrafting in such conditions. Some pigmentation may remain unless the pigmented moles are shaved at a sufficiently deep level and a thick graft is used to camouflage the remaining pigment.

E. Decorative Tattoos

The use of dermal overgrafting in camouflaging decorative tattoos has provided an excellent simple solution in most cases. Rees and Casson (7) suggested that tattoos could be removed as a thick split-thickness skin graft with a dermatome and the defect meticulously overgrafted. They could achieve almost uniform perfection in such treatment. Vecchione (11) used a handheld razor blade, secured in a curved hemostat, to shave away the pigment precisely and selectively with as little dermis as possible. The shaving continued layer by layer until all the pigment was removed. He endeavored to preserve the lower layers of the dermis or at least subdermal fibrous attachments. If the pigment was deposited below the dermis in the subdermal fat, it was selectively excised and the dermal integrity preserved with fine chromic catgut suture. A thin split-thickness skin graft was then applied. Dermal overgrafting avoids full-thickness excision of the tattoo and subsequent application of split-thickness skin grafts onto the subcutaneous fat with its inherent imperfect graft take, contracture, and, possibly, hypertrophic scarring. The net result of these sequelae can be less cosmetically acceptable than the original tattoo.

F. Leukoderma

There are several reports that vitiligo vulgaris that is resistant to conservative treatment with psoralens and subsequent exposure to ultraviolet light can be successfully repigmented with minigrafts or punch grafts placed on a deepithelialized dermal bed created in the depigmented areas (12–14). The rationale of this method depends on the ability of melanocytes to migrate centrifugally from grafts and to produce pigment in the deepithelialized leukodermic skin into which they spread or extend (13,15).

Harashina and Iso (16), in 1985, adopted the principle for the treatment of leukoderma after deep burns with significant success. The depigmented areas and the surrounding scars were widely abraded with a motor-driven dermabrader to produce a smooth, flat dermal bed. Extremely thin split-skin grafts were harvested, twice meshed, and then cut into very small pieces that they called "skin chips." These chips were evenly spread over the abraded raw surface and covered and immobilized for 7 to 10 days with nonadhesive ointment gauze. Relatively small grafts could be used in this way to cover extensive depigmented areas. The technique is easier than the punch technique. It also avoids the donor site disability and disfigurement associated with sheet grafting.

Chitale (17), in 1991, reported the successful use of dermal overgrafting for vitiligo of the lower lip in one patient. A split-thickness graft from the vitiliginous patch was removed and replaced by a split-thickness skin graft of identical thickness from the arm. A uniformly dark color developed in the lip 1.5 years later.

G. Hemangiomas

Rees and Casson (7) indicated that dermal overgrafting could be used in the treatment of hemangiomas in cosmetically critical areas. Adamson et al. (18) used the method repeatedly, three times, in a case of extensive cavernous hemangioma of the buttock, hip, and thigh with success. They concluded that repeated cutaneous dermal overgrafting could provide several layers of skin graft to protect against injury and improve appearance. However, they believed that the method was best suited for stable, nonenlarging lesions that failed to regress spontaneously.

H. Deep Dermal Burns

Janzekovic (19–21) introduced the technique of "early tangential excision and skin grafting" of deep dermal burns on the third to the fifth day after the burn. The technique entails the sequential excision of dead skin layers until the deep viable, bleeding dermis is reached. An autologous skin graft is then applied to this viable dermal bed. Janzekovic's technique is, in fact, dermal overgrafting. She demonstrated better aesthetic and functional results with the technique than by conservative treatment and grafting after 3 or more weeks. The dermis survives with early excision and skin grafting in dermal burns (22,23). With expectant treatment, the dermis may necrotize as a result of desiccation or infection. Early tangential excision of dermal and subdermal burns of the face has been used, and better aesthetic and functional results were reported for dermal burns (20,21,24–28).

I. The Donor Site of a Thick Skin Graft

A standard useful procedure well known to every plastic surgeon is to overgraft the donor site of a thick graft with a thin graft harvested from adjacent skin. The aim of the procedure is to expedite healing and prevent probable hypertrophic scarring and concomitant disfigurement.

IV. THE TWO COMPONENTS OF OVERGRAFTING: THE BED AND THE GRAFT

A. The Dermal Bed

1. Thickness

The thickness of the bed left behind depends on the nature and thickness of the lesion as well as the desired outcome. In corrugated, hypertrophic, and keloidal scars most of the bulk of the scar is removed, leaving a thin layer of deep tissue. This thin collagenous layer provides an internal biological splint as well as a vascular substrate that supports the graft. To raise, or elevate, atrophic and unstable scars, on the other hand, as much bed as possible is saved after deepithelialization. The removal of the surface epithelium must be complete, however, but with no more than minimal removal of the subepithelial tissue. The same principle applies to further operations, if applicable, so as to build up a dermal cushion.

2. Instruments

The instruments used to remove the surface epithelium vary depending on the nature of the lesion, the thinness and evenness of the surface tissue to be removed, the contour, the amount of debulking required, and the personal preference of the operator:

a. Sandpaper

See Webster et al. (2).

b. Mechanical Dermabrader (29)

Sandpapering and dermabrasion have the disadvantage of grinding epithelial cells into the bed on which the skin graft is to be placed, probably increasing the incidence of subsequent epidermoid cyst formation.

c. Dermatome and Skin Graft Knife

Rees and Casson (7) reported simple and accurate deepithelialization using an electrical dermatome such as the Brown or the Castroviejo electrokeratome. They resort to a mechanical dermabrader only when the contour of the area to be overgrafted is such that a dermatome cannot be used to denude the surface. They feel that dermabrasion is also sufficient when the surface is composed of scar epithelium with few or no skin appendages remaining in the dermis, such as a healed burn scar, to avoid formation of inclusion epidermoid cysts.

d. Large Scalpel Blade (4–6)

The present author depends mainly on large blades, no. 20, 21, and 22, on a standard no. 4 scalpel handle.

e. Large Blades on Modified Scalpel Handle

The author introduced three modifications on a no. 4 scalpel handle (Fig. 2A–C):

1. A longer angulated handle to allow a better grip and clearance of the operating hand from the surface, thus facilitating shaving
2. A thumb rest to allow a firmer grip
3. A tip on which no. 20, 21, or 22 blade can be mounted so that the cutting edge is directed to either the right or left side of the same handle (Fig. 2C).

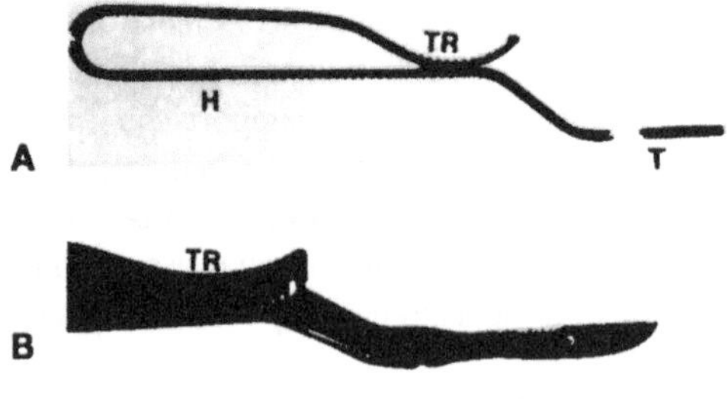

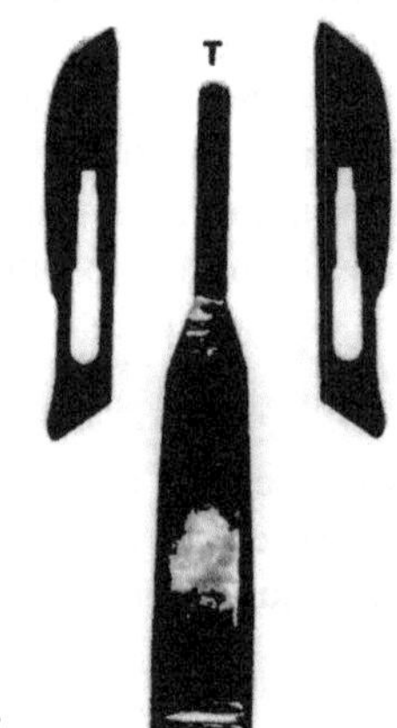

Figure 2 **(A)** Side view of the author's modified scalpel handle or "shaving knife." H, Handle; TR, thumb rest; T, tip. **(B)** Oblique view of the knife showing the thumb rest and the blade in place. **(C)** Undersurface of the tip showing that the blade can be fitted so that the cutting edge can face either right or left.

f. Carbon Dioxide Laser

The efficacy of the carbon dioxide laser for skin deepithelialization in humans was initially demonstrated using reduction mammaplasty as a clinical model (30,31). This use has been extended to include other flap transposition and overgrafting of skin grafts (32).

The carbon dioxide laser can play a role in skin deepithelialization, where it provides an advantage when rigid skin immobilization is impossible. It can allow rapid deepithelialization with minimal subsequent hemorrhage and preservation of the subdermal vascular plexus (31,33). The latter advantage is due to the fact that the zone of coagulative necrosis is limited by a constant, predetermined power density, which allows controlled serial removal of epidermis or dermis as required. This will prevent inadvertent damage to underlying structures, as might occur when a scalpel alone is used (32).

Minor complications such as the subsequent development of inclusion cysts and more alarming complications such as wound dehiscence of minor or major degrees make the indiscriminate use of the carbon dioxide laser for every situation requiring skin deepithelialization not justifiable (34). However, in selected situations such as dermal overgrafting, it appears to be safe, reasonable, and expedient option.

3. Smoothing the Bed

This can be carried out using a no. 15 blade on a no. 3 scalpel handle or by a mechanical dermabrader (7). The author prefers a 5 3/4 in., curved Metzenbaum scissors.

4. Hemostasis

Hemostasis must be absolute if the graft "take" has to be complete. This can be achieved by traditional methods such as topical thrombin, pressure with a gauze sponge moistened with topical adrenaline solution (1:200,000), followed by careful electrocoagulation of any persistent bleeding points.

The present author uses a different technique that proves very effective every time. He spreads the freshly cut skin graft over the dermal bed and applies pressure with a gauze pad for 5 minutes. The graft is then carefully removed and a widely spread sheet of blood and fibrin clots is revealed on the dermal bed. This is delicately pealed off using a non-toothed Adson dissecting forceps.

By convention, two pathways of blood coagulation are recognized: extrinsic and intrinsic. The extrinsic system is initiated by exposure of blood to injured tissue via the release of tissue thromboplastin (35). This seems to be the mechanism underlying hemostasis in the author's method.

B. The Graft

1. Donor Site

The location of the donor site might seem irrelevant as long as it can provide enough skin to resurface big lesions. However, when it comes to lesions in the face, it is essential to select a donor site that can provide the same, or the nearest, color and texture match. In this respect, the supraclavicular or lateral neck region is preferred as the donor site, unless the size of the graft required precludes using this area. A surprisingly large split-thickness graft can be harvested from these areas if depressions in contour are filled out by subcutaneous infiltration with saline to obtain a flat surface upon which the Reese drum dermatome can be applied (36). Retroauricular skin is excellent for small lesions on the face (8).

The present author finds the inner side of the upper arm the next most suitable donor site for the face. Besides being flat, which allows the use of Watson's modified Braithwaite's skin grafting knife or the like, this site can provide a relatively big sheet of hairless graft that can cover a whole forehead or a similar area.

2. *Graft Thickness*

The graft thickness depends on the lesion. Sometimes thin grafts (about 0.015 inch) are selected for scars with a tenuous blood supply. It is usually believed that thin grafts survive better than thick grafts when blood supply at the host site is poor.

An intermediate-thickness skin graft (about 0.018 inch) is suitable, however, in most cases, and allows uneventful, primary, scarless healing of the donor site. Thicker grafts are required to build up a dermal cushion over bony prominences and unstable scars.

3. *Suturing the Graft*

For optimal cosmetic results it is important that:

1. The graft be sutured on an exact level with the surrounding skin.
2. A moderate amount of stretch and tension is applied to the graft while suturing it in place.

However, if dermal overgrafting is used for unstable scars over bones and in venous stasis ulcers of the leg, the rules are different:

1. The shaved area must extend widely beyond all scar tissue to reach completely normal surrounding skin that should be overgrafted as well. Only by this means will anastomosis occur between the normal vascular and lymphatic elements of the graft and the host at the treated site. These vascular connections are very important in obtaining a stable repair. Lymphatic continuity between the graft and the dermal lymphatic plexus of the normal surrounding skin is important in establishing healthy drainage of the scar.
2. A thick graft should be placed on the deepithelialized site, without tension, in a state of maximal relaxation. This appreciably increases the bulk of tissue transplanted, which is the chief objective of the procedure.

V. PRACTICAL TIPS ON "ELEVATION" OF DEPRESSED SCARS

A. Anesthesia

Large lesions are surgically dealt with under general anesthesia. Small lesions could be dealt with under local infiltration analgesia with 1% lignocaine for both the scar and the donor site of the graft. Adrenaline should not be used because it obscures the bleeding points in the shaved, or dermabraded, scar, which is necessary to determine the depth of shaving, as explained in item 5 in Sect. V.B.

B. Surgical Procedure

If you have a single depressed scar, you have to focus on this area only. However, if you have a mosaic of normal skin interspersed with depressed scars of variable sizes (Fig. 3A), you had better deal with the mosaic as a whole.

In elevation of a depressed scar, or a mosaic, the author's technique is as follows:

1. Mark the scar, or the area to be shaved, with methylene blue (Fig. 3B).
2. Infiltrate the area subcutaneously with normal saline solution to make the scar, or mosaic, turgid and more prominent to facilitate shaving of the surface epithelium (Fig. 3C).
3. Incise along the marked periphery down to middermis with a no. 15 scalpel blade on a no. 3 handle.
4. During the surgical procedure, the assistant should keep the area immobilized and taut to facilitate shaving. With small scars, however, use the thumb and index finger of your nondominant hand to steady the skin until you complete the deepithelialization.
5. Start the deepithelialization from the incised margin using a no. 20, 21, or 22 scalpel blade on a no. 4 handle or the author's modified scalpel handle (Fig. 3D). The cutting blade should proceed tangentially to the surface in the same manner as you cut a skin graft. Remove a thin layer of surface tissue in the depressed scar and avoid exposure of the subcutaneous tissue. In a mosaic of depressed scars and normal skin, remove consecutive tangential layers of the normal skin to plane it and make it level with the adjacent deepithelialized depressed scars.
6. Avoid interrupting the continuity of the dermal bed. However, should this happen inadvertently, bring the disrupted dermal margins together with few interrupted, inverted 6-0 or 5-0 catgut stitches. The stitches should be inverted to place the knots deep toward the fat. This will minimize the amount of foreign material on which the graft will not take.
7. Provisional hemostasis can be achieved by applying pressure to the shaved scar, or area, with a gauze pad moistened with warm saline solution.
8. Cut an intermediate-thickness skin graft (0.018 inch approximately) using a Watson's modified Braithwaite's skin graft knife, or the like, for large grafts. Silver's miniature skin graft knife is useful for cutting small grafts. Skin graft knives, the author believes, are better for cutting grafts than scalpel blades or ordinary razors held on a hemostat, because with the former exact uniform graft thickness can easily be gauged.
9. Spread the freshly cut graft over the shaved scar or mosaic, and apply pressure with a gauze pad for 5 minutes. This will effect definitive hemostasis as explained in Sect. IV.A.4. Removing the graft will then reveal a dry surface (Fig. 3E and F).
10. Wash the graft in normal saline solution to remove any blood clots from the undersurface.
11. Lay graft over the deepithelialized scar and fix it in position with interrupted 5-0 black silk sutures, securing good coaptation with the incised periphery of the bed and applying moderate stretch to the graft while suturing it. Insert some long 4-0 black silk sutures for "tie-over" (Fig. 3G).
12. Put a single layer of petroleum jelly gauze on the graft. Then build up a mound of cotton wool over it, and secure in place with the tie-over sutures (Fig. 3H). If the shaved scar is in an anatomic site that can be securely wrapped with a bandage, e.g., forehead or a limb, you do not need to apply the relatively sophisticated tie-over technique. You need only apply the petroleum jelly gauze, a

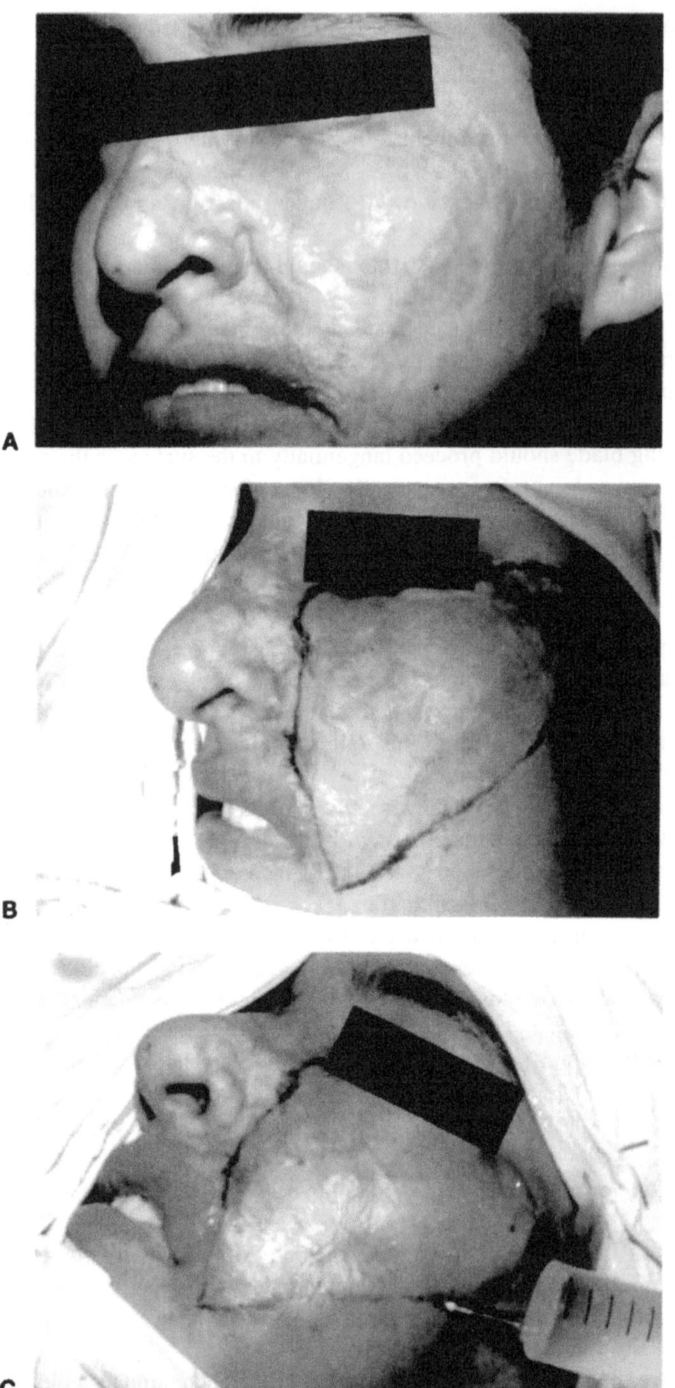

Figure 3 **(A)** Mosaic of depressed scars of the left cheek and the left side of the nose. **(B)** The borders of the mosaic to be deepithelialized are marked with methylene blue. **(C)** The mosaic is infiltrated subcutaneously with normal saline solution.

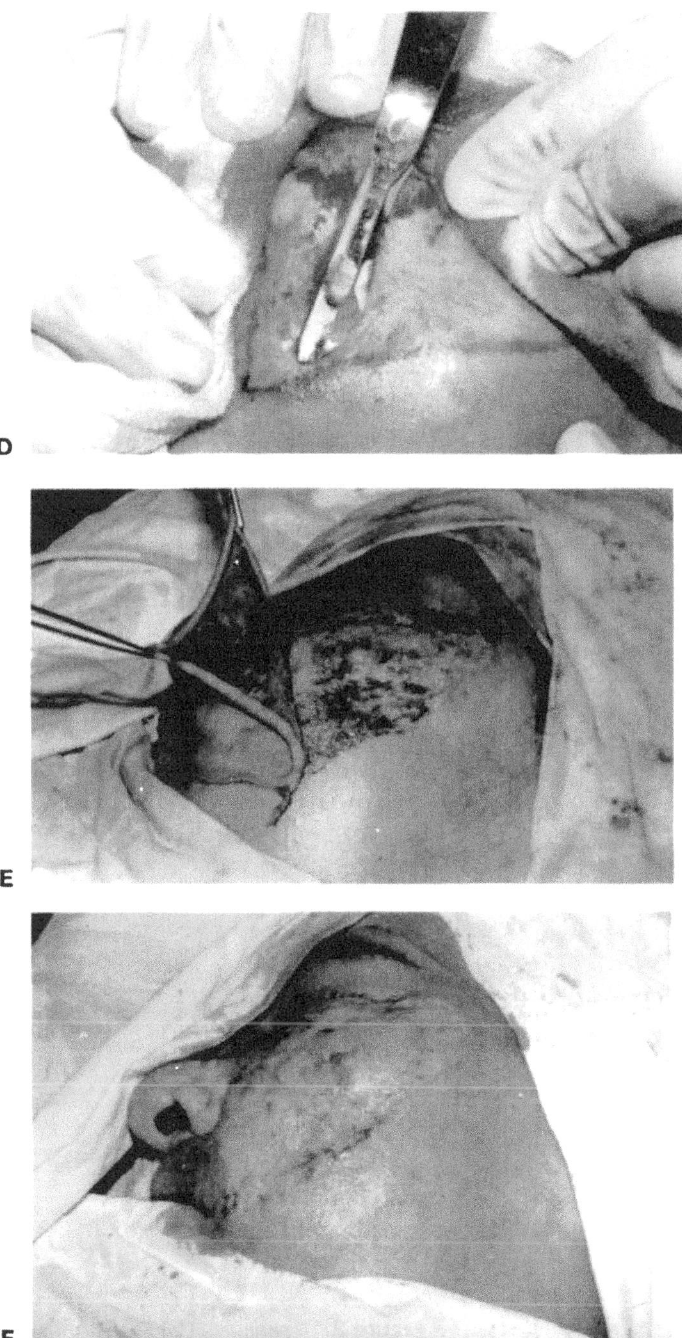

Figure 3 *(continued)* **(D)** Deepithelialization in progress. **(E)** The graft is being gently removed after allowing definitive hemostasis to occur. Note the clotted blood on both the deepithelialized bed and the undersurface of the graft. **(F)** The dry deepithelialized bed after removing the graft and clots.

(figure continues)

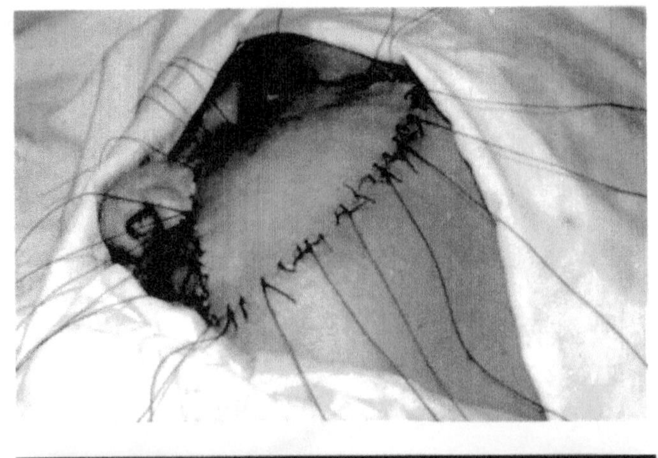

G

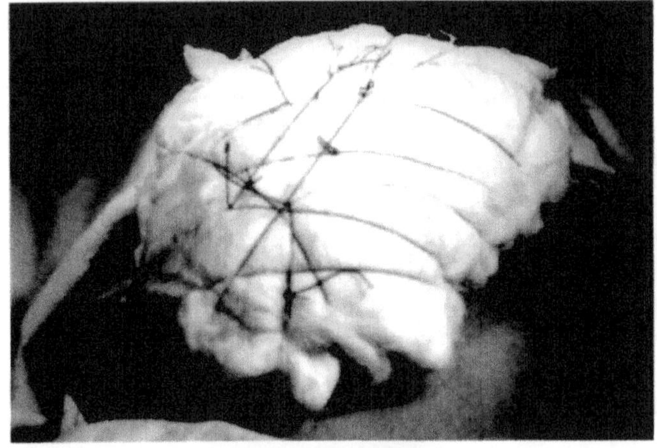

H

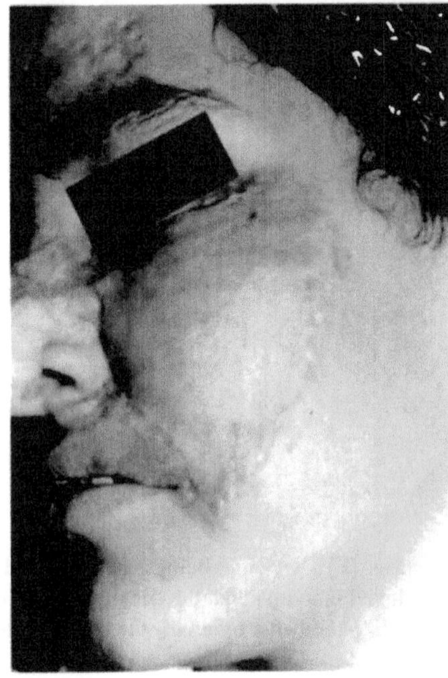

I

Figure 3 *(continued)* **(G)** The graft fixed in place with interrupted 5-0 black silk sutures and long 4-0 "tie-over" silk sutures in between. **(H)** Tie-over stitches securing the "mound" of cotton dressing in place. **(I)** An excellent result 6 weeks postoperatively.

piece of Gamgee tissue, and then secure this dressing in place over the graft with a crepe bandage.

C. Postoperative Management

The dressing is taken down and the stitches are removed on the fifth postoperative day. Thereafter, the graft and surroundings are cleansed daily with normal saline solution and then protected with a closed dressing of a single layer of petroleum jelly gauze, several layers of dry cotton gauze, and Micropore adhesive tape. This is continued for a week, when the graft will be left exposed.

Avoid exposing the graft to direct sunlight for 6 months. This is to protect against hyperpigmentation.

Keep the graft moist for the first six postoperative months until the sweat and sebaceous glands in the graft have regenerated. This is achieved by smearing the surface twice daily with a dermatologic cream for dry skin conditions. The best preparation, however, should contain white soft paraffin 14.5% w/w, light liquid paraffin 12.6% w/w, and hypoallergenic anhydrous lanolin 1.0% w/w in an emulsion base.

D. Assessment and Follow-up

Objective assessment of the result is based on graft take, improvement in the appearance in general, absence of hyperpigmentation, proper elevation of the depression to the surrounding skin level, proper merging of the margins into the surrounding skin, absence of contracture or wrinkling of the graft, and absence of inclusion epidermoid cysts under the graft. This assessment should be carried out routinely at every postoperative visit and, finally, at 1 year. Some cases, however, could be followed up for several years. Subjective assessment is based on the patient's, or parent's satisfaction.

The author achieved excellent results in almost 93% of the cases and attained the patient's or parent's satisfaction in about 91%. Figure 3I is an early satisfactory result at 6 weeks. Figure 4A–C illustrate an excellent result in another patient at 3 years follow-up.

VI. PRACTICAL TIPS ON "FLATTENING" OF HYPERTROPHIED SCARS

A. Anesthesia

The procedure for anesthesia is the same as in Sect. V.A.

B. Surgical Procedure

The assistant should immobilize the area and keep it taut throughout the shaving or "debulking." Shaving is carried out using scalpel blade no. 20, 21, or 22 on a no. 4 scalpel handle or modified handle. The author recommends the following:

1. Start shaving at the level of, and parallel to, the surrounding skin in the same manner as you cut a skin graft, leaving the peripheral 2 mm of the scar intact to hold the stitches fixing the graft to the bed. Cutting this thick chunk of scar will

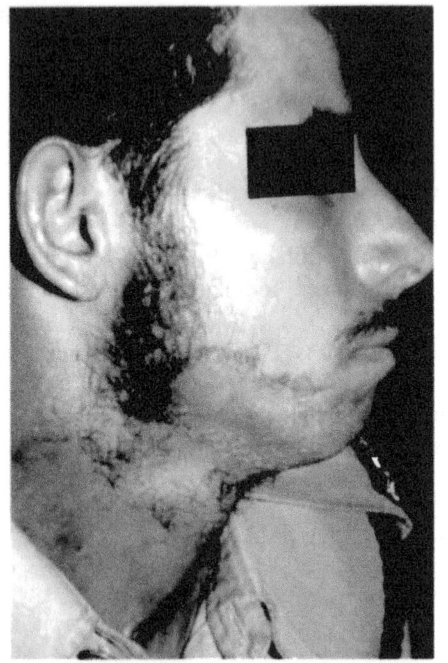

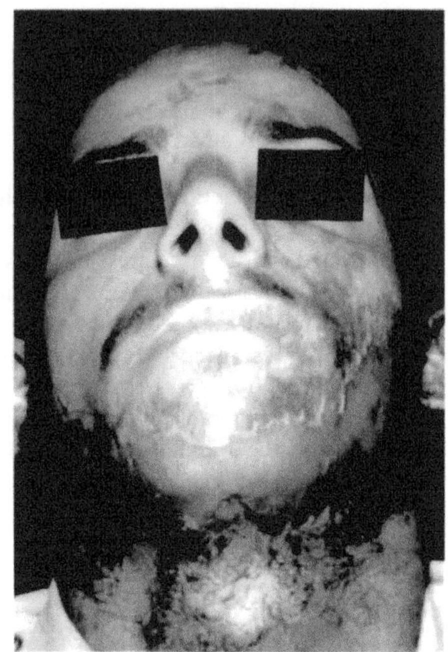

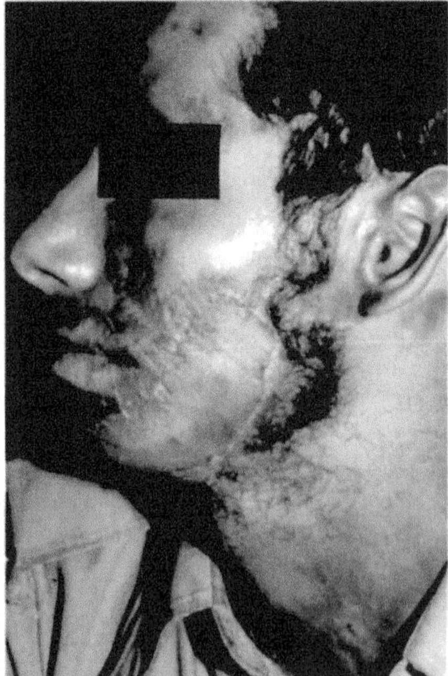

Figure 4 **(A–C)** Excellent result of dermal overgrafting of depressed, atrophic burn scars over the mandible, chin, and submandibular region, 3 years postoperatively. Note the smooth surface and excellent graft color, the perfect contour of the chin, and the "imperceptible" merging of the graft edges into the surrounding skin.

leave a surface of pearly white, whorly bundles of thick collagen interspersed with numerous punctate bleeding points. The collagen bundles will constitute a relatively uneven surface.

2. Repeat the tangential excision of thinner collagenous layers with one hand while steadying the area with the fingers of the other hand. As you excise deeper, the bleeding points become less in number, bigger in size, and bleeding becomes more profuse. The collagen bundles assume a pinkish hue as you go deeper.
3. Remove more tissue from the center so as to leave a saucer-shaped area at the end of the procedure. This is because the hypertrophied, or keloid scar, is usually thicker at the center. Do not breach the continuity of the collagen and do not expose the subcutaneous fat.
4. Keep pinching a fold of the collagenous bed between thumb and index finger before each tangential excision to gauge the bed thickness. You will have reached the proper depth and will have to end the shaving if you can lift a thin fold of the pinkish collagen and the bleeding becomes profuse (see item 2 above).
5. Smooth the uneven surface by trimming some of the bulging collagen bundles using a curved Metzenbaum scissors.
6. Provisional and definitive hemostasis, care of the bed, thickness and fixation of the graft, and dressing are the same as with the elevation technique (see Sect. V.B, items 6–12). The only difference is that you suture the graft to the peripheral 2-mm rim left from the outset of the procedure and do not puncture the normal skin outside the rim. This is to avoid the development of hypertrophied stitch marks.
7. If you have a mosaic of hypertrophied scars interspersed with islands of normal skin, you should shave the whole area and not just the scars. The 2-mm scar border described in item 1 above should be left only at the periphery of the mosaic and not each scar. This method will yield a far more superior cosmetic result (Fig. 5A and B).

C. Postoperative Management

This is the same as in Sect. V.C.

D. Assessment and Follow-Up

The outcome of the procedure is assessed objectively depending on improvement in appearance and contour and smooth texture of a normally pigmented graft on a thin collagenous bed that is level with the surrounding skin at every follow-up visit and at 1 year. Some cases can be followed up for several years postoperatively. Subjective assessment is based on the patient's, or parent's, satisfaction.

The state of growth of the hypertrophied scar at operation is as important as the perfection with which the surgical technique and postoperative management are executed. It is important to select a mature scar. Maturity can be reached in quite young scars, whereas activity is perpetuated in others for a longer time. The author finds that pale, nontelengiectatic hypertrophic scars that have ceased to produce symptoms for at least 3 months yield the best results. Avoid grafting actively growing hypertrophic scars. In these in-

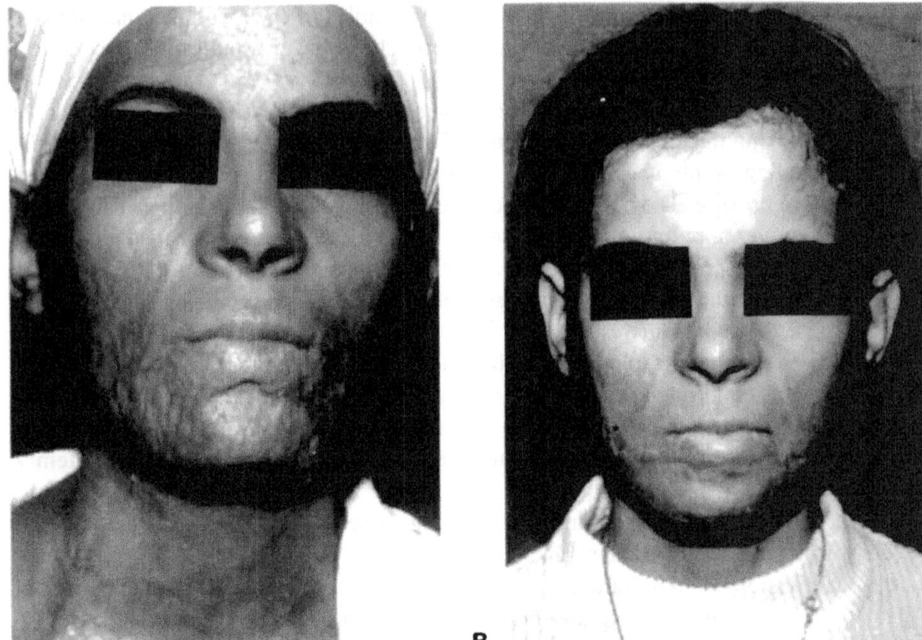

Figure 5 **(A)** Mosaic of hypertrophied burn scars of the chin, lower lip, and lower jaw. **(B)** One year after the operation. Note the smooth surface and normal color of the graft. Also note the excellent lip and chin contours.

stances, the graft will take but recurrence and a hypertrophic graft will inevitably result because of the increased connective tissue synthesis.

In the author's experience, a 97% objectively excellent result can be achieved in well-selected mature scars and the patient's satisfaction in almost every case. Figures 5, 6, 7, and 8 illustrate excellent results.

VII. A PITFALL OF OVERGRAFTING IN ELEVATION OF DEPRESSED SCARS

Perceptible elevation of the graft edge above the surface of the surrounding normal skin is one problem of the procedure that can happen in three situations:

1. A thick graft applied to the shaved, or dermabraded, scar only. The present author avoids this pitfall in such a situation by using an intermediate-thickness skin graft (approximately 0.018 in.) that, almost invariably, suffices to elevate the shaved scar and level it with the adjacent skin. This, together with meticulous suturing and coaptation of the graft at the level of the surrounding skin margins, gives excellent results (Fig. 4A–C).
2. Overgrafting a shaved, or dermabraded, scar and the surrounding skin, which together constitute an "aesthetic unit" of the face. This is resorted to in certain situations to improve the aesthetic outcome (37–40).

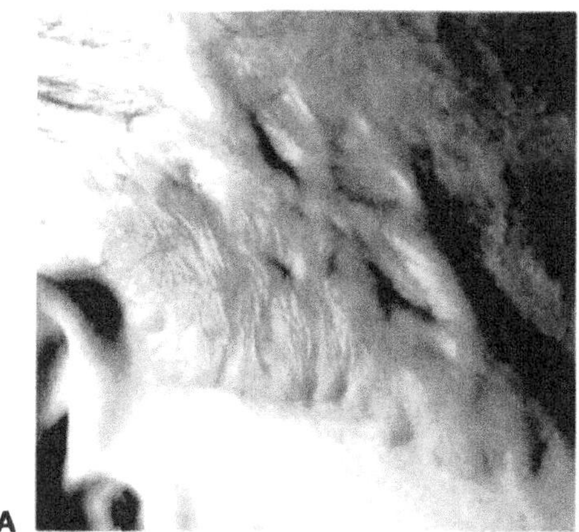

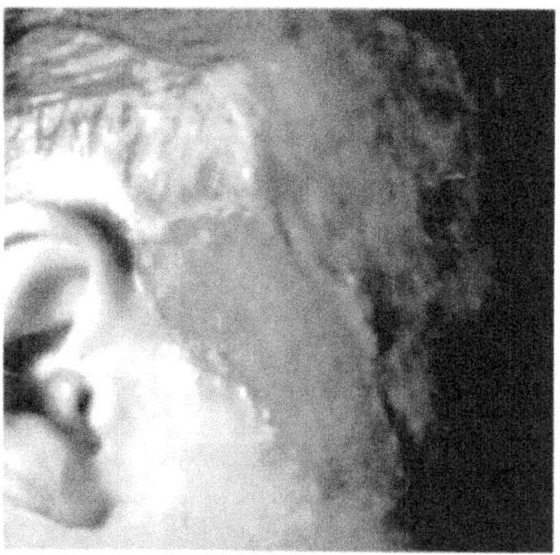

Figure 6 **(A)** Hypertrophic scar in the preauricular region. **(B)** Two years after shaving and skin grafting. (From Ref. 9.)

3. Overgrafting a strip of normal skin around the scar as in Hynes' technique in unstable scars and chronic venous ulcers (5).

Hynes claimed that he could manipulate the donor site while harvesting the graft so as to produce a graft much thicker in the center than at the periphery. The very thin periphery would make the edges of the graft "merge imperceptibly" with the normal skin.

This sounds easy but in reality it is not, as Pigott (41) pointed out. He reviewed 50 scars treated by this method and discovered that although the color and texture problems of the scar were often improved, those with extreme contour defects were not greatly improved. Furthermore, it was difficult to hide the borders of the graft and obtain "invisible" mending.

Faced with such a problem, the present author believes that dermabrasion of the graft edges at a subsequent stage, in 3 months, would help level out the contour.

VIII. COMPLICATIONS

Complications of dermal overgrafting are few and can be easily avoided in most instances. In that respect, a gospel of prevention rather than cure may be preached. The complications can be divided into:

A. Complications Due to the Procedure

1. Formation of Epidermoid Inclusion Cysts

These cysts develop from epithelial remnants of skin appendages, usually hair follicles, under the graft (42). These inclusion cysts are most commonly seen when the graft is placed on normal skin or a previous thick graft. They appear during the early weeks after dermal overgrafting as minute "pinhead" miliary cysts on the graft surface (Fig. 9). They respond to simple unroofing of the cysts by scraping with a sharp scalpel without anesthesia. They show no tendency to recur after 6 months have passed (10).

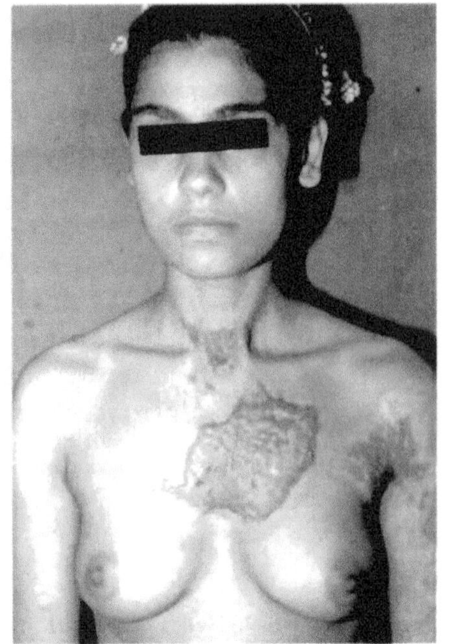
A

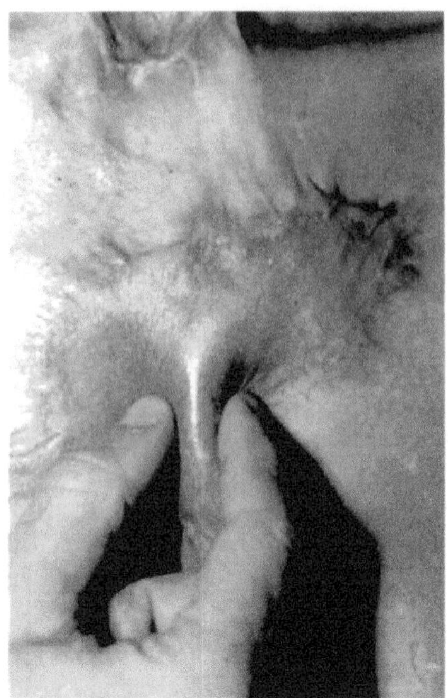
B

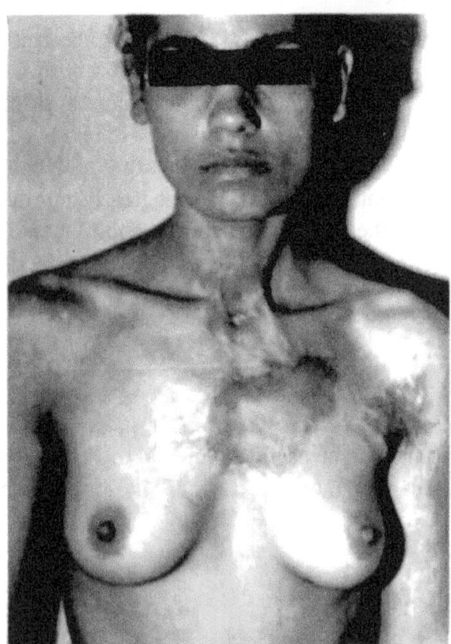
C

Figure 7 **(A)** An extensive hypertrophic burn scar of the anterior chest wall. **(B)** The thin bed of the scar under the skin graft, 3 months postoperatively. **(C)** Five years after shaving and skin grafting. (From Ref. 9.)

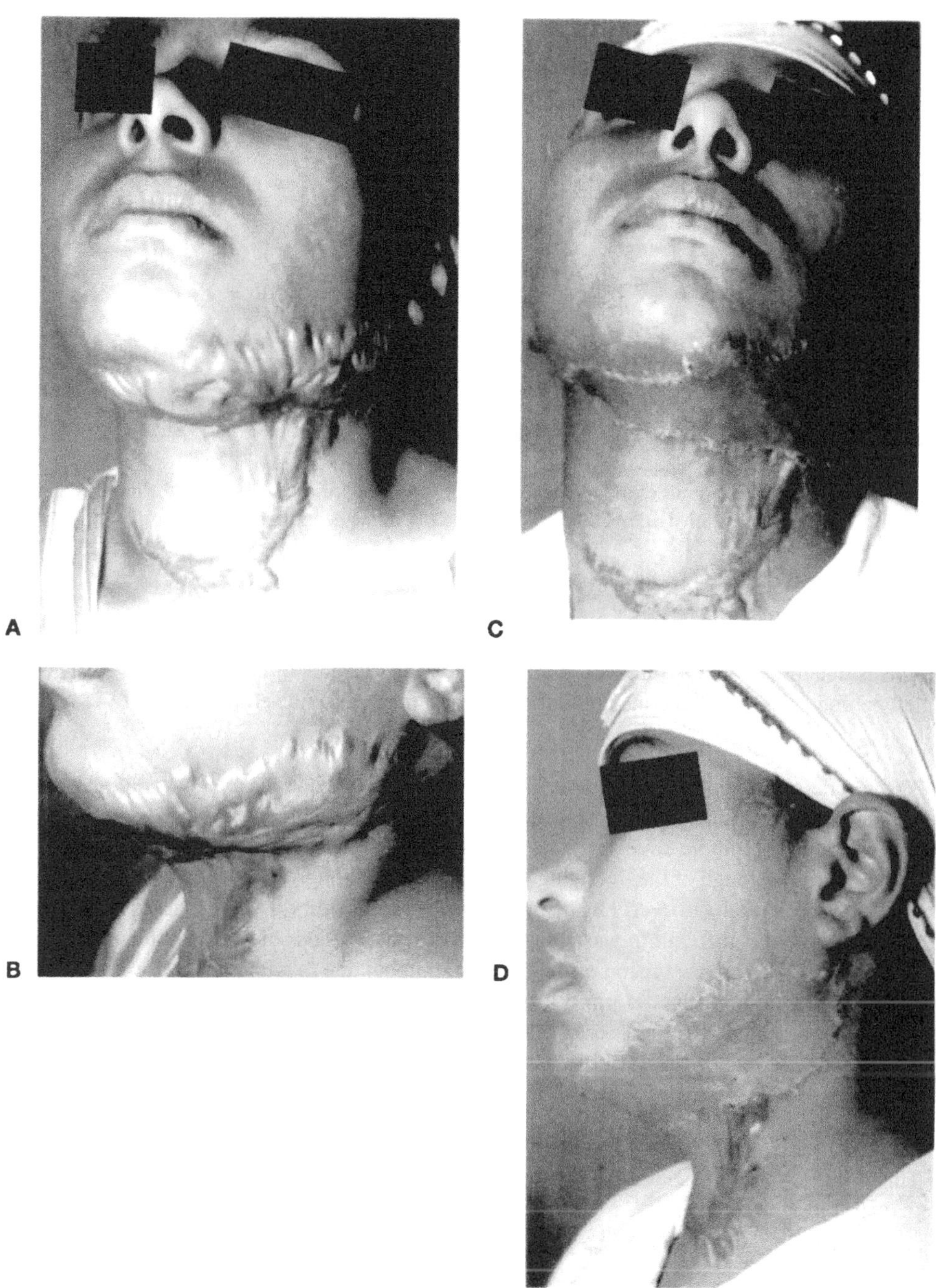

Figure 8 **(A)** Hypertrophic burn scar. **(B)** Lateral, close-up view. **(C)** Two and a half years later, showing an excellent result of shaving and skin grafting. **(D)** Lateral view of **(C)**. (**(A)** and **(C)** from Ref. 9.)

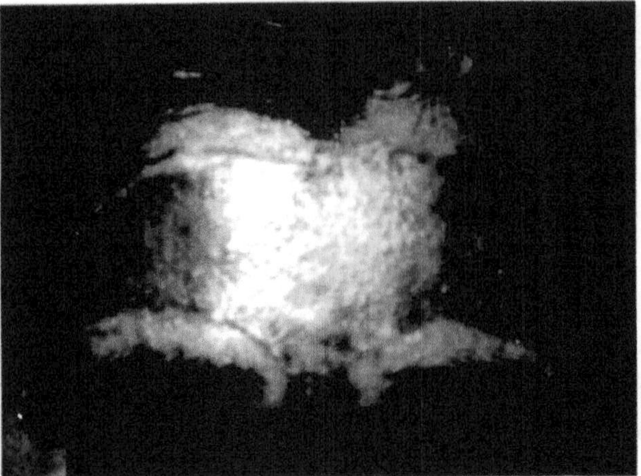

Figure 9 Dermal overgraft of the forehead for a mosaic of depressed scars. Note the minute "pin-head" miliary cysts scattered all over the graft and mainly in the central zone.

2. *Partial or Complete Graft Failure*

This is due to incomplete removal of all the epidermis. Islands of epithelium can easily be left behind and will regenerate under the graft and may cause the entire graft to fail (8).

3. *"Sponge" Deformity*

This is a deformity that has been described in relation to tangential excision and grafting in burns, which is considered one type of dermal overgrafting (see Sect. III.H). The deformity occurs when in multiple small parts of a grafted area, the bed heals underneath the graft with or without slough of the overlying graft. If the graft sloughs, a pockmark forms. If the graft does not slough, an overlying bridge forms. The deformity is very troublesome to patients because it is difficult to wash, catches on objects, bleeds, and looks quite unsightly. Treatment is by simple excision of the bridges and pockmarks with a curved iris scissors. Perhaps prevention of the deformity is easier; this is done by excising the wound deeper and by applying thinner grafts, or by applying allografts or xenografts, expecting that the area will heal promptly and will not require autografting (43).

4. *Remnants of Pigment in Shaved, or Abraded, Nevi or Tattoos*

This is due to failure to shave at a sufficiently deep level to remove the pigment and failure to overgraft with thick grafts.

B. Complications Similar to Those of Any Grafting Procedure

1. *Partial or Complete Failure of the Graft to Take*

This is due to either infection or hematoma or seroma formation under the graft. This complication can be avoided by aseptic surgical technique and by thorough hemostasis.

2. *Hyperpigmentation*

This can be largely minimized by avoiding direct exposure of the graft to sunlight for 6 months. Should hyperpigmentation develop, it can be largely ameliorated by dermabrasion at a later date.

3. *Hypertrophic Healing Particularly in Originally Hypertophic or Keloidal Scars*

This can be avoided if only mature, pale, nonsymptomatizing scars are selected for the procedure. (See Sects. III.A.3 and VI.D.)

IX. ADVANTAGES OF DERMAL OVERGRAFTING

Dermal overgrafting, in general, is a relatively simple technique that requires no special equipment or elaborate preparations, and the failure rate is very low. The postoperative complications are minimal. The cosmetic outcome is quite adequate from both the patient's and surgeon's points of view. Color and surface texture problems are almost always overcome, and the contour problem can be resolved to an appreciable extent. Specific advantages are the following:

1. Graft take is so certain that elaborate immobilization is necessary only when direct, simple bandaging cannot be applied because of the nature of the anatomic site.
2. The procedure avoids the following possible untoward effects of scar excision down to subdermal tissues and grafting (9):
   (a) The spreading edges of the wound make the raw surface two or three times as large as the original scar. Thus, a recurrence would be more extensive than the original lesion.
   (b) The soft lobulated fatty bed, with its meager blood supply, allows hematomas to form, and these could result in a poor graft take.
   (c) The soft bed yields to any forces of contracture that arise, and the graft can crumple rapidly, resulting in a poor cosmetic appearance.
3. The technique is more advantageous in elimination of decorative tattoos and pigmented skin lesions than excising them for the reasons given in Sect. IX.B.
4. No graft contracture is noticed, particularly if the procedure is carried out on hypertrophic and keloidal scars, because the tough collagen bed is already well contracted and tethered to its surroundings and resists the centripetal contractural power inherent in the graft (9).
5. If mature pale, nonsymptomatizing hypertrophic scars are selected for the procedure, recurrence is almost unknown. Should recurrence happen during pregnancy (44), for example, it will be minimal and within the confines of the original lesion (Fig. 10A–C).
6. Repeated dermal overgrafting, to build up a pad of normal dermal tissue, in unstable ulcers over bony prominences and in chronic venous stasis ulcers of the legs offers a method simple in technique and economical of tissue and hospital time. It is a method that can be safely applied to old patients without the gruesome complications of prolonged immobilization (see Sect. III.C).

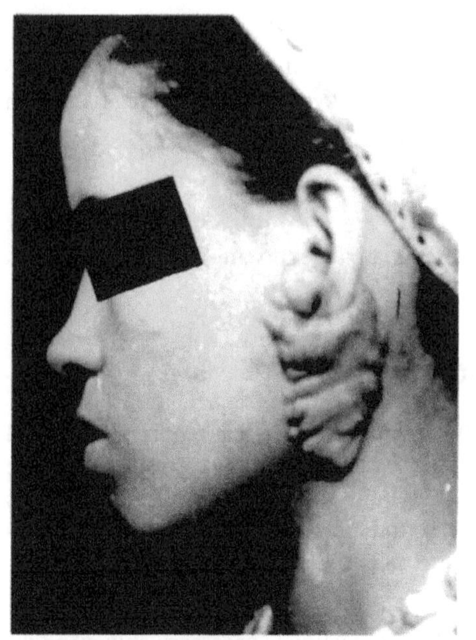

A

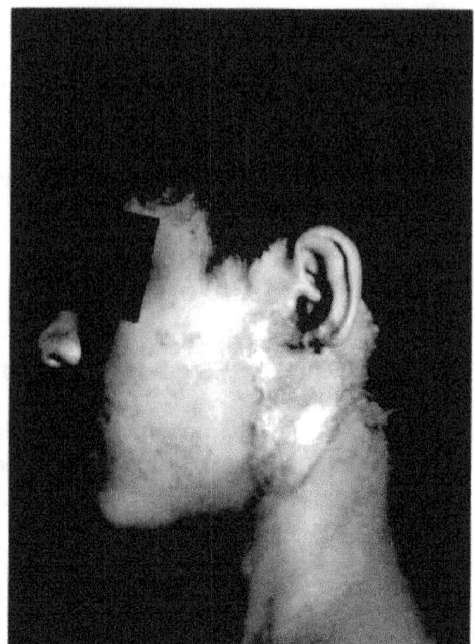

B

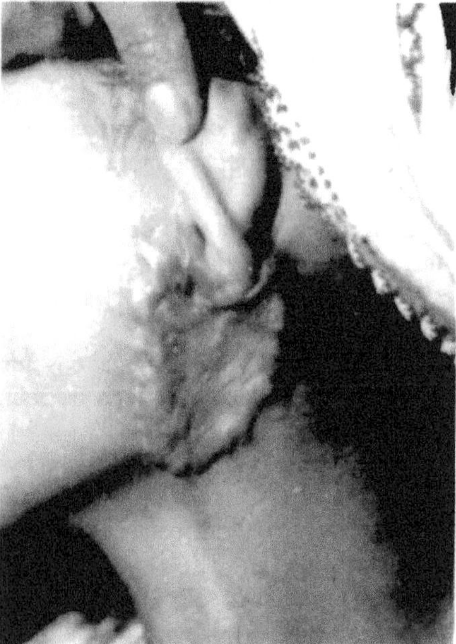

C

Figure 10 **(A)** Recurrent earlobe keloid. **(B)** Three months postoperatively, showing a satisfactory result. **(C)** Marginal hypertrophy of the border scar on the left ear 2 years later during pregnancy. (**(A)** and **(B)** from Ref. 44.)

REFERENCES

1. Webster GV. Report at the Annual Convention of the American Society of Plastic and Reconstructive Surgeons, Hollywood, FL, Oct 1954.
2. Webster GV, Peterson RA, Stein HL. Dermal overgrafting of the leg. J Bone Joint Surg Am 1958; 40A:796.
3. Iverson PC. Surgical removal of traumatic tattoos of the face. Plast Reconstr Surg 1947; 2:427.
4. Hynes W. The treatment of pigmented moles by shaving and skin graft. Br J Plast Surg 1956; 9:47.
5. Hynes W. The treatment of scars by shaving and skin graft. Br J Plast Surg 1957; 10:1–10.
6. Hynes W. Shaving in plastic surgery with special reference to the treatment of chronic radiodermatitis. Br J Plast Surg 1959; 12:43.
7. Rees TD, Casson PR. The indications for cutaneous dermal overgrafting. Plast Reconstr Surg 1966; 38:522–528.
8. Trimble JR. Dermal overgrafting in dermatology. J Dermatol Surg Oncol 1983; 9:987–993.
9. Moustafa MFH, Abdel-Fattah A-FMA. A reappraisal of shaving and skin grafting in hypertrophic burn scars. Plast Reconstr Surg 1976; 57:463–467.
10. Thompson N, Ell PJ. Dermal overgrafting in the treatment of venous stasis ulcers. Plast Reconstr Surg 1974; 54:290–299.
11. Vecchione TR. Tattoo removal using precise shave excision and dermal overgrafting. Ann Plast Surg 1988; 20:443–446.
12. Selmanowitz VJ, Rabinowitz AD, Orentreich N, Wenk E. Pigmentary correction of piebaldism by autografts: procedures and clinical findings. J Dermatol Surg Oncol 1977; 3:615.
13. Falabella R. Repigmentation of leukoderma by minigrafts of normally pigmented, autologous skin. J Dermatol Surg Oncol 1978; 4:916.
14. Selmanowitz VJ. Pigmentary correction of piebaldism by autografts: pathomechanism and pigment spread in piebaldism. Cutis 1979; 24:66.
15. Billingham RE, Silvers WK. Studies on the migratory behaviour of melanocytes in guinea pig skin. J Exp Med 1970; 131:101.
16. Harashina T, Iso R. The treatment of leukoderma after burns by a combination of dermabrasion and "chip" skin grafting. Br J Plast Surg 1985; 38:301–305.
17. Chitale VR. Overgrafting for leukoderma of the lower lip: a new application of an already established method. Ann Plast Surg 1991; 26:289–290.
18. Adamson JE, Wysocki JP, Ashbell TS. Treatment of a large hemangioma by dermal overgrafting. Plast Reconstr Surg 1978; 62:902–904.
19. Janzekovic Z. The dermal burn. In: Derganc M, ed. Present Clinical Aspects of Burns: A Symposium. Maribor: Mariborski Tisk, 1968:215–227.
20. Janzekovic Z. A new concept in the early excision and immediate skin grafting of burns. J Trauma 1970; 10:1103–1108.
21. Janzekovic Z. The burn wound from the surgical point of view. J Trauma 1975; 15:42–62.
22. Jackson DM. Second thoughts on the burn wound. J Trauma 1969; 9:839–862.
23. Jackson DM, Stone PA. Tangential excision and grafting of burns. The method and a report of 50 consecutive cases. Br J Plast Surg 1972; 25:416–426.
24. Feldman JJ. Reconstruction of the burned face in children. In: Serafin D, Georgiade NG, eds. Pediatric Plastic Surgery. St Louis: Mosby, 1984:552.
25. Baxter CR, Burke JF, Curreri PW, Heimbach D. Excisional therapy in burn injury: who, when, how. A panel discussion. J Burn Care Rehabil 1984; 5:430.
26. Briic A, Zdravic F. Lessons learnt from 2409 burn patients operated by early excision. Scand J Plast Reconstr Surg 1979; 13:107.
27. Engrav LH, Heimbach DM, Walkinshaw MD, Marvin JA. Excision of burns of the face. Plast Reconstr Surg 1986; 77:744.
28. Jonsson C-E, Dalsgaard C-J. Early excision and skin grafting of selected burns of the face and neck. Plast Reconstr Surg 1991; 88:83–92.

29. Serafini G. Treatment of burn scars of the face by dermabrasion and skin graft. Br J Plast Surg 1962; 15:308.
30. Becker DW, Bunn JC. Laser deepithelialization: an adjunct to reduction mammaplasty. Plast Reconstr Surg 1987; 79:754–758.
31. Hallock GG. Laser deepithelialization: an adjunct to reduction mammaplasty (Discussion). Plast Reconstr Surg 1987; 79:759.
32. Hallock GG. Extended applications of the carbon dioxide laser for skin deepithelialization. Plast Reconstr Surg 1989; 83:717–721.
33. Hallock GG, Rice DC. Skin deepithelialization using the carbon dioxide laser. Ann Plast Surg 1987; 18:283.
34. Puckett CL. Laser deepithelialization. Plast Reconstr Surg 1987; 80:867.
35. Cuschieri A, Giles GR, Moossa AR, eds. Essential Surgical Practice. Oxford: Butterworth-Heinemann, 1995:9.
36. Edgerton MT, Hansen FC. Matching facial color with split-thickness skin grafts from adjacent areas. Plast Reconstr Surg 1960; 25:455.
37. Gonzalez-Ulloa M, Castillo A, Stevens E, Alvarez FG, Leonelli F, Ubaldo F. Preliminary study of the total restoration of the facial skin. Plast Reconstr Surg 1954; 13:1951.
38. Gonzalez-Ulloa M. Restoration of the face covering by means of selected skin in regional aesthetic units. Br J Plast Surg 1956; 9:212.
39. Stark RB. Resurfacing of the face. Clin Plast Surg 1982; 9:27.
40. Millard DR Jr. Principalization of Plastic Surgery. Boston: Little, Brown, 1986.
41. Pigott RW. A review of 50 cases of skin scarring treated by shave and split skin graft. Br J Plast Surg 1968; 21:180–187.
42. Thompson N. A clinical and histological investigation into the fate of epithelial elements buried following the grafting of "shaved" skin surfaces. Br J Plast Surg 1960; 13:219.
43. Engrav LH, Gottlieb JR, Walkinshaw MD, Heimbach DM, Grube B. The "sponge deformity" after tangential excision and grafting of burns. Plast Reconstr Surg 1989; 83:468–470.
44. Moustafa MFH, Abdel-Fattah A-FMA. Presumptive evidence of the effect of pregnancy estrogens on keloid growth. Plast Reconstr Surg 1975; 56:450–453.

17

Autologous Fat and Dermal Grafting for the Correction of Facial Scars

Greg J. Goodman
Skin and Cancer Foundation of Victoria
Melbourne, Victoria, Australia

I. INTRODUCTION

The search for the ideal filler material seems an endless one. The substance needs to be cheap and readily available. It should not be capable of rejection and should have a low incidence of allergy and other adverse tissue reactions. It should be easy to work with and be permanent without risk of inducing communicative disease. Many of these requirements are met by the use of dermis and fat as grafting agents. The issue of permanence remains unresolved, but with refinement this parameter may also be met. The use of the patients' own tissues, like a spare parts factory, is of course not new. We all accept without reservation that skin, cartilage, and bone grafts once taken will remain, yet we have trouble accepting the same about fat and dermis. It awaits further studies and possibly refinement in techniques to see whether these grafts are likewise able to stand the test of time.

It is common in the treatment of mature scars to deal with atrophy rather than hypertrophy. Deep dermal atrophy may be aided by dermal grafting, and subcutaneous atrophy may be helped by replacing fat. The deeper forms of atrophic scarring and their correction by the deeper filling associated with dermis and fat grafts form the essence of this chapter.

II. HISTORY

Corrections of contour defects by the use of deep filling agents such as fat and dermis grafts are old techniques. Dermal grafting and dermofat grafts date back 60 years (1). They have found use in ophthalmology for orbital implantation (2,3) and in oral surgery for temporomandibular joint disease (4,5). They have been limited in their success over this time by problems such as cyst formation and unpredictable resorption characteristics. However, increased interest was shown in the behavior and longevity of these grafts in the 1960s (6,7). These grafts again appear to be attracting interest as an alternative filler material with some improvements being made in their harvesting methods (8–10).

Fat has been transplanted for over 100 years (11) and has waxed and waned in popularity. Since the mid-1980s (12,13), it has been possible to aspirate and reinject fat. Before this time fat grafts were harvested as solid grafts, requiring significant wounds for both harvesting and implanting the graft. Fat grafting was used in many surgical and cosmetic disciplines (14–16). It has tended to be maligned as a temporary technique (17,18), but improvements in technique have suggested that perseverence with fat transfer may produce accurate, long-standing, autologous correction (19–22).

III. SUMMARY OF RECENT IMPROVEMENTS IN TECHNIQUE IN DERMAL AND FAT GRAFTS

Both these old procedures have been rejuvenated by changes in the techniques. Dermal grafts have suffered from problems with graft resorption and cyst formation (10). However, use of a deepithelializing technique to a level below the sebaceous glands by either dermabrasion (8) or CO_2 laser (10) may help obviate the problem of cyst formation. Most appendageal structures can be removed by removing or destroying the epidermis and papillary dermis. Thus, deep dermis and associated fat may be transferred without this risk of cyst formation. Careful placement and handling of the graft have translated into better graft survival and longevity. The patient is also instructed to be still for 1–2 days after the procedure to maximize graft survival, as one would immobilize any grafted tissue. The other problem when dealing with scarred tissues is malposition of the graft or graft shift. Pretunneling the recipient site, breaking down the scar tissue where the dermal graft is to sit, helps this. This undermining has been termed Subcision (23,24). This also, as Swinehart (8) has stated, achieves an effect of placing a permanent "spacer" between the overlying skin and the scar so that tissues do not reattach.

Fat transfer has been through many changes in technique. This technique, like dermal grafting, consists of two phases: procurement of the graft and placement of this graft. Both phases are critical for the survival of the grafted tissue. Largely Ilouz (12,13) and Fournier (25) have modified the procurement phase. High-pressure removal of the fat by machine aspiration has been replaced by careful and gentle aspiration with specially designed aspiration cannulas, tumescent anesthesia to limit blood contamination, and less open and interventionist handling of the extracted fat before reinjection.

There is, however, no consensus among fat transfer practitioners as to the best method of extracting fat or handling it once extracted (26). The area chosen for fat transfer has been not agreed upon, with some believing that areas that have poor vascularity will do better (27). Others believe that more fibrous areas such as the upper abdomen do better (28). Still others believe that donor areas that change little with diet, containing fat with adipocytes carrying α_2-receptors, are best. These donor fat stores are said to be antilipolytic and are more likely to be successful (26). Many suggestions have been proposed in the past for treating the fat after implantation and before injection. Vitamin E, insulin, and adenosine have been considered as important factors (27,29–34). However, opinions have been divided about the relative value of these promoting substances in the vivo environment, and many feel that increasing the metabolic activity of the fat with these substances is wrong and one should instead be minimizing their metabolic demands to maximize survival. It may also be that tampering with the fat and breaking the "closed" system are traumatic to the fat and promote the chance of infection. Techniques such as straining (35,36), whisking (18), routine washing (18,37–39), and filtering (40,41) are not probably going to stand the test of time. It was said as far back as 1921 by Lexer (42) that "it is necessary that the fat tissue is not damaged at the moment of its removal nor at the moment of its implantation." To this it could be added that it should probably not be damaged in between. The injection phase has seen small aliquots or parcels of fat implanted in multiple tunnels, allowing the graft maximal access to available blood supply. Building the correction in a three-dimensional lattice of fat parcels allows an accuracy of sculpting not previously attainable. The lattice begins at the deepest level possible in the recipient area. This may be abutting bone in areas such as the malar region or be in muscle in the forehead. The likelihood of an increased graft take has meant that overcorrection is not desired or required. If further fat transfer is needed, additional fat may be taken at the time of original suction and stored frozen for further touch-ups as required. Subcision is also useful for breaking up the deep scar attachments before the fat is implanted.

IV. RATIONALE FOR DEEP AUTOLOGOUS FILLER AGENTS IN THE TREATMENT OF SCARS

Scarring, whether traumatic, postsurgical, or following cutaneous disease, may be present in different shapes, sizes, and at different levels within the skin. It is well to remember that scars are noted by the patient only if they exhibit a color or contour abnormality or they are more than about 1 cm in length. Color and length of scar are best dealt with by resurfacing techniques and specific visible light laser therapy (43). Contour defects may be small or reasonably superficial and respond to resurfacing procedures such as dermabrasion (44–46) or CO_2 (47,48) or possibly erbium laser resurfacing. The use of dermal filling agents, either biologic or nonbiologic in type, may supplement these. A variety of autologous filling agents are also available, such as punch grafting (49,50), autologous lipocollagen (51), autologous collagen (52), and cultured fibroblasts, for these superficial defects.

When deeper defects are the concern, dermal grafts and autologous fat transfer techniques may be useful. With deep atrophic scarring, just treating the surface will at best give a temporary and eventually incomplete result as the initial swelling and euphoria settle, revealing continuing tissue deficiency. Furthermore, dermal and fat transfer techniques may be employed at the same surgical procedure time as resurfacing techniques. By the use of such a combined approach to scarring of deep and superficial types, form and surface texture are addressed with minimization of the potential for excessive treatment and thus the risk of complications.

Some authorities feel that autologous fat transfer is not useful for the treatment of scarring (53), but I feel this may be due to inappropriate use of this material. It must be remembered that superficial scarring is not an indication for a deep filling agent. The dermis is a busy place with many tightly packed structures. Fat is a flowing, diffuse substance, which has no ability to be placed in such a tight environment. It is also true that the relatively poorly vascularized tissue of a scarred dermis will not be likely to nurture fat grafts. To place a subcutaneous filler such as fat below dermal scars still leaves the dermal scars to be attended. However, the role of fat is as a volume expander, a foundation for the tissue to sit on. This will allow a more superficial assault on the dermal component of the scar by resurfacing or superficial filler techniques.

It is also important to conceptualize from the appearance of the scar where it is occurring in the skin. A well-defined linear troughed scar is a dermal event and will benefit from dermal grafting. A large ill-defined divot is not predominantly a dermal event but is deeper and needs subcutaneous filling agents.

Table 1 Scarring Suitable for Dermal Grafting or Fat Transfer

Dermal grafting	Fat transfer
Postsurgical	Postsurgical
Traumatic	Traumatic
Postacne	Postacne
Postinfective, e.g. postviral	Deep morphea
Discoid lupus erythematosus	Discoid lupus profundus
Morphea	Idiopathic lipodystrophy

V. INDICATIONS

Usually, trauma or disease (Table 1) causes scars. Trauma may be natural or surgical, whereas dermatologic skin diseases causing scarring include scleroderma or morphea, facial hemiatrophy, idiopathic lipoatrophy, discoid lupus erythematosus, infection, or acne. Acne serves as an excellent model. In this disease, scarring processes may occupy epidermis, dermis, or subcutis or often a mixture of all three. Either dermal grafting or fat transfer with or without associated resurfacing techniques may help all these causes.

VI. ADVANTAGES AND DISADVANTAGES OF AUTOLOGOUS DERMAL AND FAT GRAFTING

As said earlier, the ideal filler material is one that is readily available, cheap to procure, readily repeatable, easy to implant, permanent or at least long lasting, exact in its placement, nonmigratory, nonreactive or allergenic, and with few complications of implantation.

Both dermal grafting and fat transfer have characteristics that fulfill some of these ideals and others that fall short. Table 2 outlines the relative merits and demerits of these agents set against a theoretical ideal substance and bovine collagen implant. A maximum

Table 2 Relative Merits and Demerits of Augmenting Materials

Parameter	Ideal agent	Injectable collagen	Dermal grafting	Free fat graft
Readily available	5	5	5	5
Cheap to procure	5	2	4	4
Readily repeatable	5	5	3	5
Easy to implant	5	5	4	4
Permanent or long lasting	5	1	4	4
Nonmigratory	5	5	4	4
Nonreactive	5	3	4	5
Nonallergenic	5	2	5	5
Exact in its placement	5	5	4	3
Few complications	5	4	4	4
	50	37	41	43

of 5 is awarded for a perfect score for a parameter and a minimum of 1 if the benefit of that parameter is not present for that agent. As is evident from Table 2, dermal grafting and fat transfer fulfill many of these dicta.

VII. TECHNIQUES

A. Dermal Grafting

1. Selection of Patients

Scars that are best dealt with by dermal grafting should be 3–6 mm wide. They should be readily distensible, able to be stretched out reasonably easily. If the scar is too bound down, it may be worth subcising without dermal grafting on one or more occasions before reassessing the scar for dermal grafting again. Sometimes the scar base will soften enough to allow dermal grafting to be advantageous.

Patients should be selected if their scars are of correct type, the patient is medically fit, and there are no contraindications to the technique. Patients should be examined in tangential or overhead light and their scars viewed by the examiner tangentially. The easiest way to view the patients is with a headlight so that the viewer and the light source are approaching the scar from the side. The scars are outlined in gentian violet (Fig. 1). Marking must be particularly exact with dermal grafting.

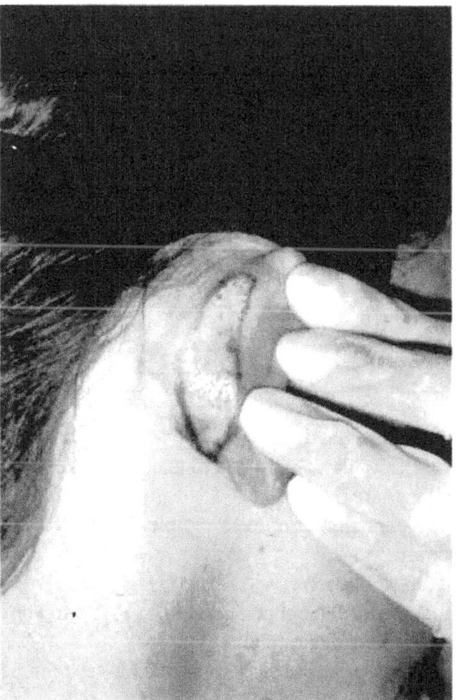

Figure 1 The dermal graft donor site marked and prepared.

Standard photography should be performed before marking and Polaroid photographs taken after the marking so that they may be referred to during the procedure and in case markings become smudged. The markings are even more important if local anesthesia is to be used. After measuring the width and length of the proposed dermal graft, the donor site is likewise measured.

2. *Equipment*

Equipment (Table 3) required for dermal grafting is quite simple. Even the deepithelialization device may be a simple bit of sandpaper or dry wall grid. A regular dermabrasion machine with wire brush or diamond fraise is also fine, as is one of the substantially more expensive infrared lasers such as the CO_2 or erbium laser.

If one is using dermabrasion or an erbium laser, routine excision of the dermal grafts is required. If one is using CO_2 lasers, the laser is usually used to excise the required tissue. Tenotomy or Gradle scissors are needed to trim the defect to shape, and a monofilament absorbable suture on a straight needle such as 4-0 Maxon or polydioxanone (PDS) is recommended for introducing the graft. A simple intravenous cannula serves as an excellent obturator for linear defects. Punch grafts of appropriate size are required if small circular grafts are required. It is best to have these in 0.25-mm increments, but one may get away with 0.5-mm increments. They should be straight walled and sharp. Probably hair transplant punches are best for the intervening sizes; the disposable punches are excellent for this purpose but do not come in all sizes.

The donor defect requires closure and sutures must be in place for 7 days (10 days with CO_2 laser excisions).

3. *Anesthesia of the Recipient and Donor Sites*

Local anesthetic, usually 1–2% lidocaine with 1:100,000 epinephrine, is injected locally both for anesthesia if the patient is awake and for hemostasis if awake or under general anesthetic. The recipient site is to be undermined, usually with a sharp instrument, and will bleed significantly without epinephrine locally. The donor site is to be deepithelialized and excised and similarly requires local anesthesia with epinephrine.

4. *Preparation of the Donor Site*

Either dermabrasion or infrared lasers (CO_2 or erbium) may be used to prepare the retroauricular donor site. Essentially, the donor site required is marked out so that enough dermal

Table 3 Equipment Required for Dermal Grafting

Suggested equipment	Comments
Dermabrasion, erbium or CO_2 laser	To deepithelialize the donor site
Excision pack	If not using CO_2 laser, will need to excise dermal graft from donor area
Marking pen	Gentian violet or similar to mark recipient site
Jeweler's forceps	To hold graft
Gradle or tenotomy scissors	To trim graft to fit defect
Suture on straight needle	Absorbable monofilament or coated, e.g., PDS, Maxon
Obturator	No. 14–16 intravenous cannula
Punches	A range of appropriate sizes 1–3mm in 0.25- or 0.5-mm increments
Suture	4/0 to close donor site

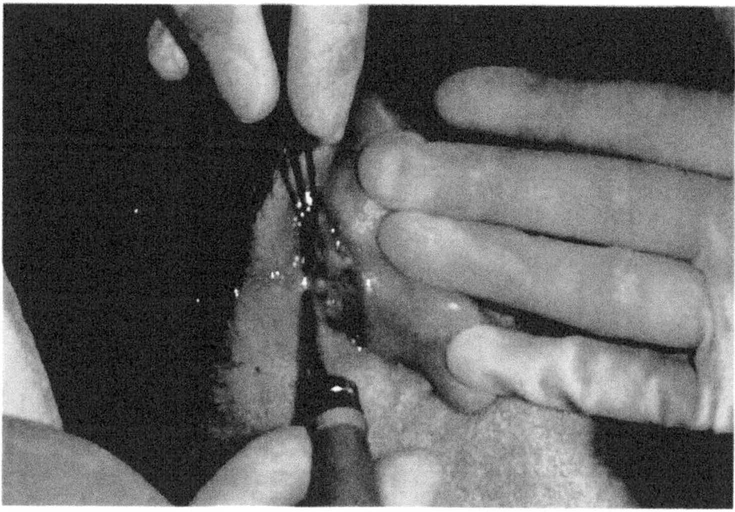

Figure 2 The graft being excised with the laser in cutting mode from the donor area.

material is harvested commensurate with primary closure of the defect to leave an imperceptible line in the retroauricular sulcus (Fig. 2).

The deepithelialization must be carried down to a level below the papillary dermis to remove the bulk of the appendageal structures (8), especially the sebaceous glands, as this seems to make a difference to the incidence of epidermal cysts. Either the dermabrasion or laser preparation of the donor site is thus taken to a level below that usually sought. With dermabrasion the appearance of coarse, frayed collagen fibers with the wire brush or removal of fine yellow dots and the appearance of coarse bleeding with the diamond fraise is the endpoint. With a CO_2 laser a number of passes are used until tissue takes on the chamois color suggestive of tissue dehydration. With the Ultrapulse laser (Coherent Lasers, Palo Alto, CA) the computer pattern generator is set so there is moderate to high overlap (about 40–50%), a relatively small pattern size, and usually a square pattern of pulses so that complete coverage of the donor zone is achieved. A 3-mm collimated handpiece may also be used. With a scanning focused laser such as the Silk Touch laser (Sharplan Lasers, Allendale, NJ) or a similar system, a short handpiece such as the 125 mm, a small spot size of 3–4 mm, and a moderate to high power of 10 W with two passes are used. In general, probably about 25–30 Js/cm^2 of total fluence to tissue should be delivered. Between passes, saline-soaked gauze is used to wipe the skin thoroughly clear of debris. This increased depth, I feel, as do others (8), is likely to leave less appendages to develop into cystic structures in the postoperative period. The erbium laser may also be used to deepithelialize the donor site, in which case the endpoint is reasonably brisk bleeding. The erbium laser has no role, however, in harvesting the graft.

5. *Harvesting the Graft*

At this stage, what is done next depends on the shape of the defect. If the defect is a linear trough–like scar, the CO_2 laser is usually set on continuous cutting mode at 7–10 W. A strip of dermis is excised by this method. If a CO_2 laser is not employed, the strip may be ex-

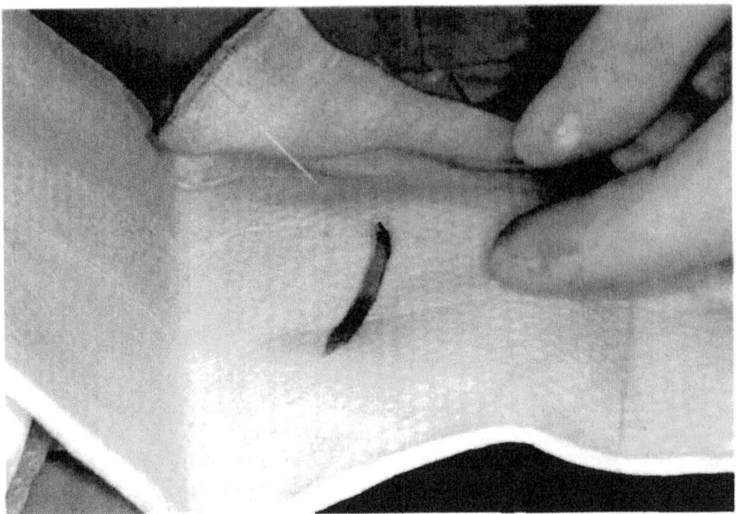

Figure 3 The graft being trimmed to size for the recipient pocket.

cised with a scalpel. It is important to trim any charred tissue from the graft if one is using a CO_2 laser. It is then trimmed with Gradle or tenotomy scissors to match the defect it is to fill (Fig. 3). It is, however, better for the graft to be just a little short for the defect rather than too long, as discussed later (see complications later). The depth of the recipient site defect will determine whether, and how much, fat is left on the base of the graft. If the defect needs more bulk, it is quite permissible to leave fat on the base of the graft, as it does not seem to hamper its survival or increase the incidence of cyst formation. If, however, the defect to be corrected is circular, it is better to size the recipient site and take an appropriate-size punch transplant of dermis. For epidermal punch grafts, an allowance is usually made for shrinkage of tissue and the donor punch graft is sized 10–20% larger than the recipient site defect. With dermal punch grafts, the size of the donor graft should be exactly matched to that of the recipient defect.

6. *Attachment of Dermal Graft for Implantation*

Some dermal grafts do not require attachment to an introducing needle, for example, most punch dermal grafts, but the linear grafts do require attachment to a suture. I usually tie this to a 4-0 PDS suture on a straight needle (Ethicon). This will be guided into the recipient pocket, usually with the help of the plastic sleeve of a 14- or 16-gauge intravenous cannula.

7. *Production of Recipient Dermal Pocket*

For circular defects that are to receive a dermal punch graft, undermining with a no. 19–21 needle or a no. 18 Nokor needle (Becton Dickinson, Cockeysville, MD) is excellent. The defect should be undermined as fully as possible, allowing the scar to “float up.” The fibrous bands of the scar base hold the scar retracted, and breaking these free helps to release this effect. The dermal graft will be placed in this pocket and act as the “spacer” to keep the skin from reattaching to the underlying tissues. For a linear defect, a 14- or 16-gauge intravenous cannula is an easily accessible instrument. A Rhytisector (Byron, Tucson, AZ) is also a useful device for producing the pocket. An advantage of the intravenous cannula is

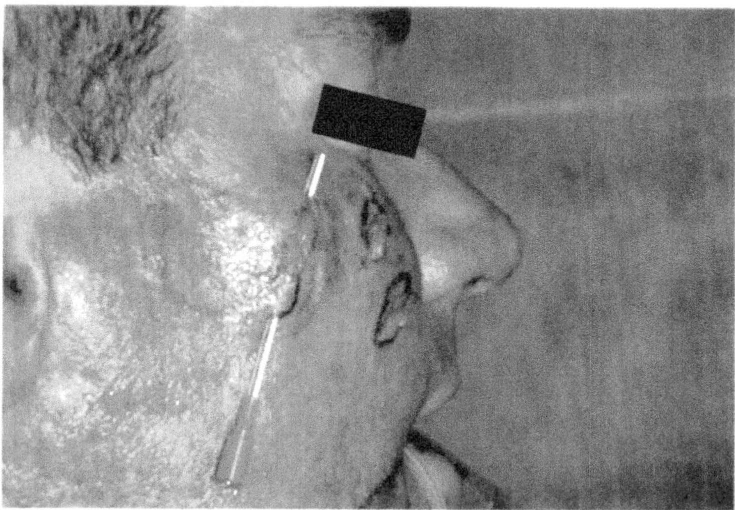

Figure 4 The intravenous cannula that has been used as an undermining tool in situ in the recipient pocket.

the plastic sheath that surrounds the introducer. Once the pocket is formed, the intravenous cannula exits at the distal end of the defect. The introducer is removed, leaving the plastic sleeve in the recipient tunnel and exiting the wound at the proximal and distal ends (Fig. 4). The PDS suture is then passed into the distal end of the wound, exiting proximally where the hub of the cannula is located (Fig. 5). This allows reuse of the cannula for other dermal

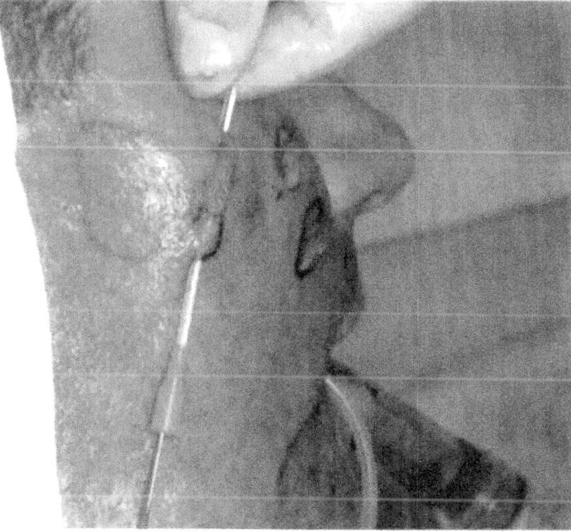

Figure 5 The 4-0 PDS needle and suture being passed into the plastic sleeve of the intravenous cannula in the recipient pocket.

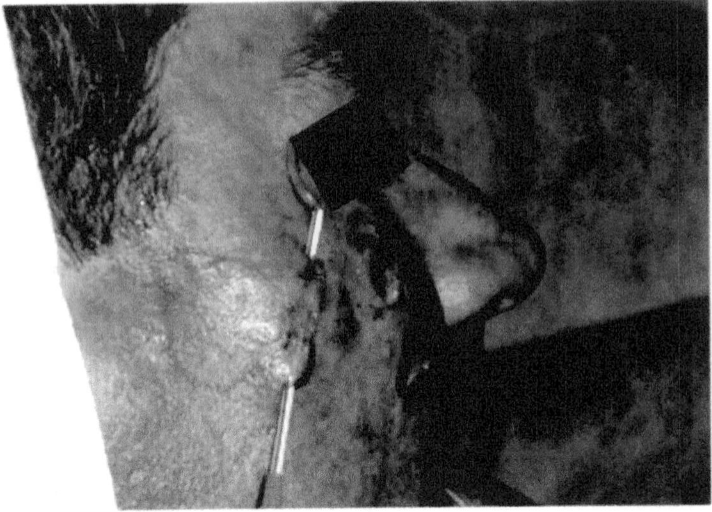

Figure 6 The graft abutting the free end of the cannula ready to be drawn into the pocket.

grafts. The PDS suture is brought out of the proximal end until the dermal graft is brought up to abut the plastic sleeve (Fig. 6). The assistant then grasps the end of the dermal graft with fine jeweler's forceps and holds the graft until final placement has occurred. The leading end of the dermal graft is passed into the beginning of the plastic sleeve, and the sleeve and trailing dermal graft are eased into position with the assistant still holding the graft. Once the position is acceptable and the sleeve has been delivered at the proximal end of the recipient site, the assistant withdraws the jeweler's forceps and the suture is cut proximally (Fig. 7). Removing the suture is not necessary, nor is any attempt at further anchoring the

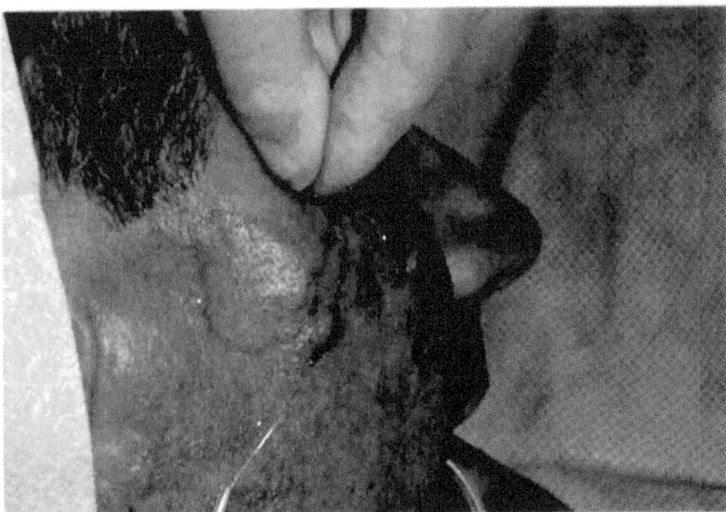

Figure 7 The graft in position just prior to severing the stitch at either end of the recipient pocket.

graft required. The ends of the wound are stretched in either direction away from the recipient site to allow the graft to sit most comfortably in the bed and avoid any tethering of the graft to one edge. This can produce skin retraction. For this reason, it is also best when trimming the graft to make it 1–2 mm shorter than the bed.

The donor site is sutured to leave the scar in the retroauricular crease. If any irregularity is left from the punch grafts, the area is further excised to produce an ellipse in the retroauricular sulcus. The resultant wound scar is usually imperceptible. A horizontal running mattress suture is excellent for closure in this location.

8. *Results and Complications*

A study was performed in 11 patients, who had a total of 32 grafts (10). Immediate complete or almost complete correction was seen in all patients. Complications were seen in five grafts. One of the infraoral grafts of one patient was poorly positioned and required correction. Resorption or partial resorption of one dermal graft was seen in two patients. Two cysts were seen, one in each of two patients, although this was not observed after the technique was modified to take deeper donor grafts. The cysts were treated with intralesional steroids; one resolved but one had to be removed by excision. Tethering that required cyst removal was also seen in the same patient. One patient who had two grafts was reviewed for only 6 weeks before relocating overseas. One patient was lost to follow-up after 6 weeks.

All other grafts (27 of 32 or 84%) were successful, providing complete correction or substantial improvement with follow-up periods of between 3 months and 2.5 years. Figures 8, 9, and 10 show early results of dermal grafting, and Figs. 11 and 12 show results at 6 months. However, this patient also had fat transfer to the lateral cheeks 6 months before and laser and dermabrasion to the entire cheek subunit 3 months before the final photograph. The area of dermal grafting is in the vicinity of both melolabial folds and has continued to provide correction to this area.

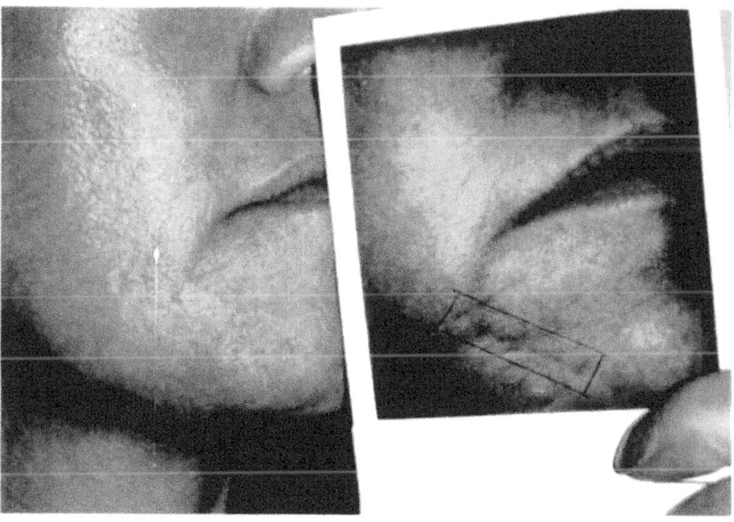

Figure 8 Early example of dermal graft result 1 month after placement.

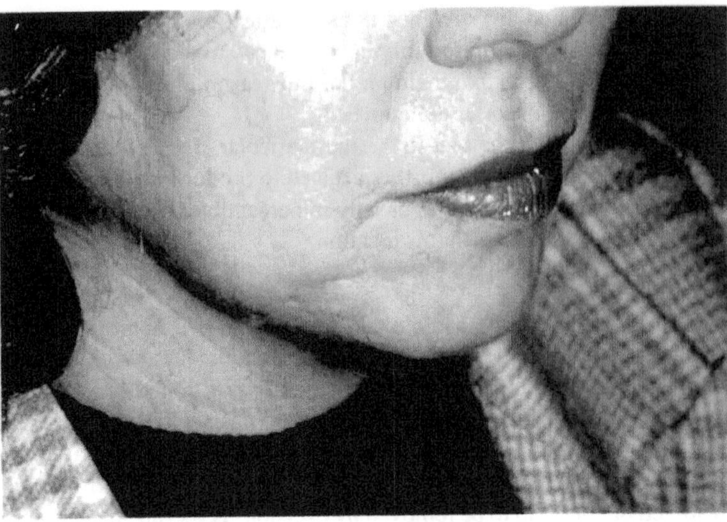

Figure 9 Preoperative traumatic contour defect.

B. Fat Transfer

There are many varied techniques for fat transfer, and one gets the impression that no matter what technique is described by the author it will be shown to be archaic in the fullness of time. Fat transfer techniques in the past seem clinically and therefore somewhat subjectively to suggest survival rates of 0–50% (17,19,20,23,54). However, fat transfer seems to work in many operators' hands (18,19,22,23,55) but with a multitude of nuances in the specific technique. In general, the similarities in the procedure are greater than the differences

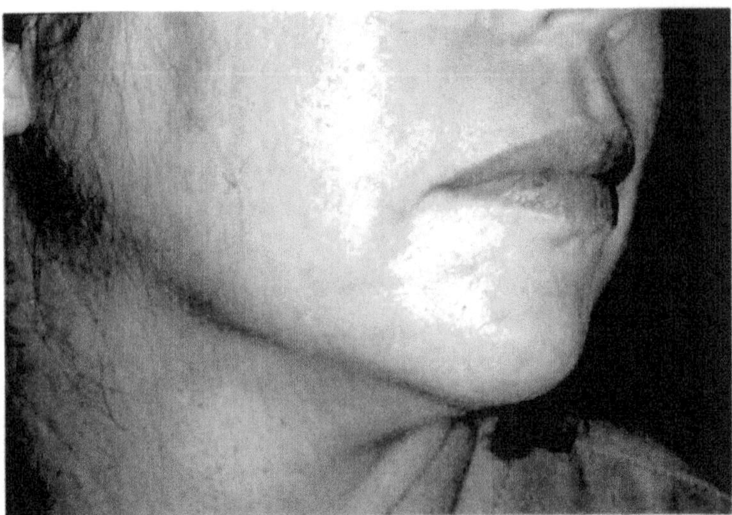

Figure 10 Early 6-week postoperative result.

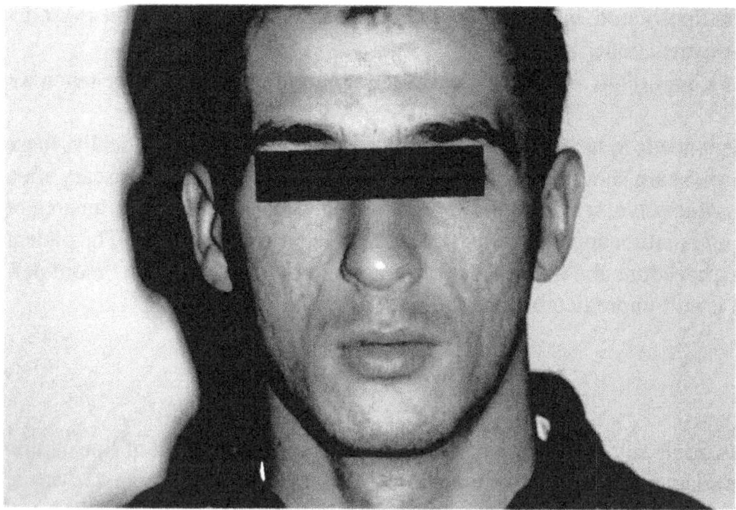

Figure 11 Preoperative contour defect, melolabial folds.

and are directed to keeping the fat graft alive and viable. Culturing and histological evaluation of low-pressure closed syringe liposuction harvest (56) have shown that mature fat cells can be harvested successfully and survive the transit.

1. Selection of Patients

As with dermal grafting, patients need to be examined in tangential lighting. The markings should be at the perimeter of the trough, and a topographic marking system, similar but in

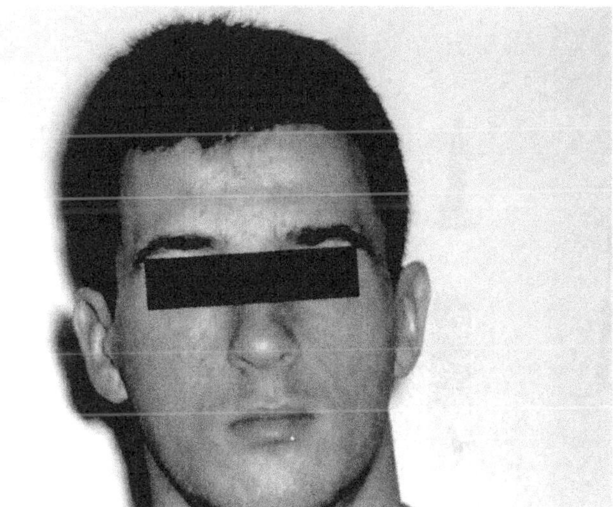

Figure 12 Postoperative result at 6 months. Note that the patient has also had laser and dermabrasion to cheeks 3 months before this photograph and fat transfer to the lateral cheeks at the time of the dermal graft 6 months before this photograph.

reverse to that used in liposuction, is useful. Here the inner markings represent the most depressed rather than elevated zones.

Photographs are important, and 35-mm and often Polaroid photographs are taken for reference.

The ideal patient needs to have defects of volume induced by scarring. Ideally, these defects should not have sharp shoulders indicating dermal pathology. However, scars often have multiple layers of involvement, and if a sharply punched-out scar lies over an area of fat atrophy, then a combination approach is indicated with fat as the base filler. The patient must understand the procedure and also accept that although fat is becoming a "more permanent" solution, it is still unpredictable and "top-ups" may be required.

2. *Technique*

a. Equipment

Although the fat was originally extracted as a solid excised graft, the advent of liposuction techniques has allowed an easier method of extraction. The next stage in fat transfer was to use a sterile collection system attached to the liposuction machinery (Figs. 13 and 14 and Table 4). However, to lessen the trauma to the fat and aid in its survival, many practitioners have taken up syringe liposuction to extract the fat for reinjection. This low pressure is thought to decrease the disruption of the delicate fat cells and maximize their viability. Usually, 10-mL Luer-Lok syringes are used for extraction and 1–3-mL syringes are used for infiltration.

Luer-Lok aspiration and infiltration cannulas are used. Although sharp cannulas have been suggested for less traumatic fat removal, the difference in viable yield is probably minimal and it is probably safer to use blunt cannulas throughout this procedure. A no. 13–14 cannula is used to extract the fat. Various cannula designs have been employed.

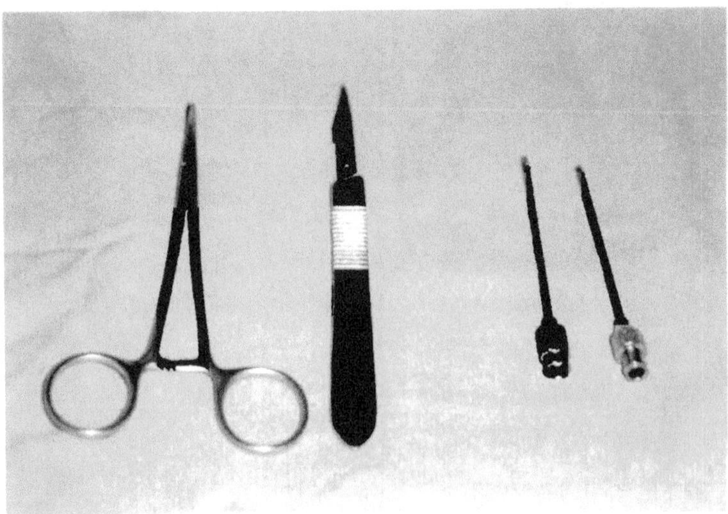

Figure 13 Aspiration equipment required for fat transfer.

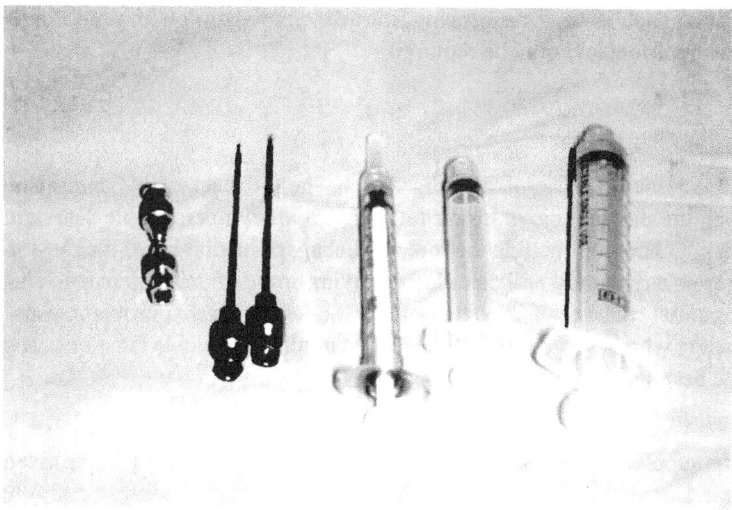

Figure 14 Transfer and infiltration equipment for fat transfer.

b. Anesthesia

The lipoaspiration begins with appropriate anesthesia of the donor site. This is best performed with a modified tumescent technique. To normal saline or Ringer's solution lidocaine is added to a concentration of 0.1% and epinephrine to 1:1,000,000. Typically, a liter of solution will contain 50 mL of 2% lidocaine and 1 mL of 1:1000 epinephrine. Other additives often used in tumescent liposuction, such as bicarbonate and steroids, are best omitted. After tumescence with pump, syringes, or other infiltration device such as a pressurized bag and lipoinfiltration cannula, the area is given time for both the anesthesia and hemostatic effects to be maximized. Intradermal anesthesia is infiltrated at sites of cannula insertion in both donor and recipient sites. If the patient is sedated intravenously, this is all that is required. However, if the patient is awake, further small amounts of local anesthetic are infiltrated into the recipient sites. The use of nerve blocks and field blocks in this setting is also laudable. A no. 30 needle is useful for the patient's comfort. If the procedure is

Table 4 Equipment Requirements

Suggested equipment	Comment
Local anesthetic solution	Ringer's or normal saline with 0.1% lidocaine and 1:1,000,000 epinephrine
Introducing cannula for tumescent anesthesia	No. 14–18 spinal needle or "shower" type
Lipoaspiration cannula	No. 13–14 blunt cannula
Syringes	1, 3, 10 mL
Rack	To hold syringes inverted after fat removal
Centrifuge	Low-revolution machine (3000 rpm) to separate fat further (optional)
Lipoinjection cannula	No. 14–19 needle for fat reinjection

part of a larger operation such as laser resurfacing, intravenous sedation with propofol or midazolam with or without fentanyl may be required.

c. Donor Site

In females the lower abdomen is a useful site (Fig. 15), as the fat is accessible and this is often an area in which the patient enjoys losing fat. One to three imperceptible scars are usually left as a legacy. Other sites include the hip, saddlebag, or medial knee. It is best in these areas to look for an asymmetry and elect for removing some of the larger side. This is important if a substantial fat transfer is contemplated. Males are often a problem, especially the asthenic patient who has a gaunt appearance and minimal available fat stores. The lower abdomen is the best bet in these patients.

3. *Procedure*

Tumescent infiltration supplemented with local anesthetic at the insertion sites is employed as described earlier. Local anesthetic consisting of 1% lidocaine with 1:100,000 epinephrine is injected at the insertion points. If this is to be a local anesthetic procedure alone, then supplemental sublingual diazepam, 5–10 mg, may be employed 30 minutes before the operation.

Once adequate local anesthesia and hemostasis with tumescence have been induced, one should wait as long as one can for the fluid to redistribute. This will decrease the fluid that will need to be decanted or centrifuged from the fat at a later stage. Waiting 15–30 minutes after infiltration is very useful.

The suction cannula is then attached to a 10-mL syringe. If the cannula is sharp, this is inserted through the skin at this point. However, if the cannula is blunt, a small nick with an awl or a blade (no. 11 or 15) is performed (Fig. 16). The cannula is inserted and the plunger is pulled back when the tip is in the correct plane. The plunger is pulled back in a fairly gentle fashion with the forefinger and thumb (Fig. 17) and maintained in this re-

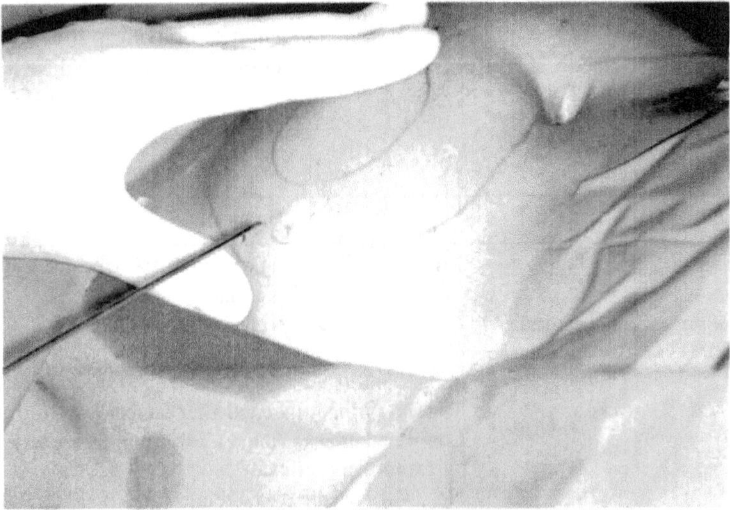

Figure 15 Lower abdominal donor site tumesced.

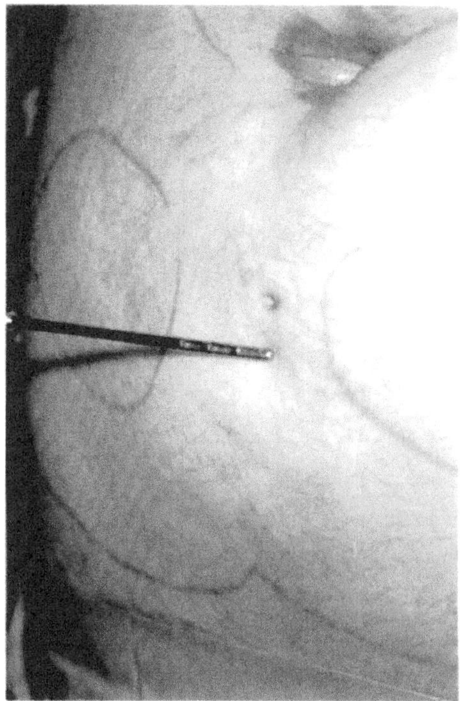

Figure 16 Nick in skin for aspiration cannula insertion.

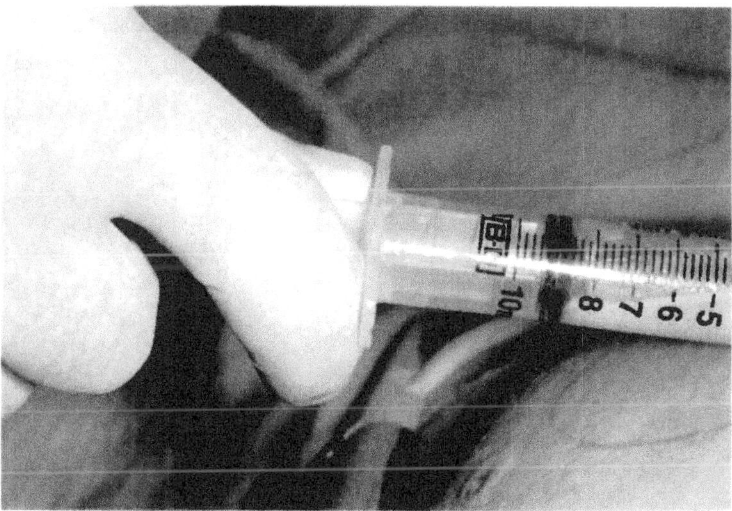

Figure 17 Syringe being retracted with forefinger and thumb.

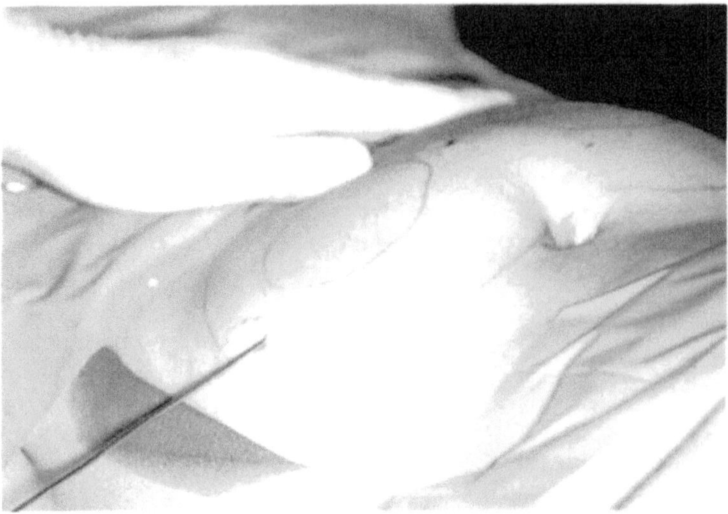

Figure 18 Nondominant "smart" hand in position.

tracted position, exerting mild negative pressure. The cannula is moved backward and forward as in a normal liposuction procedure with the nondominant hand in a position to know at all times where the tip of the cannula lies (Fig. 18). The nondominant hand is also responsible as in usual liposuction for assessing the evenness of the procedure and any local fat pockets that may need addressing. The late Sam Stegman appropriately termed the nondominant hand the smart hand. One should aim to keep the donor area smooth and ripple free and the area should be crisscrossed from two directions. In a short period of time, 10 mL of yellow fat and fluid will be collected (Fig. 19). The syringe is detached and another

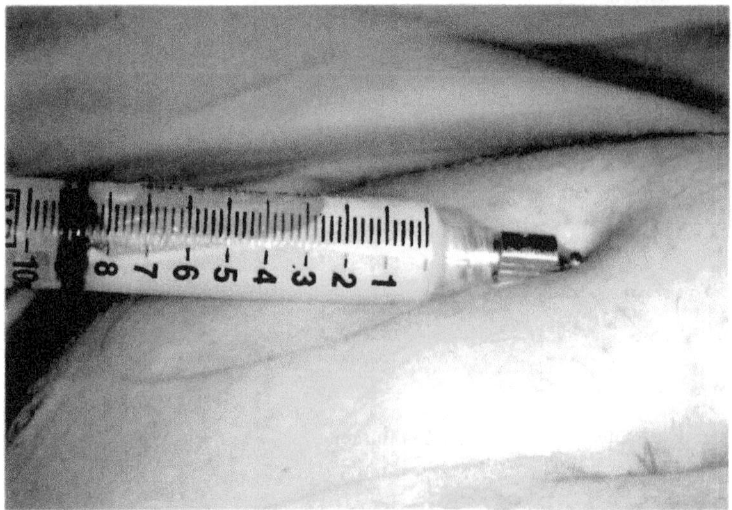

Figure 19 Fat being collected in 10-mL syringe.

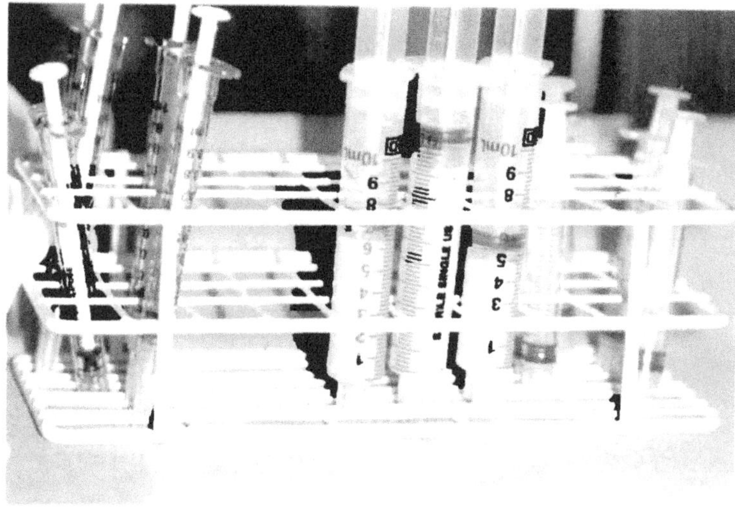

Figure 20 Inverted syringes containing fat standing in rack ready for transfer.

empty 10-mL syringe substituted. This is repeated until adequate fat is harvested for the procedure. A reserve amount of fat is also harvested and is frozen for any touch-ups that may be necessary.

The individual syringes are capped and inverted in a rack so that their tips are pointing down (Fig. 20). Alternatively, they may be centrifuged with a low revolutionary rate of approximately 3000 rpm, although the author prefers to keep the trauma and the steps in this procedure to a minimum and rarely uses this machine for the procedure. It is useful, however, if one has a great deal of blood in the aspirate or for separation of the material before freezing.

After some 5 minutes, the fat has separated from the fluid in the rack and is ready for transfer to smaller syringes. The infranatant fluid comprises local anesthetic solution and occasionally some blood-tinged fluid and is simply squirted out of the syringe into a collecting bowl after the cap is removed and discarded (Fig. 21). Remaining in the syringe are fat and a small amount of oil from disrupted adipocytes (Fig. 22).

The transfer is performed best by a closed system via a Luer-Lok–to–Luer-Lock adaptor (Byron, Tucson, AZ). Others have suggested that the fat should be washed with various substances either in the syringe or laid out on gauze. I feel that a sensitive graft tissue such as fat should not be traumatized, exposed to desiccation or the risks of infection. With the tumescent technique the fat is automatically being washed in the process of extraction and would appear not to require any more washing than this. If the fat is quite blood tinged, it is possibly an indication for washing gently within the syringe with some sterile saline or Ringer's lactate solution. The procedure should remain a closed transfer from the donor site to the recipient site. There appears little evidence at present to support any extra processes beyond what is described here. The fat is transferred via this adaptor into smaller 1- and 3-mL syringes for reinjection. Again, these are left to stand inverted and the infranatant decanted. A small amount of oil will be seen in the top of the fat column as a glistening yellow substance. This is left in the 10-mL syringe and discarded. Similarly, if any

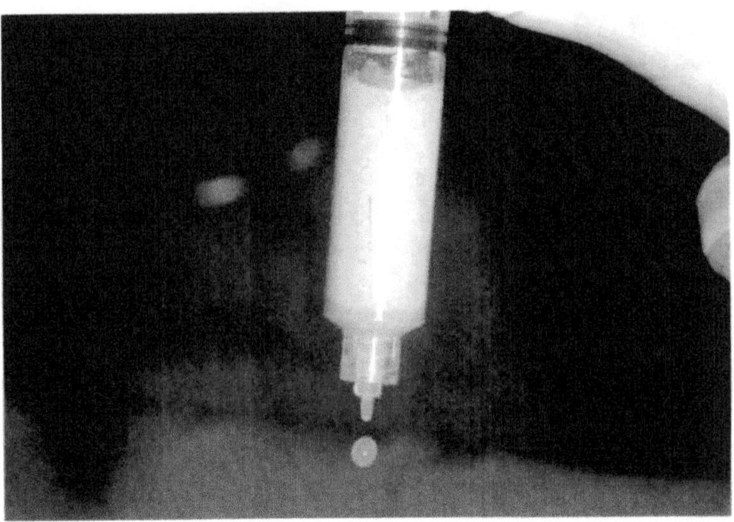

Figure 21 Separated contents of syringe being expelled from syringe.

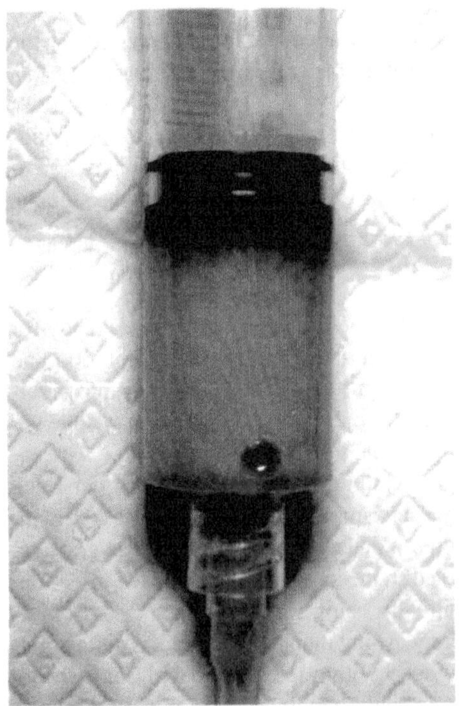

Figure 22 Fat after removal of fluid.

oil is seen in the top of the 1- or 3-mL syringe, this is not injected into the patient. It is my policy not to inject the last 5–10% of the syringe contents, so this oil, which has been said to be an irritant, is not injected.

Fat is injected into the premarked injection sites (Fig. 23) from a sensitively selected insertion site in a natural skin crease or fold. The nick can be very small and is made with a no. 11 blade or similar instrument. The cannula or another blunt instrument may be used at this point as an undermining or "Subcision" (24) tool to break up the scar tissue and release it from its attachments to deeper tissues (Fig. 24). Sharp undermining instruments are probably best avoided, especially if one is undermining larger areas. Besides the inadvertent injury to facial structures, the bruising that may occur may be cosmetically unacceptable. This bruising may also interfere with graft survival.

The lipoinjection may be fed through a small no. 18 cannula as long as a 1- or 3-mL syringe is used. Guns and other injection devices are not ideal for this procedure, as they are too unpredictable in their injection pressures and volumes. Fat is best injected as a three-dimensional lattice of 0.1–0.3-mL aliquots built up to support the more superficial skin layers. This insertion of small amounts of fat is more likely to survive than a large bolus, as it remains closer to its available blood supply. The smaller syringes, especially the 1-mL tuberculin-type syringe, allow the finest control of the injection volume (Fig. 25). The smaller volume syringes are especially well suited to filling smaller defects.

Postoperatively the patient should immobilize the augmented area, refraining from eating, drinking, smiling, and talking for 3–4 hours. Patients are given antibiotics for 6 days

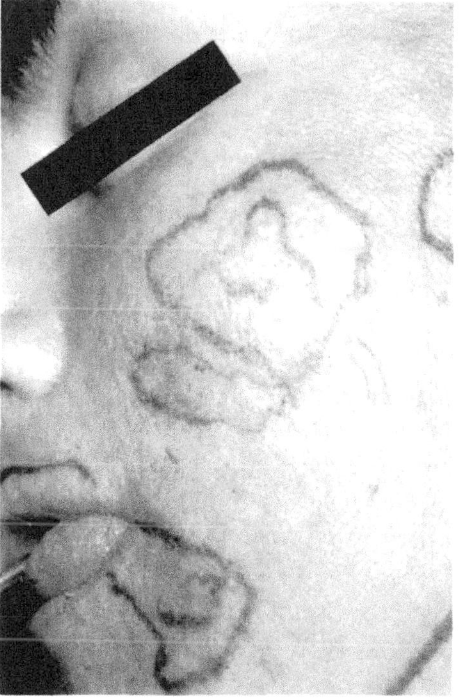

Figure 23 Preoperative recipient site markings.

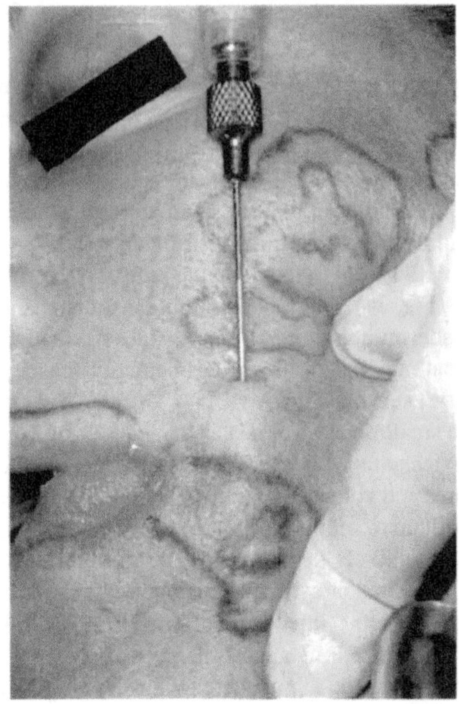

Figure 24 Subcision of scars with the blunt lipoinfiltration cannula.

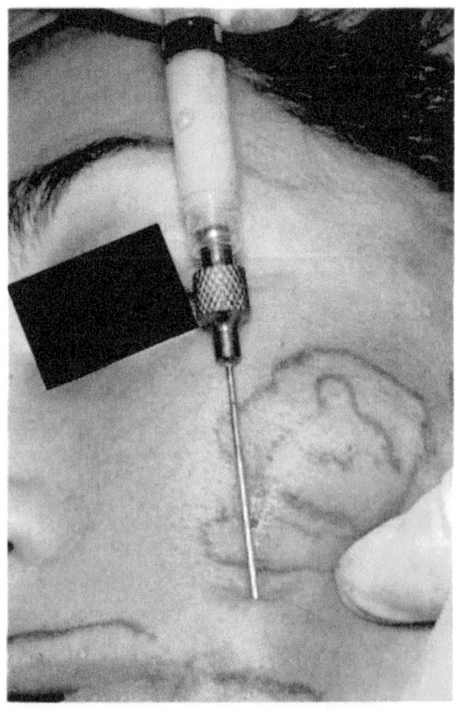

Figure 25 Insertion of fat via small syringes allows most accurate placement.

beginning 1 day preoperatively. Some authors use ice packs, but I do not find the incidence of ecchymosis high enough with blunt cannulas to require these.

4. Results and Complications

Nonsurvival of the grafted fat may be expected to occur to some degree in most if not all fat transfers. Some fat is disrupted, unable to recover; some just fails to develop a blood supply. This percentage seems technique and practitioner sensitive. In general terms, 40–80% survival would appear to be the general range of expectations. Coleman (19) noted no fat resorption in 400 patients whose nasolabial folds were injected with many years of careful follow-up study. This is in contrast to the experience of Ersek (18), who found the longevity of fat transfer disappointing with possibly only 10% survival being noted at 2 years and virtually no survival in acne pits after 6 weeks. It would be prudent for the fat transferrer to suggest to his or her patients that some fat may disappear and some will be permanent and that some further fat transfers may be required to top up the result. In the author's experience approximately 10–20% of patients require further top-up procedures.

Overcorrection should be kept to a minimum, certainly no more than 10–20% above the desired correction. There will be some loss of volume as the fluid and oil not removed during the separation process are lost. Above this fat is quite often a long-term corrective implant and overfilling can become a difficult problem. One cannot just suction the extra fat, as it does not exist as a single bolus but is a lattice among the host tissues. So undercorrection is probably a safer endpoint than overcorrection. The residual fat may always be frozen, and this frozen fat may be used for up to 6 months after the procedure for any residual or resorbed areas. Prolonged storage may risk infection and the fat must be at least visually inspected before use. If the fat is discolored, it should be discarded.

Complications are few. Swelling is virtually universal and usually mild. However, swelling is more prominent with the multiple tunneling technique. Bruising is not very common with the blunt technique. Infection has not been seen, but asepsis and a closed transfer technique are recommended. Antibiotics should also be used. Blindness has been reported with glabellar fat transfer (57), presumably following inadvertent intravascular injection of vessels communicating with the retinal vasculature. When injecting in this area it would thus seem prudent to use blunt cannulas, to use low-pressure injections of small aliquots of fat, and to inject on withdrawal of the cannula.

Some results are shown in Figs. 26–31 for patients who have had fat transfer for scarring.

VIII. COMMENTS ON COMBINING TECHNIQUES

With scarring, techniques are often combined, with CO_2 or erbium laser resurfacing, dermal grafts, fat transfer, and punch grafting and excisions being useful together. These procedures may be performed in a single operative session, but a logical sequence is best followed.

The steps required are as follows:

1. Relevant marking and anesthesia.
2. While waiting for tumescence to take effect, dermal grafts may be inserted.
3. Fat transfer is then performed to premarked areas.

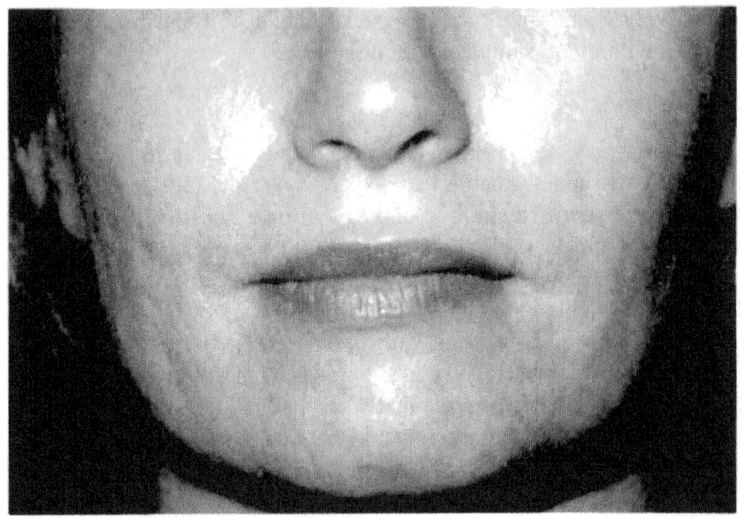

Figure 26 Patient before fat transfer.

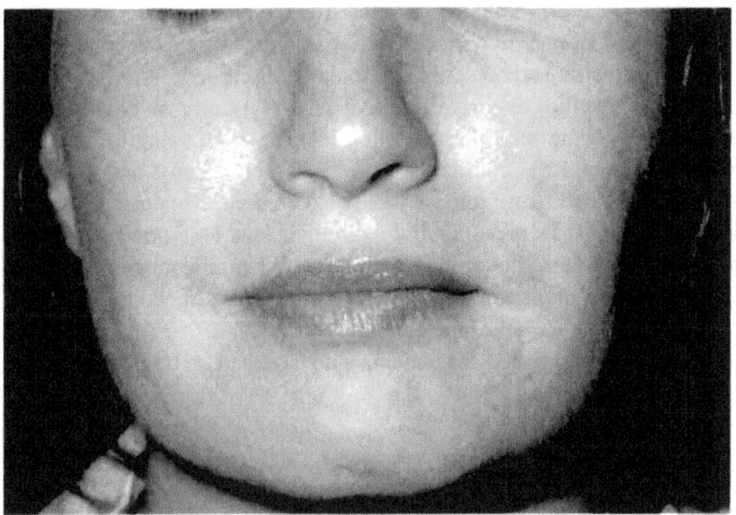

Figure 27 Patient 3 months after fat transfer.

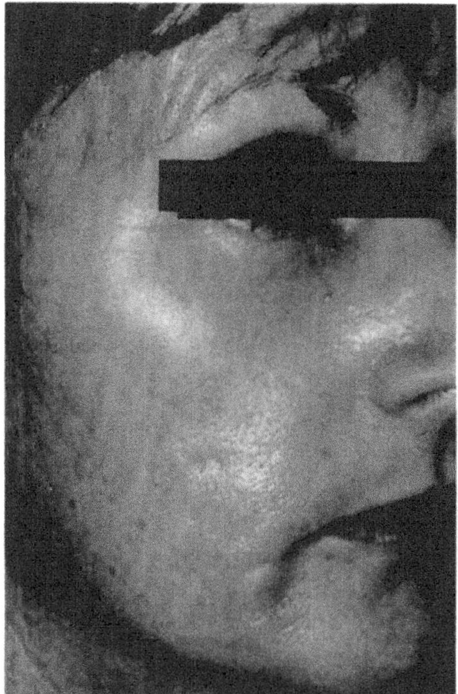

Figure 28 Patient before fat transfer.

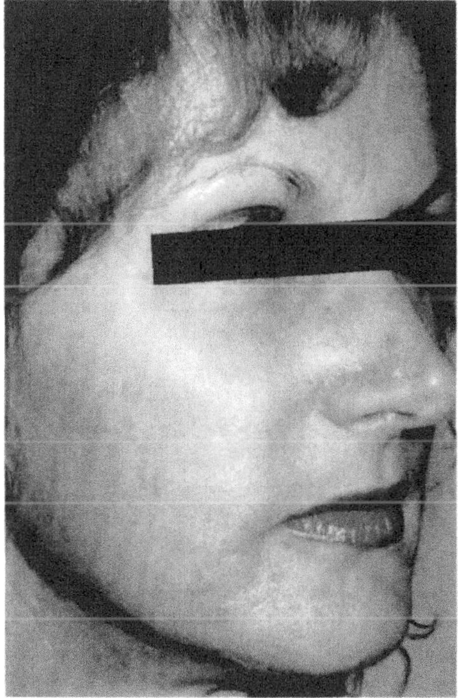

Figure 29 Patient 6 weeks after fat transfer.

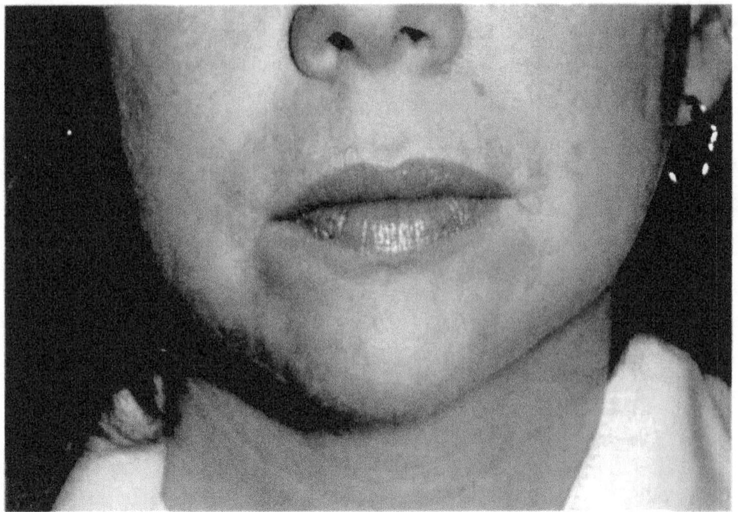

Figure 30 Patient before fat transfer.

4. CO_2 or erbium laser resurfacing is then performed.
5. At the end of this stage remaining punched-out scars are sized and appropriate punch grafts or excisions are employed if required.

Some patients who have had a combination of fat and/or dermal grafting with resurfacing performed are shown in Figs. 31–43. Figures 44–47 show the desired amount of correction one should aim for at the 5-day mark (Figs. 43 and 44) and the 3-week mark (Figs. 46 and 47) after a combination of resurfacing and fat transfer.

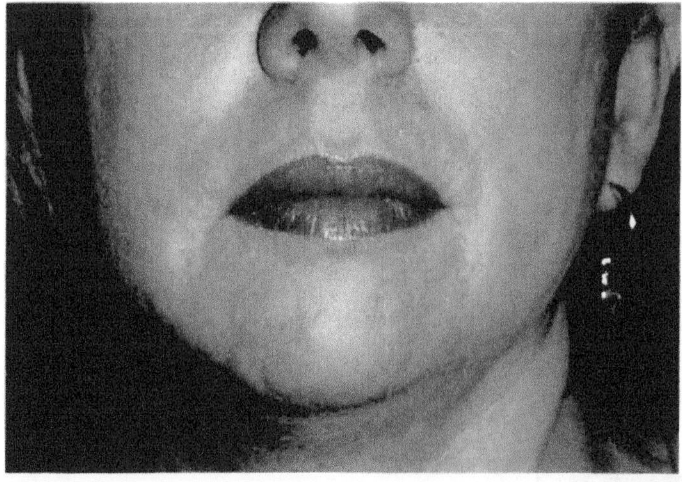

Figure 31 Patient 3 months after fat transfer.

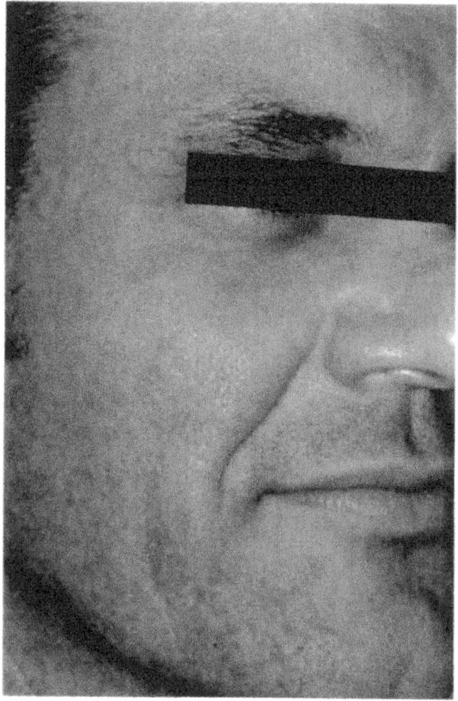

Figure 32 Patient before dermal graft to cheek line and CO_2 laser resurfacing.

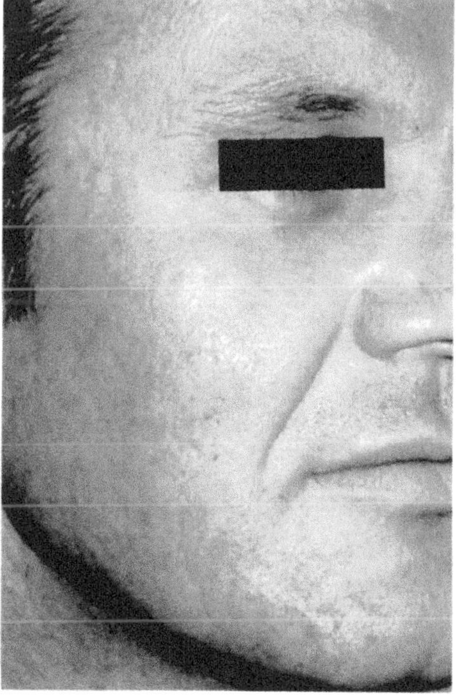

Figure 33 Patient 3 months after dermal graft and resurfacing.

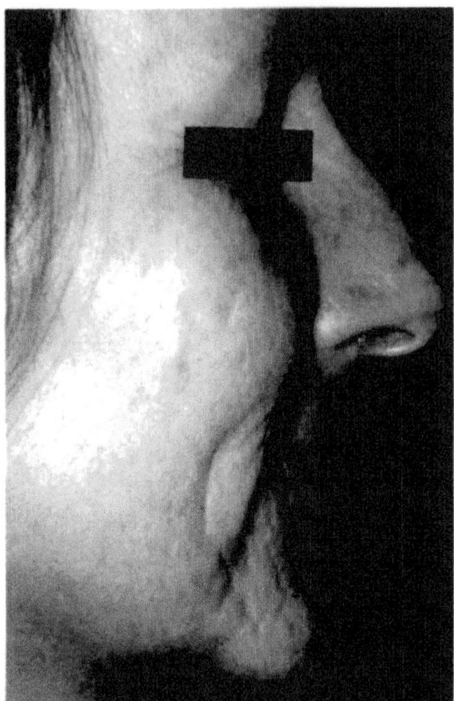

Figure 34 Patient before fat transfer and CO_2 laser resurfacing.

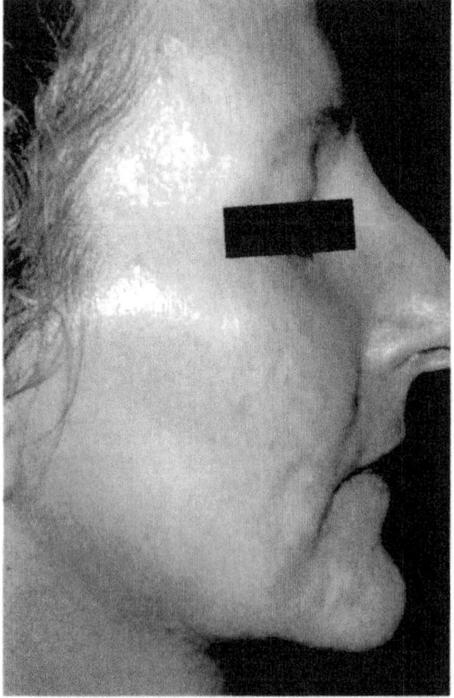

Figure 35 Patient 2 months after fat transfer and CO_2 laser resurfacing.

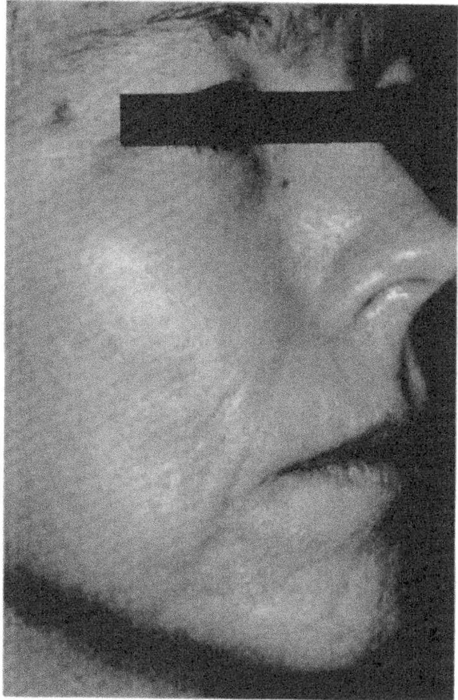

Figure 36 Patient before fat transfer and CO_2 laser resurfacing.

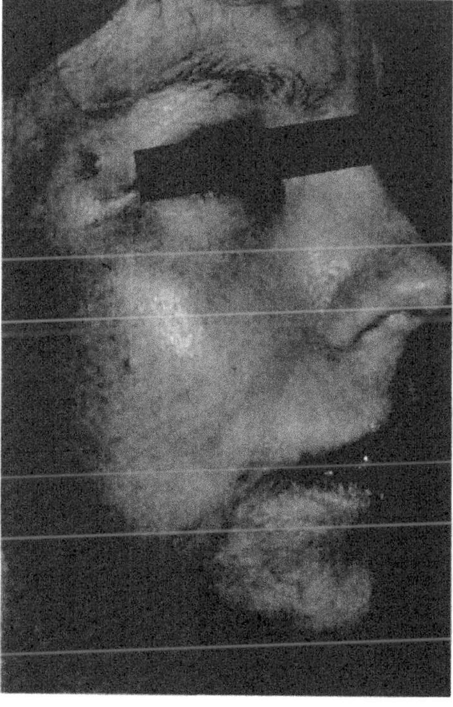

Figure 37 Patient 6 weeks after fat transfer and CO_2 laser resurfacing.

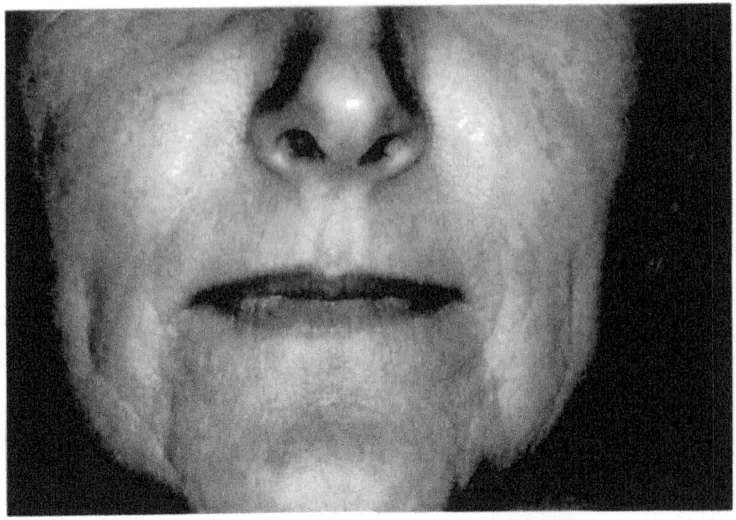

Figure 38 Patient before fat transfer and CO_2 laser resurfacing.

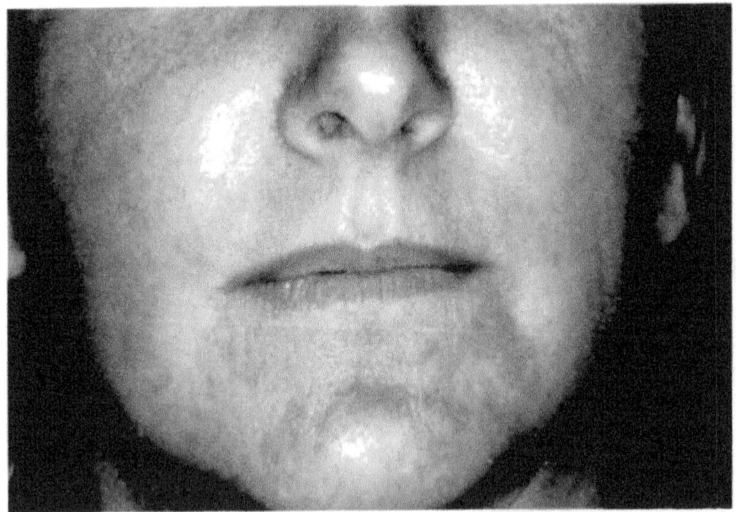

Figure 39 Patient 6 weeks after fat transfer and CO_2 laser resurfacing.

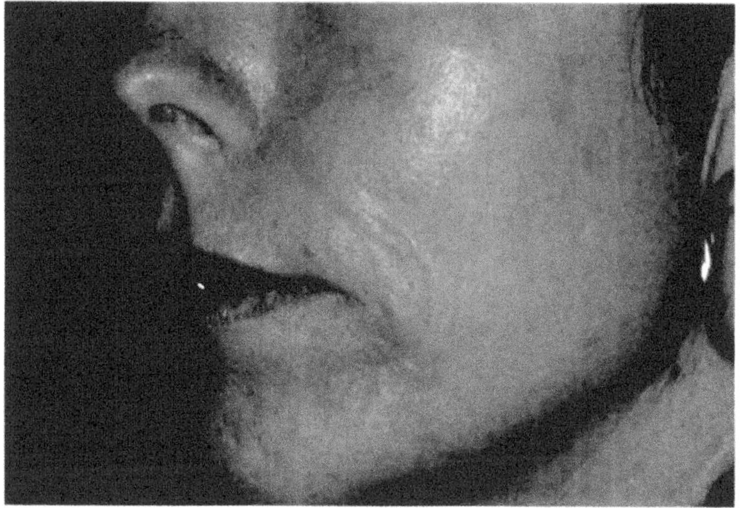

Figure 40 Patient before fat transfer and CO_2 laser resurfacing.

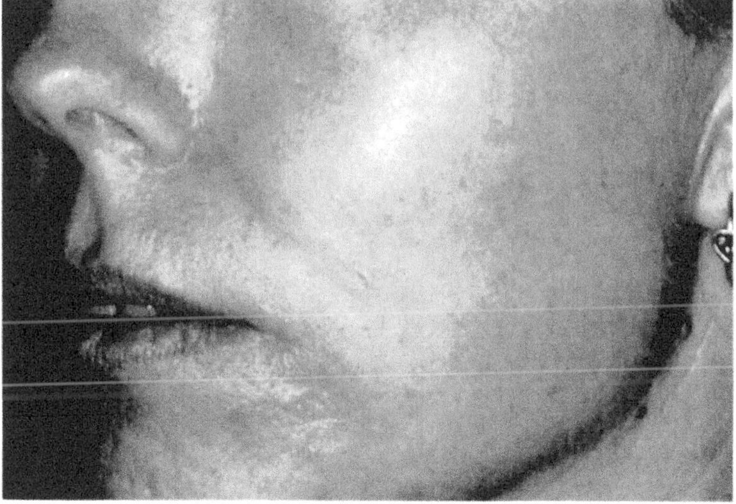

Figure 41 Patient 3 months after fat transfer and CO_2 laser resurfacing.

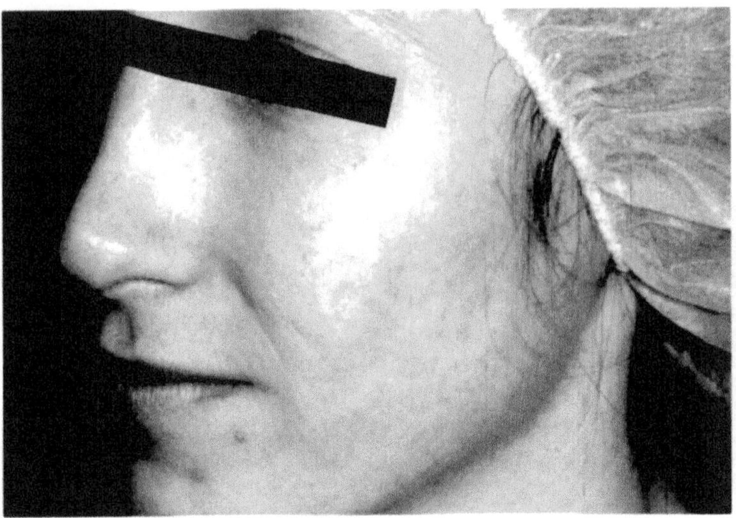

Figure 42 Patient before fat transfer and CO_2 laser resurfacing.

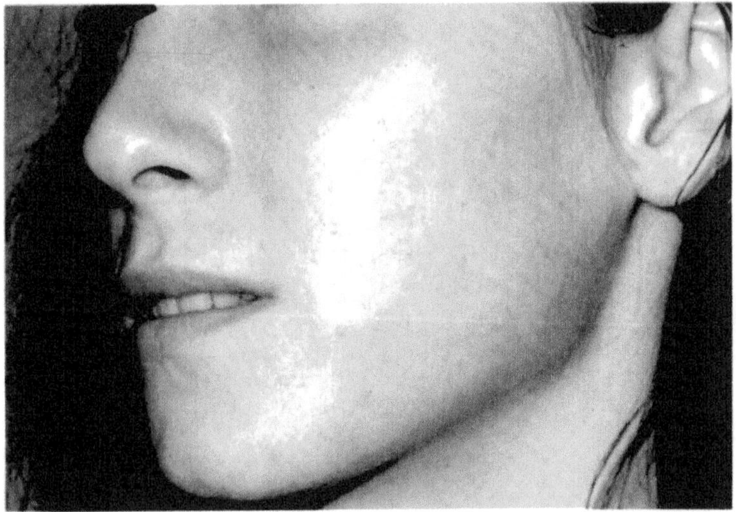

Figure 43 Patient 14 months after fat transfer and CO_2 laser resurfacing.

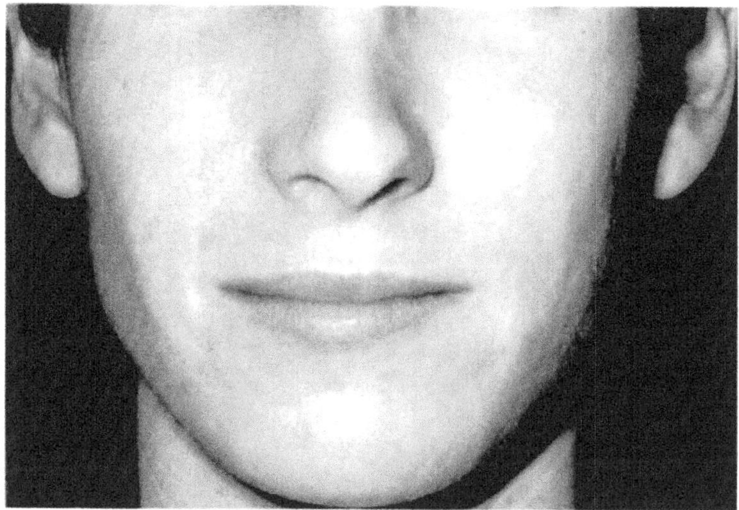

Figure 44 Patient before fat transfer and CO_2 laser resurfacing.

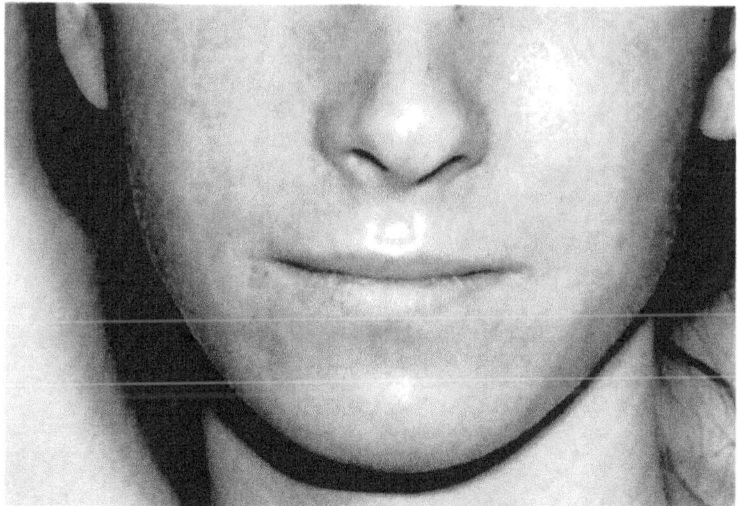

Figure 45 At dressing removal (5 days postoperatively); note lack of overcorrection employed.

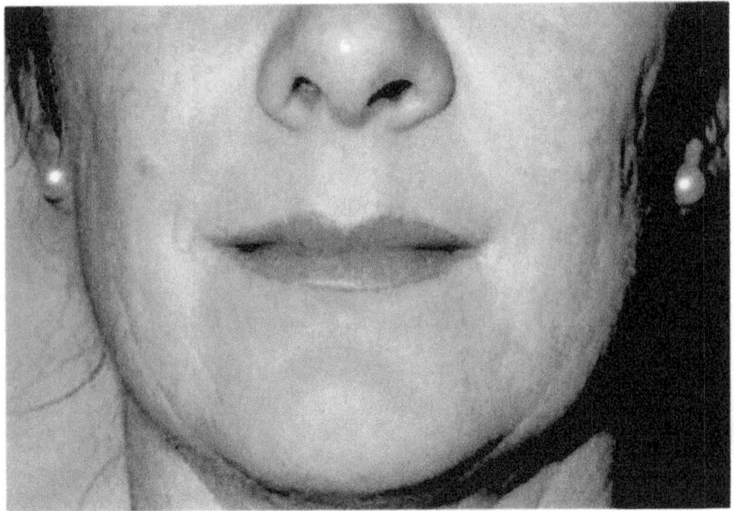

Figure 46 Patient before fat transfer and CO_2 laser resurfacing.

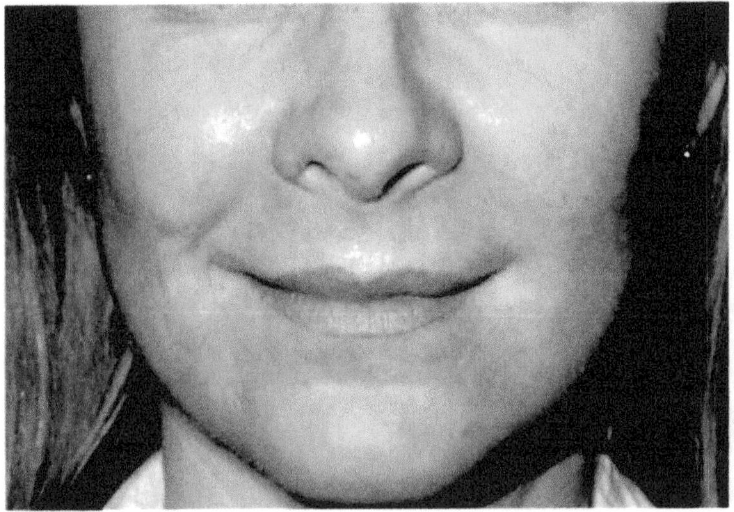

Figure 47 Desired level of correction at 3 weeks postoperative stage.

IX. CONCLUSIONS

Fat transfer and dermal grafting are useful additions to an expanding armamentarium of dermatologic techniques in the treatment of scarring. The scarring and the patient must be appropriate. These substances are grafts, once living tissues that must be nursed back to health. They should be treated gently and carefully to ensure their viability. Some loss of graft tissue may occur, but these procedures show some promise of permanence once true take of the graft occurs. There are some refinements that we hope will further develop these techniques, but they already show many of the characteristics of the perfect filler materials.

REFERENCES

1. Peer LA, Paddock R. Histologic studies on the fate of deeply implanted dermal grafts: observations on sections of implants buried from one week to one year. Arch Surg 1937; 34:268.
2. Bosniak SL. Avoiding complications following primary dermis-fat orbital implantation. Ophthalmol Plast Reconstr Surg 1985; 1:237–241.
3. Wojno T, Tenzel RR. Dermis grafts in socket reconstruction. Ophthalmol Plast Reconstr Surg 1986; 2:7–14.
4. Stewart HM, Hann JR, De Tomasi DC, Neville BW, et al. Histologic fate of dermal grafts following implantation for temporomandibular joint meniscal perforation: a preliminary study. Oral Surg Oral Med Oral Pathol 1986; 62:481–485.
5. Steinberg MJ, Hohn FI. Procurement of dermal graft from the suprapubic or inguinal fold region with primary linear closure. J Oral Maxillofac Surg 1994; 52:813–816.
6. Boering G, Huffstadt AJ. The use of derma-fat grafts in the face. Br J Plast Surg 1965; 20:172.
7. Sawhney CP, Banerjee TN, Chakravarti RN. Behaviour of dermal fat transplants. Br J Plast Surg 1969; 22:169.
8. Swinehart JM. Pocket grafting with dermal grafts: autologous collagen implants for permanent correction of cutaneous depressions. Am J Cosmet Surg 1995; 12:321–331.
9. Abergel RP, Schlaak CM, Garcia LD, et al. The laser dermal implant: a new technique for preparation and implantation of autologous dermal grafts for the correction of depressed scars, lip augmentation, and nasolabial folds using silk touch laser technology Am J Cosmet Surg 1996; 13:15–18.
10. Goodman GJ. Laser assisted dermal grafting for the correction of cutaneous contour defects. Dermatol Surg 1997; 23(2):95–99.
11. Neuber F. Fettransplantation. Bericht uber die Verhandlugen der Deutscen Gesellschaft fur Chrurgie. Zbl Chir 1893; 22:66.
12. Ilouz YG. De l'utilization de la grasse aspiree pour combler les defects cutanes. Rev Chir Esth Langue Fr 1985; 10:13.
13. Ilouz YG. The fat cell graft. A new technique to fill depressions. Plast Reconstr Surg 1986; 78:122.
14. Czerny A. Plastischer Ersatz der Brustdruse durch ein Lipoma. Chir Kongr Verh 1895; 2:216.
15. Cabezudo JM, Lopez A, Bacci F. Symptomatic root compression by a free fat transplant after hemilaminectomy:case report. J Neurosurg 1985; 63:633.
16. Devine HB. Free fat and fascia transplantation in the treatment of ankylosed joints and diseases of the bone. Med J Aust 1914; 1:123.
17. Ellenbogen R. Invited comment on autologous fat injection. Ann Plast Surg 1990; 24:297.
18. Ersek RA. Transplantation of purified autologous fat: a 3-year follow up is disappointing. Plast Reconstr Surg 1991; 87:219–227.
19. Coleman SR. Long-term survival of fat transplants: controlled demonstrations. Aesthetic Plast Surg 1995; 19:421–425.

20. Eppley BL, Snyders RV Jr, Winkelmann T, Delfino JJ. Autologous facial fat transplantation: improved graft maintenance by microbead bioactivation. J Oral Maxillofac Surg 1992; 50:477–482.
21. Pinski KS, Roenigk HH Jr. Autologous fat transplantation. Long term follow-up. J Dermatol Surg Oncol 1992; 18:179–182.
22. Coleman SR. The technique of periorbital lipoinfiltration. Oper Tech Plast Reconstr Surg 1994; 1:120.
23. Orentreich DS. Soft Tissue Augmentation Seminar, Aad, San Francisco, Dec 1992.
24. Orentreich DS, Orentreich N. Subcutaneous incisionless (subcision) surgery for the correction of depressed scars and wrinkles. Dermatol Surg 1995; 21:543–549.
25. Fournier PF. Facial recontouring with fat grafting. Dermatol Clin 1990; 8:523–537.
26. Shiffman MA. Autologous fat transplantation. Am J Cosmet Surg 1997; 14:433–442.
27. Skouge JW. Autologous fat transplantation in facial surgery. Presented at meeting of American Academy of Cosmetic Surgery: Controversies in Breast and Facial Augmentation, Philadelphia, Aug 7–9, 1992.
28. Asken S. Autologous fat transplantation: micro and macro techniques. Am J Cosmet Surg 1987; 4:111–121.
29. Meschik Z. Vitamin E and adipose tissue. Edinburgh Med J 1944; 51:486.
30. Katoes AS Jr, et al. Perfused fat cells: effects of lipolytic agents. J Biol Chem 1933; 248–289.
31. Sidman RL. The direct effect of insulin on organ cultures of brown fat. Anat Rec 1956; 124:723.
32. Solomon SS. Comparative studies of the antilipolytic effect of insulin and adenosine in the perfused fat cell. Horm Metab Res 1980; 12:601.
33. Smith U. Human adipose tissue in culture studies on the metabolic effects of insulin. Diabetologica 1976; 12:137.
34. Solomon SS, Duckworth WC. Effect of antecedent hormone administration on lipolysis in the perfused isolated fat cell. J Lab Clin Med 1976; 88:984.
35. Berdeguer P. Five years of experience using fat for leg contouring. Am J Cosmet Surg 1995; 12:221–229.
36. Krulig E. Lipo-injection. Am J Cosmet Surg 1987; 4:123–129.
37. Lewis CM. The current status of autologous fat grafting. Aesthetic Plast Surg 1993; 17:109–112.
38. Carpaneda C, Ribeiro M. Study of the histologic alterations and viability of the adipose grafts in humans. Aesthetic Plast Surg 1990; 17:43–47.
39. Horl HW, Feller AM, Biemer E. Technique for liposuction fat re-implantation and long term volume evaluation by magnetic resonance imaging. Ann Plast Surg 1991; 26:248–258.
40. Johnson GW. Body contouring by macroinjection of autogenous fat. Am J Cosmet Surg 1987;4: 103–109.
41. Argrus J. Autologous fat transplantation: a 3 year study. Am J Cosmet Surg 1987; 4:95–102.
42. Lexer E. Correcion de los dedulos (Mastoptose) por medio de la implantacion de grasa. San Sebastian Guipuzcoa Media 1921; 63:213. Translated in Hinderer UT, del Rio JL. Erich Lexer's mammaplasty. Aesthetic Plast Surg 1992; 16:101–107.
43. Alster TS. Improvement of erythematous and hypertrophic scars by the 585nm flashlamp-pumped pulse dye laser. Ann Plast Surg 1994; 32:186.
44. Yarborough JN. Scar revision by dermabrasion. In: Roenigk RK, Roenigk HH, eds. Dermatologic Surgery. New York: Marcel Dekker, 1989:909–933.
45. Alt TH, Goodman GJ, Coleman WP, et al. Dermabrasion. In: Coleman WP III, Hanke CW, Alt TH, Asken S, eds. Cosmetic Surgery of the Skin—Principles and Techniques. 2nd ed. St Louis: Mosby-Year Book, 1997:112–151.
46. Goodman GJ. Dermabrasion using tumescent anesthesia. J Dermatol Surg Oncol 1994; 20:802–807.
47. Weinstein C. Carbon dioxide laser resurfacing. In: Coleman WP III, Hanke CW, Alt TH, Asken S, eds. Cosmetic Surgery of the Skin—Principles and Techniques. 2nd ed. St Louis: Mosby-Year Book, 1997:152–177.

48. Goodman GJ. Facial resurfacing using a high-energy, short-pulse carbon dioxide laser. Australas J Dermatol 1996; 37:125–131.
49. Solotoff S. Treatment for pitted acne scarring—postauricular punch grafts followed by dermabrasion. J Dermatol Surg Oncol 1986; 12:1079.
50. Johnson W. Treatment of pitted scars. Punch transplant technique. J Dermatol Surg Oncol 1986; 12:260.
51. Hanke CW, Coleman WP. Dermal filler substances. In: Coleman WP III, Hanke CW, Alt TH, Asken S, eds. Cosmetic Surgery of the Skin—Principles and Techniques. 2nd ed. St Louis: Mosby-Year Book, 1997:217–230.
52. Melton JL, Hanke CW. Soft tissue augmentation. In: Roenigk RK, Roenigk HHR, eds. Dermatologic Surgery. 2nd ed. New York: Marcel Dekker, 1996.
53. Skouge JW, Ratner D. Autologous fat transplantation. In: Coleman WP III, Hanke CW, Alt TH, Asken S, eds. Cosmetic Surgery of the Skin—Principles and Techniques. 2nd ed. St Louis: Mosby-Year Book, 1997:206–216.
54. Peer LA. Loss of weight and volume in human fat grafts. Plast Reconstr Surg 1950; 5:217.
55. Moscona R, Ullman Y, Har-Shai Y, et al. Free fat injections for the correction of facial hemiatrophy. Plast Reconstr Surg 1989; 84:501.
56. Jones JK, Lyles ME. The viability of human adipocytes after closed-syringe liposuction harvest. Am J Cosmet Surg 1997; 14:275–279.
57. Teimourian B. Blindness following fat injections. Plast Reconstr Surg 1988; 82:361.

18
The Overlap Technique

Marwali Harahap
University of North Sumatra Medical School
Medan, Indonesia

M. Reza Perkasa Marwali
Wayne State University
Detroit, Michigan

There is frequent demand for correction of depressed, retracted scars, particularly in the head and neck region. A depressed scar may be due to a chronic fistula resulting from infected teeth, skin infection, injury, or surgery.

I. METHODS

There are many methods for correction of depressed retracted scars. The first contribution was made in 1876 by Buck (1), who employed the following technique: The epidermis and a thin layer of dermis are excised. The wound edges are advanced over the dermal platform, and the scarred subcutaneous tissue is buried under the undermined sutured wound edges, thus correcting the depression (Fig. 1). Similar techniques were described by Poulard (2) in 1918 and Gillies and Millard (3) in 1957.

Flaps of adipose tissue can be utilized to bolster a depressed scar after excision of the scar (4) (Fig. 2) or the subcutaneous fat can be overlapped after undermining superficially and deeply (5) (Fig. 3).

Lewin and Keunen (6) described a modification of Buck's technique. Incisions are made around the scar. The circumcised island, containing the scar, is deepithelialized, and one edge of the scar itself is folded on top of the scar and sutured in place. The opposite edge is folded on top of this. The skin flaps are approximated over the bulk, which consists of scar tissue mass flipped on itself twice (Fig. 4).

To correct the depression adequately I combine the technique of Buck and the overlapping of flaps of adipose tissue so that more subcutaneous bulk is obtained (7). The following cases are illustrative.

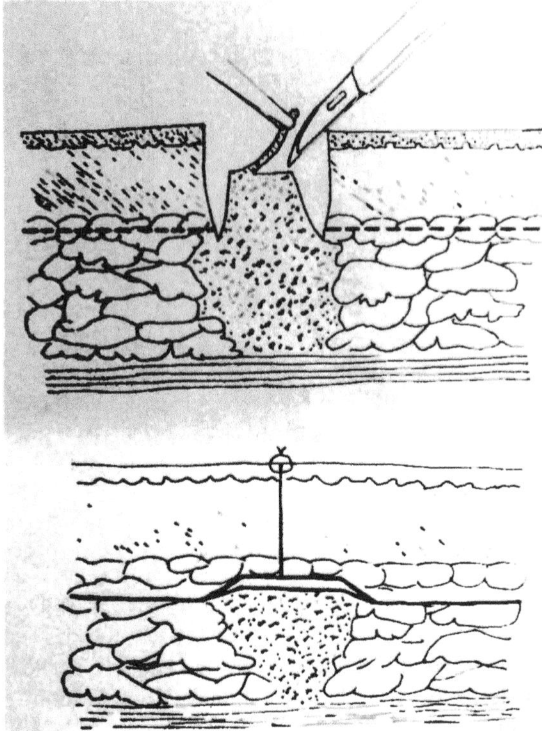

Figure 1 After the epidermis and a thin layer of dermis are excised, the wound edges are advanced over the dermal platform and the scarred subcutaneous tissue are buried under the sutured wound edges. (From Ref. 7.) (Reprinted with permission from J Dermatol Surg Oncol Vol. 10 No. 3, Harahap M: Revision of a depressed scar, pages 207–209, 1984. Elsevier Science, Inc.)

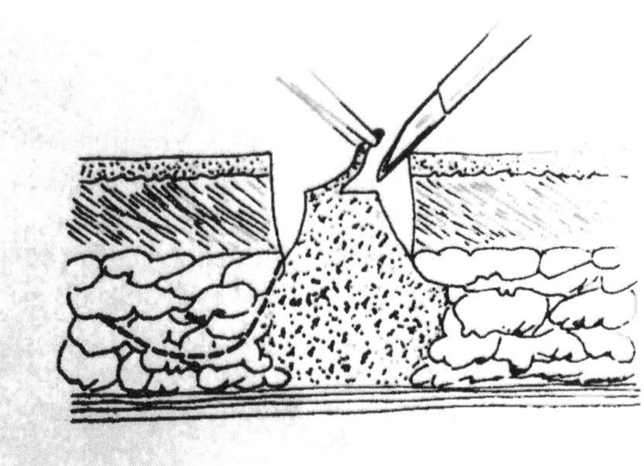

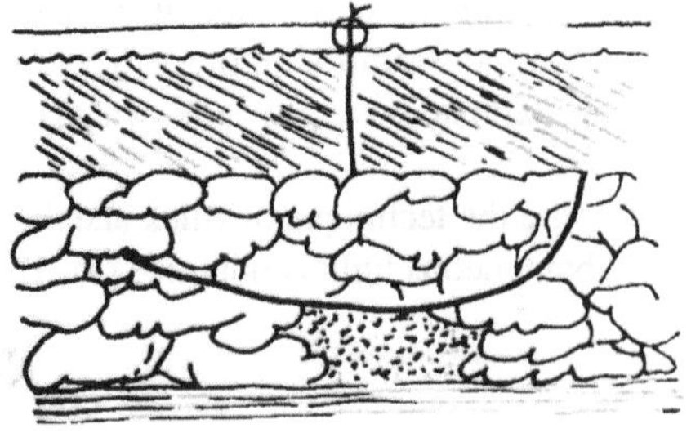

Figure 2 After the scar has been excised, flaps of adipose tissue can be utilized to bolster a depressed scar. (From Ref. 7.) (Reprinted with permission from J Dermatol Surg Oncol Vol. 10 No. 3, Harahap M: Revision of a depressed scar, pages 207–209, 1984. Elsevier Science, Inc.)

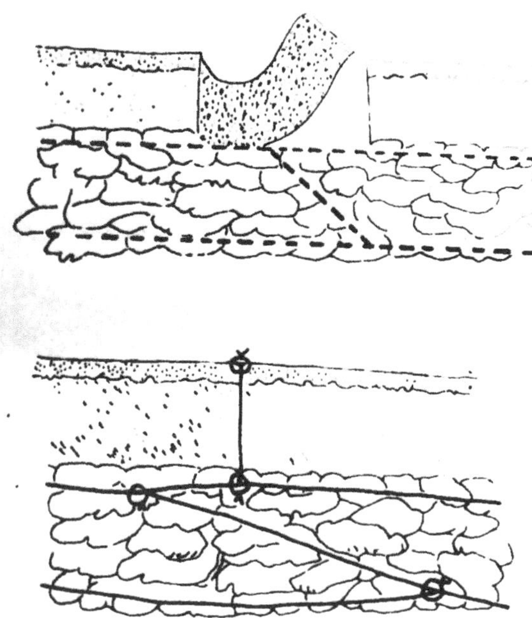

Figure 3 After the scar has been excised, subcutaneous fat is overlapped to cover up the scar. (From Ref. 7.) (Reprinted with permission from J Dermatol Surg Oncol Vol. 10 No. 3, Harahap M: Revision of a depressed scar, pages 207–209, 1984. Elsevier Science, Inc.)

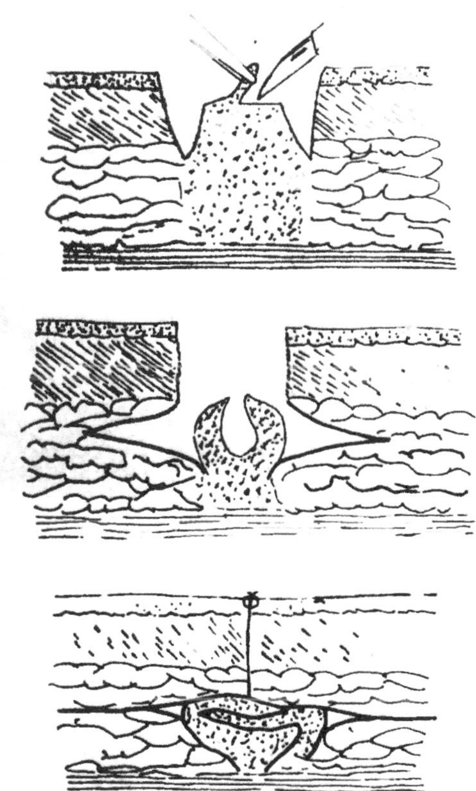

Figure 4 The circumcised island containing the scar is deepithelialized and the edges are brought together on top of one other. The skin flaps are approximated over the bulk. (From Ref. 7.) (Reprinted with permission from J Dermatol Surg Oncol Vol. 10 No. 3, Harahap M: Revision of a depressed scar, pages 207–209, 1984. Elsevier Science, Inc.)

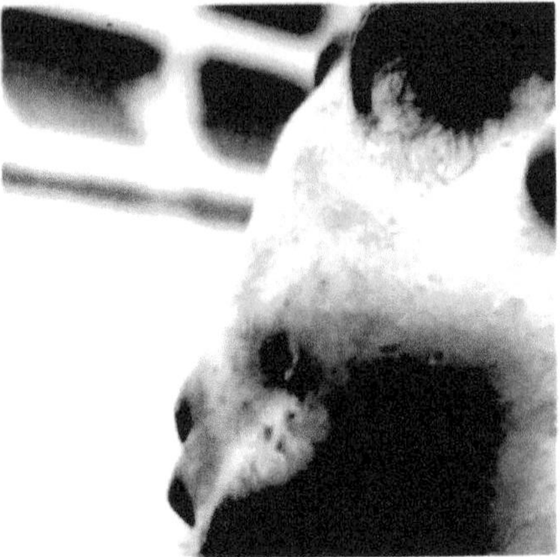

Figure 5 An unsightly dimple or depressed scar on the left cheek. (From Ref. 7.) (Reprinted with permission from J Dermatol Surg Oncol Vol. 10 No. 3, Harahap M: Revision of a depressed scar, pages 207–209, 1984. Elsevier Science, Inc.)

II. CASE REPORTS

A. Case I

The patient, a man aged 32 years, had a history of a chronic draining skin fistula for over a year. When a chronically infected mandibular molar was extracted, the sinus stopped draining. The fistula closed and contracted to the inferior border of the mandible, making an unsightly dimple or depressed scar (Fig. 5).

Fusiform incisions were made around the scar in the natural tension lines of the skin (Fig. 6). The epithelium was dissected from the scar, leaving the dermal component intact. Undermining was carried out both superficially and deeply in the subcutaneous layer. This

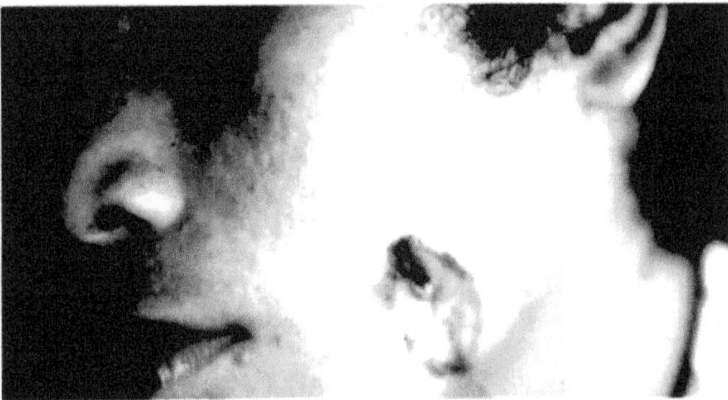

Figure 6 Fusiform incisions are made around the scar in the natural tension lines of the skin. (From Ref. 7.) (Reprinted with permission from J Dermatol Surg Oncol Vol. 10 No. 3, Harahap M: Revision of a depressed scar, pages 207–209, 1984. Elsevier Science, Inc.)

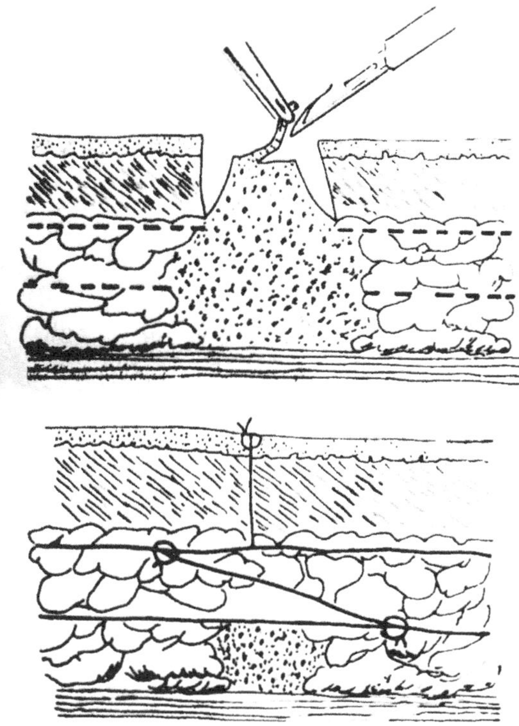

Figure 7 Both flaps of adipose tissue are advanced across the wound to overlap each other and are secured by sutures to cover up the dermal scar. (From Ref. 7.) (Reprinted with permission from J Dermatol Surg Oncol Vol. 10 No. 3, Harahap M: Revision of a depressed scar, pages 207–209, 1984. Elsevier Science, Inc.)

produced flaps of adipose tissue on both sides of the wound. Both flaps of adipose tissue were advanced across the wound to overlap each other and were secured by sutures to cover up the dermal scar (Fig. 7).

The skin edges can be approximated with a subcuticular nylon suture; an additional fine nylon suture is optional. Figures 8 and 9 show the pictures of the patient before and after the operation.

B. Case 2

The patient, a woman aged 36 years, gave a history of fistula in the left cheek over the mandible, present for 2 years. Small quantities of pus accumulated beneath the scab. The drainage ceased when a chronically infected molar was extracted. Closure of the fistula followed, and the sinus contracted to the mandible, resulting in an ugly depression in the skin (Fig. 10).

The same technique of operation was performed on this patient. Figure 11 shows the result of the operation.

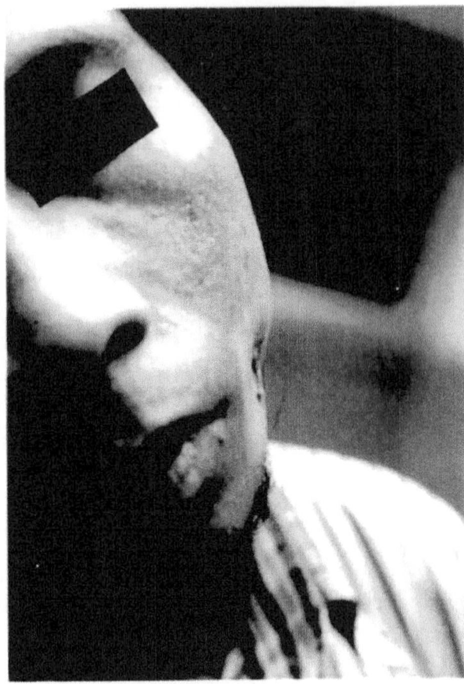

Figure 8 Before the operation. (From Ref. 7.) (Reprinted with permission from J Dermatol Surg Oncol Vol. 10 No. 3, Harahap M: Revision of a depressed scar, pages 207–209, 1984. Elsevier Science, Inc.)

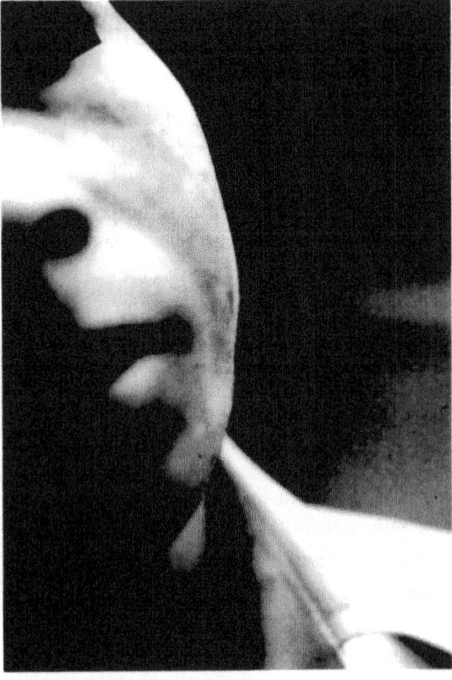

Figure 9 After the operation. (From Ref. 7.) (Reprinted with permission from J Dermatol Surg Oncol Vol. 10 No. 3, Harahap M: Revision of a depressed scar, pages 207–209, 1984. Elsevier Science, Inc.)

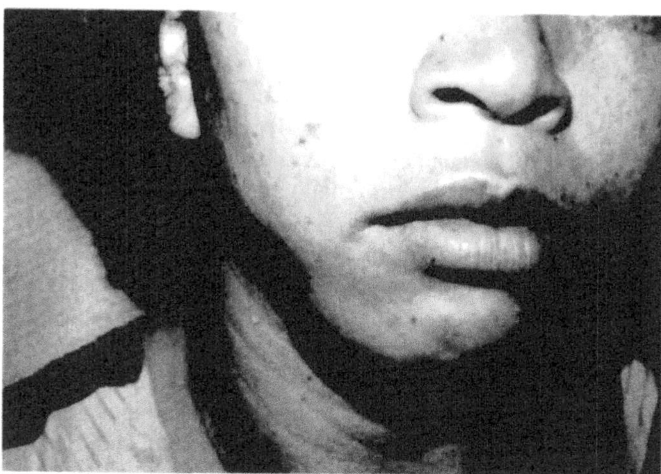

Figure 10 An ugly depression in the skin of the cheek. (From Ref. 7.) (Reprinted with permission from J Dermatol Surg Oncol Vol. 10 No. 3, Harahap M: Revision of a depressed scar, pages 207–209, 1984. Elsevier Science, Inc.)

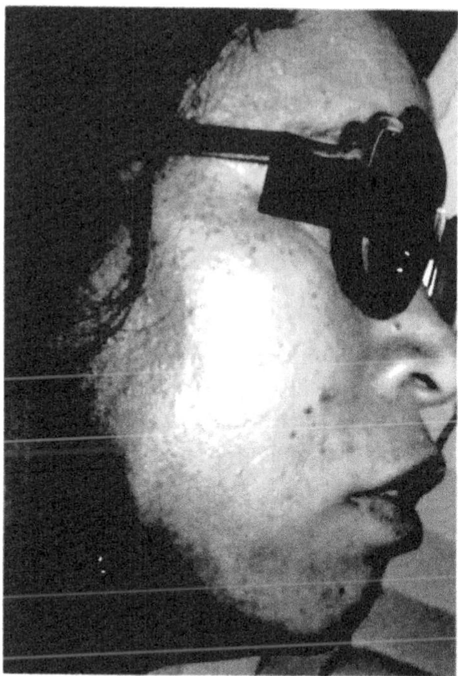

Figure 11 The result of the operation. (From Ref. 7.) (Reprinted with permission from J Dermatol Surg Oncol Vol. 10 No. 3, Harahap M: Revision of a depressed scar, pages 207–209, 1984. Elsevier Science, Inc.)

III. COMPLICATIONS

Surgical revision procedures are subject to all of the usual operative complications (8). Among the general complications, hemorrhage and postoperative hematoma occur most frequently. Good hemostasis is vital before wound closure. A small rubber band drain removed early in the postoperative period (24 to 48 hours) should be used whenever there is likely to be bleeding or seepage of serum.

Another general operative complication shared by scar revision is that of infection. Wound infections generally appear from the fifth to tenth postoperative day, although they may appear earlier. To prevent postoperative infection, the following methods should be used: support of the patient's defenses; gentle, clean surgery; reduction of contamination; and prophylactic antibiotics when indicated. For antibiotics to be effective in the treatment of wound infection, the organism must be identified and the appropriate antibiotic given.

Wound dehiscense is a partial or total disruption of the operative wound. It represents failure of the wound to gain sufficient strength to withstand stress placed upon it. Such wounds are of necessity closed under some tension. Although wound dehiscense may occur at any time following wound closure, it usually occurs between the fifth and eighth days after operation. Tying sutures too tightly strangulates wound circulation and is probably the most common technical error leading to dehiscence. Wound dehiscence is best managed by prompt elective reclosure of the incision.

Some patients are allergic to catgut following the use of subcutaneous or subcuticular catgut suture. The wound may drain from several spots and dicharge catgut from the wound in repeated chronic sterile abscesses, or catgut sutures can be extracted from beneath the draining points.

IV. DISCUSSION

Because scar tissue is devoid of sebaceous glands and hair follicles, sebaceous secretions and hair growth do not occur, complications one might expect if unscarred skin were buried.

It may be expedient to use fat as a flap that carries its own blood supply. Flaps of fatty tissue tend to retain their original bulk. Fat may be undermined and shifted with a permanent pedicle from adjacent fatty areas to fill depressions such as depressed scars; the marginal skin and subcutaneous fat are then undermined and sutured over the flap of fatty tissue to provide an even contour (9).

REFERENCES

1. Buck G. Contributions to Reparative Surgery. New York: Appleton, 1876.
2. Poulard A. Traitement des cicatrices faciales. Presse Med 1918; 26:221.
3. Gillies SH, Millard DR Jr. The Principles and Art of Plastic Surgery. Vol. I. Boston: Little, Brown, 1957:75.
4. Converse JM. Kanzanjian and Converse's Surgical Treatment of Facial Injuries. 3rd ed. Vol. I. Baltimore: Williams & Wilkins, 1974:472.
5. Lewis JR Jr. Atlas of Aesthetic Plastic Surgery. Boston: Little, Brown, 1973:8.

6. Lewin ML, Keunen HF. Revision of the posttracheotomy scar. Correction of the depressed, retracted scar. Arch. Otolaryngol 1970; 91:395.
7. Harahap M. Revision of a depressed scar. J. Dermatol Surg Oncol 1984; 10:206–209.
8. Harahap M. Fusiform excision with primary closure. In: Harahap M, ed. Complications of Dermatologic Surgery. Berlin: Springer Verlag, 1993:137–159.
9. Converse JM. Reconstructive Plastic Surgery. 2nd ed. Vol. 1. Philadelphia: Saunders, 1977:261, 472.

19

Fusiform Excision and Serial Excisions

Eckart Haneke
Wuppertal Hospitals Ltd.; Clinical Health Center, University of Witten/Herdecke; and Academic Teaching Hospital of Heinrich, Heine University of Düsseldorf
Wuppertal, Germany

Fusiform excisions are now relatively rarely discussed among the options of surgical scar revisions; however, in daily practice they are quite often used. Serial excisions, once commonplace procedures, virtually disappeared from the literature—but not in practice—after skin expansion became a more fashionable approach. However, the complication rate of skin expansion is still high, it may cause considerable morbidity during the period of inflation, and expanders are quite costly. Thus, fusiform excisions, whether performed as a one-step or multistep procedure, still occupy a very important place in dermatologic surgical scar revision. Fusiform excisions obey the rule that the simplest closure is the best and therefore scars left from fusiform excisions often have the characteristics of an "ideal" scar: they are flat and level with the surrounding skin; they are a good color match with the adjacent skin; they run parallel to the relaxed skin tension lines (RSTLs); they remain narrow; and short excisions are without straight, unbroken lines that can be easily followed with the eye (1). However, even the seemingly simplest method of surgical scar revision such as fusiform excision is not a "quick fix" for a complicated problem such as an unsightly scar (2). Scars amenable to revision by fusiform and serial excisions are widened, hypertrophied, webbed, pincushioned, and pitted. Often, a sequence of different procedures is necessary to achieve an optimal result.

I. PITTED SCARS

Pitted scars are common sequelae of acne vulgaris. They are usually not amenable to collagen injections and any ablative technique. Apart from punch elevation and transplantation techniques, fusiform excisions often give excellent postoperative results.

The skin is stretched perpendicular to the RSTL (Fig. 1a). Using a no. 11 scalpel, the scar pit is excised with stabbing motions of the pointed blade. This results in a linear excision with straight-line closure (3) being placed along the RSTL. Although using a punch is

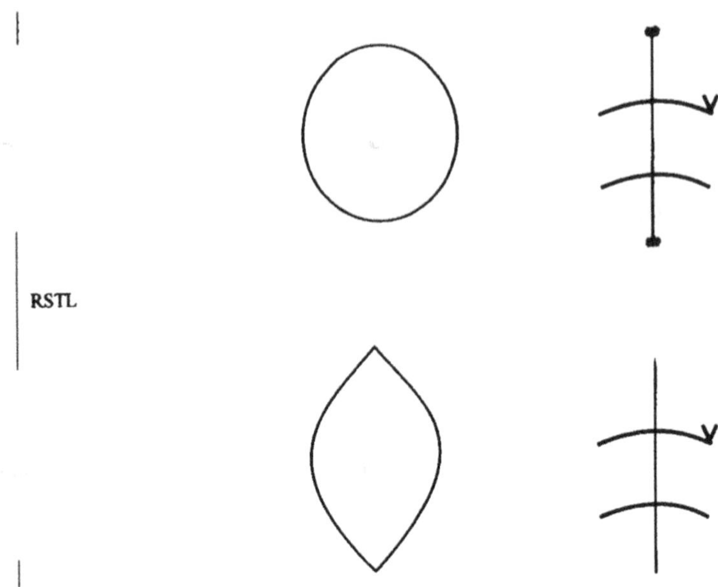

Figure 1 Punch excision versus fusiform excision of ice-pick acne scars. Upon stretching the skin perpendicular to the relaxed skin tension lines before punching the scar out, an oval defect will result, which in most cases gives a satisfactory result but may end up with tiny dog-ears. A fusiform excision prevents dog-ear formation.

usually quicker than using the scalpel, the latter ensures wound angles of approximately 30 degrees so that closure is more aesthetic (Fig. 1). The small fusiform or rhombic defect can easily be closed using 6-0 monofil resorbable material for buried dermal sutures; when the defect is very small it may be difficult to place buried stitches, and percutaneous sutures with 7-0 nonabsorbable material may be a good alternative. However, a good bite of the deep dermal layer must also be taken in order to stretch the entire dermis evenly. A buried backstitch suture has proved to be of great value because it can be used in regions or wounds where the wound edges cannot be sufficiently everted during suture to avoid wound margin inversion (Fig. 2). Care has to be taken to evert the skin and close the wound with precise alignment of tissue layers (see Fig. 5). Steri-strips support the skin suture and allow early removal of the stitches. They should be left in place for 10 days or more in order to avoid scar spread.

Often, many pitted scars lie close together. Multiple pits may be excised in the same session when the excisions can be placed along a line parallel to an RSTL. Removal of several scar pits that are situated perpendicular to the RSTL may result in skin tension and scar dehiscence. To avoid scar spread of excisions lying close together, one vertical mattress suture may be used for two parallel excisions. For this far-far-near-near suture, the needle is inserted at the outer wound margin of the first excision, runs under the bridge of skin between the excisions, exits far from the margin of the second excision, reenters the skin nearer to that margin to exit in the upper dermis of this wound, is carried through the bridge of skin at exactly the same level, and enters the outer margin of the first in the upper dermal level to exit near the wound. On tying the suture, both defects are closed and suture of

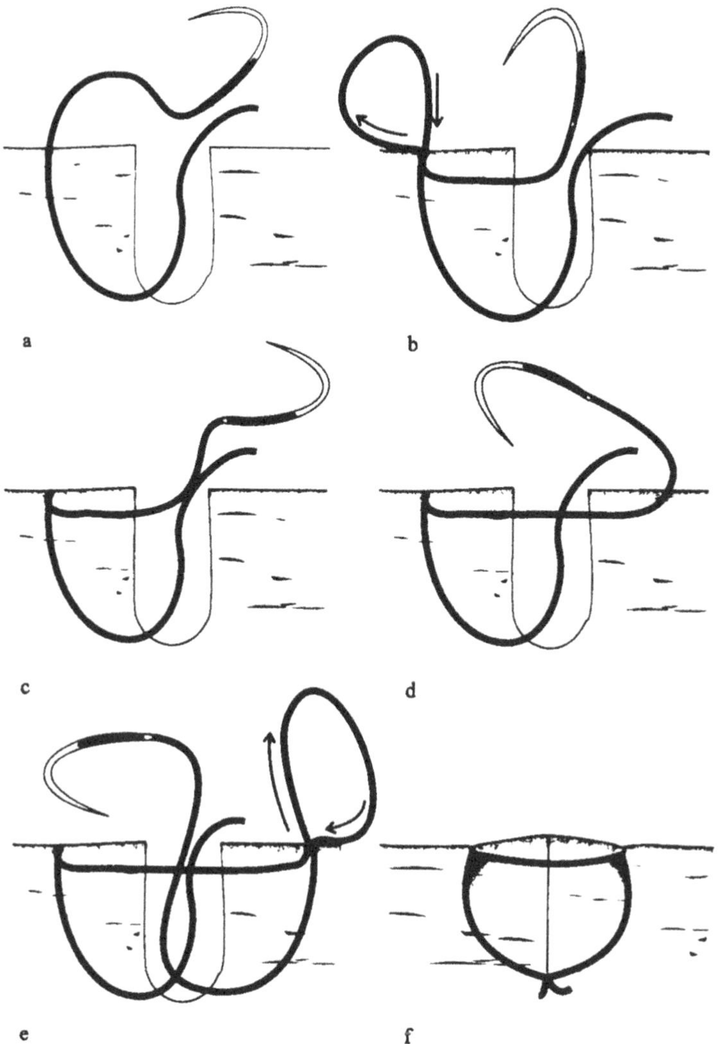

Figure 2 Buried backstitch suture for eversion of wound edges. **(a)** The needle is inserted into the dermis from its undersurface and exits about 5 mm from the wound edge. **(b)** The needle is inserted into the skin through its preceding exit point and carried to the wound margin at the border between the papillary and reticular dermis to exit in the wound edge. **(c)** The suture disappears in the papillary dermis when pulled tight. **(d)** The needle is inserted into the opposite wound margin at the same level as in the former one to exit again 5 mm from the edge. **(e)** The needle is entered into the last exit point behind the thread in order to avoid cutting it and exits at the undersurface of the dermis. **(f)** The suture is pulled tight and knotted; two little dimples on the skin surface remain for a few days but will soon disappear completely.

one excision cannot cause spread of the other one lying next to it (Fig. 3). However, a slight depression of the entire area of pitted scars may result when too many pits are excised with one procedure, thus causing a poor result. Serial excisions of pits are recommended to avoid this distortion. The speed with which the multiple-step procedure can be performed depends on the size and location of the scars and the age of the patient. It is known that in chil-

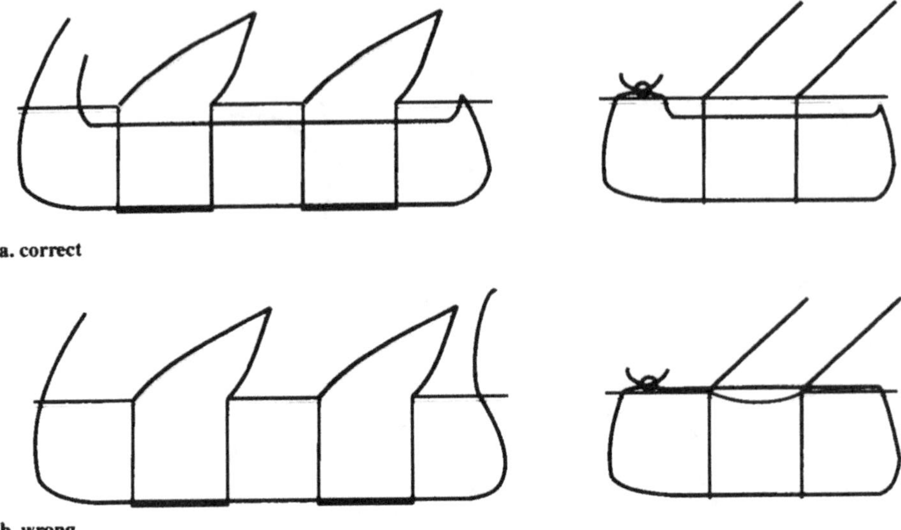

Figure 3 Suture of two small defects lying close to each other. **(a)** Correct suture keeps tissue in between the defects on the same level. **(b)** A simple suture will lower the tissue in between under the level of the two outer wound margins.

dren and adolescents who are still growing, skin under tension grows faster than normal. Allowing longer periods of time between consecutive excisions will result in better scars. However, most patients requiring revision of pitted scars are beyond their growth phase but do not yet have redundant skin as in old age. The timing of repeated serial excisions is left to the experienced assessment of the surgeon, who has to be aware that many patients tend to be persistent in their pleas to perform complete scar revision earlier than conditions would warrant.

II. LARGE ACNE SCARS

Some patients have large acne scars that are not amenable to superficial ablation techniques and small fusiform excisions. These scars, most frequently resulting from inflamed and ruptured cysts, may present features reminiscent of hypertrophic scars, although the bulging is in fact due to subcutaneous shrinkage. Large fusiform or multiple excisions are then necessary. It is crucial to respect the RSTLs. However, fortunately, most lesions are arranged along the axis of the main facial lines. Large scars are often located in the midcheek and nasomental fold area. Usually, enough skin is available for elliptical excisions. The wound edges are closed in two layers with buried dermal sutures and a nonabsorbable running dermal suture. Steri-strips are used to prevent spread and hypertrophy of the scar as well as to maintain circumscribed pressure. The advancement of the skin also accomplishes a midcheek facelift, further improving the contour of the skin (4).

III. WIDESPREAD SCARS

Widespread scars resulting from incisions and excisions are the most frequent indication for correction by fusiform excision. Scar dehiscence is usually the result of either suture under tension or continuous or repeated tension from stretching the skin; this is almost inevitable after excisions from the back, arms, legs, and abdomen. The technique described for revision of dehiscent scars is also the best approach to prevent their development; however, it has to be admitted that there is no absolutely safe procedure guaranteeing a fine scar line. Usually, the later this surgical intervention is performed the better the result (5,6).

Atrophic paper-thin scars require the same technique for revision.

A. Dehiscent Scar on the Back

Many benign and malignant skin tumors are located on the back. If they have to be removed by simple excision, they frequently leave an unsightly scar with suture marks and considerable spread. In addition, they are often hypertrophic. They are best treated with fusiform excision and closure (7). At least part of the spread may be due to too short an excision compared with its width. Very wide scars therefore require a longer axis of the spindle (Fig. 4; see also Figs. 13 (p. 374) and 14 (p. 375). Unfortunately, even the suture marks may be hypertrophic, adding to the unsightly appearance of the scar. Their inclusion in the first excision is often not possible, so serial excisions may be necessary.

Under local infiltration anesthesia with 1% lidocaine, without or with epinephrine, an incision is carried out all along the margins of the scar reaching into the subcutaneous fat

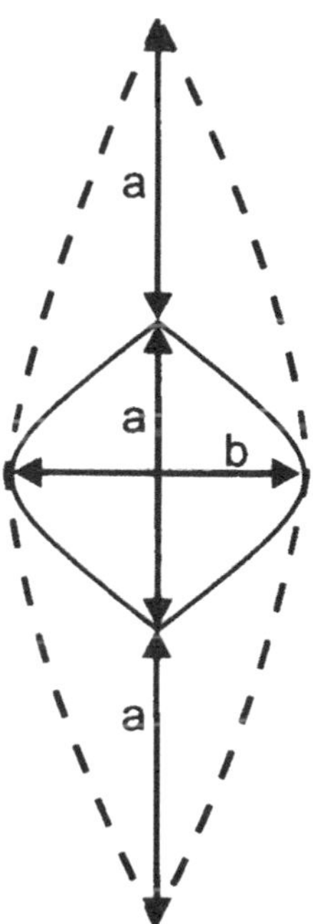

Figure 4 A wide, almost round scar has to be excised to give at least a length-to-width ratio of 3:1.

(Fig. 4). The incision may be angled at about 80 to 85 degrees to the surface, which will result in slightly more tension at the deep dermal level as compared with the upper third (Fig. 5). If the wound opens and eventually forms an angle wider than 30 to 35 degrees at its tips or has a length-to-width ratio smaller than 3 to 1, the excision has to be prolonged. Suture is the most critical point of the whole procedure. It has to remain stable as long as possible, must be well tolerated, must not cut through skin, and must not leave suture marks. Percutaneous sutures, even with atraumatic monofil material, cannot provide these requirements, and buried dermal sutures are a must. It is necessary to use either absorbable material that remains stable for several months, e.g., polydioxanone or polyglactane; permanent natural suture material such as silk, which tends to dissolve over a period of several years; or even synthetic nonabsorbable sutures. Special attention has to be paid to correct placement of the stitches. They have to include about 80% of the thickness of the dermis but must not contain adipose tissue, because subcutaneous fat is not able to resist the pressure after the knot is tied. After circumscribed fat necrosis, the stitch is no longer tight and scar spread will result. The stitch has to take a larger bite of tissue in the deep dermis; this is even more pronounced when the incision was angled at 80 to 85 degrees. This is very important, because it distributes more tension into the deep layers of the corium, and a slight spread of 1 or 2 mm will remain invisible because there is less tension in the superficial and papillary dermis (Fig. 5). Skin eversion has also been observed to give superior scar correction results by other authors (8).

A special suture technique may help to keep the wound margins close to each other. It is well known that foreign material may interfere with wound healing, and any suture

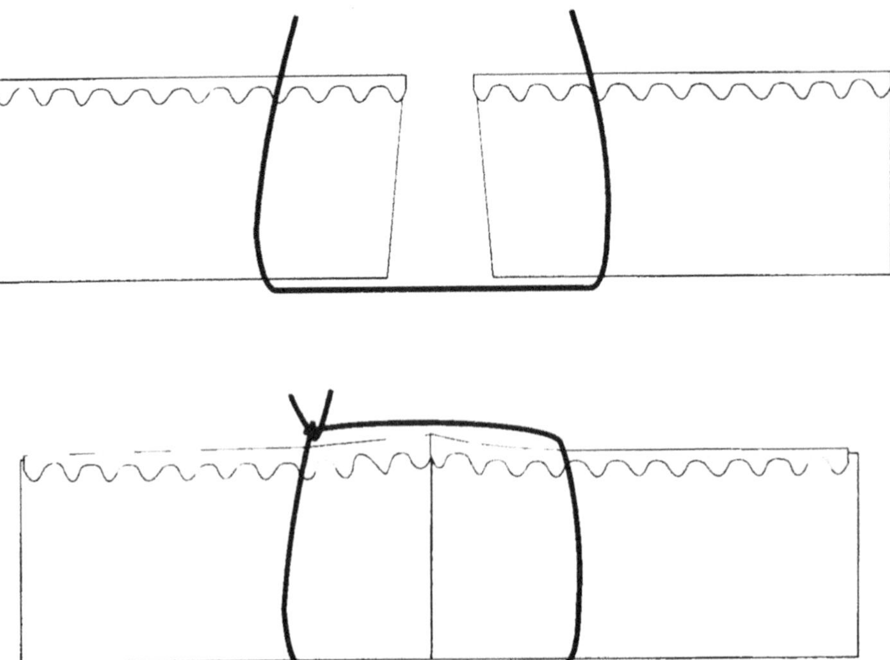

Figure 5 Eversion of the wound edges is facilitated by angling the wound edges to 80 degrees; the smaller the angle, the more eversion can be achieved.

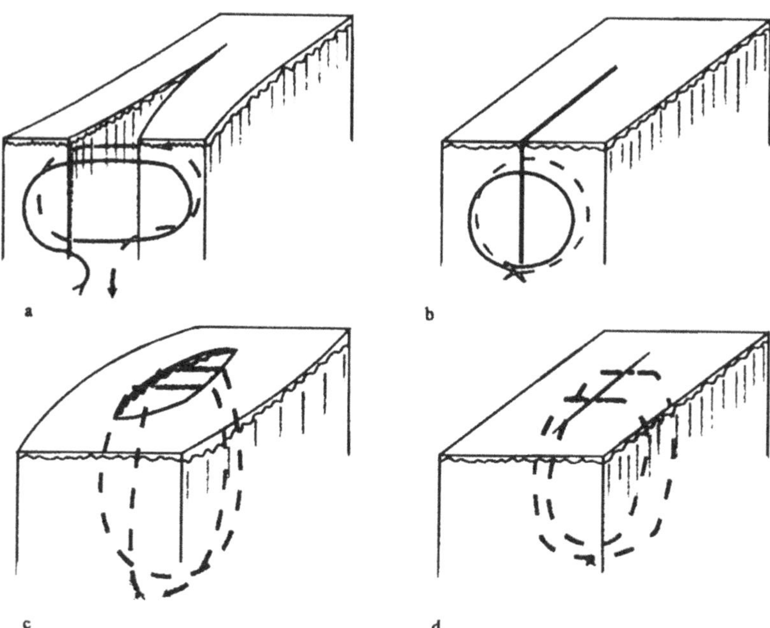

Figure 6 Buried parallel pulley suture. (**a** and **c**) A double loop is formed with the suture beginning from the undersurface of the dermis like a simple buried dermal suture; a second turned is performed about 3 to 5 mm parallel, resulting in a parallel pulley suture. Seen from the undersurface, this suture is like a buried cross-stitch. (**b** and **d**) After the knot is tied, this suture offers double strength with just one knot; thus less foreign material is buried in the surgical wound. (**a** and **b**) Side view; (**c** and **d**) oblique view.

brings foreign material into the wound. A buried vertical pulley suture was therefore developed, reducing the number of knots while increasing its stability (9,10). This suture is essentially an inverted buried cross-stitch (Fig. 6). The needle is inserted into the undersurface of the dermis without including fat, exits at the reticular dermis–papillary dermis border, and reenters at the opposing wound margin in a symmetrical fashion to exit at the undersurface of the dermis. Three to 5 mm apart, a parallel suture is performed and the knot is tied. This suture acts as a pulley, has double strength, and brings less foreign material into the wound because it requires only one knot for two stitches (9).

Tension sutures may be a very valuable adjunct to common sutures in revision of spread scars. It has to be kept in mind that in most cases the reason for scar dehiscence is still present and therefore the risk of recurrent scar spread is very high. Tension sutures should be placed well away from the wound edges in order to avoid compromise of their blood supply. They may be vertical mattress sutures or horizontal butterfly sutures (11,12) (Fig. 7); both are also useful as everting skin sutures. The vertical mattress suture is a far-far-near-near suture. The needle is inserted into the skin about 15 to 20 mm from the wound edge and carried along the dermis-subcutis border to the wound and again under the dermis of the opposite wound edge to exit away from the wound; the needle direction is reversed to enter again nearer to the wound edge, run through the dermis, and enter at the same level of the other wound margin to exit at the skin between the wound edge and the first needle

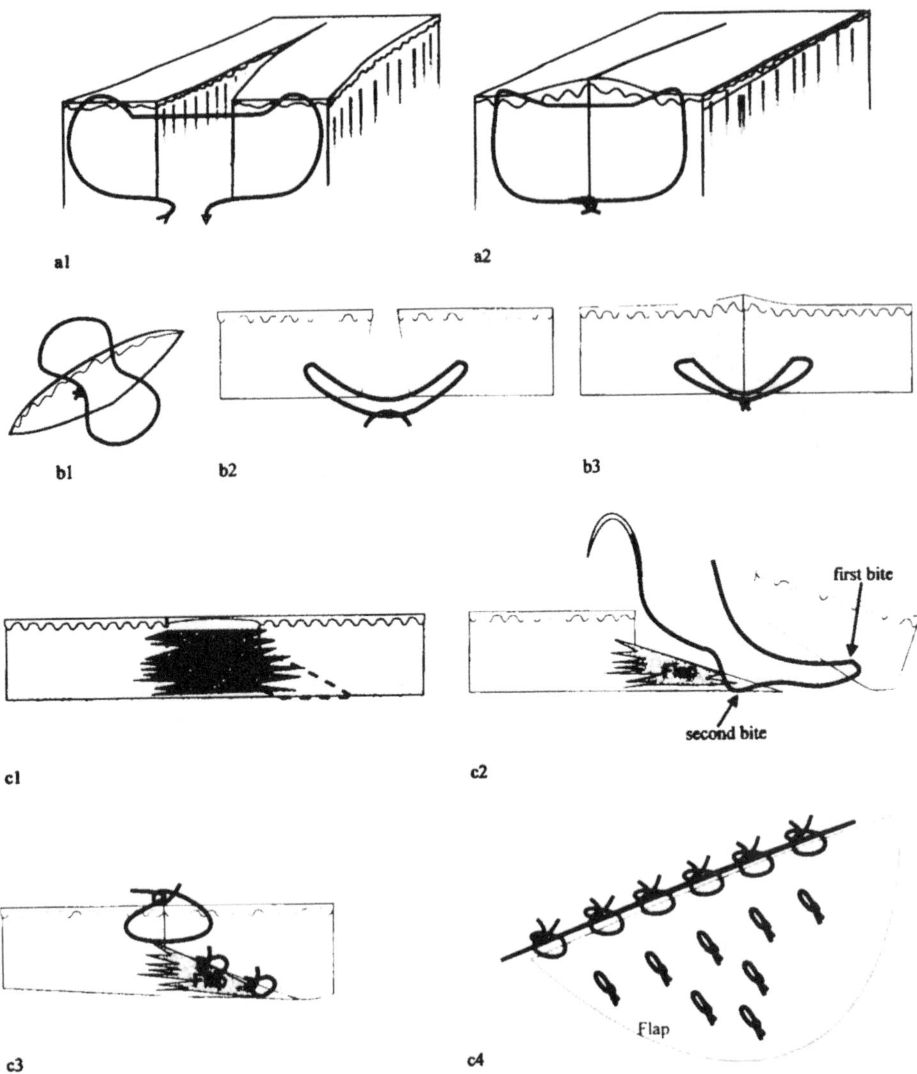

Figure 7 Tension sutures. **(a1)** Simple vertical mattress suture; the greater the distance of the suture loop from the wound edge and the deeper the backstitch is in the dermis, the more eversion can be gained. The suture may or may not remain completely subepidermal. **(a2)** After the knot is tied, the scar line is gently elevated. **(b)** Dermal-subcutaneous butterfly suture after Breuninger. **(b1)** View from above through the skin before knotting. **(b2)** Lateral view before knotting. **(b3)** Lateral view after knotting. Again, the bigger the bite of tissue, the more tension can be distributed away from the wound edge and the more eversion is possible. **(c1)** Widespread scar with excision line (broken line) marked for dermal flap. **(c2)** Excision of superficial portion of scar to form a scar flap; the opposite wound margin is elevated to allow the flap to be slipped under it and sutured. **(c3)** Dermal walking sutures fix flap to opposite dermis. **(c4)** Dorsal view of dermal walking sutures and skin sutures.

insertion (Fig. 7a). The degree of eversion can be increased by running the backstitch through middermis instead of upper dermis or by utilizing a greater distance for the stitches from the wound edges. For the horizontal tension suture, the skin is elevated and the needle inserted at the undersurface of the dermis to exit again at the undersurface; the other side of the wound is treated in a symmetrical fashion so that the suture material runs parallel to the wound margin in the dermis (Fig. 7b). Again, the farther the bite from the wound edge, the more eversion can be achieved. These tension sutures are tied only until the edges are apposed by primary sutures to prevent them from being tied too taughtly.

The horizontal bootlace pulley suture is also useful as a tension suture. The stitches are then placed similarly to those in the butterfly suture. After the first bite of dermis, the second bite on the opposite wound margin follows the same direction and the next stitches are reversed to form a horizontal eight (13). Additional interrupted buried sutures are useful for exact alignment of tissue layers.

It has not yet been confirmed that the buried dermal flap (14) is able to reduce scar dehiscence by reinforcing the closure. The spread scar is deepithelialized and a curved incision is carried out along one long side of the scar. The wound margin is undermined sufficiently to allow the flap of scar tissue to be pulled over the scar flap. A walking suture is used to move the skin over the scar flap. The first bite is taken in the deep portion of the mobilized skin and the second bite is placed in the scar flap (Fig. 7c). More sutures are performed toward the opposite side of the wound, thereby pulling the normal skin over the flap. It has to be kept in mind that scars do not withstand continuous tension, and the new scar, although reinforced with the scar flap, may not necessarily be more resistant to tension (14).

IV. DEPRESSED SCAR

Depressed scars fixed to underlying fasciae and muscles are quite commonly seen on the abdomen. Frequently, they are also widespread. They are particularly obvious in obese people, in whom they may cause large unaesthetic skin folds. The correction of these depressed scar may pose considerable problems.

The cutaneous scar is removed using a fusiform excision. The deep margins of the wound are freed from the underlying fascia to allow very careful dissection of the subcutaneous fat from the fascia to form a skin-hypodermis flap. Using blunt dissection scissors and opening them in a vertical fashion instead of a horizontal, windscreen-wiper-like fashion permits even small vessels penetrating the underlying fascia to be seen and left intact. Meticulous hemostasis is essential to avoid hematoma and/or seroma formation with the risk of postoperative infection. In order to avoid dead space formation, a subcutaneous suture with rapidly absorbing 3-0 to 4-0 material is used to approximate the adipose tissue; it is important to take a greater bite of fat in the deep than in the more superficial layer. Maximal eversion is essential for skin sutures. Horizontal tension sutures as described above are a good option for bringing both the deep dermis and the subcutaneous tissue together. These sutures are inserted about 15 mm from the wound edges so that their tension does not interfere with the blood supply of the wound margin. Buried dermal sutures and a running intracuticular suture are used for final wound closure.

V. HYPERTROPHIC SCARS

Mature hypertrophic scars may be excised and the new skin wound sutured directly when its direction is parallel to an RSTL. Atraumatic surgery is mandatory, and careful buried dermal suturing to distribute tension evenly must be performed (7,15) (see Figs. 13–15 (pp. 374–376)). However, all factors that led to scar hypertrophy are usually still active, and the patient should be counseled that proper immobilization, if possible even splinting, steri-strips, and other devices for wound support may have to be used for several months.

VI. KELOIDS

Keloids have to be seen as autochthonous proliferations of scar tissue in susceptible people. They are notorious for recurrences that each time are bigger than the lesion just treated before. Therapy of keloids is aimed at modifying them so that the region becomes more functional, better looking, asymptomatic, and not recurrent (16). At present, there is no single method guaranteeing this kind of success (17).

Surgical excision alone has a recurrence rate of 50 to almost 100%. To reduce this appalling failure rate, some preventive measures have to be respected. The actual excision must be as simple and small as possible; this is a fusiform excision along the RSTL. Local anesthesia is performed using epinephrine or ornipressin as a vasoconstrictor in order to minimize bleeding and avoid hematoma formation. The surgery must be performed atraumatically using sharp scalpels, which may have to be changed during the procedure. The use of forceps should be abandoned as much as possible; skin hooks are used instead to minimize trauma to the skin (18). Direct tension should be taken away from the wound edges by using tension sutures; they will also help to evert the wound margins. The use of percutaneous stitches is equivocal: they may cause suture marks, which grow to disastrous keloids in case of a recurrence, however, the role of even very well tolerated, inert monofil absorbable sutures left in the dermis has not yet been convincingly evaluated. If possible, skin stitches should be removed after 5 to 7 days, but this is often not possible over areas of natural skin stretch, which are particularly prone to develop keloids (see Fig. 16 (p. 377)).

Earlobe keloids, when not too large, can be excised and the defect closed directly. Sometimes the core excision (19) can be combined with a small fusiform excision. We always combine this treatment with repeated corticosteroid injections and pressure.

Keloids may also form after skin excision for correction of a projecting pinna. They may obliterate the entire postauricular fold. A fusiform excision and two-layered buried dermal and running subcuticular sutures have given excellent results in combination with injections of triamcinolone acetonide crystal suspension.

VII. DOG-EAR

Dog-ears are common sequelae of excisions with an imbalance of too short a long axis to too wide a narrow axis. Although the usual 3.5:1 ratio may be overcome when using the tissue-sparing technique (20), this is not possible everywhere on the body and is no longer applicable once a dog-ear has formed.

Several techniques can be used for dog-ear repair, most of which are fusiform excisions or modifications. If a wound has already healed and the small amount of scalloped tissue on both ends of the scar did not stretch out sufficiently, a simple elliptical excision is performed to remove the excess tissue. A few buried stitches will be sufficient to close the wound (Fig. 8a).

If a dog-ear is to be corrected at the end of operation, a small hook is used to elevate the excess skin to one side. The straight incision line is prolonged, the excess tissue is undermined, the skin is stretched to the other side using the hook, and another incision is carried out in prolongation of the wound (18). Meticulous suture completes the procedure (Fig. 8b).

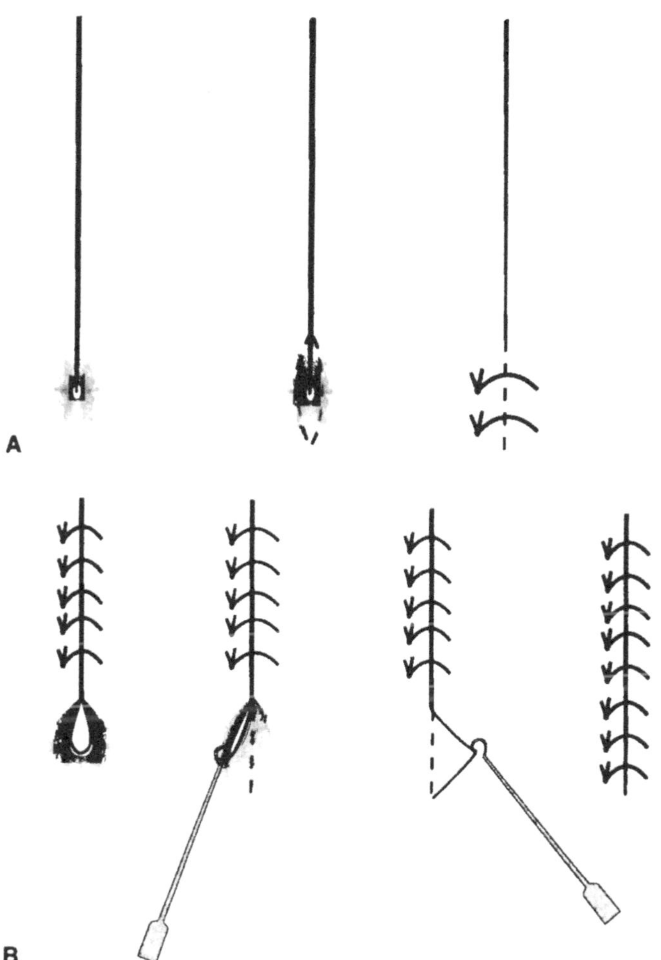

Figure 8 Dog-ear repair. **(A)** Repair of a dog-ear some time after wound healing is completed requires only a small fusiform excision. **(B)** A dog-ear at end of operation (b1) may be removed by pulling it to one side and prolonging the incision (b2), then stretching the tissue flap out and again prolonging the incision (b3), finally suturing the wound (b4).

VIII. BURN SCAR, PARTIAL EXCISION

Scars from deep second-degree and third-degree burns are usually large, often appear atrophic, may be hyper- or hypopigmented, and develop hypertrophic areas and contractures. Whereas small atrophic burn scars may be excised completely, this is not possible for large ones. A study comparing extramarginal (= complete) excision with intramarginal (= partial) excision revealed that scarring after complete scar excision was worse than after intramarginal excision. The best cosmetic results were obtained when hypertrophic scars were excised intramarginally (21–23).

The incision is placed in the RSTL if possible and carried down through the scar tissue to the subcutaneous layer. Depending on the location and extent of the hypertrophic fibrous tissue, the adjacent scar may be debulked extending to the peripheral tissue, but undermining has to be omitted or performed very cautiously because the surrounding scar tissue has altered vascularity. A two-layered suture is used to close the wounds using 4-0 or 5-0 polydioxanone or polyglactane for buried dermal sutures and 5-0 monofil simple interrupted skin sutures to be removed after 5 to 7 days (Fig. 9). Intramarginal excision resulted in virtually invisible "scars in the scar" (24), whereas extramarginal excisions gave more obvious scars.

IX. SCAR BANDS

Burns, traumatic wounds, especially infected laceration wounds, and wrongly placed surgical wounds may cause scar bands when running over the flexure of a joint. They usually require excision and broken-line scar revision in most cases. Sometimes, a scar band is like the string of an arch pulling up entirely normal skin on both of its sides. The excision of such a narrow scar band may leave a fine scar line within skin of normal flexure and may sometimes suffice for an adequate functional and cosmetic result.

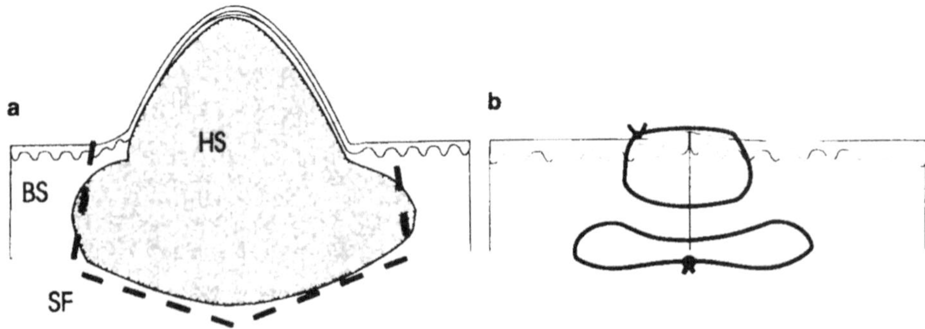

Figure 9 Intrascar excision of hypertrophic portion of burn scar. **(a)** Removal of hypertrophic scar tissue. **(b)** Suture of defect using a butterfly suture to distribute tension to tissue away from the wound edges and simple percutaneous skin suture.

X. CONTRACTURE

Scar contractures are mainly seen in the medial canthus, in the oral commissure, on the ala nasi, on the neck, and over joint flexures (15). Especially small lesions in the medial canthus may be repaired by a fusiform excision. It may be useful to tack the suture to the underlying periosteum of the side of the nose in order to avoid tenting and a recurrent contracture. If the contracture was due to a longitudinal scar over the inner eye corner, it is excised and the wound opened to redirect the scar by suturing the edges horizontally. Because the medial canthus is an ideal site for second-intention healing, it is not critical if the new defect cannot be closed completely; however, the wound edges should be fixed to the underlying periosteum.

XI. RADIATION SCAR

Until about a quarter-century ago, x-irradiation used to be a very popular treatment for basal and squamous cell carcinomas even in relatively young patients. Radiation scars, in contrast to surgical ones, have the tendency to worsen with time, to become vulnerable, to develop nonhealing ulcers, and eventually to undergo malignant degeneration. Many patients who had x-ray treatment for a skin lesion that could well have been excised surgically now present for removal of their unsightly radiation scar. Many of these treatment sequelae can be removed using a simple fusiform excision. This is done as for any other benign lesion of the same size, i.e., a total excision following the RSTL. We have not tried to use serial partial excisions for large lesions; instead, we used large fusiform excisions with either relaxing incisions or V-Y advancement to both sides of the excision. The secondary defects are located within normal, nonirradiated skin and therefore have a normal healing tendency, in contrast to the radiodermatitis.

XII. SCARS OVER CONVEX SURFACES

Scars over convex surfaces such as the cheek or the mandibular arch tend to cut into the skin like a wire stretched over the convexity. This is due to normal scar contracture that occurs from both ends of any scar. Usually, a fusiform excision has a slightly longer axis after suture than the length of the original defect, and this is sufficient to prevent obvious scar contracture. However, this may not be enough over convexities. The fusiform excision should then be slightly curved to form a lazy S; this gives a slightly longer scar and takes the tension from the scar. Beginning to suture from one end and progressing to the other will result in a perfect suture line (Fig. 10).

XIII. SCAR REDIRECTION: TRANSVERSE TO VERTICAL CLOSURE

Scar redirection to obtain an optimal arrangement along the RSTL can sometimes be achieved using a fusiform excision. A scarred frenulum is a frequent event in noncircumcised men. The scarred area is excised under local anesthesia with the spindle being in the

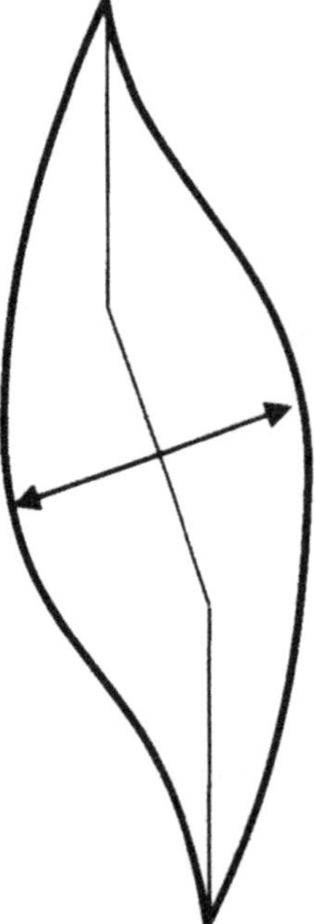

Figure 10 Lazy S excision for convex surfaces. This suture avoids the aspect of a tense wire.

horizontal direction. The fusiform defect is opened using blunt scissors and sutured longitudinally, giving extra length to the frenulum (Fig. 11) (25).

This technique may be used also for other ill-placed excisions, such as on the upper lip. It is particularly useful when there is no supporting structure that can hold any other type of scar revision.

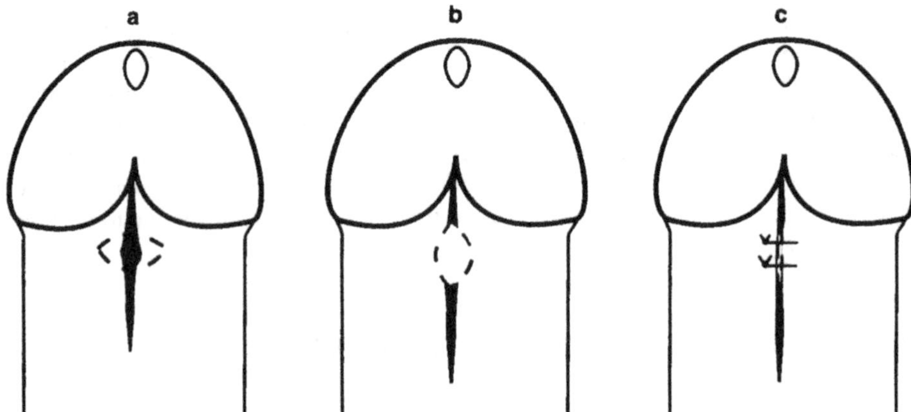

Figure 11 Scar redirection for the correction of a scarred frenulum. **(a)** The scarred portion is excised using a horizontal fusiform excision. **(b)** The horizontal spindle-shaped defect is widened vertically. **(c)** The defect is sutured in the direction of the frenulum.

XIV. SPLIT NAIL

A narrow longitudinal wound of the nail matrix will give a scar with consecutive defective nail production over the length of the scar resulting in a split-nail formation. Correction of a split nail, which, in fact, is a modification of a cicatricial pterygium, requires meticulous atraumatic surgery. The scar is excised down to the bone, either only the matrix or also the nail bed, and the soft tissue is dissected from the bone of the distal phalanx. The nail plate is cut about 1 to 2 mm to both sides from the defect. The matrix and nail bed are sutured using 6-0 polydioxanone; care has to be taken to evert the wound edges to obtain optimal wound coaption. It is wise to place all sutures first and to tie them only later, because it may be difficult to take the correct tissue bite when the wound edges are tightly knotted. The nail plate is approximated using 4-0 nonabsorbable monofil sutures after small holes have been drilled into the nail plate; this helps to keep the matrix and nail bed wound edges tightly together. Finally, the proximal nail fold is sutured. A thin plate of silicone may be inserted between the proximal nail fold and the matrix–nail plate in order to avoid scar formation between the eponychium and the matrix, which would inevitably result in a recurrence (Fig. 12) (26).

XV. SERIAL FUSIFORM EXCISIONS

Serial fusiform excisions are an optimal technique for the removal of medium-sized congenital nevi and other benign lesions that cannot be excised and closed in a single procedure. Large scar areas or hypertrophic scars within burn scars are also amenable to serial excisions. In most of these cases, skin expanders are an alternative and their pros and cons

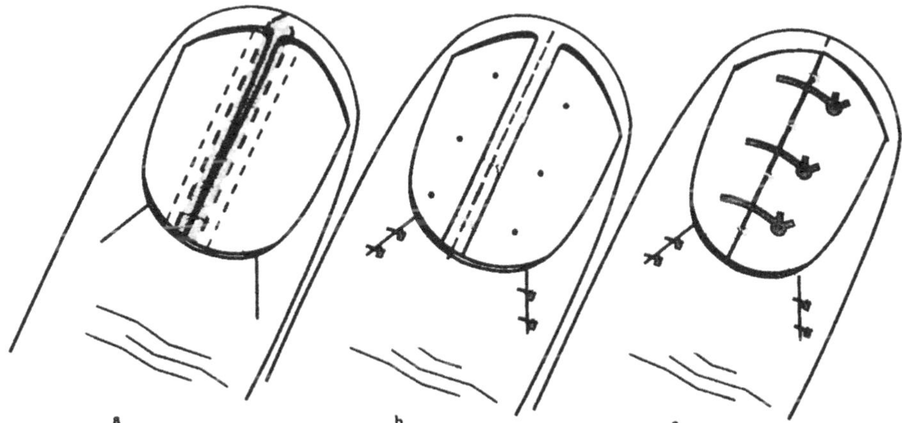

Figure 12 Split-nail correction. **(a)** The split nail is due to a scar running from the matrix through the nail bed. The proximal nail fold is incised on both sides to allow it to be reflected in order to expose the matrix. The scar is excised and narrow strips of the nail plate are removed. **(b)** The matrix and nail bed are sutured as well as the proximal nail fold. Small holes are drilled into the nail plate on both sides of the defect. **(c)** 3-0 skin sutures are used to appose the nail plate, thus relaxing the matrix and nail bed sutures.

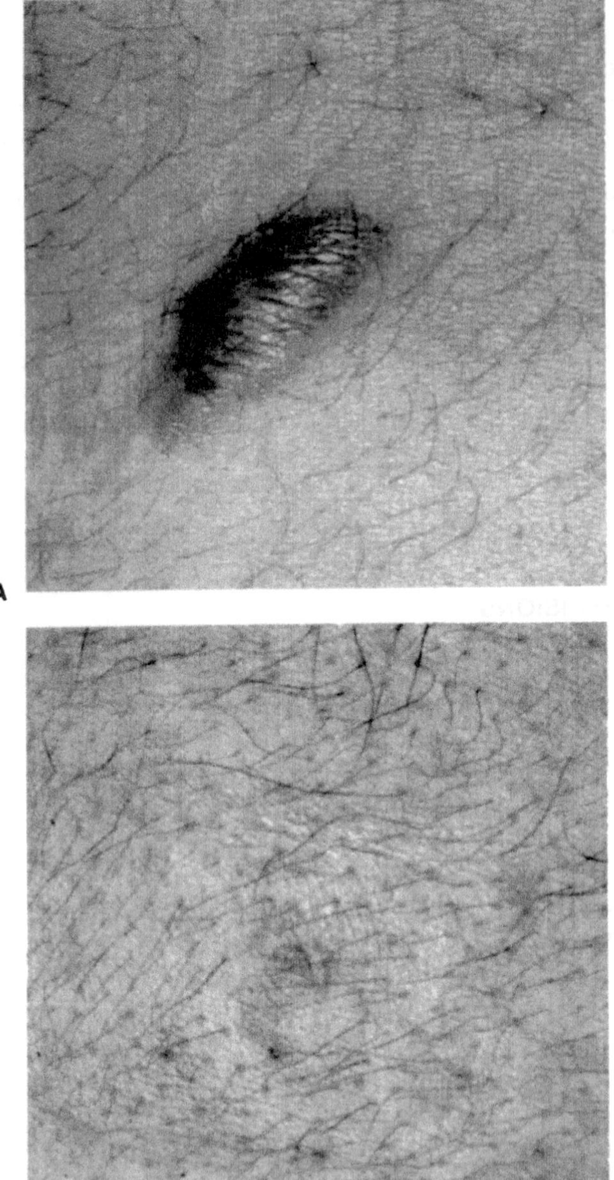

Figure 13 **(A)** Typical scar on the back with dehiscence, hypertrophy, and suture marks. **(B)** One year after fusiform excision and pulley suture.

have to be discussed with the patient before beginning serial excisions. Technically, serial excisions are not demanding and can be performed to correct large scar areas. They can be combined with preoperative suturing to allow more scar tissue to be removed. It is, however, crucial to keep in mind that serial excisions work on the same principle as skin expanders, although more biologically. Sufficient time has to be planned between the ses-

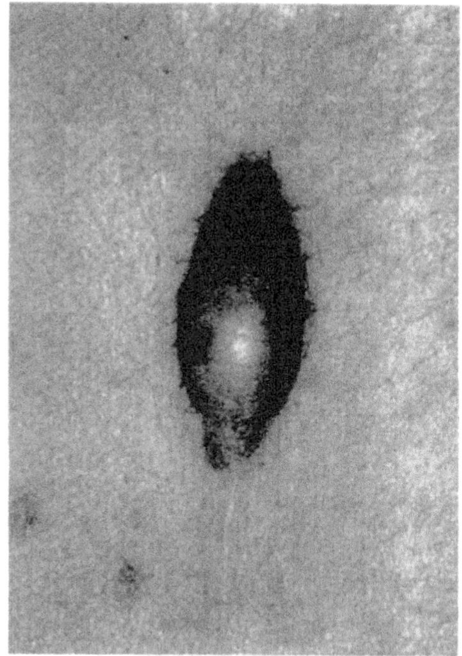

A

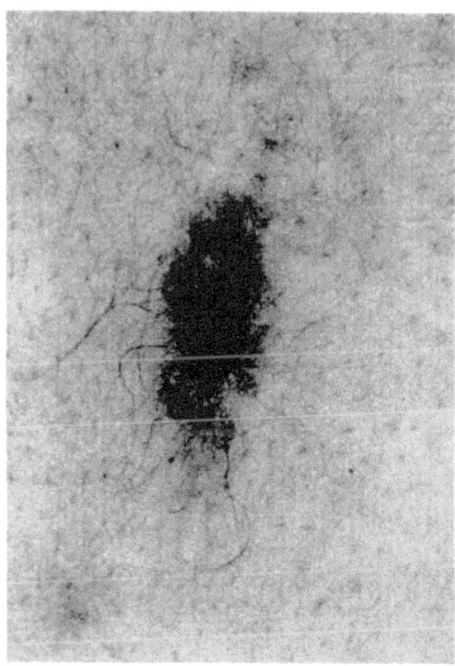

B

Figure 14 **(A)** Keloidal scar on the back. **(B)** Six months after simple excision and pulley suture.

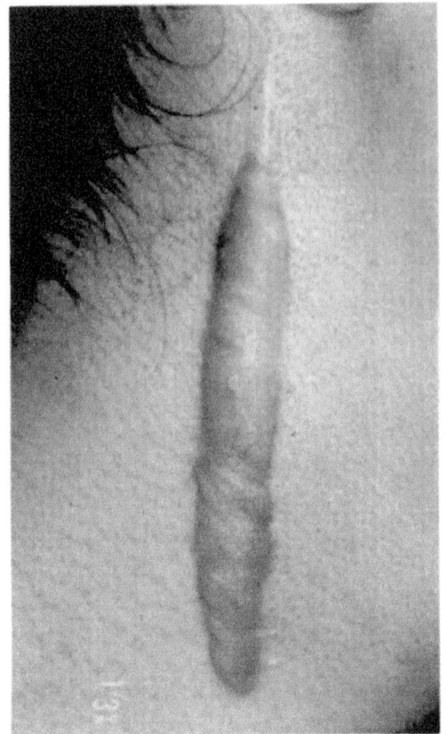

A

B

Figure 15 **(A)** Grossly hypertrophic scar on the neck. **(B)** Eleven months after fusiform excision; postoperative treatment with silicone gel sheeting.

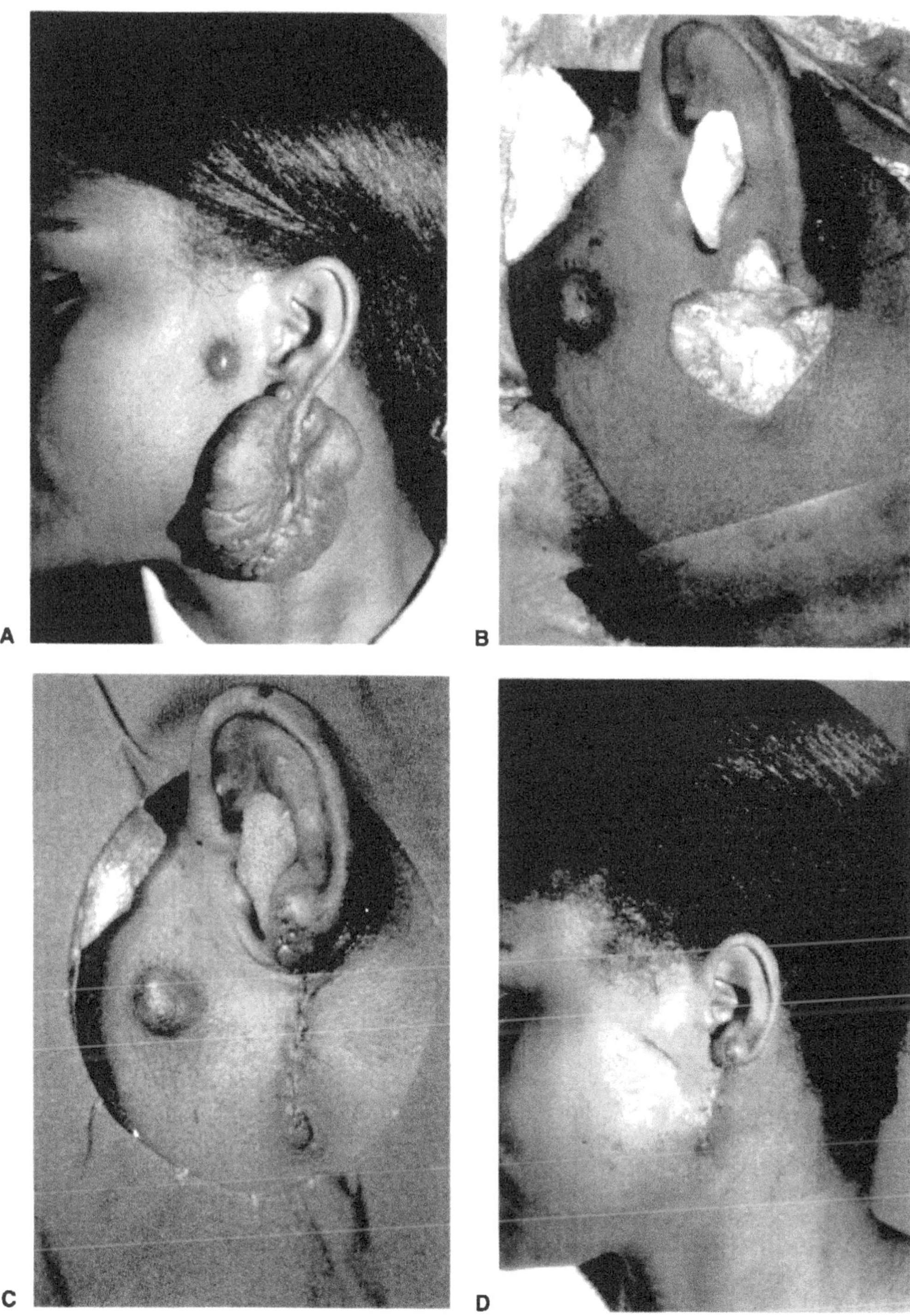

Figure 16 Large keloid that developed from successive surgical operations on an earlobe keloid. **(A)** Before operation. **(B)** Two fusiform excisions in V shape. **(C)** End of operation. **(D)** Six weeks after operation; the preauricular keloid was excised just 5 days ago.

sions, depending on the patient's age, growth phase, and localization and size of the lesion. Serial excisions expand adjacent tissue, which may result in expansion of adjacent scar. It is therefore essential to place tension sutures outside the entire area to be excised in that multistep procedure. Cosmesis of the interim scar is less important. Sutures can therefore be left in place for a longer time to avoid spread of the scar. Nonabsorbable sutures, depending on the location 3-0 or 4-0 monofil polypropylene, should be used because they will be excised with the following operation. It is self-evident that each new excision will have to take the scar from the former one in its center. When a three-step operation is planned, it is wise to excise at least 80% of the scar width with the first two operations in order to have less tension at the end of the final excision, because this will have to pay attention to both the functional and the cosmetic aspects.

Serial excisions should not be tried for the elimination of keloids.

REFERENCES

1. Tardy ME, Thomas JR, Pashcow MS. The camouflage of cutaneous scars. Ear Nose Throat J 1981; 60:61–70.
2. Thomas JR, Ehlert TK. Scar revision and camouflage. Otolaryngol Clin North Am 1990; 23:963–973.
3. Webster RC, Smith RC. Scar revision and camouflage. Otolaryngol Clin North Am 1982; 15:55–68.
4. Stal S, Hamilton S, Spira M. Surgical treatment of acne scars. Clin Plast Surg 1987; 14:261–276.
5. Härtel P. Wundheilung, Narbenbildung, Zeitpunkt zur Korrektur. Zbl Chir 1988; 113:745–750.
6. Borges AF. Timing of scar revision techniques. Clin Plast Surg 1990; 17:71–76.
7. Rudolph R. Wide spread scar, hypertrophic scars, and keloids. Clin Plast Surg 1987; 14:253–260.
8. Wolfe D, Davidson TM. Scar revision. Arch Otolaryngol Head Neck Surg 1991; 117:200–204.
9. Haneke E. Developments and techniques in general dermatologic surgery. In: Dahl MV, Lynch PJ, eds. Current Opinion in Dermatology. Vol. 1. Philadelphia: Current Science, 1993:145–151.
10. Haneke E. Variationen der Flaschenzugnaht. In: Mahrle G, Schulze H-J, Krieg T. Fortschritte der operativen und onkologischen Dermatologie 8: Wundheilung-Wundverschluβ. Heidelberg: Springer, 1994:158–164.
11. Breuninger H, Schippert W. Die intrakutane Schmetterlingsnaht mit resorbierbarem synthetischem monofilem Nahtmaterial. Z Hautkr 1991; 66(suppl 3):69–71.
12. Breuninger H, Keilbach J, Haaf U. Untersuchungen zur Wundheilung nach Verwendung resorbierbaren synthetischen Nahtmaterials bei intrakutanen Schmetterlingsnähten. In: Mahrle G, Schulze H-J, Krieg T. Fortschritte der operativen und onkologischen Dermatologie 8: Wundheilung-Wundverschluβ. Heidelberg, Springer, 1994:165–170.
13. Motley RJ, Holt PJA. Subcutaneous pulley and "boot-lace" sutures. Abstracts XIV Congress International Society Dermatol Surgery, Sevilla, 1993:117 (cited in Haneke E. Developments and techniques in general dermatologic surgery. In: Dahl MV, Lynch PJ, eds. Current Opinion in Dermatology. Vol. 2. Philadelphia, Current Science, 1995:129–136).
14. Rudolph R. Scar revision. In: Georgiade N, ed. Essentials of Plastic, Maxillofacial and Reconstructive Surgery. Baltimore: Williams & Wilkins, 1986:123–129.
15. Sherris DA, Larrabee WF Jr, Murakami CS. Management of scar contractures, hypertrophic scars, and keloids. Otolaryngol Clin North Am 1995; 28:1057–1068.
16. Brown LA Jr, Pierce HE. Keloids: scar revision. J Dermatol Surg Oncol 1986; 12:51–56.
17. Papachatzaki I, Haneke E. Combined method for the management of keloids. Hellenic J Dermatol 1995; 6:221–225.

18. Zoltán J. Atlas der chirurgischen Schnitt- und Nahttechnik zur Erzielung optimaler Wundheilung. Budapest: Akadémiai Kiadó, Basel: Karger, 1977.
19. Salasche SJ, Grabski WJ. Keloids of the earlobes: a surgical technique. J Dermatol Surg Oncol 1983; 9:552–556.
20. Stewart JB. Tissue sparing repair: a new approach to shorten excisional lines. J Dermatol Surg Oncol 1992; 18:822–826.
21. Engrav LH, Gottlieb JR, Millard ST, Walkinshaw MD, Heimbach DM, Marvin JA. Partial excision of residual burn lesions. J Burn Care Res 1987; 8:398–402.
22. Engrav LH, Gottlieb JR, Millard ST, Walkinshaw MD, Heimbach DM, Marvin JA. A comparison of intramarginal and extramarginal excision of hypertrophic burn scars. Plast Reconstr Surg 1988; 81:40–43.
23. Yang J-Y. Intrascar excision for persistent perioral hypertrophic scar. Plast Reconstr Surg 1996; 98:1200–1205.
24. Engrav LH. Discussion to J-Y Yang. Plast Reconstr Surg 1996; 98:1206–1207.
25. Haneke E. Organerhaltende operative Therapie des frühen Peniskarzinoms. In: Dummer R, Panizzon R, Burg G, eds. Fortschritte der operativen Dermatologie 11: Operative und konservative Dermatoonkologie im interdisziplinären Grenzbereich. Berlin: Blackwell Wiss Verlag, 1996:103–107.
26. Haneke E. Cirugía dermatológica de la región ungueal. Mongr Dermatol 1991; 4:408–423.

20
The Z-Plasty Technique

Hisakazu Seno and Akira Yanai
Juntendo University
Tokyo, Japan

Shinichi Hirabayashi
Teikyo University
Tokyo, Japan

The Z-plasty is a useful technique and one of the most widely employed techniques in plastic surgery. The Z-plasty was known as far back as the early 19th century (1,2). The technique was popularized by Davis (3,4), and many investigators began to devote their efforts toward theoretical aspects (5,6). Thus, the Z-plasty came to be routinely used in a plastic surgery. The technique and its application are mentioned in most textbooks dealing with specialties.

The basic shape of the Z-plasty is formed by transposition of two triangular skin flaps of equal size. Modification of the Z-plasty technique such as multiple Z-plasty, four-flap Z-plasty, and five-flap Z-plasty have been reported.

I. PRINCIPLE AND EFFECT OF THE Z-PLASTY

The basic shape of the Z-plasty is formed by two triangular skin flaps of equal size created by three incisions of equal length cut at 60-degree angles (Fig. 1). The transposition of triangular flaps results in lengthening of the central limb of the Z design and also some other effects.

One should be aware that the common statement "the three lines of the Z must always be of equal length" is not correct (7). When used to correct a contracture, the centerline of the Z should be slightly longer than the two limbs because there may be a shortening of this trunk after the contracture is released. This may be quite marked when the contracture is severe, and the design of the Z-plasty must take this into account (Figs. 2 and 3).

Principally, Z-plasty is utilized for (a) elongation of the skin in a predetermined direction, (b) changing the direction of the scar, (c) division of the scar into several portions in order to make it inconspicuous, (d) correcting the location of mispositioned tissue, and (e) alteration of three-dimensional formation.

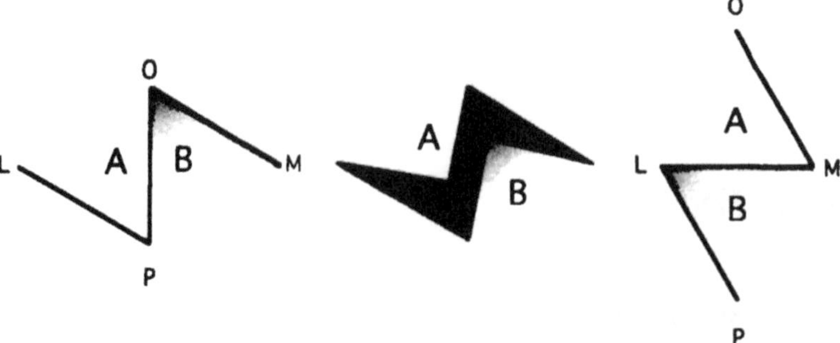

Figure 1 Typical Z-plasty. Central limb O-P is elongated by transposition of triangular flaps A and B. The Distance between L and M is compensatingly shortened.

A. Skin Elongation

The transposition of two flaps effects elongation of the scar contracture. Limitation of the elongation effect depends on the angle formed by the central limb and the other two limbs (8) (Fig. 4).

Greater elongation is obtained when the Z-plasty angle widens. Tension occurs at the triangular flap's pivot point. Great tension at the pivot point with flap rotation results in an irregular surface. In the usual clinical situation when one needs to elongate an area, one

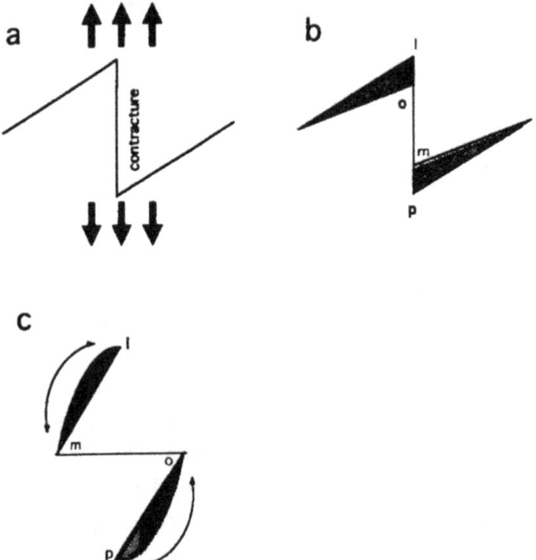

Figure 2 Design of the Z with tension in the up-down directions. **(a)** Z-plasty is positioned with three limbs of equal length. Tension is applied in up and down directions. **(b)** Contracture is released by skin incision that shortens limb length, as indicated by l-o and m-p. **(c)** Puckering is seen on both sides of the Z after transposition of the flaps.

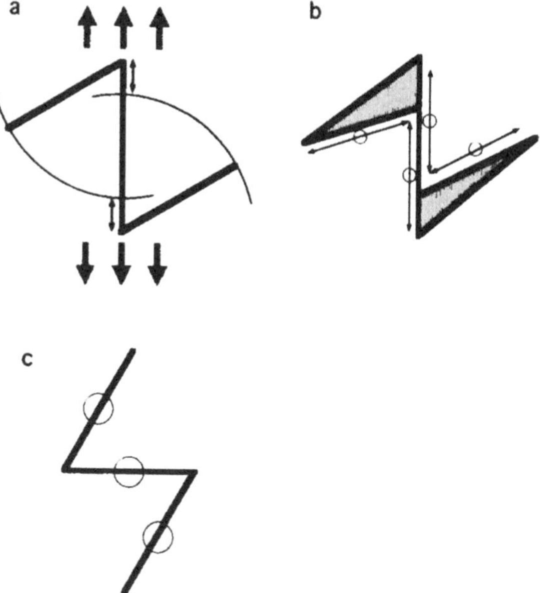

Figure 3 Design of the Z with tension in the up-down directions. In most cases of Z-plasty the central limb should be designed longer than the other two. **(a)** Design of the Z with tension in the up-down directions. Small arrows indicate shrinkage after skin incision. **(b)** Contracture release by skin incision and flap transposition results in all limbs becoming of equal length. **(c)** No distortion occurs as all limbs are of equal length after completion of flap transposition.

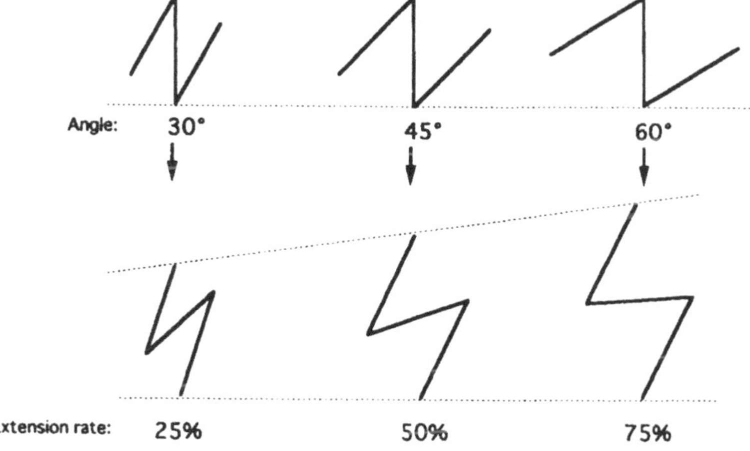

Figure 4 Rates of Z-plasty extension. (From Ref. 8.)

must consider that the resulting scar should lie along the relaxed skin tension line (RSTL), in which case the Z-plasty angle cannot always be 60 degrees.

B. Changing Direction of the Scar

The direction of each limb changes after transposition of the flaps. A scar on the limb is moved synchronously at the same time.

C. Changing Direction of Central Limb to Align with RSTL

This is a great help when a scar intersects a large wrinkle such as the nasolabial fold (Fig. 5).

Some articles appear to have misconceptions regarding the direction of the completed suture lines; in other words, the direction of the central line deviates after flap movement (9) (Fig. 6).

Even linear scars have some width in most cases, and therefore excision is required in carry out such scar revision. As shown in Fig. 7, movement of the points occurs after scar excision and temporary closure of the defect has taken place: A, B, C, and D shift to the new points A′, B′, C′, and D′. The lines A′-C′, B′-D′, and C′-D′ thus do not coincide with the primary envisioned lines A-C, B-D, and C-D. The extent of shifting of the four points may be increased the closer Z-plasty is performed to the center of the scar and the greater the scar width. Furthermore, when the two triangular flaps (Fig. 7) are transposed, the points A′ and B′ shift to become points A″ and B″, and C′ and D′ become C″ and D″. The resulting suture lines A″-C″, C″-D″, and B″-D″ lie in positions quite different from the primary envisioned lines A-C, C-D, and B-D. When a scar lies perpendicular to the RSTL and the angle of the defect for which Z-plasty is to be performed is 60 degrees, the resulting line C″-D″ coincides with the primarily envisioned C-D line.

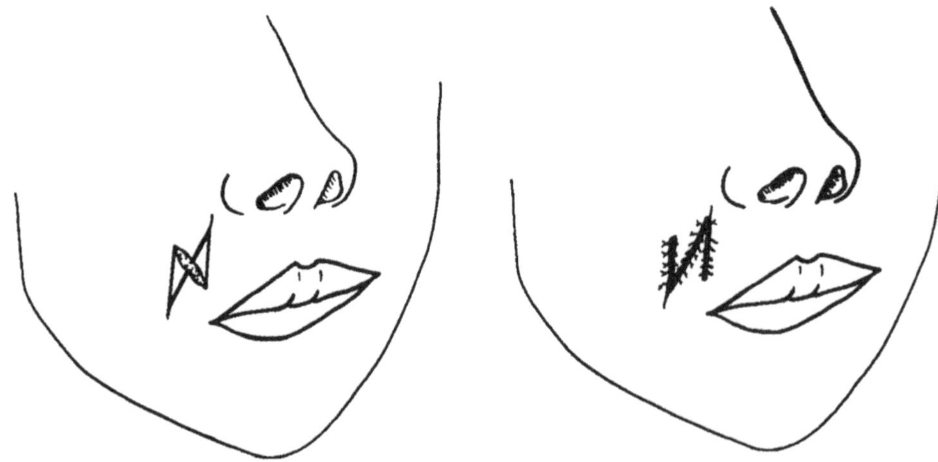

Figure 5 Z-plasty design for scar crossing nasolabial fold ensures that central limb falls into the fold.

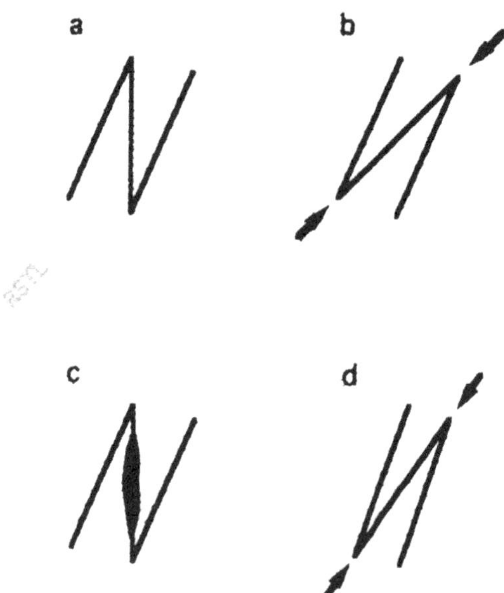

Figure 6 Change in direction of the central limb. **(a)** Z-plasty design is geometric. **(b)** Expected geometric figure. Central limb follows RSTL. **(c)** Excision of scar in central limb becomes necessary in most cases. **(d)** Direction of central limb is changed by excision of scar. Central limb doesn't follow RSTL.

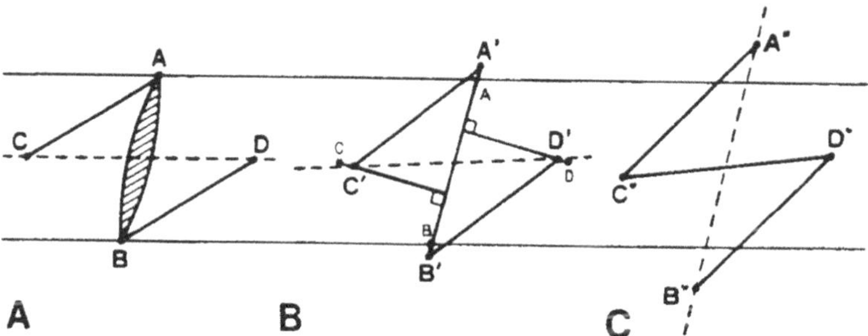

Figure 7 Shifts in positions and directions of lines. **(A)** Scar excision and design of Z. **(B)** Temporary closure of defect. **(C)** Transposition of flaps in lengthening of center line, and new suture lines. (From Ref. 9.)

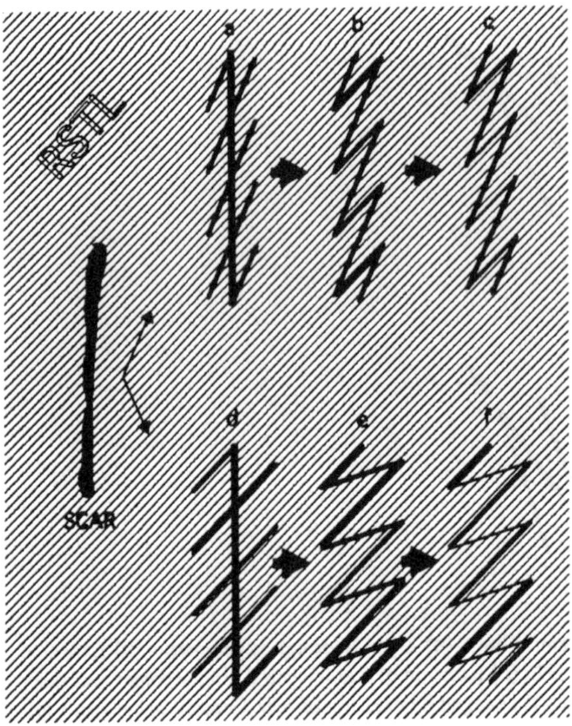

Figure 8 **(a)** Design to ensure that central limb will finally align with relaxed skin tension line (RSTL). **(b)** Result. **(c)** Completed Z-plasty. Time course results in central limb scar not becoming conspicuous as do limbs that cross RSTL. **(d)** Design in which two Z limbs follow RSTL. **(e)** Result. **(f)** Conspicuous limb scars follow RSTL. Result is less conspicuous than in **(c)**.

D. Changes in Direction of the Two Limbs to Align with RSTL

This technique is utilized when a scar transects the RSTL. It results in two linear scars meeting the RSTL and one linear scar (central limb) lying in the other direction (Fig. 8). Under ordinary conditions, hypertrophic scars tend to occur on the two limbs rather than the central limb after Z-plasty. This is because two triangular flaps tend to be pressed together at the central limb. The two flaps demonstrate a tendency to return to their original positions (Fig. 9). In many cases, two of the Z-plasty limbs should align with the RSTL (Fig. 10).

E. Correcting Location of Tissue

Triangular flap tissue can be moved through Z-plasty transpositioning of two triangular flaps. This is utilized for correcting the position of the eyebrows, outer canthus, wings of

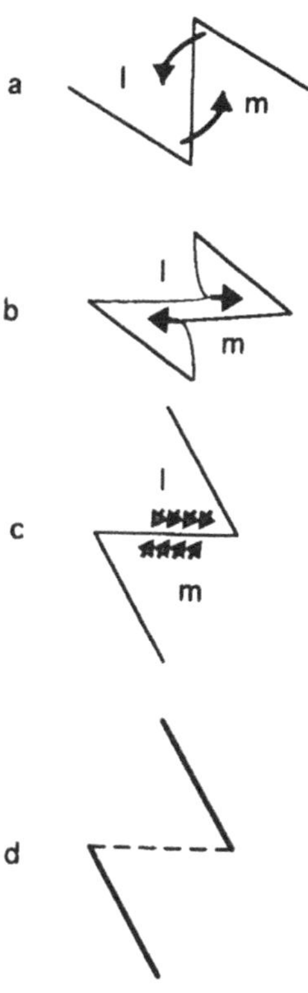

Figure 9 **(a)** Flaps are transposed in direction of arrows. **(b)** Arrows indicate directions of tension needed in flap transposition. **(c)** Pressure occurrs between flaps in direction of the arrows (the central limb) as each flap tends to return to former position. **(d)** Interflap pressure has effect of lessening scar conspicuousness.

the nose, and corner of the mouth (Fig. 11). In this method, the size and angle of each are dependent on the design required. The shape of the Z is often deformed.

F. Divide a Straight Scar into Several Parts

A straight scar on the skin surface is conspicuous and also tends to become indented. Z-plasty of a conspicuous straight scar can change it into a quiet zigzag scar. The correct design should be selected for best results. After Z-plasty the scar should connect with a wrinkle line. When Z-plasty is performed, the length of the suture line increases. It appears paradoxical that a longer scar should be less conspicuous than a short scar. The following may explain this. (a) The zigzag line freely conforms with expansion and contraction of the skin. When there is an alteration of expression, the scar is not conspicuous because of this phenomenon. (b) One limb of the Z-plasty shows improvement close to the disappearance. It is not conspicuous when it changes to a line cut up short. (c) A distinct shadow occurs

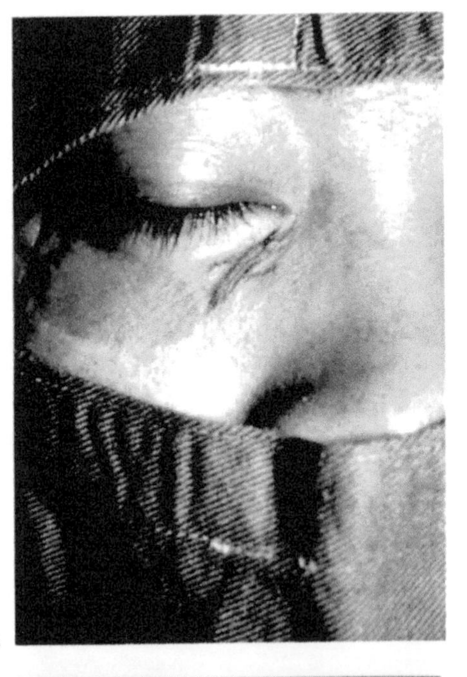

A

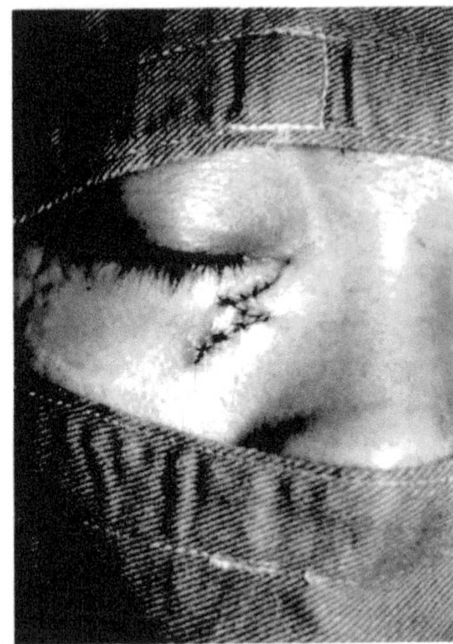

B

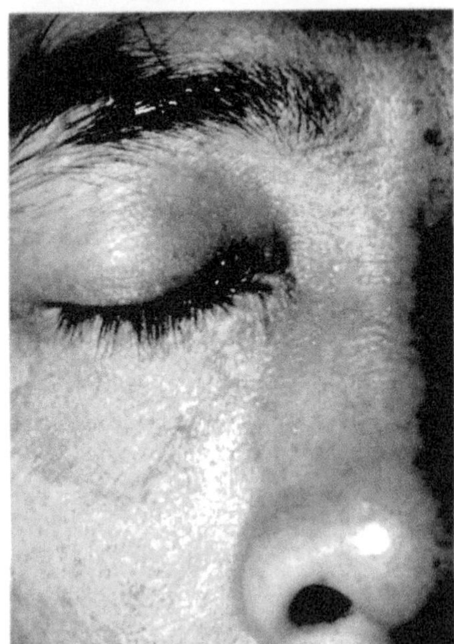

C

Figure 10 **(A)** Design of Z-plasty for scar revision at lower eyelid. **(B)** Suture lines. Two of the Z-plasty limbs align with the RSTL. **(C)** A result 3 months after the operation.

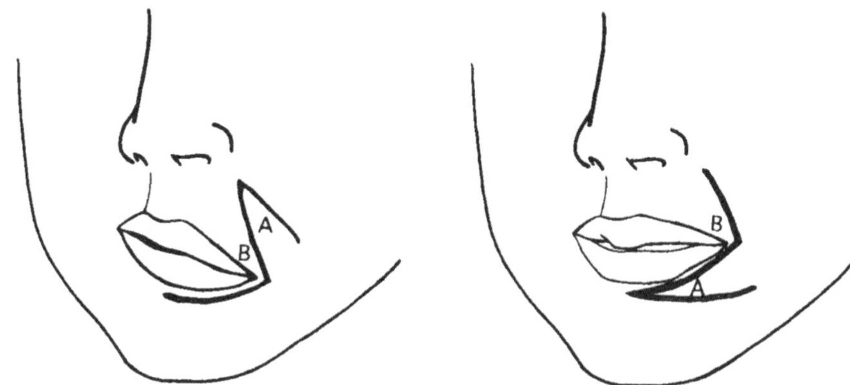

Figure 11 Z-plasty applied to construction of contracture at mouth corner.

along a straight scar when light is directed at it, making it conspicuous. A zigzag wound loses conspicuousness because the shadowing become scattered.

There is also a W-plasty for zigzag line modification of a scar. Z-plasty is especially effective when there is scar contracture or existence of a trap-door deformity. W-plasty, on the other hand, is effective when the scar direction does not align with a wrinkle and the scar is very long (Fig. 12).

G. Changing Three-Dimensional Form

It is possible for Z-plasty to change a limited area of dent deformation or deformation projection into a flat plane. A dent (or projection) area in the central limb becomes a flat plane crossing at right angles (Fig. 13). This technique is applied to webs between fingers, a cleft lobule, and web formation by scar contracture.

II. MODIFIED Z-PLASTY

A. Multiple Z-Plasty

Multiple Z-plasty is often used for long scar revision. In planning, multiple Z-plasty and single Z-plasty have the same elongation effect, but tension appears to be less in the former case. However, the actual elongation is greater in the latter case (10) (Fig. 14).

Careful consideration is especially required in designing Z-plasty for scars with few contracutures as, for example, in revision of facial scars with few contractures. Trimming of a flap is possible, and an effect of excessive elongation is lessened in this method (6) (Figs. 15 and 16).

A good application of multiple Z-plasty is in reconstruction of long facial scars and finger contracture scars. Long facial scars should be divided into several portions with as

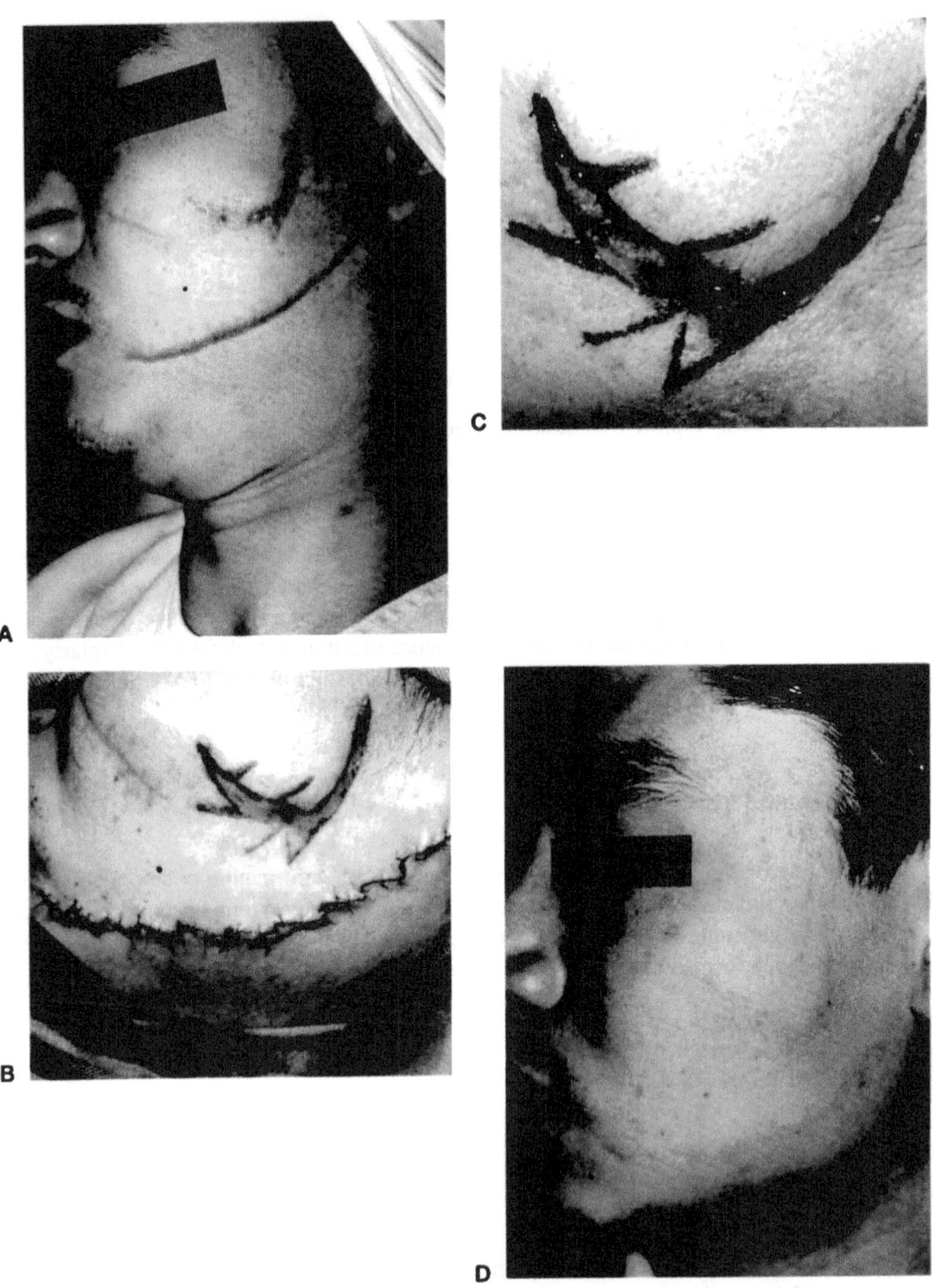

Figure 12 **(A)** Straight scar and trap-door deformity on the cheek. **(B)** Z-plasty is applied to the trap-door deformity, and W-plasty is applied to the long straight scar. **(C)** Trimming of flap. An effect of excessive elongation is lessened with this method. **(D)** A result 3 months after the operation.

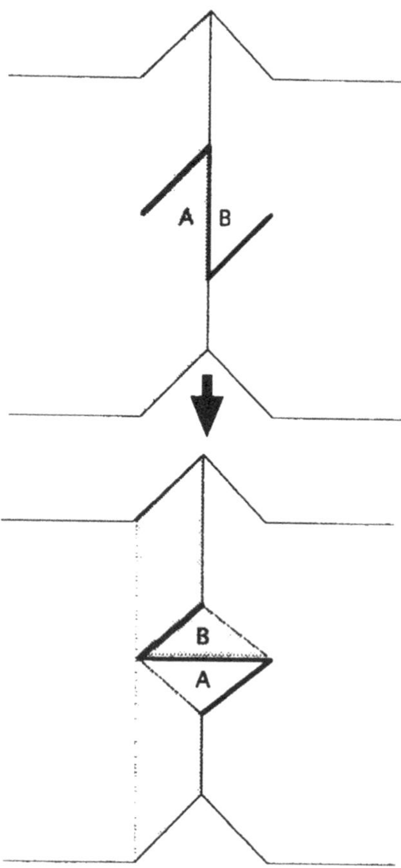

Figure 13 Dent in central limb becomes flat plane crossing at a right angle.

little elongation by Z-plasty as possible. In cases of finger scar revisions, there is no side-wise skin area, making multiple plasty the comfortable choice.

B. Four-Flap Z-Plasty

Maximum extension is effected when two triangular flaps with a 90-degree angle at the apex are utilized. Pivot point skin distortion is also greatest. The 90-degree angle flaps are therefore divided into four 45-degree angle flaps. Although there is no change in elongation effect, distortion of the skin at the flap pivot point can be reduced (Fig. 17).

C. Five-Flap Z-Plasty

One V-Y advancement flap is combined with two Z-plasty flaps. This is useful for reconstruction of contracted medial canthus and finger webs (11) (Fig. 18).

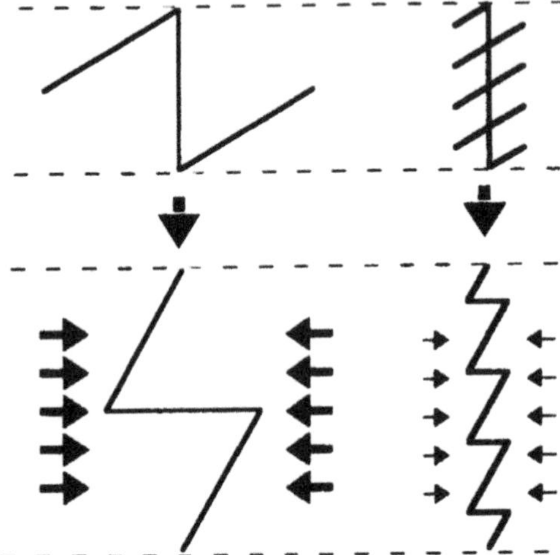

Figure 14 Comparison of single Z-plasty and multiple Z-plasty for the same scar. Although elongation is, by geometric comparison, similar, the sidewise shortening effect is quite small with multiple Z-plasty.

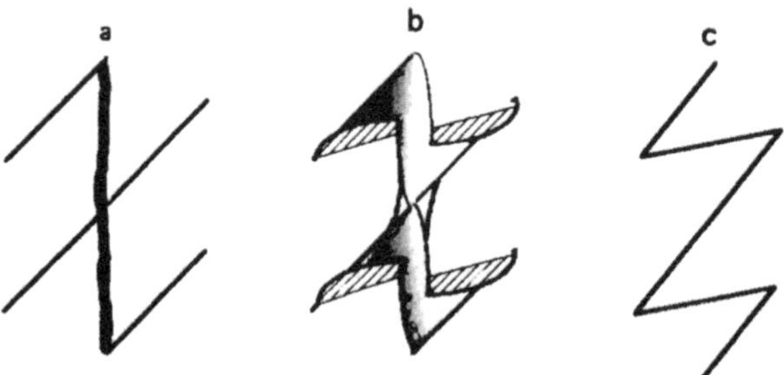

Figure 15 Z-plasty for a scar that requires little elongation. **(a)** Z-plasty design. **(b)** To reduce elongation, the shaded flap areas are trimmed. **(c)** Z-plasty is completed.

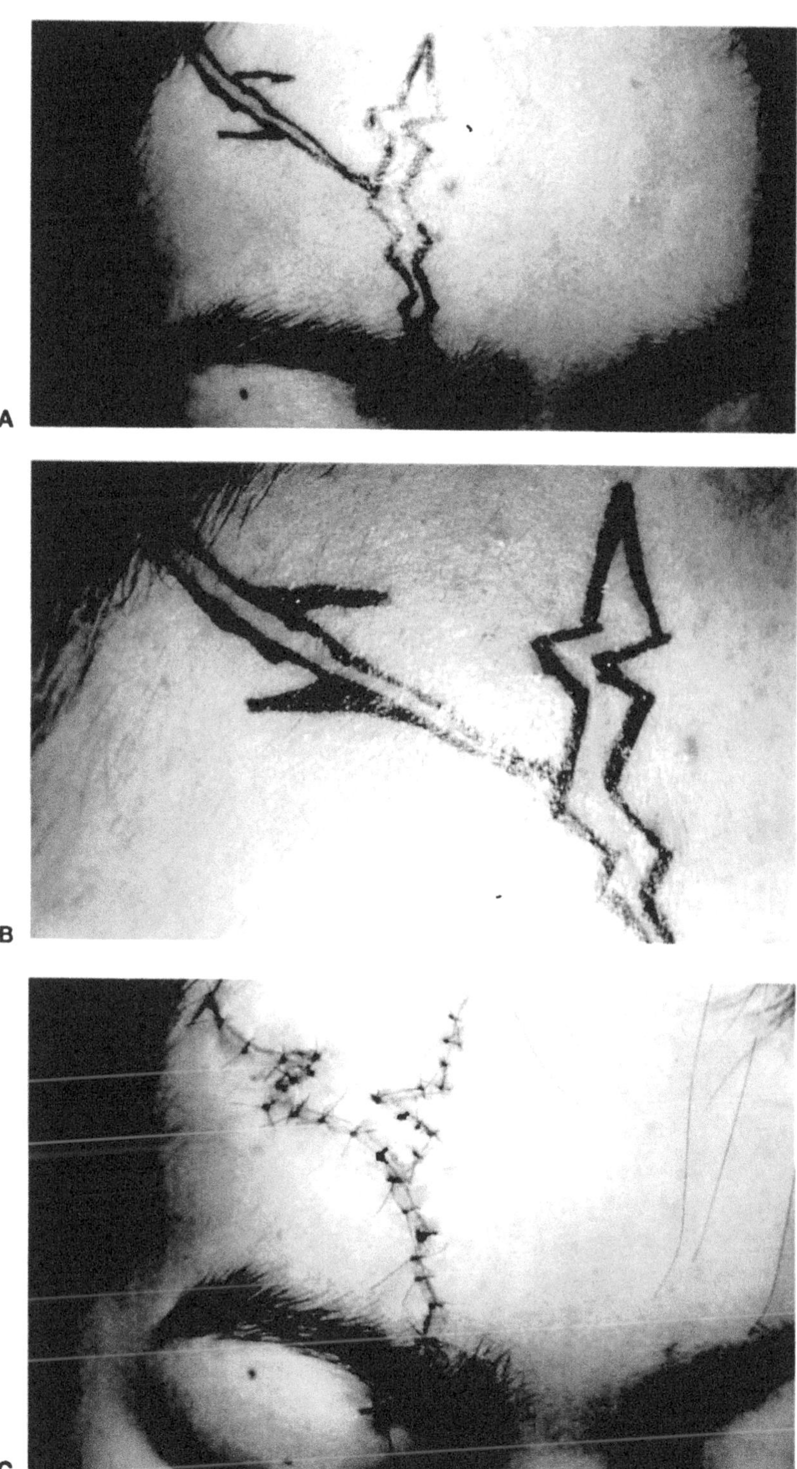

Figure 16 **(A)** Single Z-plasty and W-plasty are applied to forehead scars. **(B)** Trimming of triangular flaps. **(C)** Result.

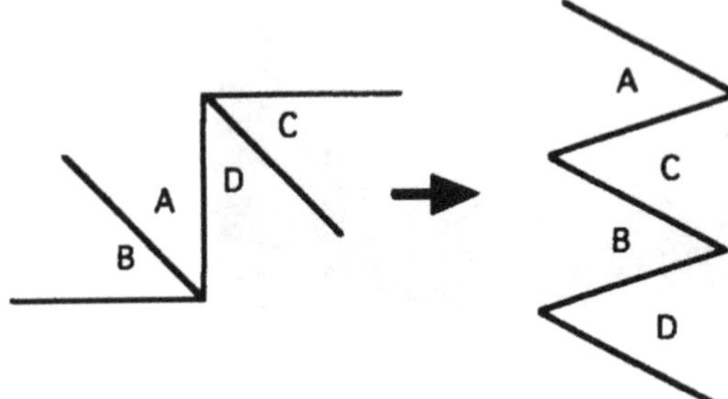

Figure 17 Four-flap Z-plasty.

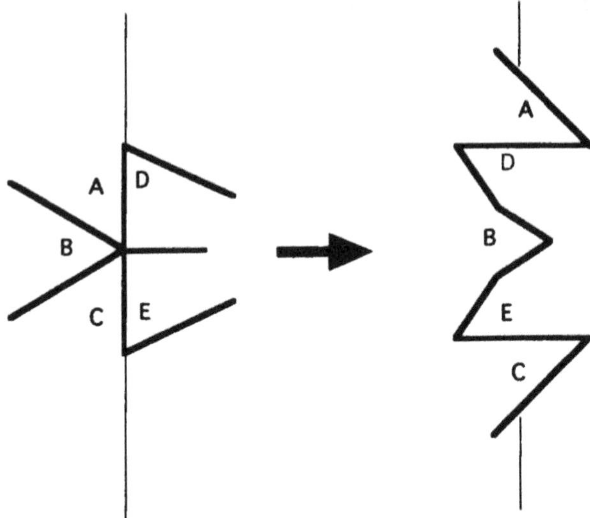

Figure 18 Five-flap Z-plasty.

REFERENCES

1. Horner WE. Clinical reports on the surgical department of the Philadelphia Hospital, Blockley for the months of May, June, and July. Am J Med Sci 1837; 21:99-112.
2. Dononvilers CP. Présentation de Malades. Bull Soc Chir Paris 1854; 5:35:118.
3. Davis JS. The relaxation of scar contractures by means of Z or Z-type incision. Ann Surg 1931; 94:871–874.
4. Davis JS. Present evaluation of the merits of the Z-plastic operation. Plast Reconstr Surg 1946; 1:26–38.
5. McGregor IA. The theoretical basis of the Z-plasty. Br J Plast Surg 1957; 9:256–259.
6. Roggendorf E. The planimetric Z-plasty. Plast Reconstr Surg 1983; 71:834–842.
7. Yanai A. The Z in Z-plasty must have a long trunk. Br J Plast Surg 1986; 39:390–394.
8. McGregor IA. The Fundamental Techniques of Plastic Surgery, 6th ed. New York: Churchill Livingstone, 1975, p. 38.
9. Yanai A. Direction of suture lines in Z-plasty scar revision. Aesthetic Plast Surg 1985; 10:97–99.
10. Furnas DW. The Z-plasty biomechanics and mathematics. Br J Plast Surg 1971; 24:144–160.
11. Mustarde JC., ed. Plastic Surgery in Infancy and Childhood, 2nd ed. Edinburgh: Livingstone, 1979, p. 223.

21
The W-Plasty Technique

Takuya Onizuka and Fumio Ohkubo
Showa University School of Medicine
Tokyo, Japan

W-plasty was first described by Ombredanne in 1937 (1) and used to correction a congenital constricting band. In 1959, "W-plasty" was reported in detail by Borges (2,3).

I. NAME

W-plasty was named as such by Borges (2,3) because of the resemblance of the preoperative incision design and the postoperative scar to the alphabetic letter "W."

II. PURPOSE

The purposes of W-plasty are (a) prevention of the bowstring effect of a long linear scar (4) and (b) illusional formation of an inconspicuous linear scar by transformation of the long linear or complicated scar to a short zigzag line (5).

III. DIFFERENCE BETWEEN W-PLASTY AND CONTINUOUS Z-PLASTY

Although both W-plasty and Z-plasty produce the same zigzag scar postoperatively, the following are points of difference.

1. Flap transplantation is unnecessary in W-plasty.
2. Elongation of the scar is minimal in W-plasty.
3. Unnecessary skin can be trimmed in W-plasty.
4. Skin is bulky at the flap pivot point in Z-plasty.

IV. INDICATION FOR W-PLASTY

W-plasty is indicated in the following cases:

1. Scar
   (a) A scar running along a natural wrinkle line. Because the natural wrinkle line itself has a smooth curve, a linear scar along this line, especially in the face,

becomes much more conspicuous by the bowstring effect of the scar when speaking or laughing.
   (b) Prevention of mild or moderate scar contracture. However, a severe scar should be repaired by W-Z plasty (2).
   (c) Conspicuous or complicated scar repair.
   (d) Depressed scar repair. However, a severely depressed scar should be repaired by Z-plasty.
   (e) Trap-door flap deformity repair.
   (f) Suture mark repair.
2. Congenital constricting band of the extremities (1,2).
3. Epicanthus (5).
4. Syndactyly (6).
5. Vaginal reconstruction (7).
6. Nostril rim deformity (5).

V. CONTRAINDICATIONS FOR W-PLASTY

W-plasty is not recommended for the following cases:

1. A scar running along the oculomalar groove. The eyelid skin is thin and pigmented, and the cheek skin is thick and white. Therefore, the postoperative scar becomes more conspicuous because of these different types of skin.
2. A severely constricted scar. For this scar, Z-plasty is necessary.
3. Ectropion of the free margin, such as a lip or lid. This deformity needs Z-plasty.
4. Taut surrounding skin.

VI. PSYCHOLOGICAL EFFECT OF W-PLASTY

When observing a point of a long line, an illusion of the line continuing beyond the end point appears, which makes the line look longer that it actually is. This illusion can be avoided by converting the linear line to a zigzag line.

A shadow caused by the direction of light, such as sunlight or electrical light, in any scar. As lines running parallel to the direction of light do not produce shadows, the short shadows of the zigzag line are not as conspicuous as a linear long shadowy scar. W-plasty has a big effect on aesthetic improvement.

VII. TECHNIQUE OF W-PLASTY

Figure 1 depicts the technique of W-plasty, as outlined below.

1. The length of the W is about 5 mm (3–10 mm) and the angle of the flap tip is approximately 60 degrees (45–90 degrees). Each triangular tip faces the midpoint of the opposing triangular base. If this angle is sharp, circulation impairment may occur; if obtuse, the jagged line would resemble a linear line, thereby losing the W-plasty effect. If the length of the W is longer than about 5 mm, the characteristics of W-plasty disappear and the postoperative line appears conspicuously long.

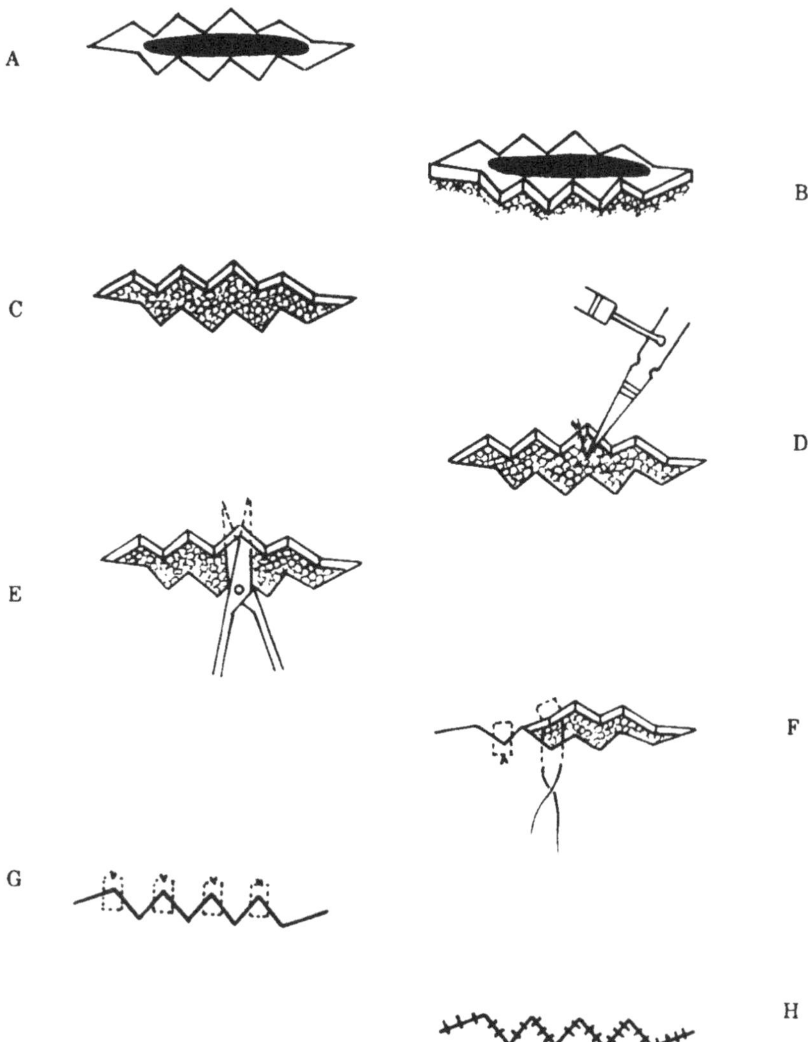

Figure 1 Technique of W-plasty. **(A)** Design of W-plasty. **(B)** Excised tissue. **(C)** Wound after scar excision. **(D)** Hemostases. **(E)** Subcutaneous undermining. **(F)** Subcutaneous sutures. **(G)** After subcutaneous sutures. **(H)** Skin sutures.

2. Incision should be done precisely with a sharp no. 11 blade. A running W knife is unnecessary.
3. Subcutaneous tissue is undermined for sufficient approximation of the wound edges.
4. Hemostasis should be amply performed. A drain is unnecessary.
5. Dermostiching is performed with Vicryl 5-0 or 6-0.
6. The skin is sutured with interrupted nylon thread. A continuous subcutaneous suture should not be used to approximate the edges, because of technical difficulties and time consumption.

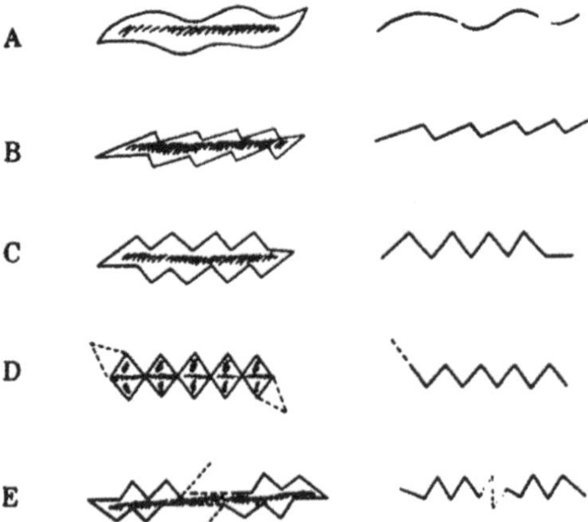

Figure 2 Modified types of W-plasty. **(A)** Wave type. **(B)** Roof tile shape. **(C)** Mountainous type. **(D)** Diamond shape. **(E)** Combination type. (From Ref. 5.)

7. If protrusion of the flap tip occurs after suturing, the tip is trimmed. A triangular suture method is not used because it is very difficult and troublesome.
8. Length and angle of the flap should be changed according to the type and shape of the scar (Fig. 2).
9. A postoperative pressure dressing is necessary for prevention of edema, hematoma, and a hypertrophic scar.

VIII. REPRESENTATIVE CASES

Representative cases of W-plasty are shown in Figs. 3–6.

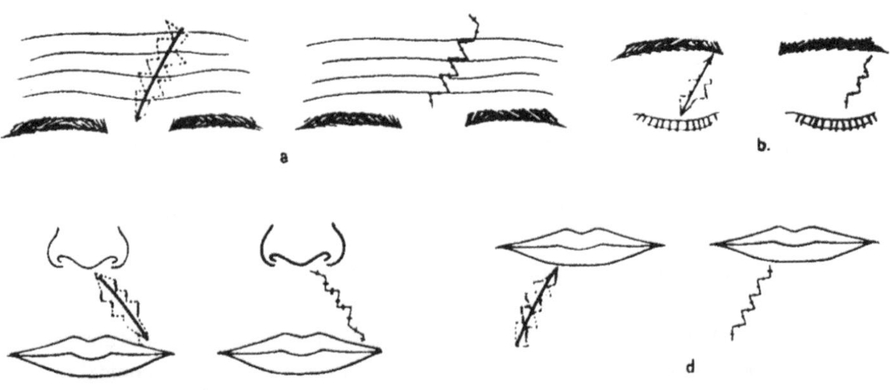

Figure 3 Examples of W-plasty. (From Ref. 5.)

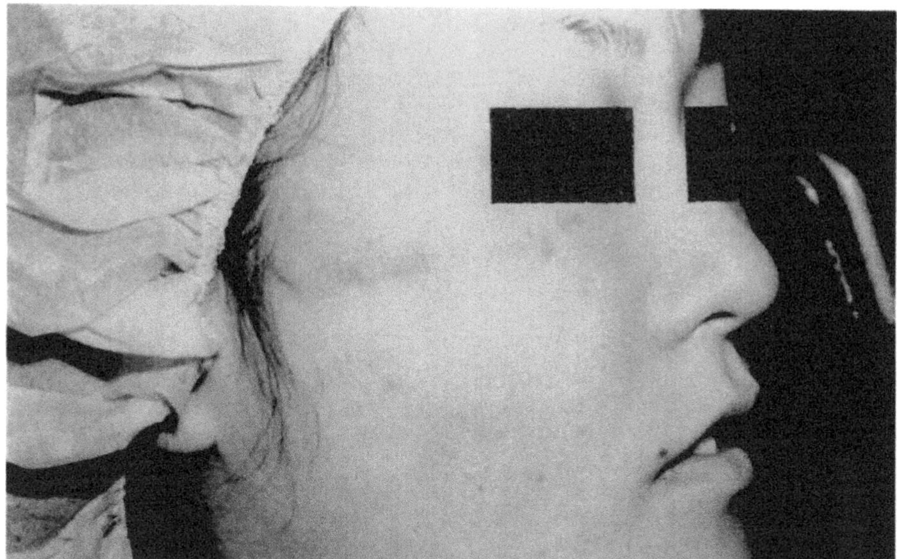
A

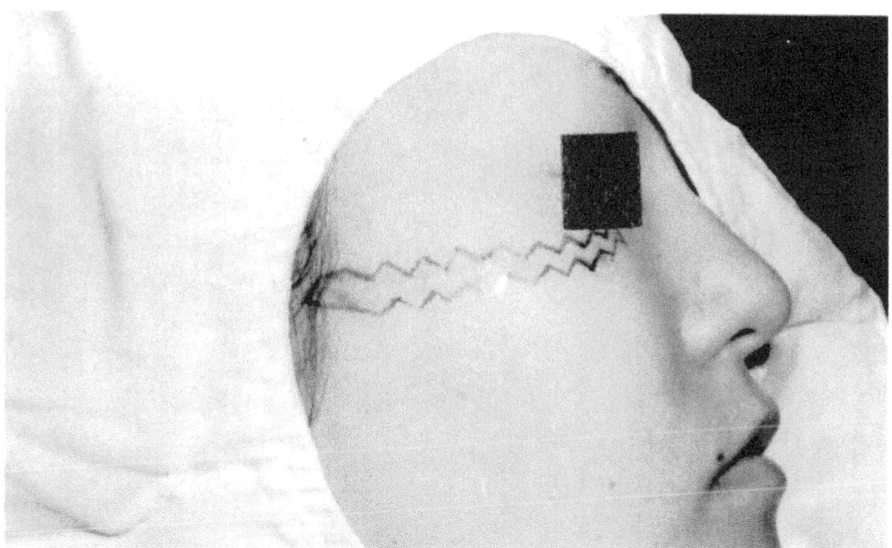
B

Figure 4 Scar of the right cheek. **(A)** Preoperative view. **(B)** Design of W-plasty. **(C)** Excision of the scar. **(D)** Subcutaneous sutures. **(E)** Skin sutures. *(figure continues)*

IX. COMBINATION USE OF W-PLASTY WITH OTHER TECHNIQUES

W-plasty is used in combination with other techniques as in the following.

1. W-Z Plasty. For severely constricted or web-type scars, W-plasty and Z-plasty are combined (5). Z-plasty elongates and changes the direction of the contractile scar to the lines of minimal tension (1).

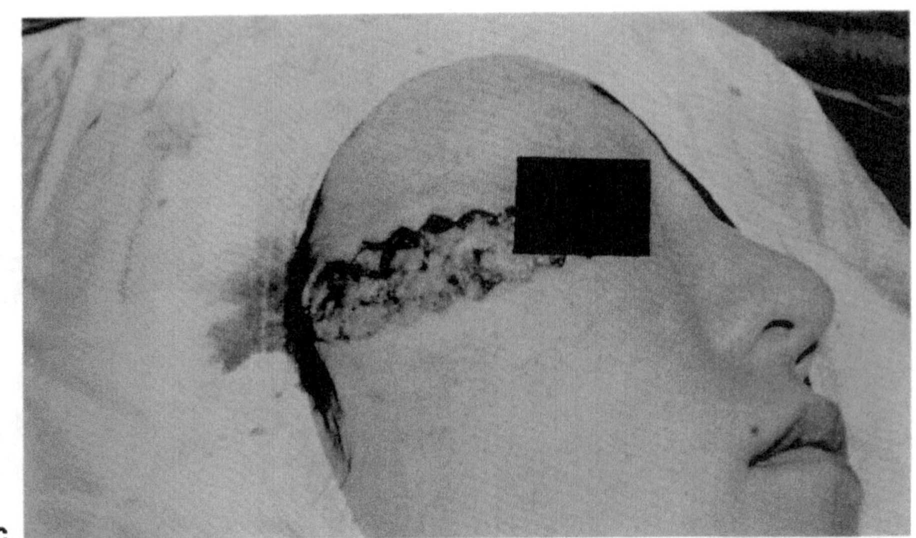
C

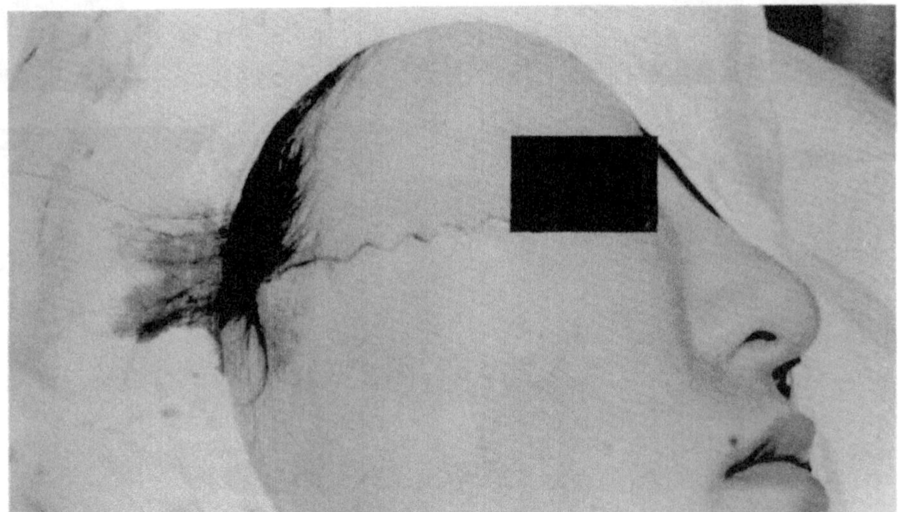
D

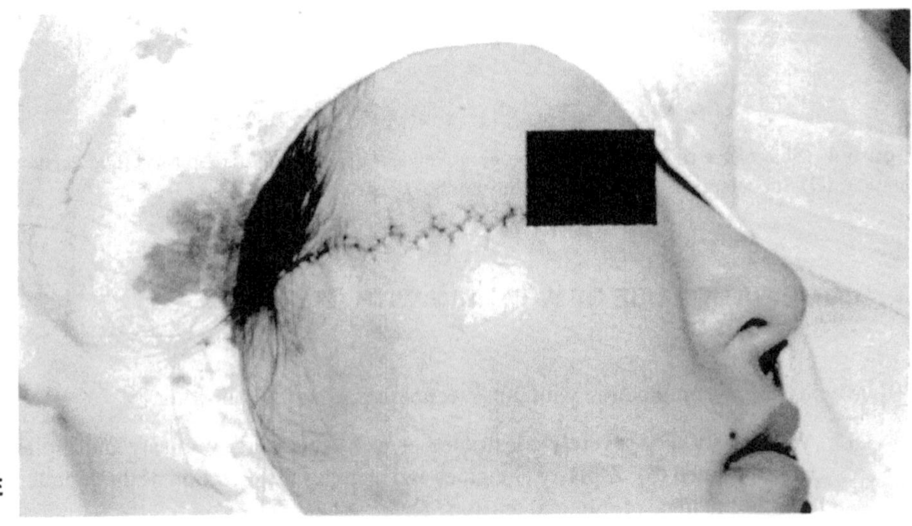
E

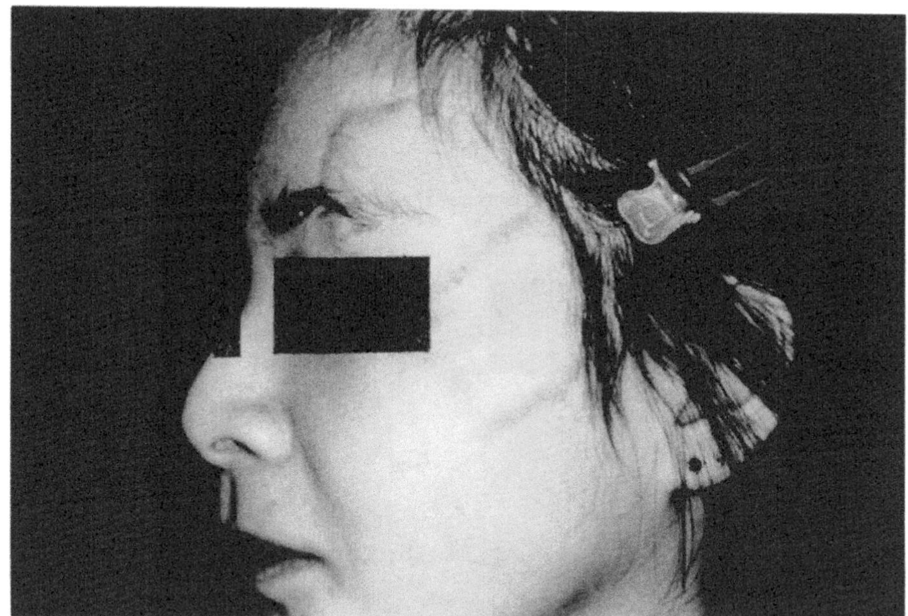

A

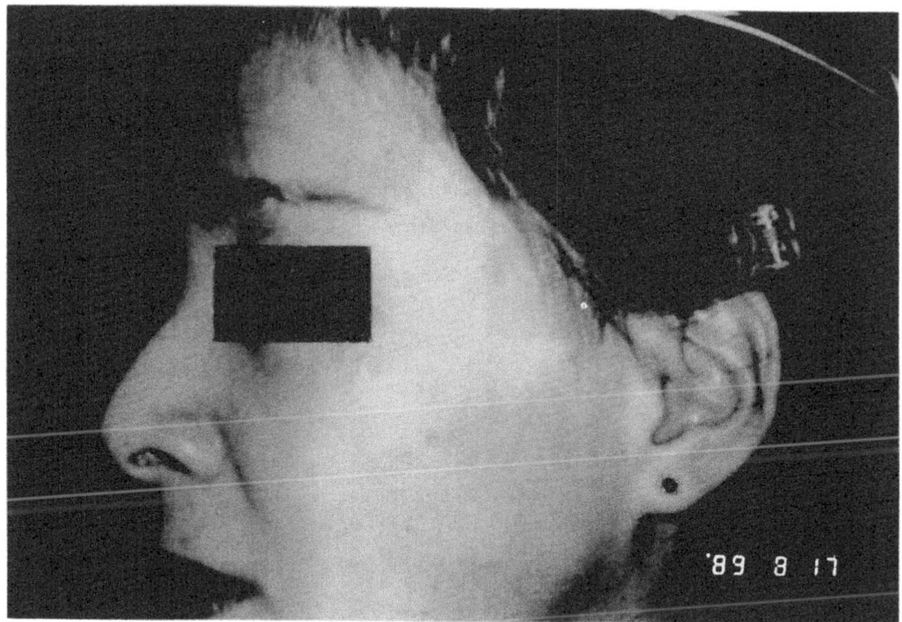

B

Figure 5 Example 1: scar of the left face. **(A)** Preoperative view. **(B)** Postoperative view.

Figure 4 *(continued)*

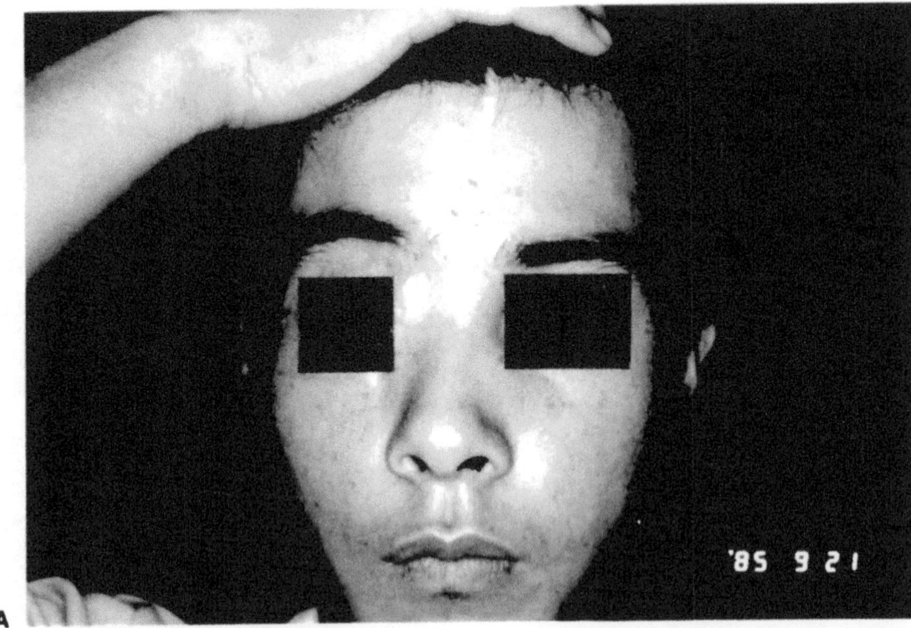

A

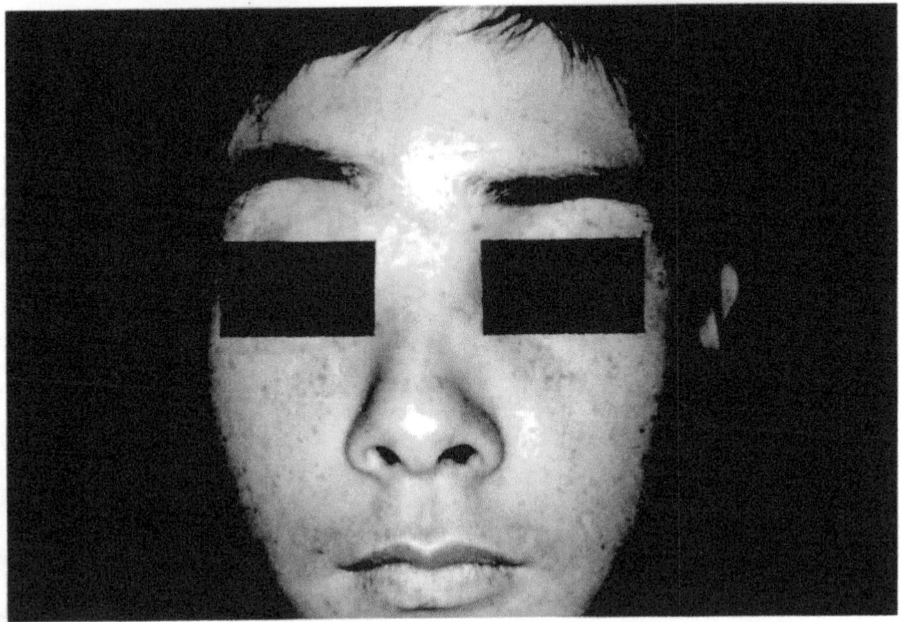

B

Figure 6 Example 2: scar of the forehead and right eyelids. **(A)** Preoperative view. **(B)** Postoperative view.

2. Rhomboid and W-plasty. This is a combination of the rhomboid flap and W-plasty (5).
3. W-M-plasty. The combination of W-plasty and M-plasty has been reported to repair syndactyly (6).
4. W-Poulard-plasty. This is a combination of W-plasty and the Poulard technique, in which dermal tissue or subcutaneous tissue is buried to improve the surface curve (5,8).

REFERENCES

1. McCarthy JB. Plastic Surgery. Vol. 1. Philadelphia: Saunders, 1990:64–65.
2. Borges AF. Improvement of antitension-lines scar by the "W-plastic" operation. Br J Plast Surg 1959; 12:29–33.
3. Borges AF. Historical review of the Z- and W-plasty revisions of linear scars. Int Surg 1971; 56:182–186.
4. Borges AF. Elective Incisions and Scar Revision. Boston: Little Brown, 1973.
5. Onizuka T. Operative Plastic and Aesthetic Surgery. Tokyo: Nankodo, 1996.
6. Karacaoglan N, Velidedeoglu H, Cicekci B, Bozdogan N, Sahin U, Turkguven Y. Reverse W-M plasty in the repair of congenital syndactyly: a new method. Br J Plast Surg 1993; 46:300–302.
7. Yueh-Bih Tang Chen, Tai-Ju Cheng, Ho-Hsiung Lin, Yuh-Shih Yang. Spatial W-plasty full-thickness skin graft for neovaginal reconstruction. Plast Reconstr Surg 1994; 94:727–731.
8. Saleh M, Howard AC. Improving the appearance of pin-site scars. J Bone Joint Surg 1994; 76-B:906–908.

22

The Geometric Broken-Line Technique

Terence M. Davidson and Drew M. Horlbeck
University of California, San Diego, and VA Health Care
San Diego, California

The concept of a broken line is simple (Fig. 1). The human eye follows a straight line, but if the line is somehow broken, in some irregular fashion, then the human eye has difficulty following it, for it picks up the straight line and follows that but fails to predict the change in direction and so wanders into free space. The eye then has to return to where it lost the line, pick up the next straight line, and follow that until that line changes direction. It then has to find the next straight line with each direction change. This is such a time-consuming, troublesome process that one does not see the scar as clearly as one sees a straight-line scar. This principle is seen in today's transposition flaps, where one can repair a small circular defect with a transposition flap with a curvilinear design or repair the same circular defect with an angulated flap, such as the design in Fig. 2, using either a 30- or even a 60-degree transposition flap. In one case you achieve a curvilinear closure and in the other case you create an angulated broken line closure. The angulated closure is aesthetically superior to the curvilinear design.

There are important principles when this concept is applied to the human face. The lines and the angles have to be defined. Any given segment should not exceed 0.5 cm and all angles must be acute. Ninety degrees works well, but angles more acute, such as 60 degrees, also work well. When the angle is oblique, the eye can pick it up and follow it continuously. It is then no longer cosmetically camouflaged.

The segment lengths change depending upon where on the body the broken-line scar revision is performed. In areas such as the back, one uses slightly longer lines, up to 0.6 cm. In cosmetically more important areas one should shorten these distances. For example, on a lower eyelid or the upper lip these lines might be as short as 0.2 and 0.3 cm. The principles of the acute angles remain the same.

Generally speaking, any scar that is longer than 2 cm, that does not fall in the junction of one aesthetic area with another, that is wider than 2 mm, or that for any other reason is not cosmetically favorable can probably be improved.

The most difficult part of the geometric broken line is its design (Fig. 3A–F). Begin by dividing the horizontal scar from left to right into a series of segments. The distance between segments is variable. For purposes of description, these planning lines are called

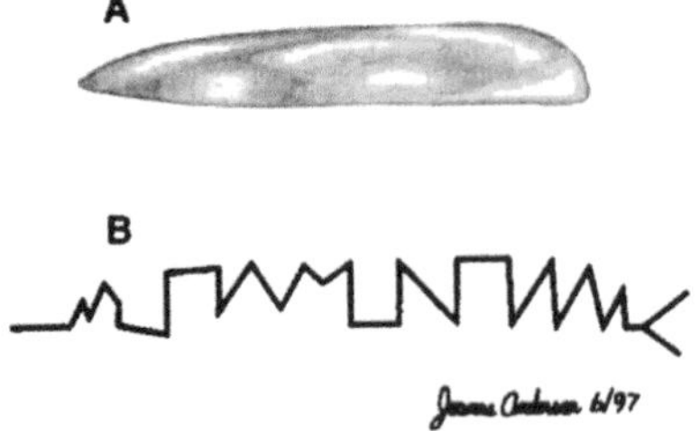

Figure 1 Geometric broken-line closure concepts. **(A)** Scar. **(B)** Excision and closure with an irregularly broken line. This broken line evades the human eye.

crosshatches. In this example the first line crosses outside the scar by 2 mm. The second line, which is 3–4 mm away from the first crosshatch, crosses the scar by 3 mm. The next crosshatch, which is any where up to 5 mm distant, now crosses the scar by 4 mm and then the next one crosses it by 5 mm.

There is then a series of 5-mm crosshatches. Their separation is variable, not to exceed 5 mm. This pattern continues until one gets to the other end, where the length process is reversed so that the crosshatch farthest from the end is 5, then the next is 4, the next one is 3, and the last one is 2 mm.

One then designs a series of interposition flaps in each of these boxes. The flaps are a variety of designs. One uses a random mixture of triangles and quadrangles (Fig. 4). First design the top using these randomly designed flap patterns. One then draws the mirror images on the bottom so that one has a series of flaps that, after excising the scar, will interdigitate.

Next create a design for the end. Typically, this will either be a 30-degree angle such as shown on the left-hand side of Fig. 3 or is designed as a 30-degree angle shown at the opposite end, but because of its length it is modified into two parallel 30-degree angle flaps called an M-plasty.

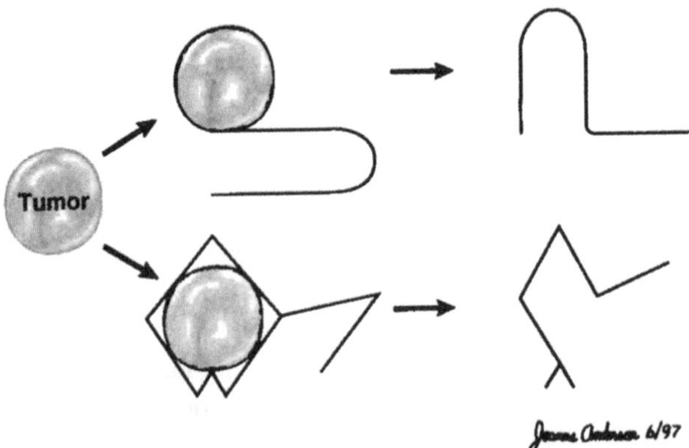

Figure 2 Transposition flap closure of a circular defect. According to the principles of a geometric broken line, the curvilinear closure is far more easily noticed and preceived than the angulated excision and closure.

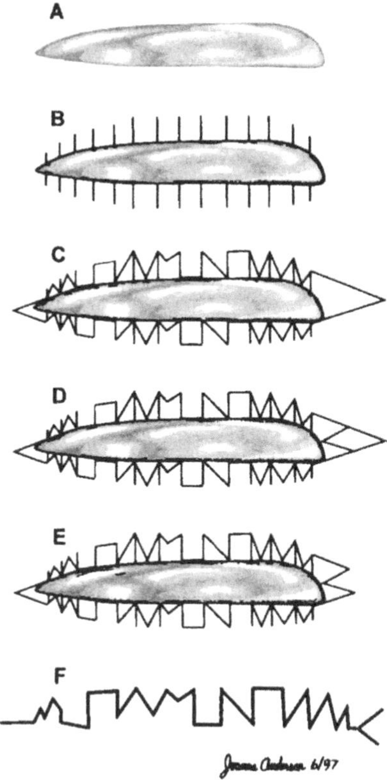

Figure 3 Design of a geometric broken line closure. **(A)** The scar. **(B)** Crosshatching. **(C)** Flap design. **(D)** Addition of an M-plasty. **(E)** Completion of an M-plasty. **(F)** Final closure.

Triangular Flaps

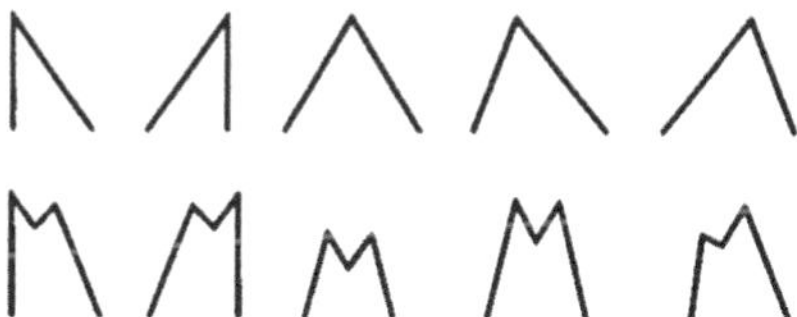

Quadrangular Flaps

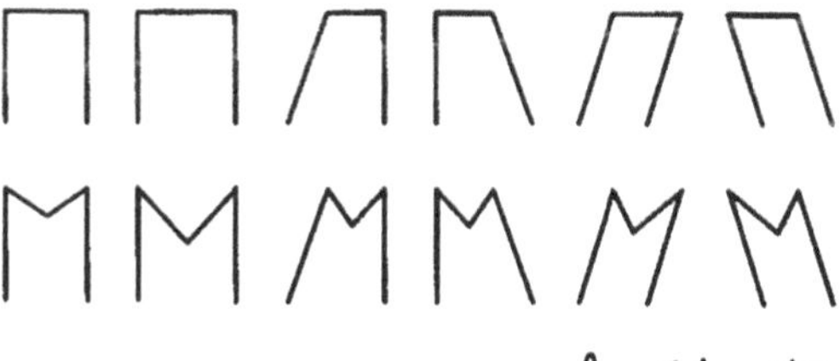

Figure 4 Variations in flaps used in geometric broken-line surgery.

The rules of restricting the line length to 5 mm or less dictate whether a single 30-degree angle or an M-plasty will be utilized.

Figure 3F shows the finished design. One now excises the scar. The scar revision surgery typically uses a no. 11 blade. This is invariably performed by holding the scalpel in a vertical direction, putting the no. 11 blade into the apex of each flap, and cutting centrally toward the scar. Therefore, if one slips, one cuts into the scar and not into the normal skin. One does this with a series of saw cuts and when one has finished making all of the cuts, one then repeats the process, typically with a new blade, cutting each corner, completing each of the cuts, and thereby excising the scar with the necessary free tissue.

The flaps are then undermined, hemostatis is achieved, and the wounds are sutured together. Several variations are important. Figure 5 shows a scar with linear and curvilinear segments. One begins at each end, again with increasing length flaps, until one is at 5 mm. When one gets to the curvilinear part, the flaps that run perpendicular to the scar are very much larger on one side than they are on the other. Hence, most of the quadrangular designs are ineffective. For the portions designed on the curvilinear part, it is standard to use triangles as would be used in a running W-plasty. Triangles will absorb the diversity of size and angles much more easily than do the quadrangular flaps.

The next concept is matching the geometric broken line (GBL) to the favorable skin tension lines. For this purpose, consider a standard scar and vary the direction of the FSTL indicated by the arrows. In any scar revision the best lines are those that parallel the FSTL and the least favorable are those that run perpendicular. It is unfortunately necessary in most geometric broken line closures to design some elements of the scar revision perpendicular to FSTLs. One can do this in a fashion that minimizes the problem (Fig. 6A and B).

In all cases there are pros and cons to how these are sloped and designed. There are pros and cons to how sophisticated and complex the design should be, and sometimes one

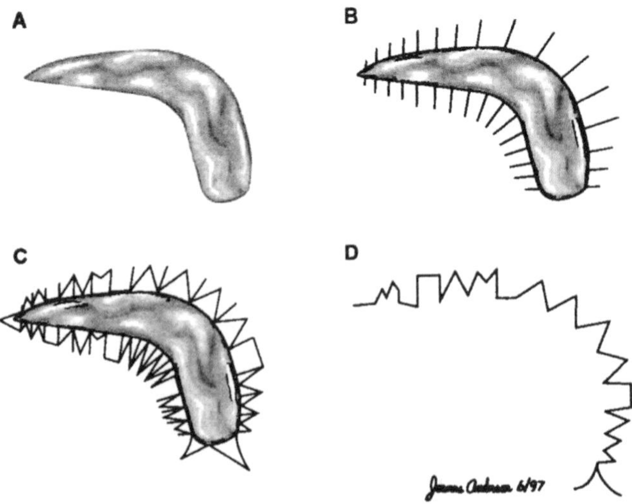

Figure 5 **(A–D)** Designs of a geometric broken-line closure around a curvilinear scar. For this portion the running W-plasty has a great advantage.

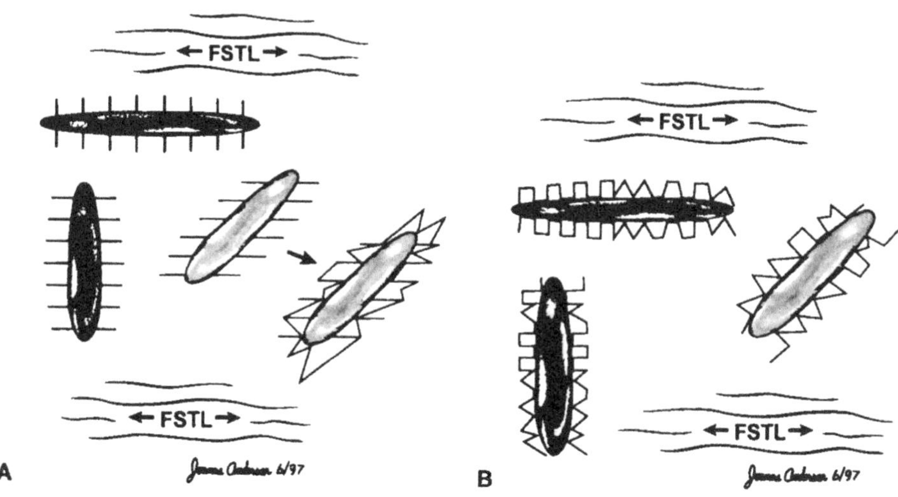

Figure 6 Modifying the geometric broken-line closure for surrounding favorable skin tension lines. **(A)** Crosshatch design. **(B)** Geometric broken-line design.

ends up with more scar and an inferior result by trying to be too fancy. In addition, GBL techniques can be time consuming and each angle, each complexity, each change of direction is another minute cutting and another minute suturing. These minutes add up to hours.

It should be clear that the geometric broken line closure is really a combination of quadrangles and triangles. As opposed to the classic running W-plasty, these little flaps are not all oriented similarly. Even the running W-plasty becomes a broken-line closure, albeit a broken line running W-plasty closure.

In some cases there is an advantage to providing lengthening along the scar line. This can be done in one of two fashions. The standard, as is used for revising a vertical tracheostomy scar, would be to design a running W-plasty. To achieve lengthening one employs Y to V maneuvers so that each of the little Ys is converted into a V. When these expand as shown in Fig. 7 and the flaps are interpolated, the tissue is borrowed from horizontally and expanded vertically. Lengthening is therefore achieved.

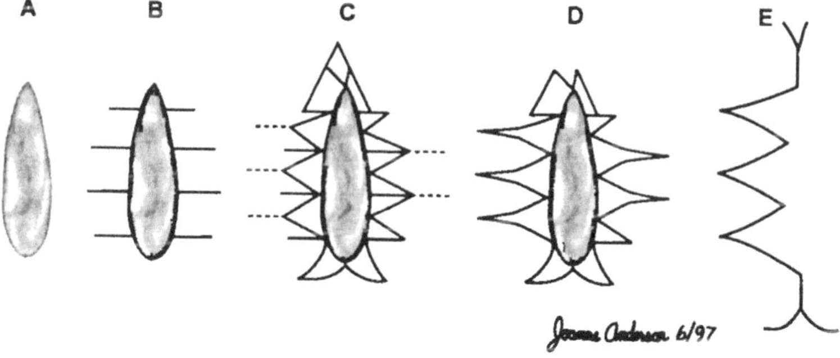

Figure 7 **(A–E)** Designs of a geometric broken line to close a vertical tracheostomy scar. The Y-to-V maneuver is an excellent lengthening maneuver.

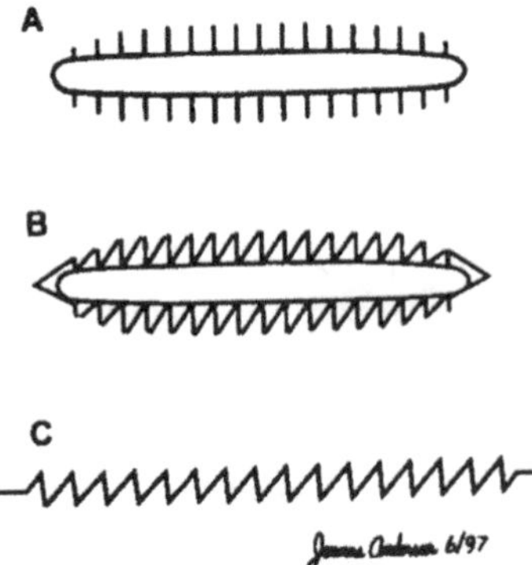

Figure 8 Z-plasties and scar revision. **(A)** Usual crosshatch design. **(B)** Use of a Z-plasty. **(C)** Final closure showing both the lengthening and the predictable regularity of a conventional serial Z-plasty.

The other technique to achieve lengthening is to use a Z-plasty. Z-plasties can be used alone for scar revision. The problem with the running Z-plasty scar revision is that it may cause unsightly lengthening, i.e., may cause too much lengthening; or, if the Zs are not used in some randomized design, then just like the running W-plasty, this can become a regular predictable pattern (Fig. 8).

To get lengthening one begins with the usual crosshatching into segments and then uses one or two of the segments and converts them into a Z-plasty. In the standard Z-plasty, the central limbs and the lateral limbs are of similar lengths. In this example there are two alternatives. The first would be to leave these as 5-mm limbs and to create a series of Z-plasties (Fig. 9A–C). The alternative is to increase the lengthening by using a single, albeit longer, Z-plasty design. Combining two crosshatch segments, there are now 10-mm limbs and the design is one that looks like Fig. 10. Note that we use triangles close to areas that

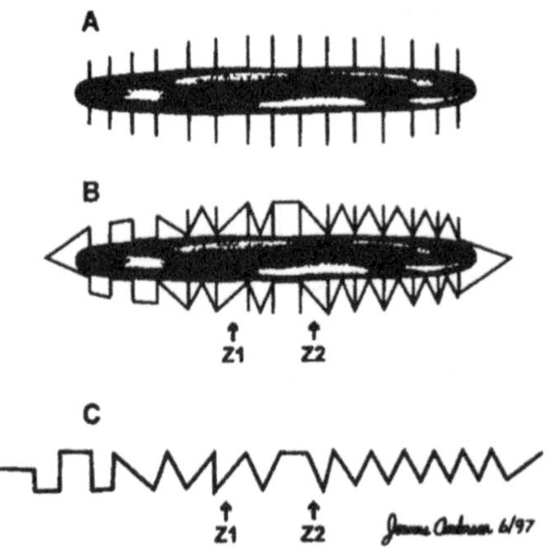

Figure 9 **(A–C)** A Z-plasty in a geometric broken line closure. This figure shows how a Z-plasty can be used in a standard geometric broken line closure.

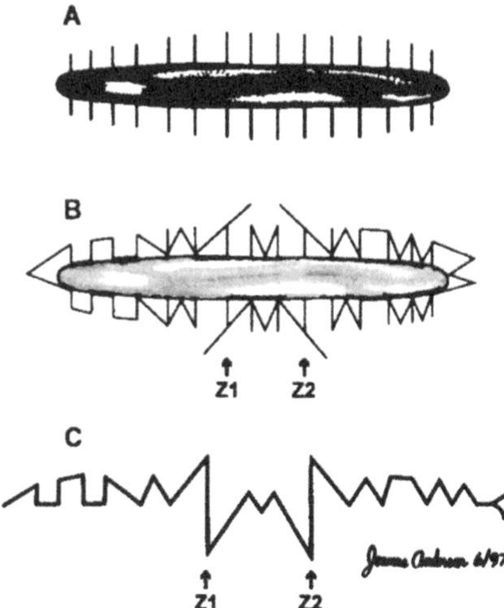

Figure 10 Z-plasty in a geometric broken line closure. Z-plasties are difficult to use. Greater lengthening is achieved in this design by using a twice normal size Z-plasty, thereby gaining greater lengthening than would have been achieved with smaller Z-plasties.

are difficult, because it is often easier to take up tissue length and angle discrepancies in triangular flaps than it is with rectangles, squares, or other designs.

Another scenario is one in which a scar crosses a natural boundary, such as a scar that runs perpendicular to the junction of cheek with lip. In these cases a Z-plasty is used to change the direction of the scar. One begins by drawing the standard Z-plasty that one would use to accommodate that direction change. The lateral limbs are drawn so that they run parallel, not perpendicular to the favorable skin tension lines. The crosshatch segments are drawn and the remainder of the GBL is designed as shown in Fig. 11A–E. This closure is then incorporated into the scar revision with a final design shown in Fig. 11E.

Running Z-plasties and serial Z-plasties can also be used. Incorporating these complex Z-plasties into a GBL may not have a great deal of cosmetic or functional advantage and has significant potential for error and difficulties with closure.

Techniques for repairing the most common GBL mistakes are important to know. The first involves having a disparate number of triangular flaps on the opposite scar sides. For purposes of demonstration, consider three flaps on top and two on the bottom as drawn in Fig. 12. To correct this, one divides one of the triangular flaps into two and ends up with three triangular flaps. Because of the ability of the running W-plasty to absorb variations in length and angles, the error is easily corrected. A more difficult error to correct is one in which a disparate number of quadrangular flaps are cut. The concept is shown in Fig. 13 with two flaps drawn on top and three drawn on the bottom. For purposes of demonstration, the flaps are redrawn so that the central quadrangle is abnormally long. The extra rectangular flap is converted into a triangle and a defect is made by cutting a vertical line in one of the upper rectangular flaps. This trimmed rectangular flap (now a triangle) fits into this triangular defect. Now there is the correct number of flaps and the opposing sides are easily juxtaposed.

The next topic requiring discussion is techniques for closure. In the old days it was said that "scar revision required an hour per inch for the cutting and closure." With today's materials and techniques, the surgical time is greatly shortened.

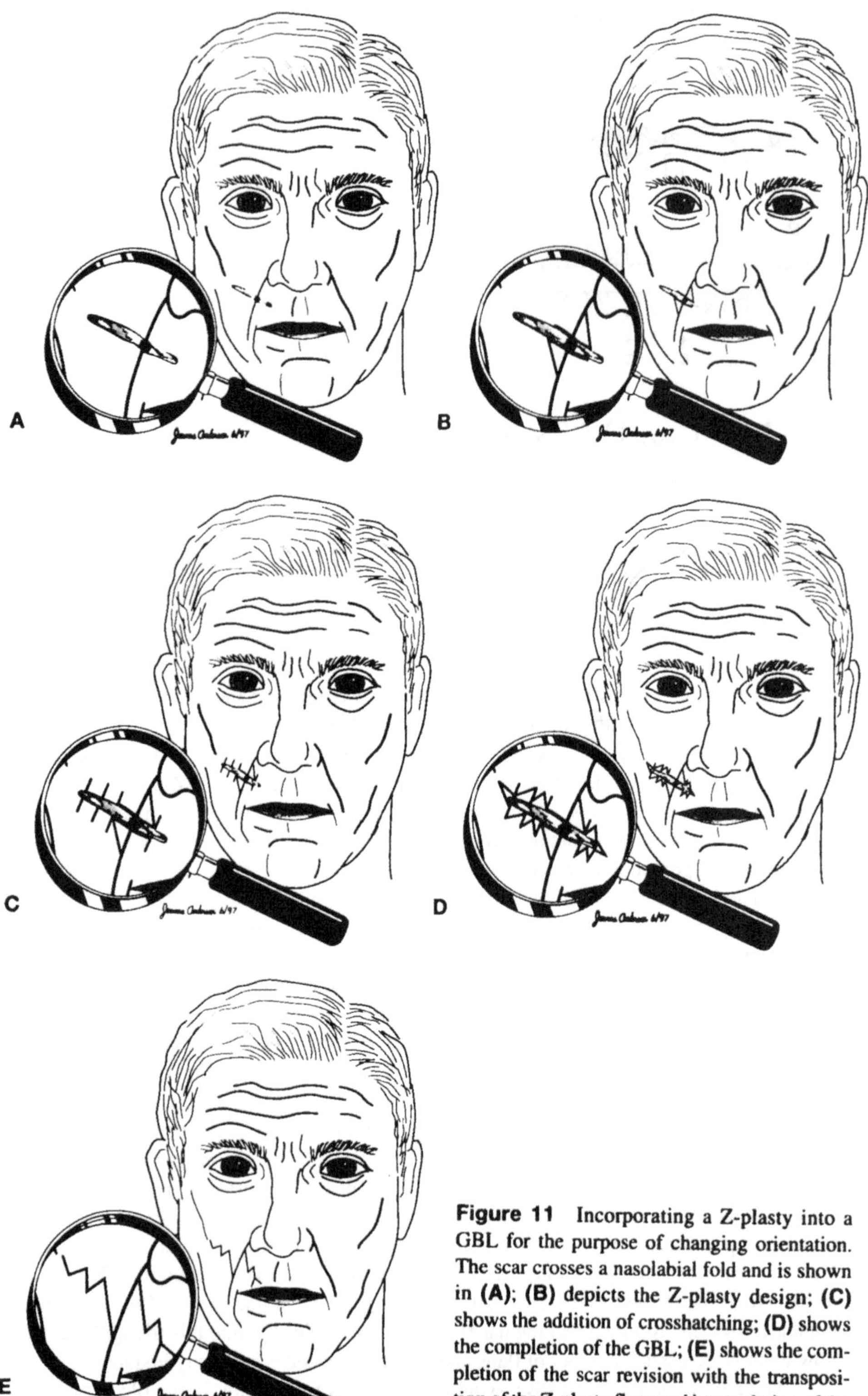

Figure 11 Incorporating a Z-plasty into a GBL for the purpose of changing orientation. The scar crosses a nasolabial fold and is shown in **(A)**; **(B)** depicts the Z-plasty design; **(C)** shows the addition of crosshatching; **(D)** shows the completion of the GBL; **(E)** shows the completion of the scar revision with the transposition of the Z-plasty flaps and interpolation of the GBL flaps.

Disparate Triangles

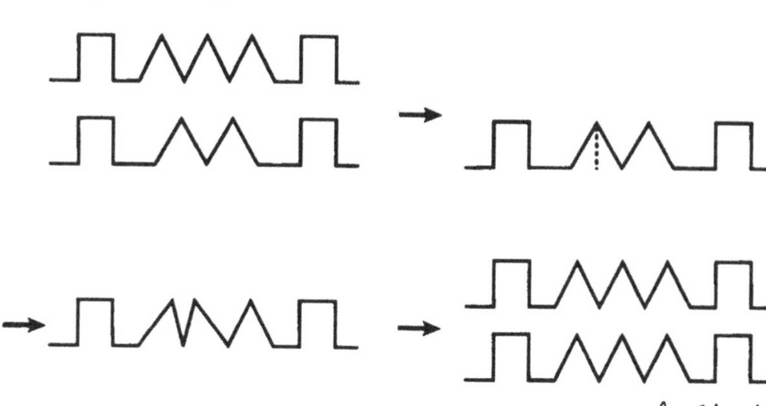

Figure 12 Disparate triangles. Occasionally one errors by cutting a disparate number of triangles. This can be corrected by dividing one of the triangular flaps into two.

Once the tissues are excised, they are undermined for a distance of 1–2 cm on either side, the distance being dictated by the size of the scar and the tension of the tissue. Hemostatis is achieved and then the subcutaneous-dermal sutures are placed. The standard dermal closure involves suturing dermis as shown in Fig. 14. The problem with this is that if one were to do this with every single flap (a) it would be time consuming and (b) it would virtually strangulate the entire blood supply to the geometric broken-line closure and potentially result in a poorly oxygenated, devitalized piece of skin. One could end up with a scar even worse than the original.

One solution is to use dermal sutures placed farther back from the wound edge, thereby gaining greater tissue influence. This has been previously published. The drawings depict the technique in Fig. 15 and 16.

Disparate Quadrangles

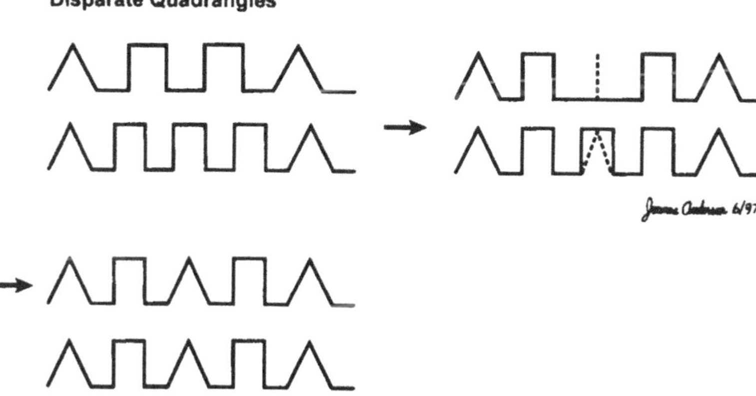

Figure 13 Disparate quadrangles. One occasionally designs a disparate number of quadrangular flaps and defects. This is corrected by converting one of the quadrangular flaps into a triangular flap and inserting it into a divided quadrangular flap on the opposing side.

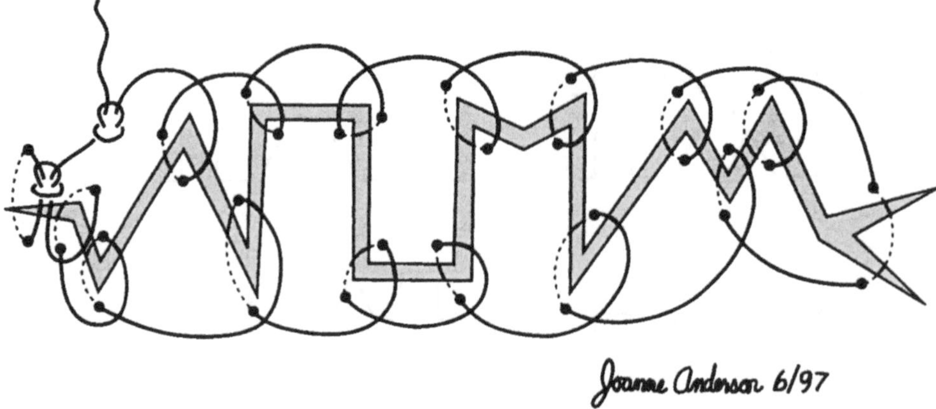

Figure 14 Technique for closing a geometric broken line closure. Subcutaneous closure is performed and then the skin is closed with a running locking fast-acting chromic suture.

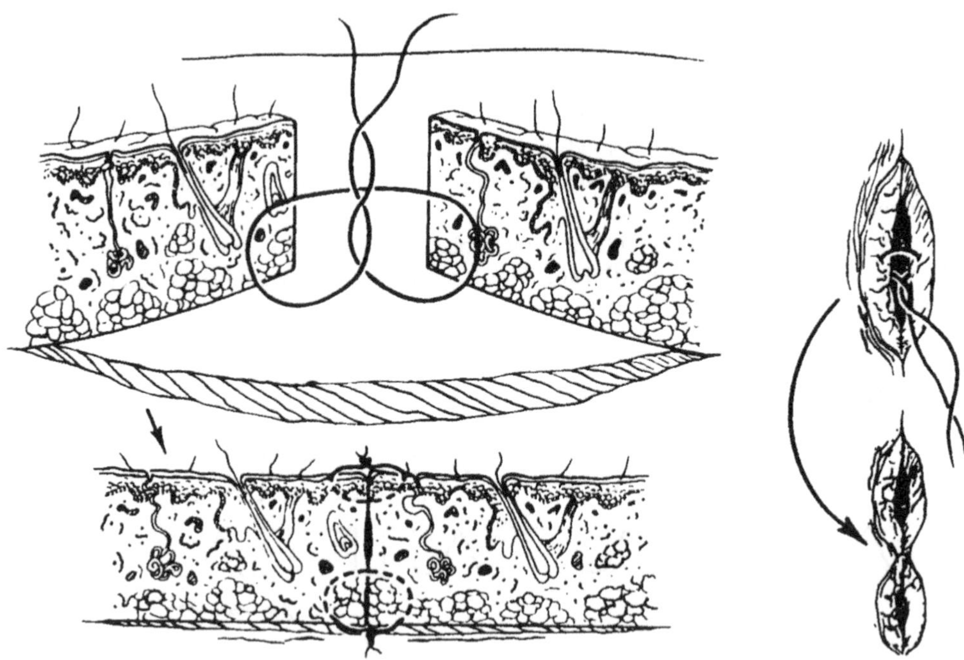

Figure 15 Classic placement of dermal subcutaneous stitch. (From Davidson TM. How I do it—head & neck and plastic surgery—subcutaneous suture placement. Laryngoscope 1987; 97:501–504.)

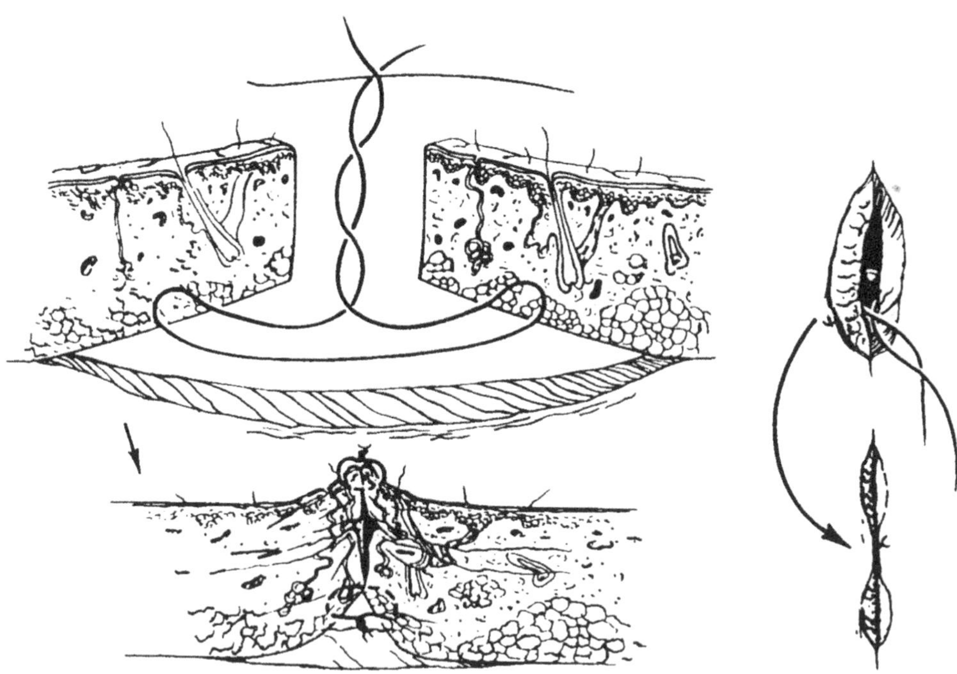

Figure 16 Dermal subcutaneous stitch to create an everted closure. (From Davidson TM. How I do it—head & neck and plastic surgery—subcutaneous suture placement. Laryngoscope 1987; 97:501–504.)

The farther the suture is placed from the wound edge, the greater the pull and the fewer the sutures needed.

The skin closure is a second issue. Standard teaching is to use a half-buried horizontal mattress (Gilles tip stitch) at every corner of every flap. These unfortunately compromise the blood supply. Simple sutures are preferred.

Placing all of these very fine little sutures is time consuming. The current technique for closure is to use a running stitch, typically with a fast-acting gut. The suture is begun at one end and then runs along one side in a locking fashion, locking each of the little apices on one side into their respective defects. At the other end, in this case, a half-buried horizontal mattress suture is used so that the tip of the M-plasty is pulled inward. At the same time, the suture is crossed over to the opposite side and run in a fashion similar to that on the first side. When it comes back to the end, the suture is tied to itself. One would typically have a few little gaps left in the middle of some of these flaps and one must remember not to suture these, for if one does, one invariably ends up with two additional sutures and invariably ends up necrosing the blood supply to the tip of the flap.

The wound is then typically Steri-stripped, in part to keep it as a moist wound and in part to assist in dissolving the fast-acting suture.

In the old days, the wound was Steri-stripped for weeks, often months, with the idea that antitension taping would prevent scar widening. With today's polyglycolic acid dermal sutures and with the realization that the antitension taping did not do much for the wound, this practice is rarely employed.

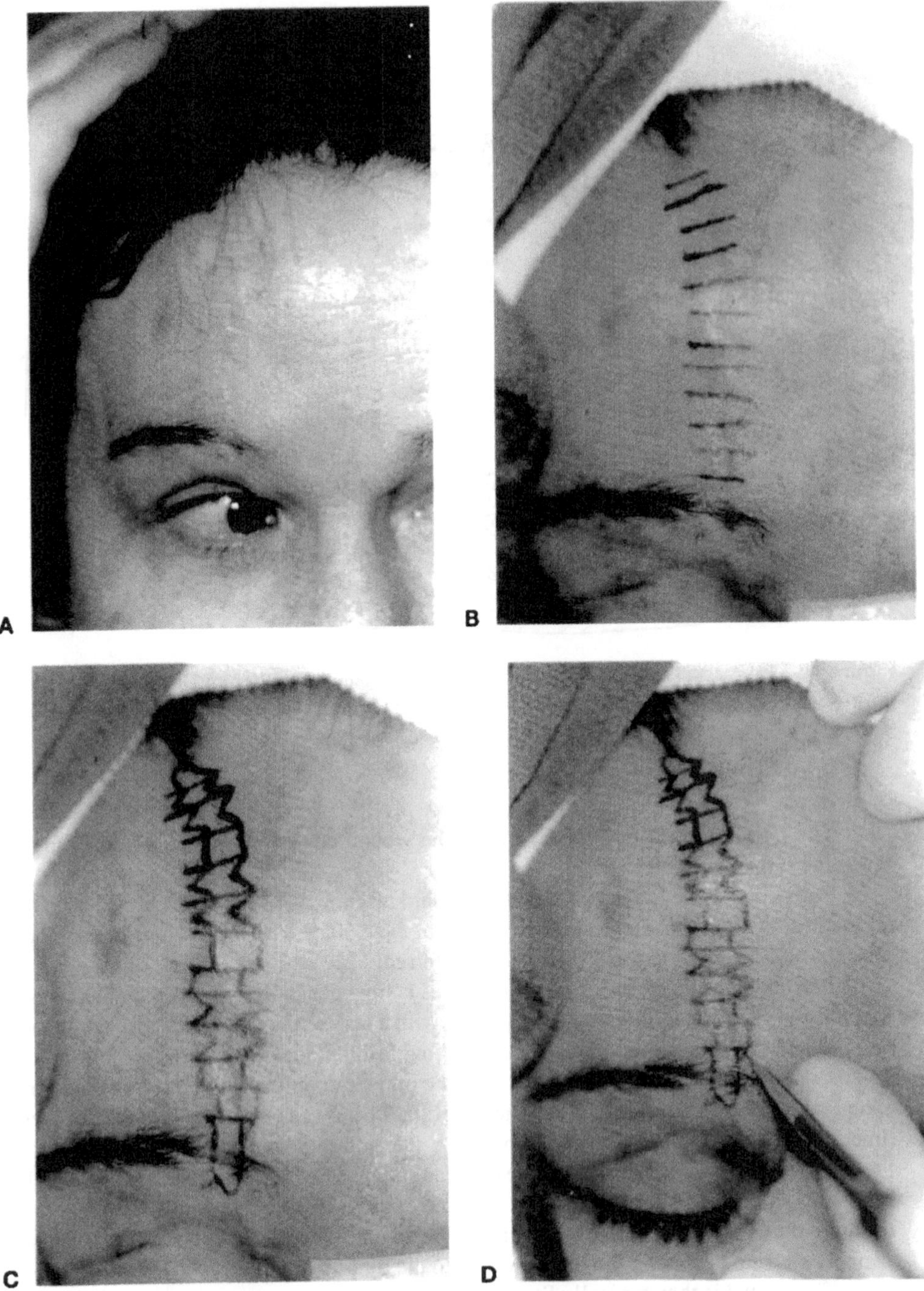

Figure 17 A case example demonstrates the technique. **(A)** A vertical forehead scar extending from the hairline through the eyebrow. **(B)** Crosshatching. **(C)** The GBL design. **(D)** Technique for a no. 11 blade incision. **(E)** All incisions made. **(F)** Scar and GBL design excised as a single piece and laid to the side. **(G)** Wound is undermined with a scissors. **(H)** Wound undermining with a scalpel. **(I)** The wound after closure. **(J)** The wound is Steri-stripped. *(figure continues)*

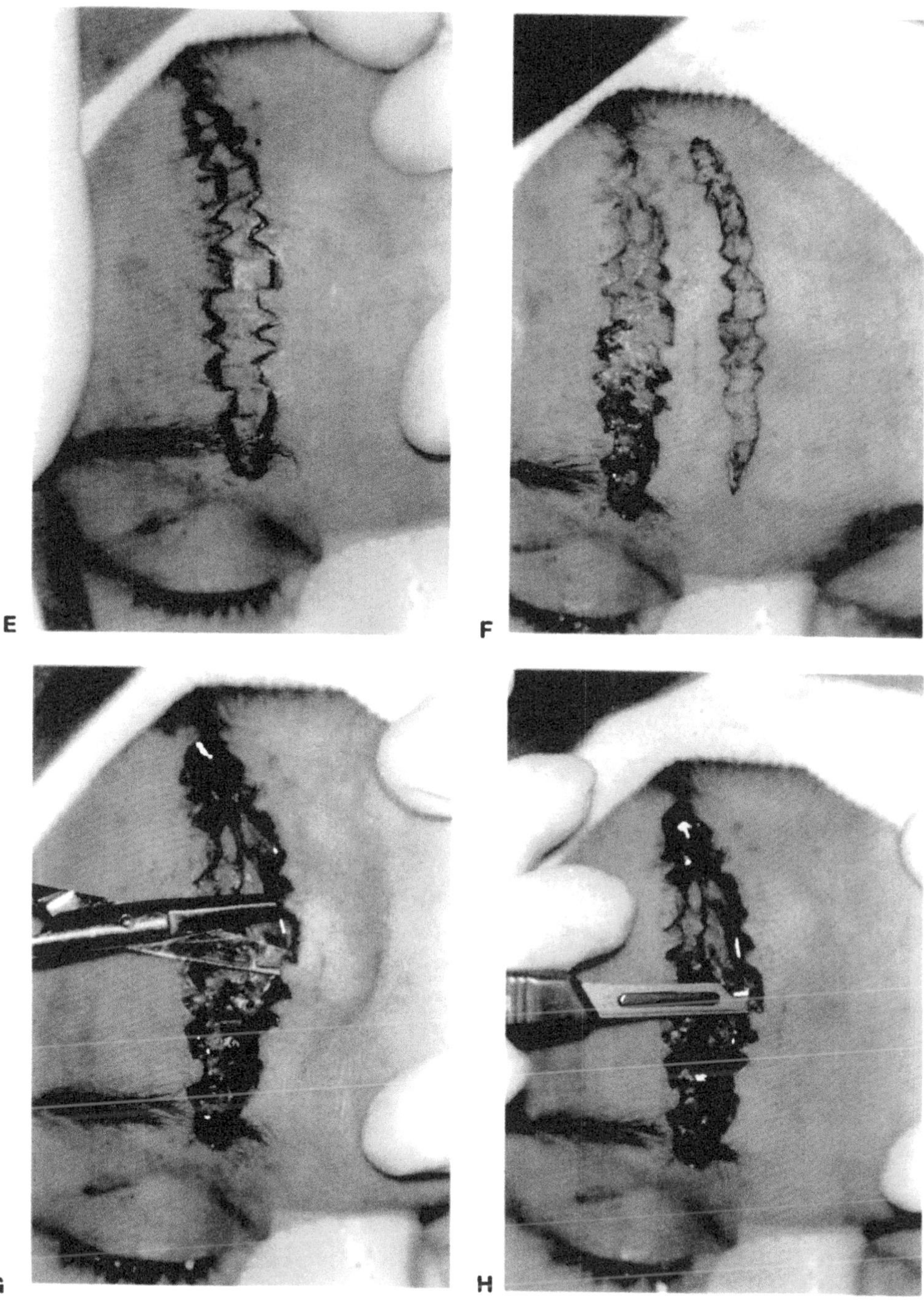

Figure 17 *(continued)*

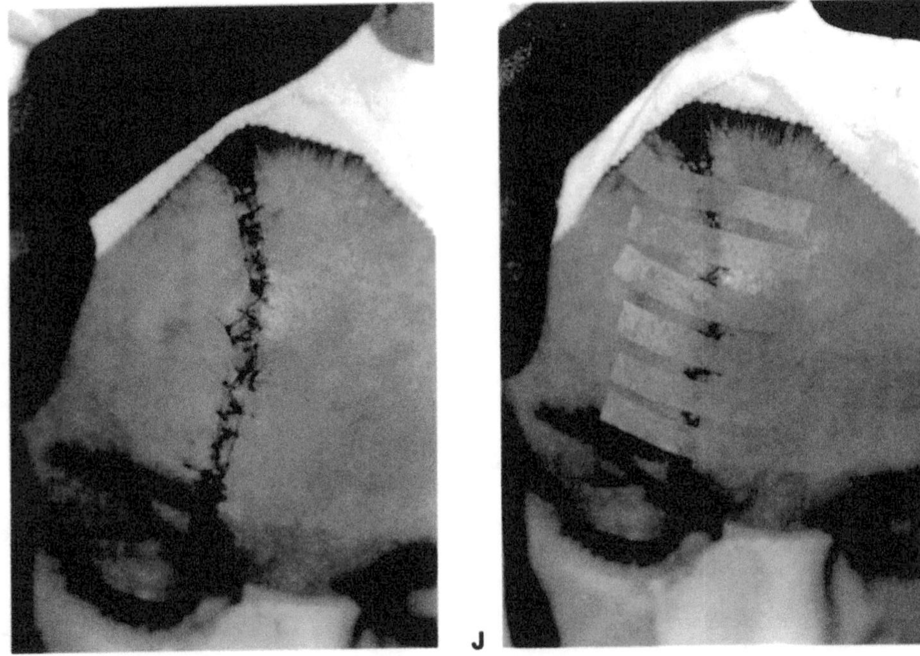

I J

Figure 17 *(continued)*

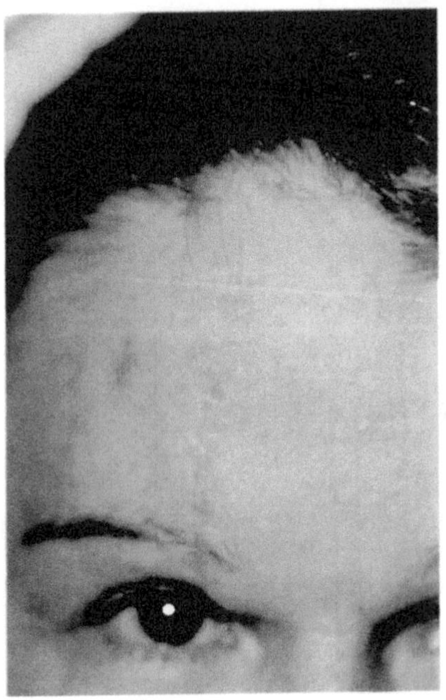

Figure 18 Postoperative healing at 4 months.

The scar is now allowed to heal. There will invariably be irregularities and texture discrepancies. These can be improved with dermabrasion. While other chapters in this book deal with dermabrasion, our philosophy is to abrade somewhere between 6 and 12 months. This may seem long but is done for two reasons: (a) That which seemed to require abrasion at 3 months may no longer warrant abrasion at 6 months. Hence, the patient is saved an unnecessary surgery. (b) Scar revision surgery makes improvement and does not make perfection. The patient needs to become comfortable with the scar and then, when an improvement is made, to recognize and appreciate it. This waiting period gives the patient time to accommodate and settle with the scar. Abrasions separated by 6–12 months not only facilitate the physiologic healing but also enhance the psychologic healing.

Certain principles of wound closure need to be kept in mind. If one has an open incision that is distance X long, then one can place a single suture that same distance X back from the wound and literally close the entire wound with a single suture. Alternatively, one can place the sutures $1\frac{1}{2}$ X back from the wound and use two of them spaced by $\frac{1}{2}X$ and close the entire wound. Alternatively, one can divide the wound into smaller and smaller units. Generally speaking, sutures are as far back from the wound as they are far apart from each other. The same principles hold for the subcutaneous closure. In fact, the dermal stitch can be placed back in the dermis 5–10 mm from the cut dermal edge. When these pull together they pull together a much longer length of the wound, and because they are fewer and some what distant from the wound edge, they are less compromising to the blood supply.

Typically, on facial skin, we will place one of these dermal sutures as far apart as $2\frac{1}{2}$ to 3 cm, whereas if we were using fine dermal stitches we would have to use one as close as every 5 to 7 mm. When these are pulled tightly, there is some apparent extreme version. This invariably dissipates with time. The extreme version does remove a little tension from the wound, but being overaggressive is also discouraged.

The history of surgical scar revision dates back to Horner's description of a Z-plasty technique in 1837 (1). He did not describe a true Z-plasty with two transposed flaps. His technique involved raising a single triangular transposition flap, with primary closure of the donor site. The first true Z-plasty, in which both triangular flaps were transposed, was described by Berger in 1904. His flap was not intended to improve cosmesis but used to treat axillary burn synechia (2,3). It was not until 1954 that Covarrubias described the use of a running Z-plasty solely for the purpose of making facial scars less noticeable (4). In the 1940s Webster, in an attempt to improve the use of Z-plasties for cosmetic purposes, increased the number and diminished the size of the individual transposition flaps. As more experience was gained using Z-plasties, they were noted to have the disadvantages of lengthening the scar and creating bulges and depressions (5).

To rectify the shortcomings of Z-plasty, Borges introduced the running W-plasty in 1959 (6). He found the W-plasty technique provided a more favorable scar than the standard Z-plasty technique, especially those that crossed the FSTLs perpendicularly or obliquely and measured over 1.5 cm in length. He found them to be less advantageous with scars close to the vermillion border, eyelid, or nose (7,8). Running W-plasties have the advantage of creating a random pattern scar revision, which is difficult for the eye to follow. However, it became apparent that the running W-plasty, with its sequential use of triangular flaps, produced a regular pattern that was more conspicuous than was desirable.

At the same time Webster began experimenting with combinations of triangular, square, and rectangular interposed skin flaps, termed geometric broken lines. His results were published in the late 1960s. Geometric broken-line closures, like running W-plasties, were found to produce less contour disparity than did multiple small Z-plasties. The more random pattern of the geometric broken line is less perceptible than that of the running W-plasty (9). Tardy et al. (10) stated this best when they referred to the geometric broken line's "irregular irregularity" as the atrial fibrillation of the scar surgeon!

REFERENCES

1. Horner WE. Clinical Report on the surgical department of the Philadelphia Hospital, Blockley for the months of May, June and July, 1837. Am J Med Sci 1837; 21:99–112.
2. Borges AF. Historic review of Z-plasties techniques. Clin Plast Surg 1977; 4:207–216.
3. Berger P. Autoplasties par dédoublement de la palmure et échange de la lambeaux. In: Berger P, Manzet S, eds. Chirurgie Orthopédique. Paris: Steinheil, 1904.
4. Covarrubias-Zenteno R. Nuevi concepto para el tratmiento de las cictrices. Presented at the Seventh Latin-American Congress of Plastic Surgery, Mexico City, Mexico, 1954.
5. Webster RC, Davidson TM, Smith RC. Broken line scar revision. Clin Plast Surg 1977; 4:263–274.
6. Borges AF. Improvement of antitension-line scars by the W-plastic operation. Br J Plast Surg. 1959; 12:29.
7. Borges AF. Elective incisions and scar revision. Boston: Little, Brown, 1973.
8. Borges AF. The w-plasty vs. Z-plastic scar revision. Plast Reconstr Surg 1969; 44:58–62.
9. Wolf D, Davidson T. Scar revision. Arch Otolaryngol Head Neck Surg 1991; 117:200–204.
10. Tardy EM, Thomas RJ, Pashcow MS. The camouflage of cutaneous scars. Eur Nose Throat J 1981; 60:61–70.

ADDITIONAL READINGS

1. Webster RC, Davidson TM, et al. Cosmetic blepharoplasty evaluation. Aesth Reconst Facial Plast Surg (microfiche) 1975; 3(2):1–120.
2. Davidson TM, Webster RC. Scar Revision. A Self-Instructional Package from the Committee on Continuing Education in Otolaryngology (SIPac). 4th ed. American Academy of Ophthalmology and Otolaryngology, AAO-HNS, 1998.
3. Webster RC, Davidson TM, Smith RC. How I do it. Practical suggestions on facial plastic surgery: wound closure with absorbable sutures. Laryngoscope 1976; 86:1280–1284.
4. Webster RC, Davidson TM, Smith RC. Treatment of scars. In: Conley J, ed. Complications of Head and Neck Surgery. Philadelphia: Saunders, 1979:472–496.
5. Davidson TM. Lacerations and scar revisions. In: Cummings, Fredrickson, Harker, Krause, Schuller, eds. Otolaryngology-Head and Neck Surgery. St. Louis: Mosby, 1st ed. 1984, 2nd ed. 1991, 3rd ed. 1996.
6. Webster RC, Davidson TM. M-plasty techniques. J Dermatol Surg 1976; 2:393–396.
7. Webster RC, Davidson TM, Smith RC. How I do it. Practical suggestion on facial plastic surgery: external marking in rhinoplasty planning. Laryngoscope 1977; 87:126–133.
8. Nahum AM, Bone RC, Davidson TM. Case for prophylactic neck dissection. Laryngoscope 1977; 87:588–599.
9. Webster RC, Davidson TM. Broken line scar revision. Clin Plast Surg 1977; 4:263–274.
10. Wolfe D, Davidson TM. Scar revision. In: Roenigk R, Roenigk H, eds. Dermatologic Surgery: Principles and Practice. New York: Marcel Dekker, 1989:935–958.

11. Wolfe D, Davidson TM. Facial scars. In: Gates G, ed. Current Therapy in Otolaryngology—Head & Neck Surgery. 4th ed. Philadelphia: Decker, 1990:91–97.
12. Wolfe D, Davidson TM, Low W. Scar revision, In: Roenigk R, Roenigk H, eds. Dermatologic Surgery: Principles and Practice. 2nd ed. New York: Marcel Dekker, 1996:923–945.
13. Webster RC, Davidson TM, Nahum AM. San Diego Classics Scar Revision Videotapes: # 34–36 Parts I–III, 1977.

23

Topical Silicone Gel Sheeting

Michael H. Gold
Gold Skin Care Center
Nashville, Tennessee

Hypertrophic scars and keloids are very different lesions to treat, and many modalities have emerged to aid clinicians in dealing with them. Topical silicone gel sheeting is a noninvasive product for treating hypertrophic scars and keloids. The first descriptions of the use of these products mentioned their effectiveness in treating hypertrophic scars as the result of burn injuries. In 1982, Perkins et al. (1) reported the use of topical silicone gel sheets in 42 patients with hypertrophic burn scars. The burns involved newly healed lesions on scars 12 years old. Twenty of the 42 patients had been using pressure therapy prior to their use of the silicone gel sheets. All 42 reported significant improvement in their scars; pain associated with the lesions also disappeared. One patient in the original series had no flexion of the metacarpophalangeal joints prior to the use of the sheets and noted full flexion within 30 minutes of use with the treatment. In 1985 Quinn et al. (2) reported on 40 patients with thermal injury using the silicone gel sheets. All reported improvement within 2 months. By 1987, Quinn's series had 129 patients and it was noted that there was an 80% improvement at 2 months (3).

Various mechanisms of action for the topical silicone gel sheets have been proposed. In 1985, Quinn et al. found no effects with regard to pressure, no change in scar temperature, and no differences in the oxygen tension within the scars. They noted that the hydration of the skin was altered within the gel sheets and there was an evaporative water loss one-half that of normal skin, and they concluded that the stratum corneum provided a reservoir for fluid (2). In 1987, Quinn (3) felt that there was slow release of a low molecular weight silicone that would enter the stratum corneum and affect the chemical structure of the scar. Other investigators, including this author, have noted no release of silicone material into the skin. According to another possible mechanism, proposed by Davey in 1986 (4), the silicone gel is impermeable and acts like stratum corneum in reducing hemostasis and decreasing hyperemia and fibrosis, leading to the alteration of the final scar result. In 1989, Ahn et al. (5) reported the use of topical silicone gel sheets in 14 patients (12 burn injuries, 2 others) and noted improvement in all at 4 months. This was the first report of patients in a nonburn setting. Mercer (6), in 1989, described the use of the material for 22 nonburn keloids and noted 86% improvement at 2 months.

Thus, from the early investigations, topical silicone gel sheeting showed its potential to improve hypertrophic scars and keloids. This author then studied and reported the first use of this material in the dermatologic literature (7). The topical silicone gel sheet material known as Silastic was supplied by Dow Corning Wright (Arlington, TN). The material itself is a soft, adherent, semiocclusive covering fabricated from medical grade silicone polymers. The silicone material is a cross-linked polydimethylsiloxane polymer with no fillers added. Polyester fabric, polyethyleneterephthalate mesh, is incorporated for added strength.

An open-label first clinical dermatologic trial was performed to study the effectiveness of the material on nonburn hypertrophic scars and keloids in a dermatologic setting. The scars studied were secondary to either a surgical procedure or traumatic insult. Sixteen scars were initially studied. Each of the participants wore the topical silicone gel sheet for a minimum of 12 hours per day for up to 3 months. The following parameters were evaluated: change in scar thickness, change in scar color toward normal, and overall effectiveness. All study participants noted that the material was easy to use and there were no adverse reactions. Moderate improvement in the thickness of the scar was noted in 81.25% and in scar color toward normal skin in 75%. Physician evaluation revealed complete resolution or moderate improvement in thickness in 56.25% and color change in 75%. In a comparison of hypertrophic scars and keloids, the keloids were more apt to be reduced in thickness according to the patients' evaluations. Color changes were fairly constant between the two groups. Positive changes were noted in all the scars both by the patients and by physician evaluation (Fig. 1–4).

The original dermatologic evaluation had several built-in inherent biases. It was an open-label trial; no controls were utilized. Subjective analysis of photographs and questionnaires was used. Therefore, a controlled trial was planned. At almost the same time, Katz (8) reported his dermatologic experience using the topical silicone gel sheets. He found that of 15 scars treated with the topical silicone gel sheeting, 9 improved during the treatment course. Also, fresh scars (those younger than 3 months) treated with the sheet (8 out of 8) did not develop into hypertrophic scars during the study.

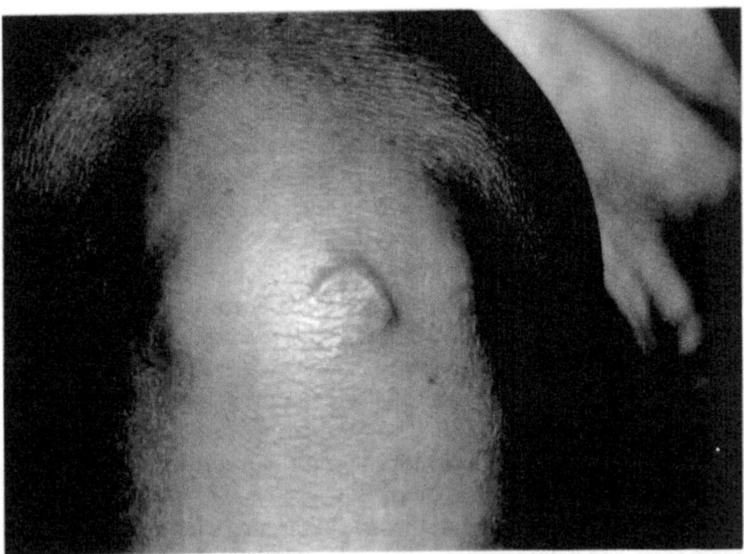

Figure 1 Baseline 1-year-old scar from a motor vehicle accident.

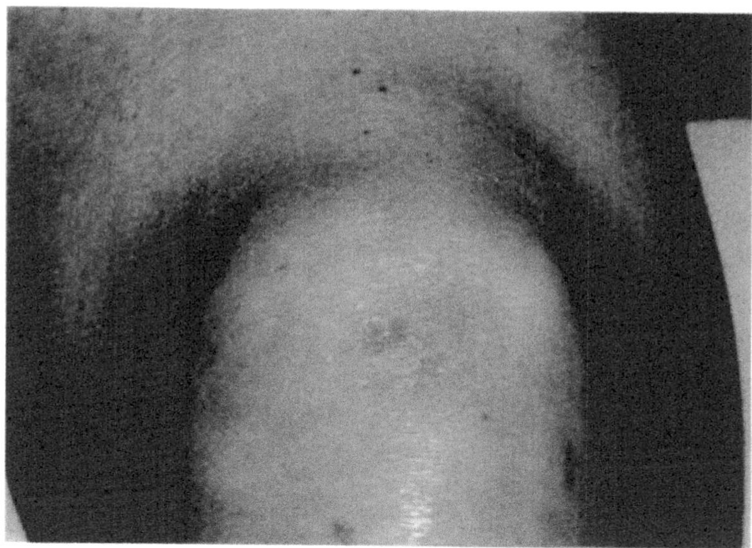

Figure 2 The same scar as in Fig. 1 after 3 months of silicone gel use.

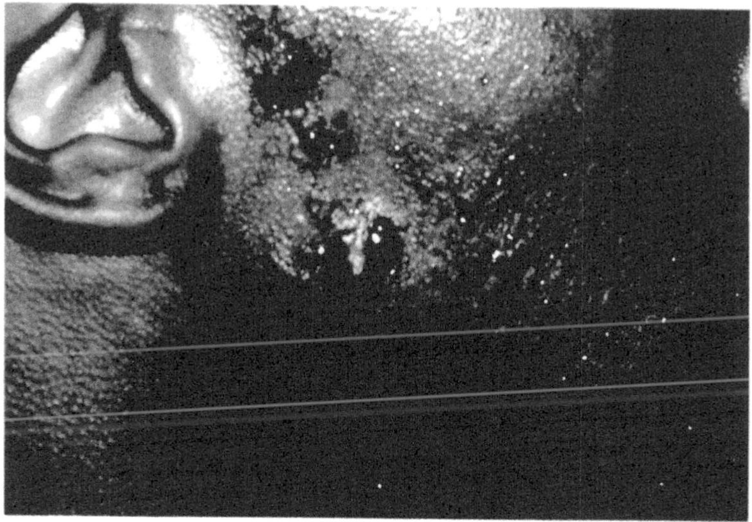

Figure 3 Keloidal scar on cheek that has been present for many years.

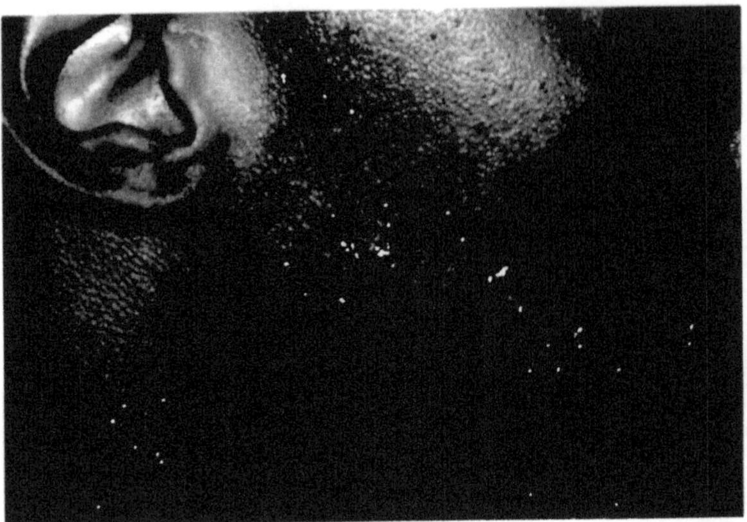

Figure 4 Three months after silicone gel sheet to right cheek keloid.

This author then reported the first controlled dermatologic clinical trial of the topical silicone gel sheets (9). The study was divided into three distinct phases. Phase I included patients who had hypertrophic scars or keloids as a result of a surgical procedure or traumatic event. Twenty-one patients were entered, 17 with hypertrophic scars and 4 with keloids. The scars to be treated were divided into two equal halves by having a tattoo mark placed in the middle of the scar. The areas that were treated were to have the topical silicone gel applied for a minimum of 12 hours per day for up to 3 months. Monthly visits allowed the following observation to be made: change in scar thickness, change in scar, color toward normal, and overall effectiveness of the product.

Phase II was designed to study the effect of the topical silicone gel sheeting in preventing recurrences after surgical removal of a keloid scar with a CO_2 laser. Two keloids were treated with the CO_2 laser in the same anatomic site. Eight patients were entered into this phase of the study. Twenty-four hours postoperatively, one of the two treated areas had the topical silicone gel sheet applied. The instructions were similar to those in phase I, and similar parameters were followed. Phase III was designed to study the effects of the topical silicone gel sheeting on hypertrophic scars resulting from a thermal burn injury. Five patients were in this phase; again, instructions and parameters followed were the same.

Phase I results showed an improvement in scar thickness in 76.2% of the treated half of the scar compared with the nontreated half of the scar. Scar color improved in 76.2%, and 81.9% noted a significant overall improvement in the treated half of the scar by the conclusion of the study (Fig. 5 and 6). Physician evaluation yielded the following results: 90.5% improvement in scar thickness, 91.5% improvement in scar color, and 95.2% overall improvement. Comparable results were seen in a direct comparison of the keloids versus the hypertrophic scars. The results from phase II showed that 12.5% of the keloids treated with the topical silicone gel sheet recurred, whereas 37.5% of the nontreated keloids recurred in the treatment period. Phase III patients noted 100% improvement in scar thickness, 80% improvement in scar color, and 100% overall effectiveness.

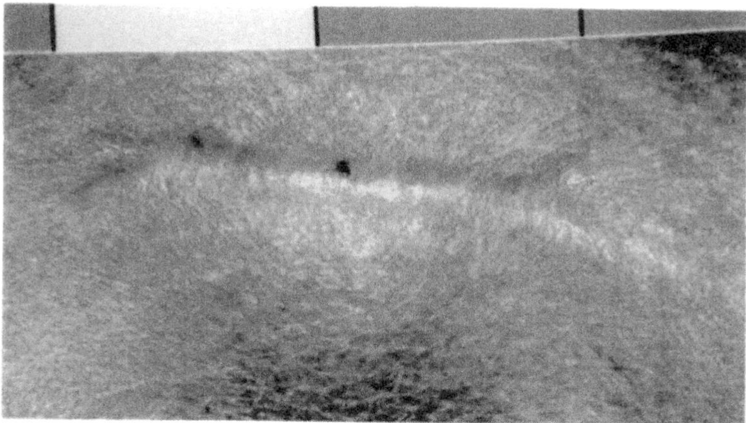

Figure 5 Pretreatment scar.

The results of both of this author's clinical trials show that topical silicone gel sheets are a useful therapeutic modality for the treatment of hypertrophic scars and keloids. The material itself is rather inexpensive and painless to wear. It reduces scar thickness in a significant majority and returns the color of many toward normal. It may also help prevent future recurrences. More research in this area is required and is ongoing at this time.

Since Silastic appeared on the market, numerous other products have come on the scene. All of these products claim to have effects similar to those of Silastic; clinical studies with regard to most of these products are, at this time, lacking. In a study by Hirshowitz et al. in 1993 (10), 88% of the lesions treated with Morelle SOS improved. The authors speculated that a static electrical field was created by friction on the silicone material surface. The passage of static electricity over a prolonged period of time is felt by these authors to be important for scar inhibition. More research, as well, into this theory is needed. Fulton (11) reported in 1995 an 85% improvement rate in 20 cases treated with Epiderm.

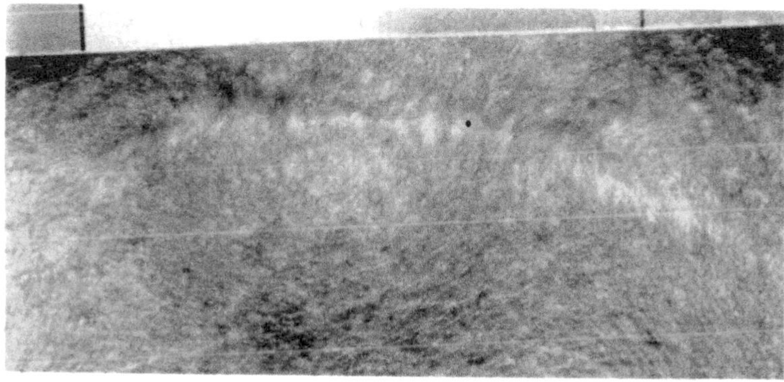

Figure 6 Silicone gel sheeting to right side of scar for 3 months.

Some of the other topical silicone gel sheeting products are:

Topigel, CUI Corporation
Epiderm, Biodermis
Silon SES, Bio Med Sciences, Inc.
WonderFlex, Silopos, Inc.
Dermasof, McGhan Medical
Morelle SOS, Pitt Enterprises
SilK, Degania
New Beginnings, PMT Corporation
NovaGel, Brennan Medical, Inc.

A silicone cream containing 20% silicone oil was studied in 1990 by Sawada and Sone in Japan (12). Forty-seven patients applied the silicone cream with an occlusive dressing over the scar. "Remarkable'' improvement was reported in 82%; only 22% improved with the oil alone. They postulated that occlusion and hydration are part of the principal modes of action of both the silicone oil and the topical silicone gel sheets. The occlusion and hydration theory is a main conception of how these materials might work. A topical cream called Kelocote is currently available in the United States. It is extremely useful for use areas of the body where using a topical covering is not acceptable.

In 1994, the marketing rights of Silastic were sold by Dow Corning Wright to Smith and Nephew Corporation, Hull, England, and a new Silastic product, Cica-Care, was introduced. This material is more adherent than the original Silastic and has replaced it in the marketplace. A European study reported by Carney et al. in 1994 (13) confirmed the effectiveness of Cica-Care. Forty-two patients were randomly assigned to either Silastic or Cica-Care; the scars treated were controlled as in previous trials. No differences in the sheets were observed, and significant improvement was noted in all the treated areas. Because Cica-Care was more adhesive and more comfortable to wear, the authors reported its usefulness in the treatment of hypertrophic scars and keloids (Fig. 7–12, all used with permission of Smith and Nephew).

On the premise that occlusion and hydration are principal factors in the mode of action of topical silicone gel sheets, the NDM Company began studying the effects of a saline-based hydrogel wound dressing in treating hypertrophic scars and keloids. The material is known as Clearsite, and preliminary results have been promising (14). Future research will determine whether saline sheeting is comparable to the silicone gel sheets.

Also, research needs to define the differences between the gel sheets (including the exact makeups of the silicone and polyester mesh) to allow the clinician to decide which product is best for his or her practice. In preliminary studies performed thus far (Smith and Nephew, personal communication, 1996), Cica-Care has had comparisons performed with regard to stretch and moisture vapor permeability. Dermasof, Topigel, and Epiderm have lower elongation at break (stretch) than Cica-Care, confirming that Cica-Care's extensibility was greater than that of Dermasof, Topigel, and Epiderms and that Cica-Care is more comfortable to have on scars. In moisture vapor permeability (a measure of occlusive property), Cica-Care was similar to Dermasof, Topiderm, and Epiderm. SilK's moisture vapor permeability is approximately 24% less than that of Cica-Care. Work is ongoing to evaluate further the currently available topical silicone gel sheets.

Clinicians cannot be experts on all of the possible treatment options available to them when confronted with a patient with a hypertrophic scar or keloid. It is prudent for the treating physician to be comfortable with a specific routine and use this in the majority of cases.

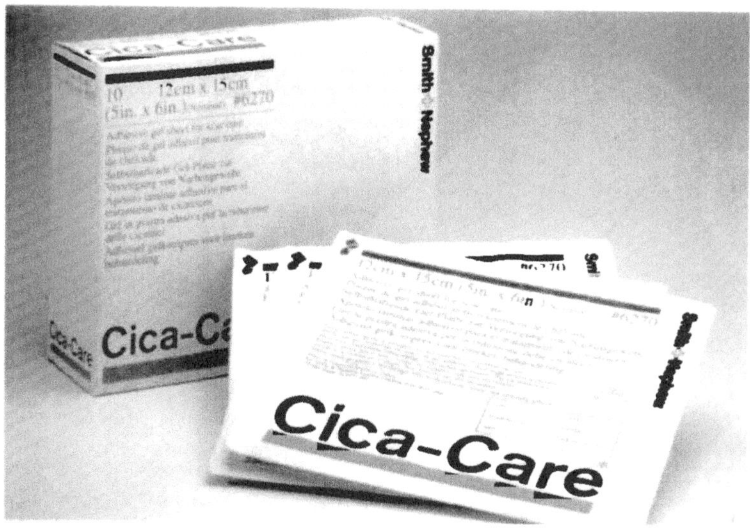

Figure 7 Cica-Care product identification.

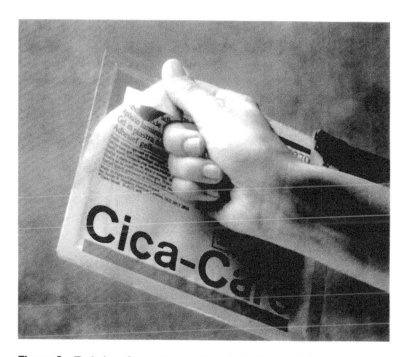

Figure 8 Technique for opening sterile topical silicone gel sheet.

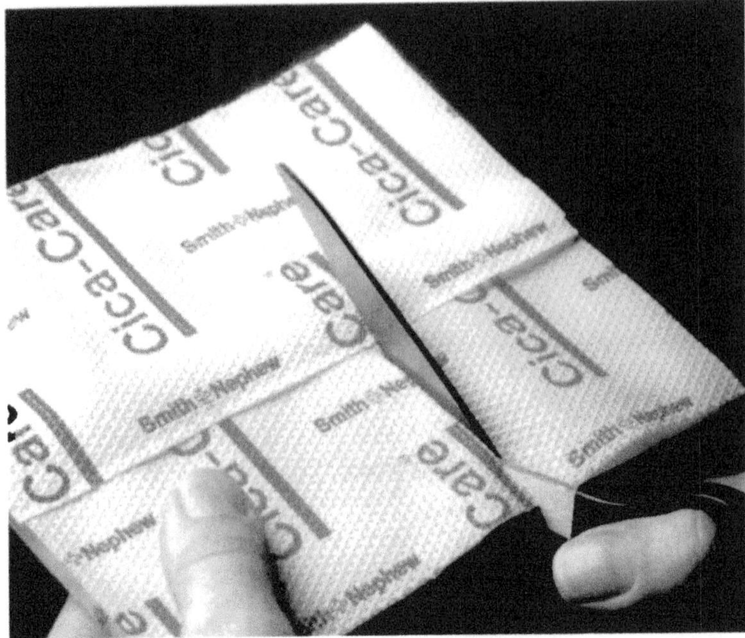

Figure 9 The Cica-Care is cut into the size of the scar.

This author commonly uses intralesional corticosteroids and Cica-Care as first-line agents. The intralesional injections are given at 2 to 4 week intervals and the Cica-Care is worn for a minimum of 12 hours per day. If, after several months of this treatment, no appreciable difference is observed, the lesion is then removed either with a simple surgical excision or with the carbon dioxide laser. Immediately after surgery, the treated area is treated intrale-

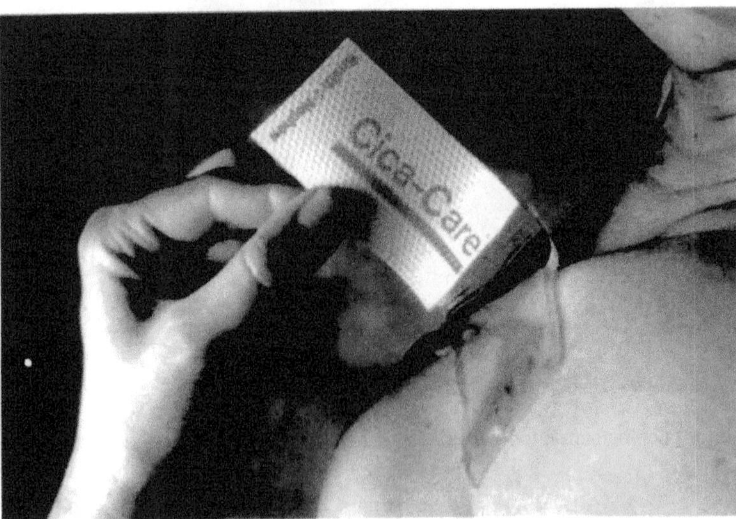

Figure 10 The Cica-Care is applied to the scar.

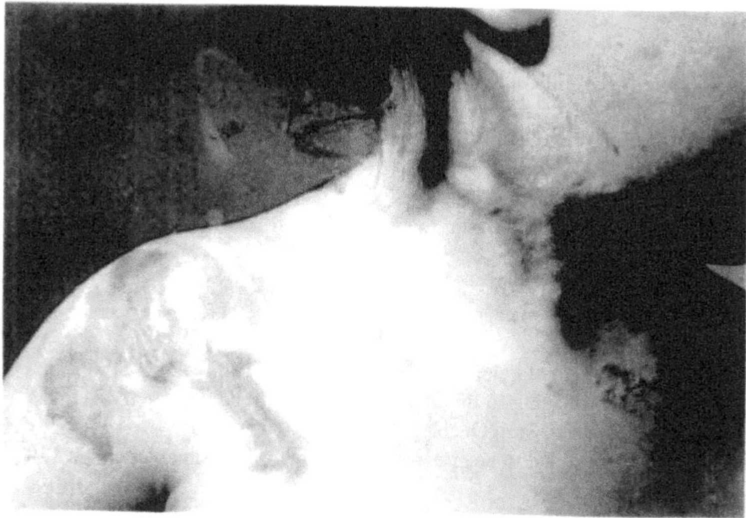

Figure 11 Pretreatment scar on right shoulder.

sional corticosteroids, and Cica-Care is applied 24 hours postoperatively (the U.S. Food and Drug Administration approval at this time for application is only on healed lesions). Intralesional corticosteroid injections are performed at 3- to 4-week intervals. Keloids on the earlobe are usually treated initially with a surgical procedure, followed by the intralesional cortisteroids and Cica-Care as described. This routine has produced highly successful results in the treatment of these potentially difficult clinical lesions.

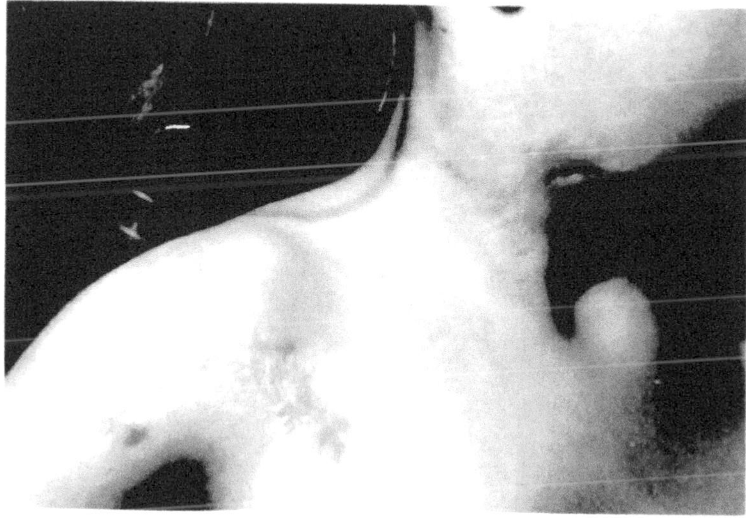

Figure 12 Result after 12 weeks of Cica-Care to right shoulder scar.

REFERENCES

1. Perkins K, Davey RB, Wallis KA. Silicone gel: a new treatment for burn scars and contractures. Burns 1982; 9:406–410.
2. Quinn KG, Evans, JH, Courtney JM, Gaylor JDS, Reid WH. Non-pressure treatment of hypertrophic scars. Burns 1985; 12:102–108.
3. Quinn KG. Silicone gel in scar treatment. Burns 1987; 13:S33–S40.
4. Davey RB. The use of silicone gel and Silastic foam in burn scar management—how does it work? Presented at the 7th Congress of the International Society for Burn Injuries, Melbourne, Feb 1986.
5. Ahn ST, Monafo WW, Mustoe TA. Topical silicone gel: a new treatment for hypertrophic scars. Surgery 1989; 4:781–787.
6. Mercer NSG. Silicone gel treatment of keloid scars. Br J Plast Surg 1989; 42:83–87.
7. Gold MH. Topical silicone gel sheeting in the treatment of hypertrophic scars and keloids: a dermatologic experience. J Dermatol Surg Oncol 1993; 19:912–916.
8. Katz BE. Silastic gel sheeting is found to be effective in scar therapy. Cosmet Dermatol 1992; 5:32–34.
9. Gold MH. A controlled clinical trial of topical silicone gel sheeting in the treatment of hypertrophic scars and keloids. J Am Acad Dermatol 1994; 30:506–507.
10. Hirshowitz B, Ullmann Y, Har-Shai Y, Vilenski A, Peled IJ. Silicone occlusive sheeting (SOS) in the management of hypertrophic and keloid scarring, including the possible mode of action, by static electricity, Eur J Plast Surg 1993; 16:5–9.
11. Fulton JE. Silicone gel sheeting for the prevention and management of evolving hypertrophic and keloid scars. Dermatol Surg 1995; 21:947–951.
12. Sawada Y, Sone K. Treatment of scars and keloids with a cream containing silicone oil. Br J Plast Surg 1990; 43:683–688.
13. Carney SA, Cason CG, Gower JP, Stevenson JH, McNee J, Groves AR, Thomas SS, Hart NB, Auclair P. Cica-Care gel sheeting in the management of hypertrophic scarring. Burns 1994; 20(2):163–167.
14. Ricketts CH, Martin L, Faria DT, Saed GM, Fwenson OP. Cytokine mRNA changes during the treatment of hypertrophic scars with silicone and nonsilicone gel dressings. Dermatol Surg 1996; 22:955–959.

24

Surgical Excision, Radiotherapy, and Intralesional Steroids

John C. Murray, Mitchell S. Anscher, Aaron J. Mayberry, and L. Scott Levin
Duke University Medical Center
Durham, North Carolina

I. SURGICAL EXCISION

A. Clinical Definition

Keloids are characterized by exuberant proliferation of collagen that extends beyond the confines of a wound. Growth of the lesion may continue for years without evidence of regression. Histologically, keloids display increased mucinous ground substance, disarrayed eosinophilic collagen sheets, and relatively smaller quantities of fibroblasts (1–4). Hypertrophic scarring is also characterized by exuberant production of collagen but does not extend beyond the confines of the wound into adjacent normal skin. Hypertrophic scars have less mucinous ground substance and fewer fibroblasts. Furthermore, hypertrophic scars may resolve over time. Acne keloidalis nuchae is a related chronic inflammatory condition that is characterized by lesions in the occiput and nape of the neck with keloid-like lesions and often with purulent draining sinuses and fistulous tracts. Both acne keloidalis and true keloids are difficult problems to cure and often result in significant morbidity for the patient. There is no established animal model for keloid study, which further confounds potential human investigational trials.

Keloids gradually develop into large unsightly masses that can cause pain, pruritus, and, if associated with acne keloidalis, localized abscesses. Typical areas of formation include the earlobes, chest, shoulder, back, and sternum. Precise etiologies are not known, but keloid scarring is most often associated with trauma. Immunologic factors and familial predisposition are also implicated (5).

B. Treatment Options

Management of keloid scarring is one of the most problematic issues in skin surgery. Many techniques are utilized with varying degress of success. The most reliable techniques are surgical excision, external beam radiation therapy, mechanical pressure, triamcinolone injection, and silicone gel sheeting. Recently, tissue expansion has also proved efficacious.

1. Surgery

Surgical excision remains the primary mode of keloid treatment. Some authors have proposed excision of the keloids leaving a rim of perimeter scar tissue to limit the amount of reaction of adjacent tissue. This is an attractive thought but has not been reliably substantiated statistically (6). Success with surgical therapy alone is variable, with recurrence rates in excess of 50%. Combination modalities have somewhat improved recurrence rates. Preferred combinations include external beam radiation therapy, intralesional steroid injection, mechanical pressure, and silicone gel.

a. Surgical Technique

The lesion should be properly prepared and draped. Local infection must be adequately treated with incision and drainage in combination with local antibiotics until resolved. Small to moderate-sized lesions can be primarily excised in a fusiform manner.

Large lesions and those that are not amenable to primary closure without undue tension can be closed utilizing tissue expander placement with sequential expansion adjacent to the keloid. Tissue expander placement is performed via dissection of a subcutaneous pocket under normal skin large enough to accept the expander. Traditionally, tissue expansion is begun after a wound healing period of 2 weeks. This healing time was essential to prevent incision necrosis and extrusion of the expander. The expansion is performed on a weekly basis using sterile normal saline administered through a subcutaneous port. Currently under investigation are endoscopically placed tissue expanders. This affords immediate expansion because the area of expansion is distant from the site of introduction. The discomfort to the patient is minimal and excellent tissue expansion can be seen within 1 month. Following adequate expansion, the implant is removed and the keloid excised. The unaffected tissue can then be advanced to cover the defect. Keloids may occur along advancement incision lines.

Basic surgical technique should be thoroughly emphasized. Monofilament suture is preferable to braided types. Undermining of adjacent tissues in the subcutaneous plane to effect a tensionless closure is essential. Placement of Z-plasties and W-plasties should be avoided because of the high recurrence of keloid within the incisions. An exception to this would be in treatment of contractures resulting from a scar across a concavity or flexure surface. Pressure applied over the involved area has been shown to be helpful. The patient should be seen postoperatively in 1 week. Follow-up should be conducted at 1-, 3-, and 6-month intervals thereafter. If keloid appears to recur, intralesional steroid injection could be useful. Above all, the patient should be informed of the high likelihood of recurrence despite the technique(s) chosen.

C. Case Studies

B.Z., a 33-year-old Hispanic woman, sustained a laceration on her left foot that healed with keloid scarring. This was initially treated by her physician with excision and skin grafting. The graft did not "take" and the keloid recurred. She was seen in our clinic, where she was scheduled for excision, grafting, and postoperative radiation treatment. The patient tolerated these procedures well and has not had a recurrence.

L.M., a 57-year-old black female, had a history of recurrent severe keloid formation involving bilateral ears, neck, back, buttocks, and thighs. She was initially treated with excision, primary closure, and methotrexate. She developed liver failure and the methotrexate was discontinued. She presented with exuberant recurrence and was treated with staged resection, skin grafting, and radiation therapy to the ears and abdominal wall. The patient tolerated these procedures well and has not had a recurrence in the regions treated.

E.O., a 34-year-old black woman, presented with recurrent plantar keloids following multiple primary excisions and closure. She was treated with excision, skin grafting, and postoperative radiation therapy. She has not developed recurrence.

R.R., a 49-year-old black male, presented with a history of recurrent keloids on the dorsum of his right foot (Fig. 1A). He was treated with excision, placement of a split-thickness skin graft, and postoperative radiation therapy. He tolerated these procedures well and had continued viability of the skin graft following radiation therapy (Fig. 1B).

T.G., a 30-year-old black male, presented with a history of recurrent acne keloidalis nuchae previously treated with multiple excisions without success (Fig. 2A). He was evaluated by our group and was deemed a suitable patient for placement of a tissue expander (Fig. 2B). After absence of an active nuchal infection was confirmed, a tissue expander was placed in the subgaleal plane with endoscopic assistance. The wound was irrigated with an antibiotic solution and closed in a multilayered fashion. Staged tissue expansion was started approximately 2 weeks postoperatively. The implant was inflated with normal saline on a weekly basis using 25 to 50 mL per session. Adequate tissue expansion was noted within 1 month. The tissue expander was removed, followed by excision and advancement of tissue. The patient tolerated these procedures well and has not had a recurrence (Fig. 2C).

D.C., a 49-year-old black woman, presented with a complaint of severe left wrist and hand pain. She was initially treated by her primary physician with cortisone and prednisone injections. She was diagnosed with carpal tunnel syndrome and underwent a left carpal tunnel release. Approximately 1 year after operation, she developed significant keloid scarring resulting in pain and a 10-degree flexion contracture (Fig. 3A). She was evaluated by our group, and a treatment plan involving keloid excision, decompression of the left median nerve and palmar cutaneous nerve, and a reverse radial forearm flap was outlined. Postop-

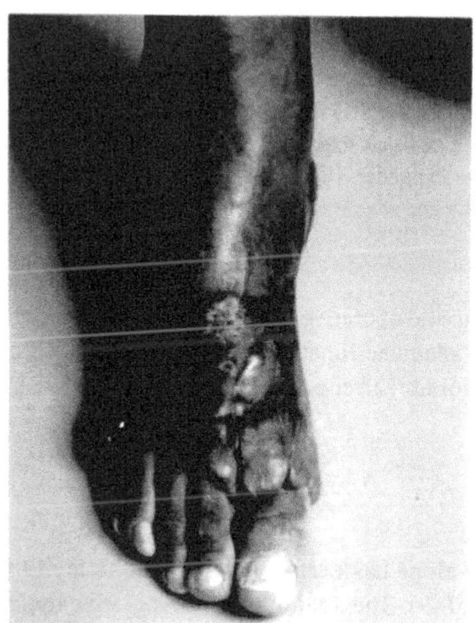

A

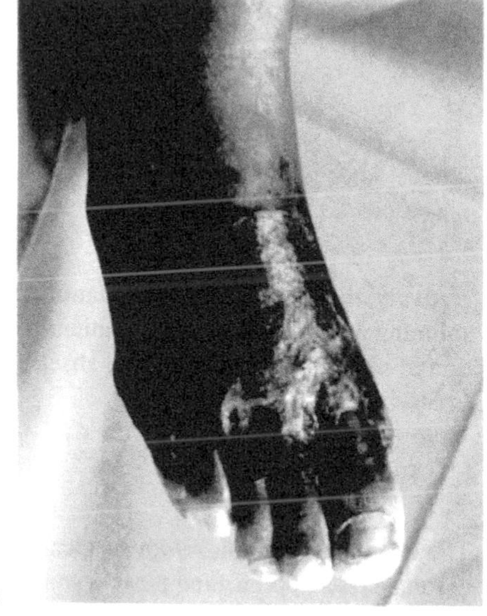

B

Figure 1 **(A)** Dorsum of right foot exhibiting severe keloid formation. **(B)** Dorsum of right foot following excision and replacement of split-thickness, meshed skin graft. Note skin graft and lateral aspects of the lesion.

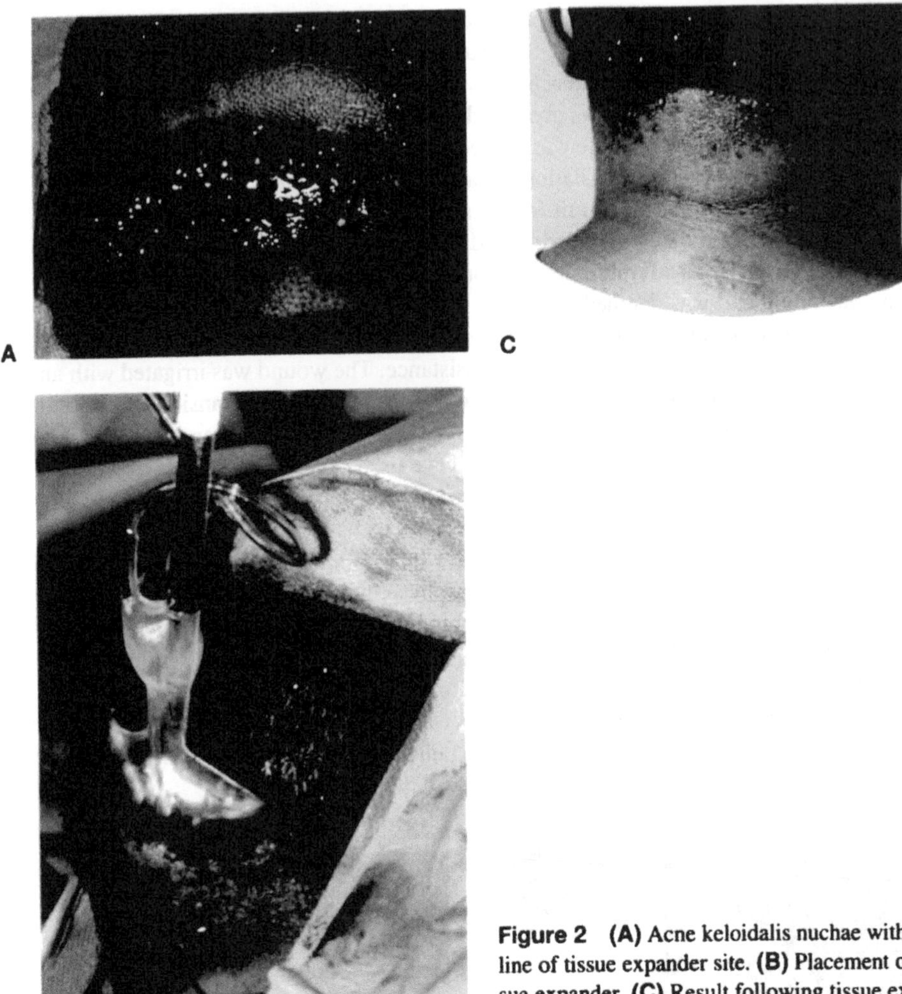

Figure 2 **(A)** Acne keloidalis nuchae with outline of tissue expander site. **(B)** Placement of tissue expander. **(C)** Result following tissue expansion and advancement after excision of the lesion.

eratively, the patient received radiation therapy to the operative site. Following appropriate splinting and hand therapy, the patient regained adequate function at the wrist with resolution of neurologic symptoms and absence of keloid recurrence (Fig. 3B and C).

II. RADIOTHERAPY

The treatment of keloids with surgical excision alone has been associated with a high recurrence rate, approaching 80% in some series (7–9). The addition of postoperative radiation therapy improves the control rate to 70–90% (10–18). Most radiation oncologists treat these patients with either low-energy photons or electrons in order to confine the radiation dose to the skin while sparing the underlying tissues and organs. Alternatively, treatment using temporary implantation of radioactive sources directly in the tissues (interstitial

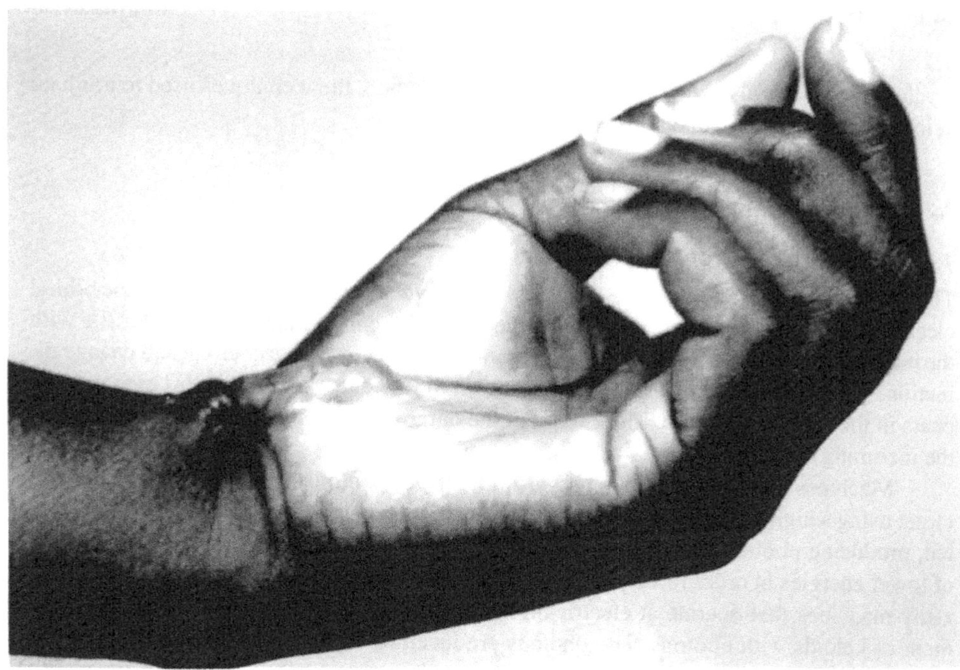

A

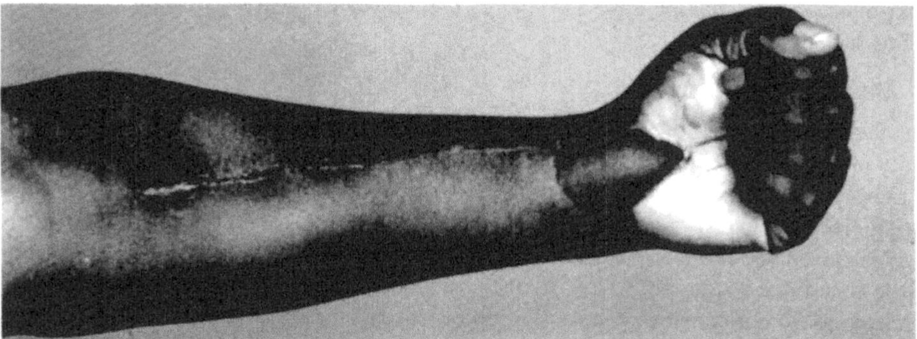

B

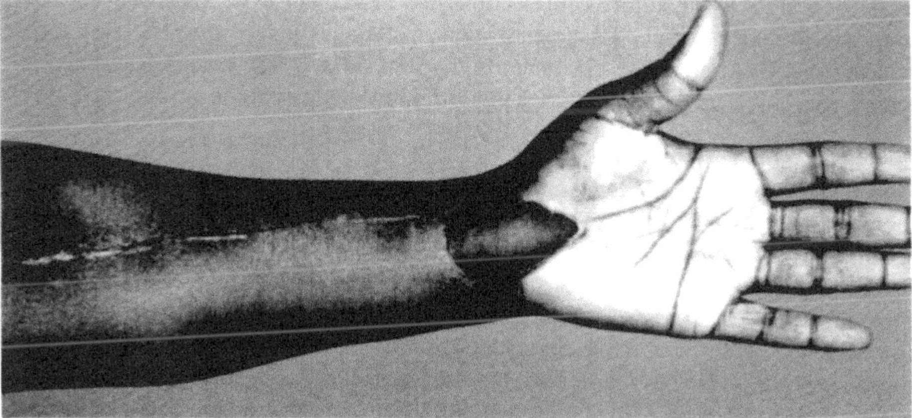

C

Figure 3 **(A)** Keloid scar causing a flexion contracture of the left wrist. **(B)** Resolution of flexion contracture following a reverse radial forearm flap. **(C)** Note mild hypertrophic scarring at the radial and ulnar aspect of the flap.

brachytherapy) has also been reported (19). In this section, the techniques used to irradiate keloids are described in detail.

A. External Beam Irradiation

1. *Low-Energy Photons*

The production of x-rays involves the interaction of an accelerated electron with the orbital electrons or the nuclei of the atoms in a target (20). If the incoming electron interacts with the nucleus, the electric field of the nucleus causes the electron to decelerate and change direction. The deceleration of the electron causes it to lose energy, and this lost energy reappears in the form of a photon. The energy of the outgoing photon depends on the energy of the incoming electron.

Machines that produce low-energy (kilovoltage) photons accelerate electrons into a target using a high-voltage electric field. The electrical potential across the field can be varied, producing photons of different energies. Metal filters can be added to absorb photons of lower energies in order to vary the effective depth of penetration of the beam. Typically, x-ray machines that operate at electrical potentials of 50–250 kVp are used for the treatment of keloids with photons. The photons produced by these machines deposit their energy maximally at the skin surface (Fig. 4). The dose drops off rapidly with increasing depth in tissue (21), making these low-energy photon beams ideal for treating superficial lesions such as keloids.

2. *Megavoltage Electrons*

With the development of the linear accelerator for medical purposes in the 1950s, the availability of low-energy photon machines for radiation therapy declined. The linear accelerator uses a more complex system to produce high-energy photons (megavoltage) by accelerating electrons into a target using high-frequency electromagnetic waves (21). If the target is moved out of the path of the electrons, the electrons themselves can be used to irradiate superficial lesions such as skin cancers and keloids. Unlike megavoltage photons, the electrons do not penetrate deeply (Fig. 5) because of the differences in the way electrons and photons interact with tissue (20). In contrast to the situation with low-energy photons, the dose at the tissue surface with electrons may be as much as 20% less than the maximum dose in deeper tissue. Tissue-equivalent material is placed over the skin to be irradiated in order to move the maximum to the skin surface. The results achieved with electrons are equivalent to those reported with very low energy photon irradiation (10).

3. *Treatment Technique*

Following excision of a keloid, the radiation field should encompass the incision and sutures with a small margin, usually 2 to 5 mm. If skin grafting is required, it is not necessary to irradiate the entire graft; only the incision line and sutures need to be treated (12). Beam-shaping devices, custom made for each patient, are used to have the radiation beam conform to the desired shape. For low-energy photons, this device consists of a thin piece of lead with a hole conforming to the size and shape of the area to be irradiated in its center. This device is placed directly on the skin; the radiation beam passes through the hole in the shield while the rest of the skin is protected. For electron beams, a similar device is constructed and is placed in a special tray in the head of the machine in order to achieve the desired beam shape. When treating very thin, irregularly shaped surfaces with electrons, such

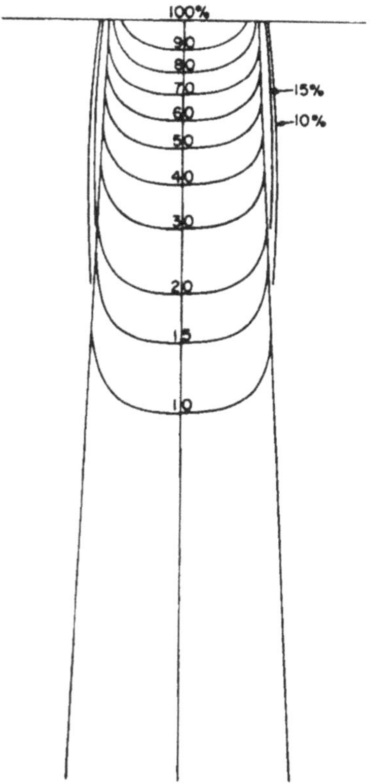

HVL 0.25 MM CU (5.0 MM AL) 40 CM S-TD
FIELD-4.0 CM DIA METAL SPECULUM

Figure 4 Dose distribution profile in tissue of a typical low-energy photon beam used for the treatment of keloids. Note that the dose is maximal at the surface (represented by the solid black line at the top of the figure). The dose falls off rapidly and is reduced to 50% of the surface dose at a depth of 3.4 cm. (Courtesy of General Electric Company.)

as the earlobe or nasal ala, it may be necessary to also utilize small lead shields (behind the ear or in the nasal cavity) to protect the underlying skin or mucosa from radiation exiting through the posterior surface of the irradiated structure. An eye shield, resembling a contact lens made of lead, may be needed to protect the lens to prevent cataract formation. When irradiating larger lesions, it may be necessary to use adjoining fields. Because of the characteristics of the deposition of electron radiation in tissue, it is more difficult to match adjacent electron fields than photon fields without producing areas that are underdosed or overdosed (Fig. 6). Care must be taken to ensure as homogeneous a dose as possible in this situation.

Doses of radiation utilized in the treatment of keloids postoperatively are generally in the range 900–1500 centigray (cGy) at the skin surface in one to three fractions. The success rates are quite high (Table 1). With these doses and techniques, the complication rates

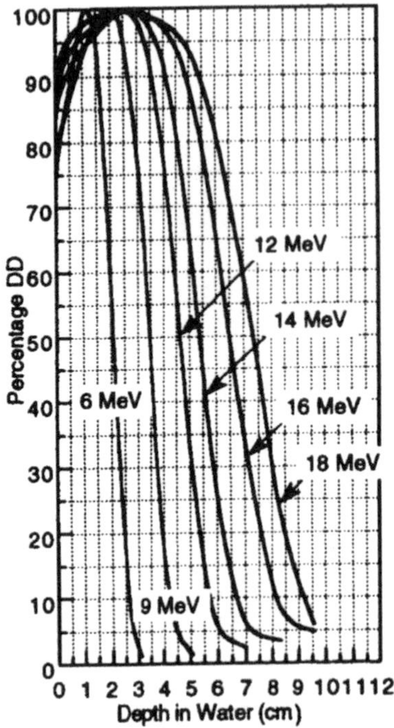

Figure 5 Dose distribution profile for electron beams of different energies. Note that the maximum dose falls below the surface, in contrast to that of the low-energy photon beam in Fig. 1. Also note that the dose falls rapidly. For example, for the 6-MeV beam, the dose is reduced to 50% of maximum at 2 cm below the surface. The percentage depth dose (percentage DD) is the dose at any given depth relative to the maximum dose, which is set at 100%. (From Ref. 21.)

are extremely low (11,16,18). Mild hyperpigmentation and telangiectasias are occasionally seen but require no treatment (18,22,23). These side effects appears to be more common if high-dose single fractions (>1000 cGy) are used (22). Wound dehiscence is rare. Radionecrosis has also been reported after single high-dose fractions ≥1000 cGy (24). This complication may require surgical resection of the affected tissue. Hyperbaric oxygen therapy (25) or pentoxifylline (26) may also be effective in the treatment of soft tissue necrosis after radiation. No cases of radiation-induced malignancy have been reported after keloid treatment.

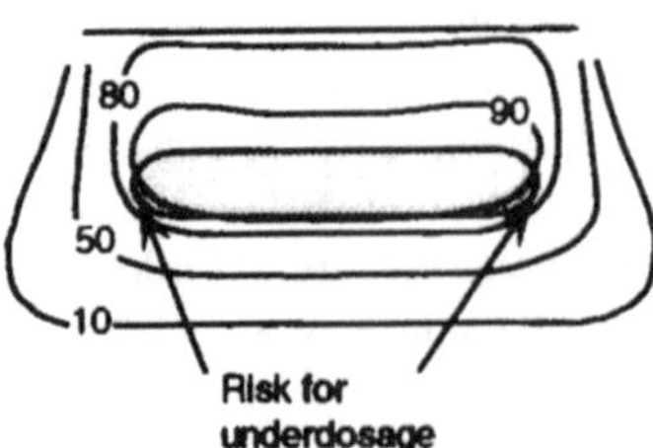

Figure 6 Dose distribution profile of an electron beam. Note that the region corresponding to 90% of the maximum dose narrows with increasing depth in tissue. Care must be taken to avoid underdosage in this region. (From Ref. 21.)

Table 1 Results of Radiation Therapy Following Surgery for Keloids

Author	Control rate (%)
Klumpar	83
Lo	82–90
Doornbos	90
Kovalic	73
Enhamre	88
Chaudhry	97
Borok	98
Inalsingh	77

Temporary interstitial implantation with the isotope iridium-192 has also been used to treat keloids following resection (19). A single iridium wire is loaded into a hollow plastic tube that was implanted in the edges of the wound as it was closed when the keloid was resected. A dose of 2000 cGy is delivered at a depth of 5 mm from the long axis of the iridium wire over 24–48 hours. The main complications related to this technique is hypopigmentation (14%). The success rate is similar to that reported with external beam techniques (79%).

III. INTRALESIONAL STEROIDS

Among the multiple treatment options for keloids and hypertrophic scars, corticosteroid injections are often an initial approach. These injections may be used alone (27) or in combination with other therapies (28,29). Corticosteroid injections rarely resolve keloids or hypertrophic scars completely, but symptoms often improve and lesions soften. Investigators have reported variable results, which may reflect differences in treatment protocol and lesion location or type. Kiil (30) reported a 50% recurrence rate over 5 years, and Griffith et al. (28) reported that 5 of 56 keloids recurred after 4 years with intralesional triamcinolone injections. Lawrence (31) reported 30% cure rate of keloids treated with surgery and perioperative triamcinolone injection.

Various corticosteroid preparations have been used for intralesional therapy. These preparations include hydrocortisone, triamcinolone, and dexamethasone. No particular advantage of any one preparation has been clearly demonstrated. Our clinic and most recent publications use triamcinolone acetonide for intralesional therapy. Because individual response is highly variable, the dosage and administration should be individualized. The individual response can be determined by using varying concentrations of triamcinolone acetonide, 10, 20, 30, and 40 mg/mL, as trial injections (29). These different concentrations are injected into different sites in a total volume at 0.05–0.1 mL. These test sites are followed to determine the optimal clinical response using the minimal concentration of triamcinolone acetonide. Following administration of these test doses, the patient may return in 3–4 weeks and repeated injections may be continued to maximize the clinical effect with minimal adverse steroid side effects.

Adverse effects of intralesional corticosteroid injection are usually local. The most common side effect is hypopigmentation, whose risk increases when the steroid concentration is greater than 5 mg/mL. With continued injection and higher total volumes of steroid, there are other adverse effects, including atrophy, telangiectasia, necrosis, ulceration, and cushingoid habitus. The risk of steroid atrophy and hypopigmentation increases if the steroid is injected inadvertently into surrounding dermis and subcutaneous tissue. Some corticosteroid may be detected in the systemic circulation, but a systemic effect of intralesional therapy has not been widely reported. Because the corticosteroid preparation is a suspension, it should be well mixed before use. If insoluble material is deposited beneath the epidermis, a collection of corticosteroid may appear as a pale or yellow material along the needle track line. This collection of corticosteroid may result in steroid atrophy and hypopigmentation. To ensure that the steroid preparation is well mixed, the corticosteroid preparation may be placed in an ultrasound or sonication device before injection. Another side effect of intralesional corticosteroid injection has been focal accumulation of mucins on histopathologic examination (32). Other reports describe focal accumulations of foreign body–type giant cells along with histiocytic reactions.

The initial injections of corticosteroid preparations are often painful. Patients may benefit from the use of a topical anesthetic such as Emla cream applied with occlusion before injection. Local anesthesia may be provided by injecting xylocaine solutions beneath keloids or hypertrophic scars prior to corticosteroid intralesional injection. Of the various delivery systems available for injecting corticosteroids, a mechanical syringe has been most useful. Syringe injection is the most efficient method of delivering a known quantity to a specific location. Because these lesions are dense fibrous tissue, needles should securely lock into the syringe. A 25- or 30-gauge needle may be used, but a 30-gauge needle may often be clogged by a 40 mg/mL triamcinolone acetonide preparation. Intralesional injections are placed at 0.5–1.0 cm intervals around the entire lesion as the volume of injection is placed into the bulk of the lesion. The injection is continued until the tissue expands, and care is taken to deposit the corticosteroid preparation in the bulk of the lesion to avoid deposition in the epidermis or the subcutaneous tissue. After the initial injection, which is often difficult, lesions frequently soften and subsequent injections are less painful. Patients are often seen in our clinic at 3- to 4-week intervals as symptoms of pruritus and discomfort often extend at least 3–4 weeks from the previous injection. Treatment intervals may be individualized and adjusted according to the therapeutic response. Some patients may experience symptomatic relief and clinical response if the treatment interval is prolonged to every 2–4 months.

Various mechanical injectors such as spring- or CO_2-powered devices may deliver intralesional corticosteroids (33,34). Mechanical injectors may be less painful for some patients, such as adolescents, who dislike the notion of needle injection. Mechanical injectors are also useful for single lesions. The mechanical injector must be used with care to avoid inadvertent infiltration of surrounding dermis. The mechanical injectors may waste a significant amount of corticosteroid preparation, as needle and syringe infiltration is more efficient. Other mechanical syringes such as the dental intralig syringe (Miltex, NY) are useful. This mechanical syringe provides a mechanical advantage requiring less effort to infiltrate firm, fibrous tissue. Other clinicians prefer 1-mL glass syringes that can be fitted with metal finger handles to apply extra exertion. Leur-Lok needles and syringes can be attached to repetitive pipette instruments to deliver calibrated doses. Of these methods of injection, the dental mechanical intralig syringe is the most efficient and least painful injection device.

Other treatment modalities such as cryotherapy are often combined with intralesional corticosteroid injection (35,36). Ceilley and Babin described cryotherapy before intralesional injection in order to facilitate infiltration after the edema and cellular destruction of cryotherapy. The cellular change and edema resulting from cryotherapy may facilitate injection by allowing injected material to penetrate more easily, and cryotherapy may provide some degree of anesthesia. Some authors have described cryotherapy as a treatment for keloids. Zacarian (37) reported good results with cryotherapy for newly formed keloids. Another study described newly formed keloids of less than 2 years' duration responding better with cryotherapy (38). In this study there was a 73.8% good response and 16.9% fair response in a series of 65 lesions. The study emphasizes the importance of repeated therapy, as some lesions were treated 10 times before the scar completely flattened. Hypopigmentation may be a side effect with cryotherapy, and it should be used for selected patients.

Corticosteroid injections are often combined with surgery, either preoperatively, perioperatively, or postoperatively. The keloid may be injected several times initially to determine its response. Some lesions may respond acceptably and the patient's satisfaction may reduce the need for further surgery, as lesions may be controlled using cortisone injection alone. For lesions that do not respond after multiple injections, surgery may be considered. Following the excision, the wound edges may be injected with corticosteroid and sutures left in place for an extra week to minimize the potential for wound dehiscence. Corticosteroid injections are then repeated every 3–4 weeks postoperatively. Treatment intervals and duration are individualized according to the lesion response.

REFERENCES

1. Blackburn WR, Cosman B. Histologic basis of keloid and hypertrophic scar differentiation. Arch Pathol 1966; 82:65.
2. Lever WF. Histopathology of the Skin. 6th ed. Philadelphia: Lippincott, 1983:604–605.
3. Mancini RE, Quaile JV. Histogenesis of experimentally produced keloids. J Invest Dermatol 1962; 38:143–149.
4. Cohen IK, Keiser HR, Sjoerdsma A. Collagen synthesis in human keloid and hypertrophic scars. Surg Forum 1971; 22:488.
5. Kazem AA. The immunological aspects of keloid tumor formation. J Surg Oncol 1988; 38:16–18.
6. Cosman B, Wolff M. Correlation of keloid recurrence with completeness of local excision: a negative report. Plast Reconstr Surg 1972; 50:163.
7. Cosman B, Crikelair GF, Ju DMC, Gaulin JC, Lattes R. The surgical treatment of keloids. Plast Reconstr Surg 1961; 27:335–358.
8. Cosman B, Wolff M. Bilateral earlobe keloids. Plast Reconstr Surg 1974; 53:540–543.
9. Inalsingh CHA. An experience in treating five hundred and one patients with keloids. Johns Hopkins Med J 1974; 134:284–290.
10. Klumpar DI, Murray JC, Anscher M. Keloids treated with excision followed by radiation therapy. J Am Acad Dermatol 1994; 31:225–231.
11. Kovalic JJ, Perez CA. Radiation therapy following keloidectomy: a 20-year experience. Int J Radiat Oncol Biol Phys 1989; 17:77–80.
12. Ship AG, Weiss PR, Mincer FR, Wolkstein W. Sternal keloids: successful treatment employing surgery and adjunctive radiation. Ann Plast Surg 1993; 31:481–487.
13. Sclafani AP, Gordon L, Chadha M, Romo T III. Prevention of earlobe keloid recurrence with postoperative corticosteroid injections versus radiation therapy: a randomized, prospective study and review of the literature. Dermatol Surg 1996; 22:569–574.
14. Chaudhry MR, Akhtar S, Duvalsaint F, Garner L, Lucente FE. Ear lobe keloids, surgical excision followed by radiation therapy: a 10-year experience. Ear Nose Throat J 1994; 73:779–781.

15. Darzi MA, Chowdri NA, Kaul SK, Khan M. Evaluation of various methods of treating keloids and hypertrophic scars: a 10-year follow-up study. Br J Plast Surg 1992; 45:374–379.
16. Borok TL, Bray M, Sinclair I, Plafker J, LaBirth L, Rollins C. Role of ionizing irradiation for 393 keloids. Int J Radiat Oncol Biol Phys 1988; 15:865–870.
17. Doornbos JF, Stoffel TJ, Hass AC, Hussey DH, Vigliotti AP, Wen BC, Zahra MK, Sundeen V. The role of kilovoltage irradiation in the treatment of keloids. Int J Radiat Oncol Biol Phys 1990; 18:833–839.
18. Lo TCM, Seckel BR, Salzman FA, Wright KA. Single-dose electron beam irradiation in treatment and prevention of keloids and hypertrophic scars. Radiother Oncol 1990; 19:267–272.
19. Escarmant P, Zimmermann S, Amar A, Ratoanina JL, Moris A, Azaloux H, Francos H, Gosserez O, Michel M, G'Baguidi R. The treatment of 783 keloid scars by iridium 192 interstitial irradiation after surgical excision. Int J Radiat Oncol Biol Phys 1993; 26:245–251.
20. Johns HE, Cunningham JR. The Physics of Radiology. 4th ed. Springfield, IL: Charles C Thomas, 1983:167–211.
21. Bentel GC. Radiation Therapy Planning. 2nd ed. New York: McGraw-Hill, 1992:16–31.
22. Enhamre A, Hammar H. Treatment of keloids with excision and post-operative x-ray irradiation. Dermatologica 1983; 167:90–93.
23. Arnold HL, Graver FH. Keloids: etiology and management of excision and intensive prophylactic radiation. Arch Dermatol 1959; 80:772–777.
24. Van Den Brenk HAS, Minty CCJ. Radiation in the management of keloids and hypertrophic scars. Br J Surg 1960; 4:595–605.
25. Norkool DM, Hampson NB, Gibbons RP, Weissman RM. Hyperbaric oxygen therapy for radiation-induced hemorrhagic cystitis. J Urol 1993; 150:232–234.
26. Dion MW, Hussey DH, Doornbos JF, Vigliotti AP, Wen BC, Anderson B. Preliminary results of a pilot study of pentoxifylline in the treatment of late radiation soft tissue necrosis. Int J Radiat Oncl Biol Phys 1990; 19:401–407.
27. Maguire HC. Treatment of keloids with triamcinolone acetonide injected intralesionally. JAMA 1965; 192:325–327.
28. Griffith BH, Monroe CW, McKinney P. A follow-up study on the treatment of keloids with triamcinolone acetonide. Plast Reconstr Surg 1970; 46:145–150.
29. Murray JC, Pollack SV, Pinnell SR. Keloids: a review. J Am Acad Dermatol 1981; 4:461–470.
30. Kiil J. Keloids treated with topical injections of triamcinolone acetonide (Kenalog). Immediate and long term results. Scand J Plast Reconstr Surg 1977; 11:169–172.
31. Lawrence WT. In search of the optimal treatment for keloids: report of a series and a review of the literature. Ann Plast Surg 1991; 27:164–178.
32. Santa Cruz DJ, Ulbright TM. Mucin-like changes in keloids. Am J Clin Pathol 1981; 75:18–22.
33. Berry RB. A comparison of spring and CO_2 powered needleless injectors in the treatment of keloids with triamcinolone. Br J Plast Surg 1981; 34:458–461.
34. Vallis CP. Intralesional injection of keloids and hypertrophic scars with the Dermojet. Plast Reconstr Surg 1967; 40:255–262.
35. Ceilley RI, Babin RW. The combined use of cryosurgery and intralesional injections of suspensions and fluorinated adrenocorticosteroids for reducing keloids and hypertrophic scars. J Dermatol Surg Oncol 1979; 5:54–56.
36. Minkowitz F. Regression of massive keloid following partial excision and post-operative intralesional administration of triamcinolone. Br J Plast Surg 1967; 20:432–435.
37. Zacarian SA. Discussion of the response of keloid scars to cryosurgery. Plast Reconstr Surg 1982; 70:683.
38. Rusciani L, Rossi G, Bono R. Use of cryotherapy in the treatment of keloids. J Dermatol Surg Oncol 1993; 19:529–534.

25
Pressure Technique

Judith A. Carr
Westchester Burn Center, Westchester Medical Center
Valhalla, New York

Scar is the inevitable final stage of wound healing. Scars that restrict joint mobility prohibit independence in self-care, influence participation in recreational and social activities, and may prevent the individual from returning to previous employment. To what degree the resultant scar affects functional and cosmetic outcomes is dependent on early and consistent treatment. Scar cannot be prevented, but it can be controlled.

Ambrose Pare first described the use of pressure as a treatment for deforming scars and contracture in the 16th century. Much has been published regarding the management of hypertrophic scar resulting from thermal injury. Although a burn-related scar may cover a larger surface area, any scar resulting from surgical incision, trauma, diabetic ulceration, or congenital disorders such as epidermolysis bullosa may benefit from scar management therapy. A rigid and raised scar, regardless of location or size, can cause considerable discomfort in the form of itching or pain. Those that cross a joint space or involve highly visible areas such as the face or hands should be aggressively treated to ensure optimal cosmetic and functional results. Factors that may predict hypertrophic scar formation were investigated by Deitch et al. These included age, race, and the location and depth of injury. Guidelines utilizing these factors were established for the use of prophylactic pressure:

1. If the wound heals in less than 10 days, no prophylactic pressure is required regardless of age or race.
2. If the wound takes 10 to 14 days to heal, prophylactic pressure is recommended for black patients only.
3. If the wound takes 14 to 21 days to heal, prophylactic pressure is recommended for patients of all ages and races.
4. If the wound takes more than 21 days to heal, prophylactic pressure is mandatory.

I. FACTORS INFLUENCING SCAR MANAGEMENT

A. Early Intervention with Appropriate Therapies

Studies by Engrav et al. showed that pressure applied at the time of grafting not only did not compromise graft take but also may have enhanced healing and reduced scar formation.

In patients identified as at risk for the development of hypertrophic scars, the application of pressure should be initiated as soon as wound closure is complete. Early pressure should be graded according to the tensile strength of the scar. The application of pressure can be initiated in the presence of open wounds, provided the wound is not located over a joint. If a significant wound is present, motion in conjunction with pressure will increase the shear force and potentially increase the wound size.

B. Education and Compliance of Patients

In order to control the development of hypertrophic scar, the clinician and the patient must work as a team. It is the clinician's responsibility to educate the patient and family regarding strict adherence to prescribed therapies. A patient who does not understand the rationale of treatment or the consequences of no treatment is less likely to be compliant.

C. Cost of Treatment

Unfortunately, the cost of treatment can be an important factor in the clinician's choice of modalities. Consideration must be given to whether the patient can afford the prescribed treatment and, if cost is an issue, whether a less expensive modality can be substituted. A more expensive modality does not necessarily produce a more desirable scar. As an example, I have witnessed a scar of the deltoid region resulting from a childhood vaccination be successfully reduced using only a coin taped with pressure applied to the scar. The patient was unable to return to the clinic and substituted a coin for the previously applied Silastic mold, which had cracked. The coin proved to be an adequate substitute, without any adverse effect on management of the scar.

D. Simplification

Treatment success relies not only on the correct choice of methods and materials but also on the patient's ability to duplicate prescribed treatments. Any treatment that requires a complex application or use of multiple products is unlikely to be used on a regular basis.

E. Frequent Monitoring

From the time of wound closure to scar maturation, the scar should be monitored on a regular basis. The initial therapy used may not be adequate for the entire period of treatment. Frequent monitoring identifies sites of inadequate intervention within a time frame when it can be easily corrected by altering the treatment. Scars should be monitored for any change in

Color
Texture
Thickness
Presence or absence of blanching
Rigidity of scar
Stage of maturation
Presence of open areas
Joint restrictions

Changes in a scar are be demonstrated by a visually apparent decrease in size and vascularity; the scar is be softer to the touch and not restricted by adhesions to underlying structures; and the patient reports a decrease in pain, increases in mobility, and improved cosmetic appearance. Ongoing assessment of a maturing scar and the success or failure of the prescribed modalities should be performed when the patient returns for follow-up care. The Vancouver General Hospital Burn Unit and the Department of Plastic Surgery devised a universal method of scar assessment: the Vancouver Scar Scale. Four criteria are evaluated and assigned a numerical value. The total of the values as determined by the evaluation of pigmentation, vascularity, pliability, and scar height is used to rate the scar. Normal skin has a value of 0. Ideally, if the prescribed treatments are appropriate for the individual, the scar should have a progressively lower score.

II. APPLICATION OF PRESSURE

Scar management in its simplest form uses the modality of pressure. Scars located over cylindrical body parts such as the extremities or trunk, when treated early, probably require only the use of pressure dressings or garments for adequate control. Concave surfaces such as the palm, joint fossa, face, and neck and well-established scars require the use of silicone molds to achieve adequate definitive pressure.

A. Pressure Wraps

A variety of compression wraps are commercially available for the application of pressure. All are readily available and low in cost. These elastic bandages can be applied over a wound with incomplete healing without the risks associated with shear and excessive pressure. When they are applied in a figure-of-8 fashion, pressure is equally distributed and can be graded depending on the tensile strength and rigidity of the scar. Patients should be cautioned against applying excessive pressure, which may lead to scar breakdown or distal edema if the entire extremity is not incorporated in the wrap. The most significant disadvantage of wraps is their bulky application, which may limit joint mobility. Where applicable, products such as Coban, a self-adherent wrap, can be used to decrease bulk and shifting of the wrap with motion. These products are especially useful for applying initial pressure to the hand. A boxer wrap style of application provides pressure over the entire hand. The fingers and body of the hand are wrapped separately, and the two regions are then joined by strips placed in the web spaces. A boxer wrap should not, however, be used for a patient who is unable to flex the fingers actively against the resistance of the wrap, as it tends to pull the fingers into extension when at rest.

B. Tubular Support Bandages

Tubular support bandages are commercially available in several sizes and can be applied in a low, medium, or high tension range by varying the size or the number of layers used. A tension guide is used to determine the proper size for either low tension (5 to 10 mm Hg), medium tension (10 to 20 mm Hg), or high tension (20 to 30 mm Hg). Studies by Judge et al. found the medium range to be most effective in reducing scars without causing distal edema or causing breakdown from excessive pressure. This pressure medium has been shown to be safely used as early as 5 to 7 days after grafting, provided care is taken to avoid shear when applying the sleeve. Although these garments are inexpensive compared with other modalities, they need to be replaced more frequently in order to maintain sufficient pressure.

C. Prefabricated Garments

In cases in which the exact fit of a garment is not essential or a lesser amount of pressure is indicated, the clinician should consider the use of a prefabricated garment (Fig. 1). Although more costly than a tubular support bandage, the prefabricated garment offers ease of application, a variety of styles and sizes, and a consistent amount of pressure. These garments retain their elasticity for a longer period of time than tubular support bandages. Most manufacturers of custom-made pressure garments also offer a selection of prefabricated garments.

D. Commercial Products

When the scar is small and located over the wrist, knee, ankle, or lower abdomen, the use of a commercially available product can be considered. When used in conjunction with a silicone interface, these products, such as athletic supports for the knee, ankle, or wrist, long-line bras, spandex shorts, or panty girdles, generally supply adequate pressure to reduce scars in the early stages of development. The relatively low cost of these products makes them a viable option for management of a small isolated scar.

E. Custom-Fitted Garments

Scars over large surface areas such as extensive burn scars or those originating from extensive soft tissue trauma are best managed with custom-fitted garments. These garments

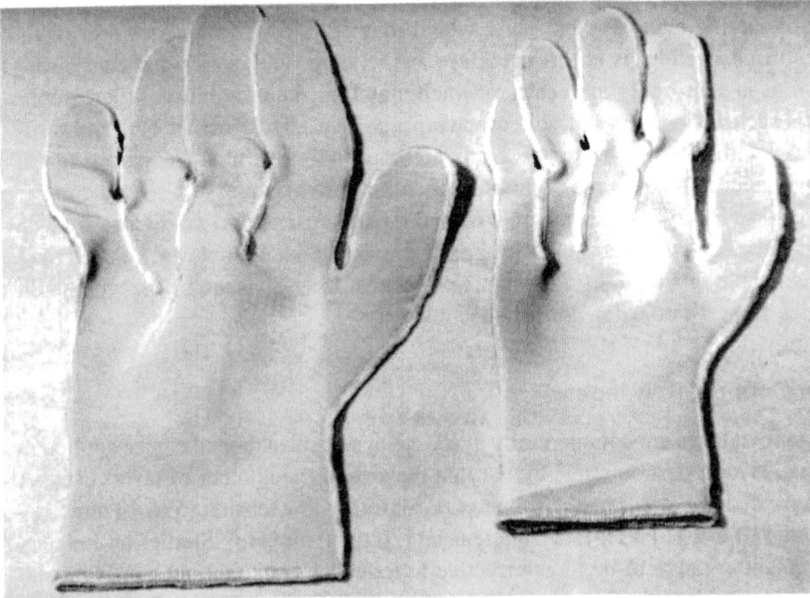

Figure 1 Prefabricated garments are available in a variety of designs and sizes.

provide optimal pressure and options in design. The garments are now available in a multitude of colors as well as having the design option of a Silastic sheeting or soft fabric liner for problem areas. To prevent excessive shear force over a friable scar, extremity zippers can be incorporated in the design of the garment for ease of application. When the tensile strength of the scar has improved, the zippers should be eliminated from subsequent orders in order to achieve optimal pressure.

III. SUPPLEMENTAL PRESSURE

Scarring over areas of natural concavity or soft tissue defects resulting from trauma require definitive pressure inserts in addition to compression for optimal scar management. Treatment modalities should be selected on the basis of extent of scarring, cosmetic and functional limitations, and the occupation or activity level of the individual.

Modalities used during waking hours should permit function. Interfaces used over joint surfaces should be thin so as not to impede function. Those used while the patient sleeps should provide maximal pressure to the scar and sustained stretch to contracted joints (Fig. 2).

Many products can be utilized for the fabrication of an interface. Of importance in the selection of the product used is the tensile strength of the scar, as newly healed areas do not tolerate the more rigid molds.

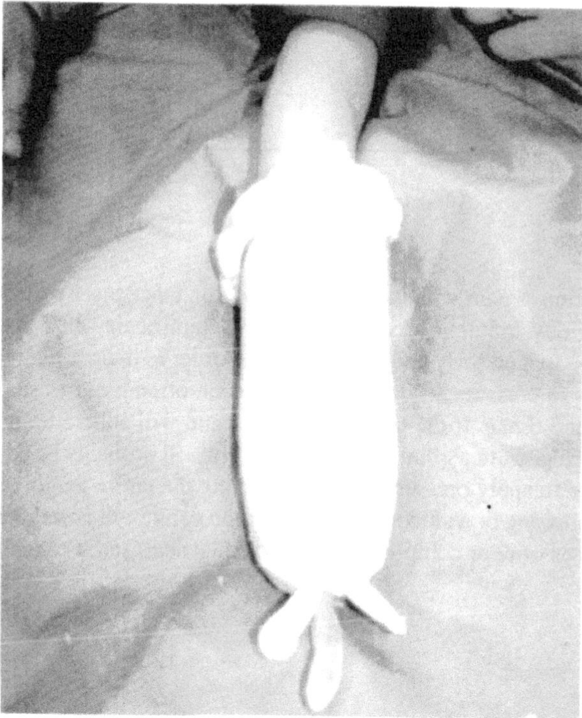

Figure 2 Full-contact definitive pressure of a child's hand can be achieved by filling a latex glove with foam elastomer.

IV. MATERIALS FOR SUPPLEMENTAL PRESSURE

Supplemental pressure inserts enhance the use of compression for the control of hypertrophic scar development. Particularly in the case of the silicone products, the benefits of the addition of supplemental pressure include a softer, more elastic scar, a decrease in scar adhesions, and a rapid improvement in range of motion of involved joints. Some of the products typically used may tend to retain moisture, which can lead to scar maceration and eventual breakdown. For this reason, whenever any of these products are utilized, the skin should be routinely monitored for signs of irritation, rash, pustules, and maceration. Good hygiene is imperative. The interface should be discontinued if evidence of any problem directly related to the use of the interface is noted.

Characteristics	Products	
Two-part base-catalyst mix	5-6-7	1. High-density foam
Soft, flexible	2-3-4-7-8	2. Mepitel
Rubberlike mold	5-6	3. Elastogel
Exact definitive mold	5-6-7	4. Dermal pads
Easily applied	1-2-3-4-5-6-7-8	5. Otoform putty
Bondable	5-6-7	6. Silastic elastomer
Adherent	1-2-8	7. Prosthetic foam
Absorbent	1-2-3-7	8. Silastic gel sheets
Washable	2-4-5-6-8	
Breathable	2-3-8	
Reduces friction	3-4-7-8	
Utilize as a graft dressing	2-3-7	
Use over fragile scar	3-4-7-8	
Use with established scar	1-4-5-6-7-8	

V. SCARRING OVER JOINTS

When located over a joint, a scar causes pain with movement. A motion that causes pain is naturally avoided, facilitating the development of scar contracture. Significant scars that cross the fold of the joint should be treated early and aggressively in order to maintain joint function and mobility. In addition to pressure, scarring in this location often requires sustained stretch to elongate contracted tissue. If the patient is reliable and will adhere to the prescribed wearing schedule, a molded gutter splint worn only at night will probably be adequate. Splints should be designed to apply pressure and stretch along the entire length of the scar band. Use of a pressure dressing or a silicone mold under the splint will speed the process of scar remodeling. In cases of poor compliance or established scar, serial casting should be considered.

VI. SERIAL CASTING

Serial casting should be considered whenever an established scar restricts joint mobility. In order to reduce a well-developed scar band, pressure and stretch should be applied in the maximal extension range that the scar will tolerate.

Using plaster for serial casting is not only economical but also highly effective. Because of the conforming nature of a plaster bandage, it provides direct contoured pressure on the scar and acts as a static force on underlying structures. Casts can be applied over areas where small open areas are present provided the cast is well padded. It is recommended that a Vaseline dressing be used over any open areas prior to the application of the cast padding. Another important feature of serial casting is that it can be used successfully on a patient who is either unwilling or unable to cooperate with traditional splinting programs or other scar management protocols. Silicone gel sheets or cast pads can be incorporated in the plaster cast as well. These sheets can be placed in direct contact with the scar, cotton webril is then applied, and the cast is fabricated. This method provides additional pressure to the joints being mobilized and is extremely beneficial in softening hypertrophic scars and scar bands. Plaster is preferred over fiberglass for outpatient use. In the event that a cast must be emergently removed, this can be accomplished by immersing the cast in water and then cutting the cast using heavy scissors.

To determine a safe range, place the scar on stretch along its entire length. The midpoint should blanch. Allow the scar to relax slightly and immobilize all affected joints in this position. Avoid sustained stretch at the endpoint of range, at the point of blanching, as scar breakdown may result. The benefits of this modality include low cost, ease of application, little need for the patient's compliance, and provision of absolute contoured pressure over virtually any scar surface.

Indications for use:

Active or maturing scar that limits joint function
Scar crossing multiple joints without interruption
Patient's noncompliance with traditional splinting regimen
Reduction of scar contracture in children

If the scar is active, initially the cast should be changed every 2–3 days. When the scar is well established, a longer period of stretch is needed to remodel the scar sufficiently to warrant a cast change. Changing the cast weekly in this case is adequate. Once maximal gains have been achieved using this modality, gains should be maintained with night splinting and the use of pressure until complete scar maturation.

General principles for cast use:

Provide adequate padding and protection of underlying skin.
Must be of sufficient length to create an equal distribution of pressure.
Distal extremity should be exposed for vascular checks.
Patient should be taught how to remove cast if neurovascular compromise occurs.
Use caution in application to avoid pressure dents in wet plaster.
Must be monitored and changed frequently to prevent skin breakdown.

VII. WELL-DEFINED SCAR

Scars formed as the result of a surgical incision should be treated prophylactically in order to prevent the development of adhesions. This is of particular importance when the incision line is located over the sternum or when hand injuries are repaired. Sternal incisions or small isolated scars can be easily treated with the application of a Silastic gel sheet and held in place with skin tape. Because some form of splinting generally follows hand surgery, a

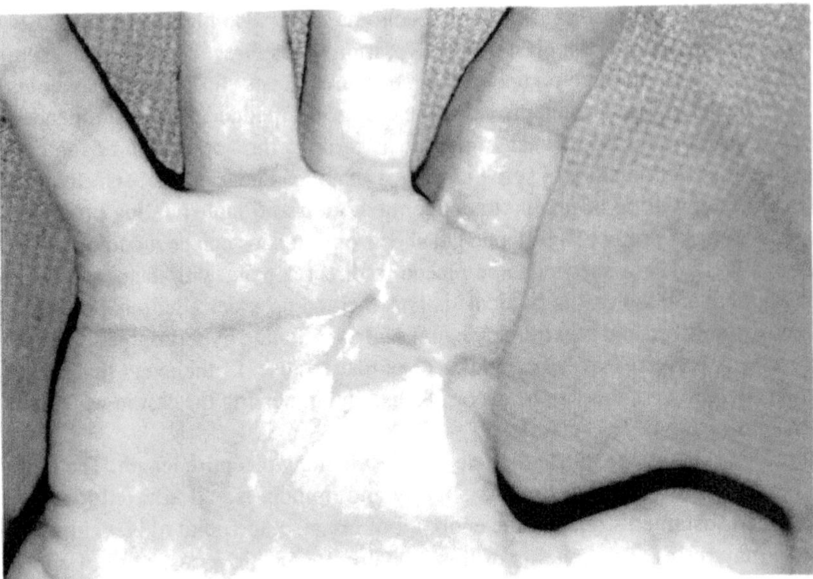

Figure 3 Adhesions formed along incision lines may ultimately affect function.

Silastic gel sheet can be easily incorporated in the splint design. If a resting splint is not necessary, the scar can be managed using a gel sheet or Silastic mold and elastic support or strap (Figs. 3 and 4).

VIII. EXTENSIVE SURFACE AREA SCAR

Extensive scarring resulting from thermal injury and massive soft tissue loss are best managed with custom-made gradient pressure garments. Patients should be measured for their garments as soon as the healed or grafted wounds are able to withstand the shearing forces that are inherent in wearing these garments. If the patient is measured too soon, friction will cause blisters and subsequent skin breakdown. This is especially disastrous when it occurs over joints and bone prominences, as the garment may have to be removed until the area is healed. The application of a pressure garment does not have to be delayed until all areas are closed. Quarter-sized or smaller areas not located over bone prominences can be safely managed with a simple dressing worn directly under the garment.

It is extremely important that the clinician monitor the garments on a regular basis to ensure that adequate pressure is being applied to all bone surfaces involved. Concave areas such as the axilla, web spaces, palm, and face as well as areas prone to scar band contracture such as joint fossae are notoriously difficult to manage properly (Fig. 5). Inserts are worn under the pressure garment and are fabricated of various materials to apply even pressure to the scar's irregular surface.

Product selection is determined by the tensile strength of the scar, the size of the area to be covered, and/or the thickness of the scar to be controlled. It is important to monitor the scar closely, as a new mold should be made whenever there is a visible reduction in the size or contour of the scar.

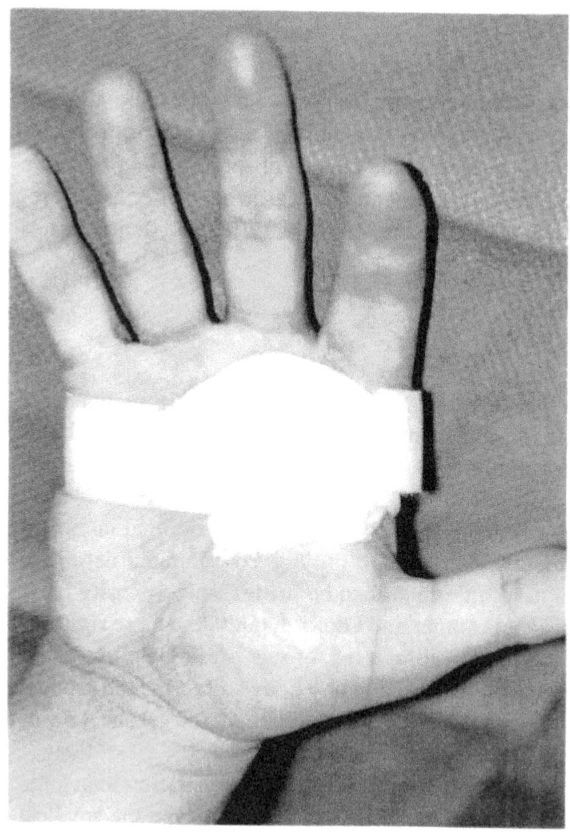

Figure 4 Simple strapping adequately secures the silastic mold and applies pressure.

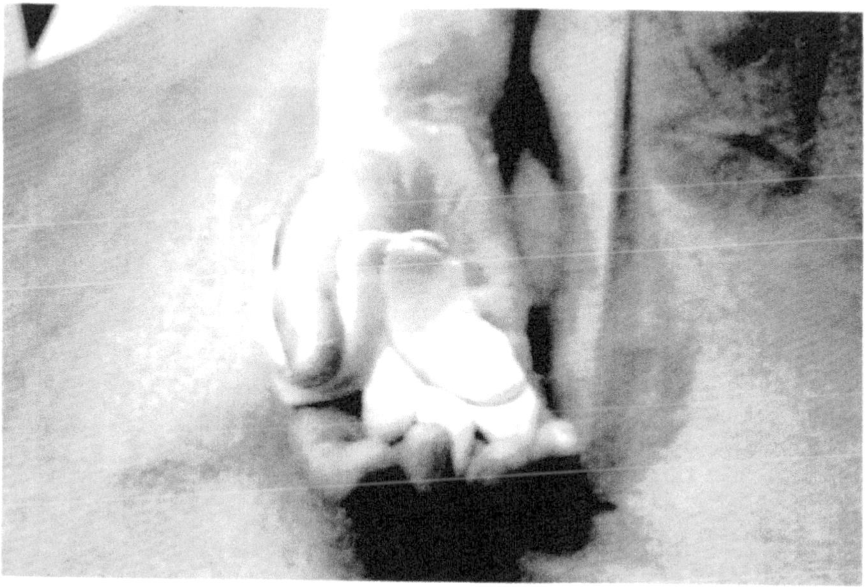

Figure 5 An Otoform mold is easily formed to fill out concave surfaces that require supplemental pressure.

In order to be effective, garments should be worn 23 hours a day for up to 12 to 18 months until the scar is mature. Patients can continue to wear their garments even after returning to work or school. The garments have the added benefit of serving as a protective shield between the healing wound and the environment. The garments can be safely removed when the scar no longer blanches with pressure and is soft, flat, and demonstrates minimal tension.

IX. ESTABLISHED SCAR

An untreated well-developed scar that is still vascularized requires aggressive treatment for possibly only minimal gains. Cosmetic improvements are likely to be little or none, but if joint function has been restricted, even minimal gains in range of motion may make the treatment worth the effort.

Custom-fitted gradient pressure garments should be ordered for optimal compression. In addition to the pressure garments, interfaces to provide concentrated definitive pressure over problem sites should be used. Interfaces can be made of high-density foam or foam elastomer for larger sites. Silastic elastomer and Otoform putty, the more rigid silicones, can be safely used for maximal pressure without risk of scar breakdown in smaller well-defined scar. Gel sheeting can be used over virtually any body surface as the product is now available in a variety of sizes and shapes. No pressure is required; the gel sheet needs only to make contact with the scar. (Figs. 6 and 7)

Attempts to remodel rigid established scars may result in more frustration than gain. However, if the patient is willing to invest the time and effort required, even the smallest of gains may improve function. If no change is seen after a month of consistent treatment, the clinician should consider forgoing any further treatment until after surgical reconstruction. Once the scar has undergone surgical correction, it is imperative to begin the application of pressure techniques as soon as the area is healed.

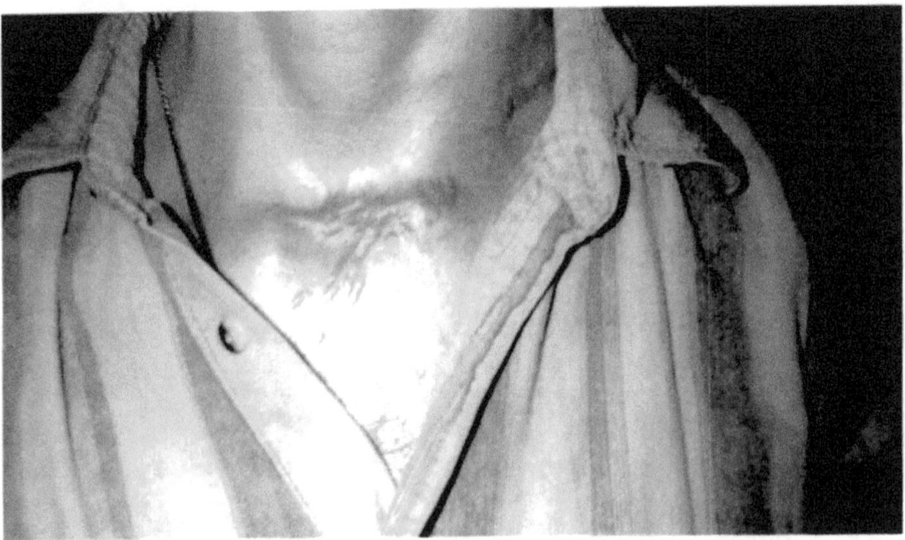

Figure 6 A small, well-defined scar can be easily managed using gel sheeting.

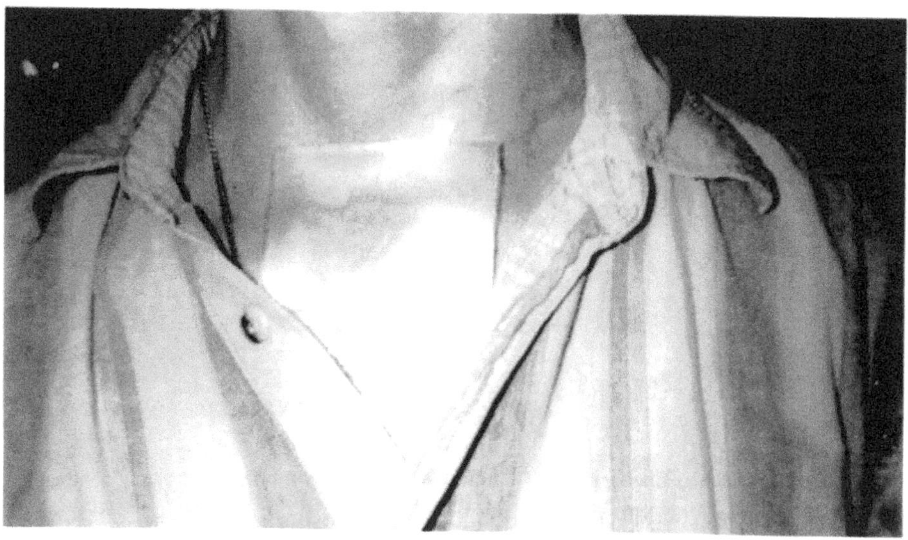

Figure 7 The gel sheeting is cut to extend beyond the scar's border and held in place with skin tape.

X. EPIDERMOLYSIS BULLOSA CONGENITA

Management of scar contractures of the hand in patients with epidermolysis bullosa, whose skin cannot tolerate the friction sustained in everyday life, poses a most difficult challenge. The objectives of scar management in these patients include not only improving function but also preventing the creation of additional areas of skin breakdown by the treatment prescribed. Most commonly, surgical correction of deformity in these patients is focused on the hands. Prevention of recontracture after surgical intervention begins in the operating room at the time of the surgical release and grafting of the fingers or palm. To facilitate graft take and to maintain the full excursion of the release, the dressing material should

- Conform to the graft surface to maintain the graft contour and graft position within the defect
- Be soft and nonabrasive to permit the application of gentle compression
- Be nonadherent and absorbent to prevent damage to surrounding tissue

The intraoperative dressing should consist of four layers. The first layer, which is applied directly over the graft, retains moisture and partially secures the graft and prevents slippage. A simple Vaseline gauze, Mepitel, or Elastogel protects the graft, facilitates healing, and is easily removed without traumatizing surrounding skin (Fig. 8). The next layer consists of an interface that acts to protect the graft as well as fill the defect created by the release. Elastogel bolsters or foam elastomer molds are ideal as nonabrasive interfaces for this layer (Fig. 9). The absorbent property of these products may also be beneficial in wicking away any wound drainage. Gentle compression is then applied using cotton webril or cast padding as a circumferential wrap. The final layer of the dressing is a thin, shelled cast. Fiberglass casting material is generally used because it is light and available in colors, which appeals to a pediatric population.

The initial dressing change is performed in 5 to 7 days. A similar dressing is reapplied until the grafts are well healed and stable in approximately 1 week. Aftercare of these

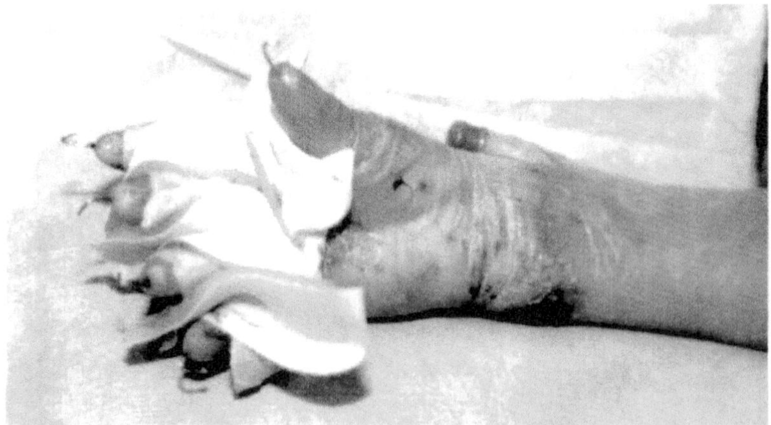

Figure 8 Products such as Elastogel act as a graft dressing and a soft bolster following contracture release.

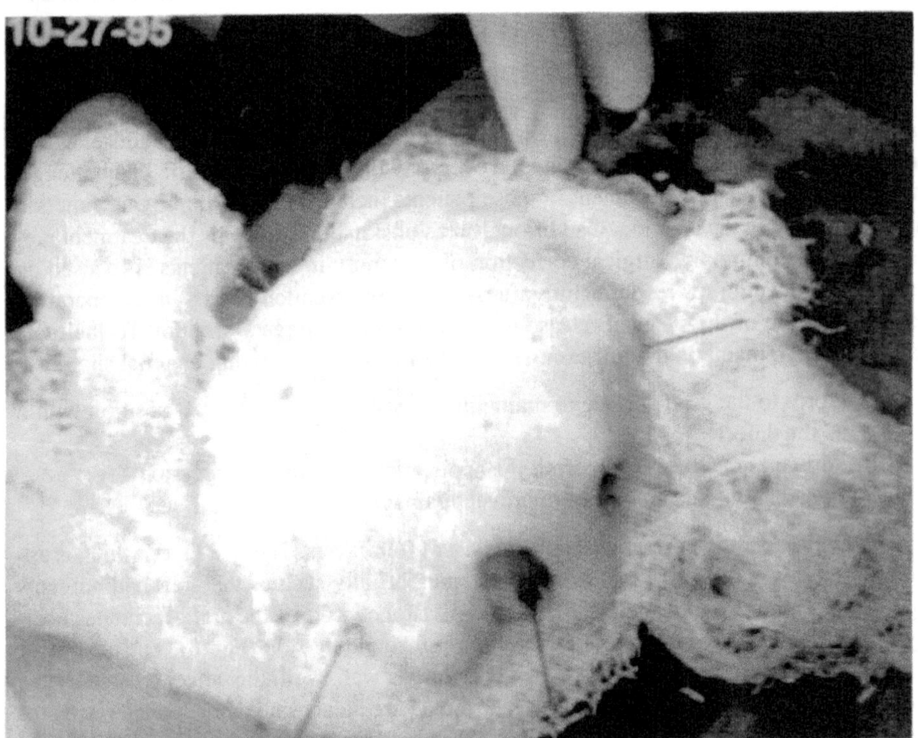

Figure 9 With the fingers positioned in maximal extension, a foam elastomer mold is poured to maintain full graft excursion.

patients focuses maximizing hand function and maintaining extension gains. Patients are encouraged to resume self-care activities within the limitations of their disability during the day and extension splinting at night to prevent recurrence for as long as possible.

The management of hypertrophic scars does not rely on one product or treatment modality. The previous suggestions are based on protocols commonly used in the treatment of burn scar hypertrophy. Most scars can be successfully managed in a cookbook fashion, provided that the intervention is initiated as soon as the wound will tolerate pressure, modalities prescribed are consistently used, and the scar is periodically monitored during the maturation process to evaluate the modality selected.

Vendors for silicone products and compression wraps:

Ali-Med (800) 225-2610
North Coast Medical, Inc. (800) 821-9319
Fred Sammons, Inc. (800) 323-5547
Smith & Nephew Rolyan (800) 558-8633

Vendors for pressure garments:

Jobst Institute, Inc. (800) 537-1063
Bio-concepts, Inc. (800) 421-5647
Barton Carey Compression Garments (800) 421-0444
Medical Z (800) 368-7478
Gottfried Medical, Inc. (800) 537-1968

BIBLIOGRAPHY

Ahn ST, Monafo WW, Mustoe TA. Topical silicone gel for the prevention and treatment of hypertrophic scar. Arch Surg 1991; 126:499–504.

Alston DW, et al. Materials for pressure inserts in the control of hypertrophic scar tissue. J Burn Care Rehabil 1981; 2:40–43.

Barillo DJ, et al. Prospective outcome analysis of a protocol for the surgical and rehabilitative management of burns to the hands. Plast Reconst Surg 1997; 100:1442–1451.

Carey SA, et al. Cica-Care gel sheeting in the management of hypertrophic scarring. Burns 1994; 20:163–167.

Carr-Collins JA. Pressure techniques for the prevention of hypertrophic scar. Clin Plast Surg 1992; 19:733–743.

Daugherty MB, Carr-Collins JA. Splinting techniques for the burn patient. In: Richard RL, Staley MJ, eds. Burn Care and Rehabilitation: Principles and Practice. Philadelphia: Davis, 1994:242–321.

Deitch EA, et al. Hypertrophic burn scars: analysis of variables. J Trauma 1983; 23:895–898.

Engrav LH, et al. Do splinting and pressure devices damage new grafts? J Burn Care Rehabil 1983; 4:107–108.

Evans EB, et al. Prevention and treatment of deformity in burned patients. In: Herndon DN, ed. Total Burn Care. Philadelphia: Saunders, 1996:455–472.

Greider JL, Flatt AE. Care of the hand in recessive epidermolysis bullosa. Plast Reconstr Surg 1983; 72:222–227.

Jensen LL, Parshley PF. Postburn scar contractures: histology and effects of pressure treatment. J Burn Care Rehabil 1984; 5:119–123.

Johnson CL. Physical therapists as scar modifiers. Phys Ther 1984; 64:1381–1387.

Judge JC, et al. Control of hypertrophic scarring in burn patients using tubular support bandages. J Burn Care Rehabil 1984; 5:221–224.

Kirn TF. Silicone gel appears inexplicably to flatten, lighten hypertrophic scars from burns. JAMA 1989; 261:2600.

Linares HA, et al. Historical notes on the use of pressure in the treatment of hypertrophic scars or keloids. Burns 1993; 19:17–21.

Malick MH, Carr JA. Flexible elastomer molds in burn scar control. Am J Occup Ther 1980; 34:603–608.

McCauley RL, Holloak M. Medical therapy and surgical approach to the burn scar. In: Herndon DL. Total Burn Care. Philadelphia: Saunders, 1996:473–478.

Mullett FLH, Smith PJ. Hand splintage following surgery for dystrophic epidermolysis bullosa. Br J Plast Surg 1993; 46:192–193.

Perkins K, et al. Current materials and techniques used in burn scar management programme. Burns 1987; 13:406–410.

Quinn KJ. Silicone gel in scar treatment. Burns 1987; 13:S33–S40.

Richard RL, Staley MJ. Scar management. In: Richard RL, Staley MJ, eds. Burn Care and Rehabilitation Principles and Practice. Philadelphia: Davis, 1994:381–415.

Rivers E. A compression hand wrap. J Burn Care Rehabil 1984; 5:291–293.

Sullivan T, et al. Rating the burn scar. J Burn Care Rehabil 1990; 11:256–260.

Van den Kerckhove E, et al. Silicone patches as a supplement for pressure therapy to control hypertrophic scarring. J Burn Care Rehabil 1991; 12:361–369.

Ward RS. Pressure therapy for the control of hypertrophic scar formation after burn injury. J Burn Care Rehabil 1991; 12:257–262.

Watson SB, Miller JG. Optimizing skin graft take in children's hand burns—the use of Silastic foam dressings. Burns 1993; 19:519–521.

Wessling N, et al. Evidence that use of a silicone gel sheet increases range of motion burn wound contractures. J Burn Care Rehabil 1985; 6:503–505.

Index

About the Editor

MARWALI HARAHAP is Professor of Dermatology at the University of North Sumatra Medical School, Medan, Indonesia. The author of numerous professional publications and the editor or coeditor of eight books, including Skin Changes and Diseases in Pregnancy (Marcel Dekker, Inc.), Dr. Harahap is a Fellow of the American Academy of Dermatology and a member of the Indonesian Society of Dermatology and Venereology; the International Society of Dermatology: Tropical, Geographic and Ecologic; the International Society of Dermatologic Surgery; and the Medical Society for the Study of Venereal Diseases; among others. He received the M.D. degree (1960) from the University of Indonesia, Jakarta.

About the Editor

Printed and bound by CPI Group (UK) Ltd, Croydon, CR0 4YY
17/10/2024
01775659-0004